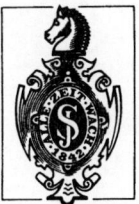

T. F. H. Schmidt B. T. Engel
G. Blümchen (Eds.)

Temporal Variations of the Cardiovascular System

Foreword by S. Julius

With 185 Figures and 42 Tables

Springer-Verlag Berlin Heidelberg GmbH

Privat-Dozent Dr. med. Thomas F. H. Schmidt
Präventiv- und Verhaltensmedizin
Abteilung für Epidemiologie und Sozialmedizin
Medizinische Hochschule Hannover
Konstanty-Gutschow-Straße 8, 3000 Hannover 61, FRG

Professor Dr. Bernard T. Engel
National Institute on Aging, Laboratory of Behavioral Sciences
Gerontology Research Center, 4940 Eastern Avenue,
Baltimore, Maryland 21224, USA

Professor Dr. med. Gerhard Blümchen
Klinik Roderbirken
5653 Leichlingen/Rhld. 1, FRG

ISBN 978-3-662-02750-9   ISBN 978-3-662-02748-6 (eBook)
DOI 10.1007/978-3-662-02748-6

© Springer-Verlag Berlin Heidelberg 1992
Originally published by Springer-Verlag Berlin Heidelberg New York in 1992
Softcover reprint of the hardcover 1st edition 1992

Typesetting: Fotosatz-Service Köhler, Würzburg, FRG

27/3145 – 5 4 3 2 1 0 – Printed on acid-free paper

Foreword

Significance of Temporal Variation in Cardiovascular Function

Research is an art of the possible; areas that are easy to investigate receive more attention than fields requiring cumbersome methodology. Temporal variations in cardiovascular function are considered a nuisance, they are the "diabolus experimentalis" waiting in the wings to affect the reproducibility of the data and spoil ones research report. In the traditional research every effort is made to standardize the conditions and minimize variability. Complex statistical techniques have been developed to remove the effects of variability, and for "smoothing" off the data. Long periods of rest to obtain proper baseline have become the rule in clinical research. These methods so overwhelmed the research that many investigators, accustomed to ignore the variability, engage in a bit of circular thinking: What cannot be measured ought to be ignored and in as much that something had been ignored, it follows that it is also unimportant. A virtue has been made out of necessity; what is easy to assess becomes the only thing worth exploring.

This preference for steady state measurements in cardiovascular research is hard to understand. When it comes to cardiovascular damage why should the average or baseline blood pressure be the most important factor? What is the basis of such thinking? One would never question, that for the same mileage, a car exposed to frequent stop and go, will be more damaged. Cardiovascular complications are likely to happen at the peaks and valleys of the blood pressure and heart rate and yet the majority of scientists continue to insist on the average value.

Against this trend it is truly refreshing to see that a substantial number of investigators has taken a keen interest in variable phenomena. The Symposium in Celle from which the present volume evolved, clearly indicates that temporal variations in cardiovascular function are an important field. Out of the apparent randomness one can start recognizing an order; there is short term, medium term (diurnal/circadian) and long term (around a year) variability. New information about the organization of the autonomic control can be gained from analysis of short term heart rate rhythmicity. Medium term, diurnal oscillations of the blood pressure and heart rate are also well documented, and new epidemiologic information strongly suggests that these oscillations might also have an important impact on the health. The preponderance of cardiac events in the early morning hours is most impressive and sets new agenda. Is this reflecting the steep morning increase of the blood pressure? What is the mechanisms of this increase and what might affect it? How important is hypotension during the sleep, does it explain some of the so called "I" curve relating hypotensive treatment and morbidity? Finally interesting data has been presented at the meeting about the long term seasonal variations in the blood pressure.

Scanning this book the reader will realize that the Symposium opens the way to asking some very important basic questions. Are the mechanism that regulate the average level of the heart rate and blood pressure and those that regulate their intrinsic rhythmicity similar? My personal bias is that these aspects of the autonomic control of the circulation are quite independent and may be regulated from different areas in the central nervous system. If this is true, and if further analysis shows that various reoccurring peaks and valleys of the pressure and heart rate are reliably related to morbidity, than treating the average blood pressure might not be the right goal. Drugs might have to be developed to preferentially affect various peaks and valleys. However such a development might not be feasible until the underlaying pathophysiology is fully understood. In the meantime evaluation of existing drugs for their effect on blood pressure variability is in order.

It is not the purpose of this preface to fully describe the content of the book. Rather I wish to pass on the reader the notion that the book has new and unique information about many hitherto ignored aspects of circulation and that variable phenomena can be systematically and usefully investigated. It requires perseverance to obtain a movie instead of a snapshot and even more to analyse the large amount of collected data. However the reward is in the emergence of entirely new views and horizons.

S. Julius

Preface

This volume has emerged from an international conference held in Celle, Lower Saxony, Germany, in 1990. A broad spectrum of eminent scientists from Europe and the USA studying cardiovascular rhythms came together to discuss various lines of their research. The contributions start with historical notes about day-night variations in the cardiovascular system and with a more general chapter on basic principles of human circadian rhythms. The two major parts of the book deal with diurnal variations in cardiac rhythms and in blood pressure rhythms. In both these areas the problems were approached in short and long term time frames, not only in humans but also in animals, and range from laboratory to field studies. In particular the interactions between behavioural and cardiovascular changes in health and disease are studied. The last section deals with diurnal variations in drug actions and investigates the chronopharmacologic and chronopharmacokinetic aspects as well as nocturnal hemodynamic effects of commonly used cardiovascular active drugs.

Rhythms synchronized to the 24 hour environmental cycle are called "diurnal". The use of the term "circadian" was introduced to indicate those "diurnal" rhythms which under constant conditions free-run with a period deviating from 24 hours. Later on it has become use to speak of a "circadian system" which may either free-run under constant conditions or be entrained to 24 hours by environmental cues (zeitgebers). The term "diurnal" for entrained rhythms is more conservative as long as it has not been demonstrated that this system can free-run under constant conditions. For many cardiovascular variables the experiments have not yet been carried out to demonstrate that they are free-running under constant conditions. In this volume we decided therefore to use preferably the term "diurnal" when dealing with rhythms synchronized to the 24 hour environmental cycle. Blood pressure variations may be circadian, although not independent from the wake-sleep rhythm. At the present it seems that the masking effect of physical activity mainly determines the diurnal variation of blood pressure. However, including the investigation of blood pressure in the "constant routine" paradigm, especially with the new noninvasive continuous methods which even allow the determination of hemodynamic components, might give us in the near future more insight into the diurnal or, more specifically, circadian organization of the cardiovascular regulatory mechanisms.

The research on diurnal rhythms of the cardiac cycle are largely stimulated by the epidemiological findings that the incidence of clinically significant events such as angina pectoris, "silent ischemia", myocardial infarction, and sudden cardiac death are not randomly distributed throughout the day. Rather, there is a marked tendency for these events to occur during the morning hours, after awakening. In addition, there are numerous human and animal studies that show that various hemodynamic patterns vary significantly throughout the day. One of the papers in this symposium (Engel) has raised the interesting notion that the heart rests overnight, and that if this is prevented, there can be a significant decline in ventricular function. The long term success of this stimulating conference is yet to be seen. Future developments are sure to show the influence of the invigorating presentations and discussions.

The conference as well as the publication of the present volume were both financially and technically supported by Hoffmann-La Roche AG, Germany. All the authors join us in extending our heartfelt gratitude to the team of Hoffmann-La Roche for such generous hospitality and exceptional technical support, which made the conference such a successful and memorable occasion. Here we particularly thank Dr. László Bethlen for supporting the organization of this conference with his great experience and skills. We are also grateful to the patient help of Hazel Schmidt in the preparation of this volume. Finally we thank Dr. Dr. Volker Gebhardt and Heike Schmitt-Spall, Springer-Verlag, as well as Klemens Schwind, Pro Edit, for their experienced editorial assistance in the publication process.

Thomas F. H. Schmidt
Bernard T. Engel
Gerhard Blümchen

Contents

Diurnal Variations – Circadian Rhythms

Day-Night Variations in the Cardiovascular System.
Historical and Other Notes by an Outsider 3
J. Aschoff

Basic Principles of Human Circadian Rhythms 15
R. A. Wever

Diurnal Variations in Cardiac Rhythms

Temporal Variations in Cardiac Rhythms in Rodents 87

Diurnal Heart Rate Rhythms in Small Mammals:
Species-Specific Patterns
and Their Environmental Modulation 87
K. Eisermann and W. Stöhr

Long-Term Changes of Heart Rate in Tree Shrews:
Indicators of Social Stress? 92
W. Stöhr

Regulation of Cardiac Performance Throughout the Day . . 99

Spectral Analysis of Heart Rate During Different States
of Activity 99
H.-H. Abel, D. Klüßendorf, E. Koralewski, R. Krause,
and R. Droh

The Neurovegetative System as a Link
Between Internal and External Environments 117
M. Pagani and A. Malliani

The Relationship Between Cardiovascular Responses
in the Laboratory and in the Field:
The Importance of "Active Coping" 127
D. W. Johnston, P. Anastasiades, C. Vögele, D. M. Clark,
C. Kitson, and A. Steptoe

Diurnal Rhythms and Heart Disease 145

Diurnal Variation and Triggers of Onset
of Cardiovascular Disease 145
G. H. Tofler and J. E. Muller

Daily Variations in ST Segment Depression in Patients
with Coronary Heart Disease 159
G. Blümchen and M. Jetté

Nocturnal Hemodynamic Responses to Chronic,
Mild Atrial Demand Pacing in Nonhuman Primates 164
B. T. Engel

Diurnal Variations in Blood Pressure Rhythms

New Techniques of Blood Pressure and Hemodynamic
Measurements in Vivo 173

Feasibility of Continuous Noninvasive 24-h Ambulatory
Finger Blood Pressure Measurement with Portapres:
Comparison with Intrabrachial Pressure 173
G. J. Langewouters, B. de Wit, G. M. A. van der Hoeven,
B. P. M. Imholz, G. Parati, G. A. van Montfrans,
and K. H. Wesseling

A New Dimension of Blood Pressure Measurement in Man:
24-h Ambulatory Continuous Noninvasive Recording
with Portapres 181
T. F. H. Schmidt, T. Steinmetz, J. Wittenhaus, P. Piccolo,
and H. Lüpsen

Peripheral Resistance Changes upon Stand-up Compared
to Those upon Tilt-up and Onset to Cycling:
Implication of the Cardiopulmonary Reflex 222
K. H. Wesseling, R. L. H. Sprangers, and W. Wieling

Diurnal Variations in Blood Pressure Regulations 240

Blood Pressure Control by Day Versus Night 240
J. Conway

Dynamic Evaluation of Neural Cardiovascular
Regulation Through the Analysis of Blood Pressure
and Pulse Interval Variability over 24 Hours 246
G. Parati, M. Di Rienzo, S. Omboni, S. Trazzi,
and G. Mancia

Field Assessment of Blood Pressure 258

Sources of Variability and Methodological Considerations
in Ambulatory Blood Pressure 258
M. D. Gellman, G. H. Ironson, N. Schneiderman,
M. M. Llabre, and S. B. Spitzer

Factors Associated with Differences in the Diurnal
Variation of Blood Pressure in Humans 272
G. A. Harshfield

Behavioral Factors in Blood Pressure Throughout the Day . 283

Effects of Behavioral Rhythms
on Blood Pressure Rhythms 283
L. F. Van Egeren

The Relationship Between Self-Reported Emotional Strain
and Ambulatory Blood Pressure and Heart Rate 297
H. Schächinger, W. Langewitz, H. Rüddel, and W. Schulte

The Effect of Occupational and Domestic Stress
on the Diurnal Rhythm of Blood Pressure 305
T. G. Pickering, W. Gerin, G. D. James, C. Pieper,
Y. L. Schlussel, and P. L. Schnall

Impact of Shifted Sleeping and Working Phases
on Diurnal Blood Pressure Rhythm 318
P. Baumgart

Assessment of Blood Pressure Variations in Hypertension . . 324

How and How Often Should Blood Pressure
Be Measured for Optimum Hypertension Control? 324
S. Eckert, H. Mannebach, H. Ohlmeier, J. Volmar,
and U. Gleichmann

Sleep-Related Breathing Disorders
and Nocturnal Hypertension 332
J. Mayer and J. H. Peter

Longterm Variation in Blood Pressure 344

Seasonal and Environmental Temperature Effects
on Arterial Blood Pressure 344
S. Giaconi and S. Ghione

Age-Dependent Variation of Diurnal Blood Pressure
Profile in Normotensive Subjects 351
G. Prager, R. Prager, and P. Klein

Diurnal Variations in Drug Actions

Recent Advances in the Chronopharmacology
of Cardiovascular Active Drugs 361
B. Lemmer

Chronopharmacokinetic Aspects with Special Reference
to Cardiovascular Drugs 371
B. Bruguerolle

Nocturnal Hemodynamic Effects of Commonly Used
Cardiovascular Drugs: Possible Implications
for Clinical and Pharmacological Management 382
M. I. Talan

Subject Index 389

List of Contributors

Abel, H.-H.
Institut für Physiologie
der Freien Universität Berlin,
Arnimallee 22, 1000 Berlin 33, FRG

Anastasiades, P.
Department of Psychiatry,
University of Oxford, Warneford
Hospital, Oxford OX3 7JX, UK

Aschoff, J.
Max-Planck-Institut für
Verhaltensphysiologie,
8138 Andechs, FRG

Baumgart, P.
Medizinische Poliklinik,
Universität Münster,
Albert-Schweitzer-Straße 33,
4400 Münster, FRG

Blümchen, G.
Klinik Roderbirken,
5653 Leichlingen/Rhld. 1, FRG

Bruguerolle, B.
Université d'Aix-Marseille II,
Faculté de Medecine, Laboratoire
de Pharmacologie Médicale,
27, Boulevard Jean Moulin,
13385 Marseille Cedex 5, France

Clark, D.M.
Department of Psychiatry,
University of Oxford, Warneford
Hospital, Oxford OX3 7JX, UK

Conway, J.
John Radcliffe Hospital,
Headington, Oxford, OX3 0DU, UK

Di Rienzo, M.
LaRC, Centro di Bioingegneria,
Fondazione "Juventute",
Via Gozzadini 7, 20148 Milan,
Italy

Droh, R.
Sportkrankenhaus Hellersen,
Paulmannshöher Weg 17,
5880 Lüdenscheid, FRG

Eckert, S.
Kardiologische Klinik,
Herzzentrum NRW,
Klinik der Ruhruniversität Bochum,
4970 Bad Oeynhausen, FRG

Van Egeren, L.F.
Department of Psychiatry,
Michigan State University,
East Lansing, MI 48824, USA

Eisermann, K.
Beringstraße 6, 8580 Bayreuth, FRG

Engel, B.T.
National Institute on Aging,
Laboratory of Behavioral Sciences,
Gerontology Research Center,
4940 Eastern Avenue, Baltimore,
MD 21224, USA

Gellman, M.D.
University of Miami,
Behavioral Medicine Research Center
(D-110), 1500 N.W. 12th Avenue,
Jackson Medical Towers, 14th Floor,
Miami, FL 33136, USA

Gerin, W.
The New York Hospital –
Cornell Medical Center,
525 East 68th Street, Starr-4,
New York, NY 10021, USA

Ghione, S.
C.N.R., Institute of Clinical
Physiology, Hypertension Unit,
Via Savi 8, 56100 Pisa, Italy

Giaconi, S.
Cardiologia, Ospedale Civile
di Volterra, 56100 Volterra (Pisa),
Italy

Gleichmann, U.
Kardiologische Klinik,
Herzzentrum NRW,
Klinik der Ruhruniversität Bochum,
4970 Bad Oeynhausen, FRG

Harshfield, G. A.
Department of Pediatrics,
Division of Cardiology,
University of Tennessee,
848 Adams Ave, Memphis,
TN 38103, USA

van der Hoeven, G. M. A.
TNO Biomedical Instrumentation,
Academic Medical Centre,
Suite 0-002, Meibergdreef 15,
1105 AZ Amsterdam,
The Netherlands

Imholz, B. P. M.
Department of Internal Medicine,
Academic Medical Centre,
Meibergdreef 9, 1105 AZ Amsterdam,
The Netherlands

Ironson, G. H.
University of Miami, Behavioral
Medicine Research Center
(D-110), 1500 N.W. 12th Avenue,
Jackson Medical Towers, 14th Floor,
Miami, FL 33136, USA

James, G. D.
The New York Hospital –
Cornell Medical Center,
525 East 68th Street, Starr-4,
New York, NY 10021, USA

Jetté, M.
Faculty of Health Sciences,
University of Ottawa,
125 University St., Ottawa,
Ontario, K1N 6N5, Canada

Johnston, D. W.
Department of Psychology,
University of St. Andrews,
St. Andrews, Fife KY16 9JU, UK

Kitson, C.
Department of Psychology,
St George's Hospital Medical School,
Cranmer Terrace,
London SW17 0RE, UK

Klein, P.
Institut für Kardiologie
und Klinische Forschung,
Emmeramsplatz 2,
8400 Regensburg, FRG

Klüßendorf, D.
Institut für Physiologie
der Freien Universität Berlin,
Arnimallee 22, 1000 Berlin 33, FRG

Koralewski, E.
Institut für Physiologie
der Freien Universität Berlin,
Arnimallee 22, 1000 Berlin 33, FRG

Krause, R.
Leistungszentrum Berlin
Sportmedizin, Forckenbeckstraße 21,
1000 Berlin 33, FRG

Langewitz, W.
Psychosomatische Abteilung,
Kantonspital Basel,
Petersgraben 4, 4031 Basel, CH

Langewouters, G. J.
TNO Biomedical Instrumentation,
Academic Medical Centre,
Suite 0-002, Meibergdreef 15,
1105 AZ Amsterdam,
The Netherlands

Lemmer, B.
Zentrum für Pharmakologie,
Klinikum der J. Wolfgang
Goethe-Universität,
Theodor-Stern-Kai 7,
6000 Frankfurt/M 70, FRG

Llabre, M. M.
University of Miami, Behavioral
Medicine Research Center
(D-110), 1500 N.W. 12th Avenue,
Jackson Medical Towers, 14th Floor,
Miami, FL 33136, USA

Lüpsen, H.
Rechenzentrum der Universität Köln,
Berrenratherstraße 136,
5000 Köln 41, FRG

Malliani, A.
Istituto Ricerche Cardiovascolari,
Via Bonfadini 214, 20138 Milano,
Italy

Mancia, G.
Ospedale Maggiore di Milano,
Centro di Fisiologia Clinica
e Ipertensione, Università di Milano,
Via Francesco Sforza 35,
20122 Milano, Italy

Mannebach, H.
Kardiologische Klinik,
Herzzentrum NRW,
Klinik der Ruhruniversität Bochum,
4970 Bad Oeynhausen, FRG

Mayer, J.
Klinikum der Philipps-Universität,
Zentrum für Innere Medizin,
Abteilung Poliklinik,
Baldingerstraße,
3550 Marburg, FRG

van Montfrans, G. A.
Department of Internal Medicine,
Academic Medical Centre,
Meibergdreef 9,
1105 AZ Amsterdam,
The Netherlands

Muller, J. E.
Institute for Prevention
of Cardiovascular Disease,
1 Autumn St, Boston,
MA 02215, USA

Ohlmeier, H.
Kardiologische Klinik,
Herzzentrum NRW,
Klinik der Ruhruniversität Bochum,
4970 Bad Oeynhausen, FRG

Omboni, S.
Ospedale Maggiore di Milano,
Centro di Fisiologia Clinica
e Ipertensione, Universitá di Milano,
Via Francesco Sforza 35,
20122 Milano, Italy

Pagani, M.
Istituto Ricerche Cardiovascolari,
Via Bonfadini 214, 20138 Milano,
Italy

Parati, G.
Ospedale Maggiore di Milano,
Centro di Fisiologia Clinica
e Ipertensione, Universitá di Milano,
Via Francesco Sforza 35,
20122 Milano, Italy

Peter, J. H.
Klinikum der Philipps-Universität,
Zentrum für Innere Medizin,
Abteilung Poliklinik,
Baldingerstraße,
3550 Marburg, FRG

Piccolo, P.
Abteilung für Epidemiologie
und Sozialmedizin,
Medizinische Hochschule Hannover,
Konstanty-Gutschow-Straße 8,
3000 Hannover 61, FRG

Pickering, T. G.
The New York Hospital –
Cornell Medical Center,
525 East 68th Street, Starr-4,
New York, NY 10021, USA

Pieper, C.
The New York Hospital –
Cornell Medical Center,
525 East 68th Street, Starr-4,
New York, NY 10021, USA

Prager, G.
Institut für Kardiologie
und Klinische Forschung,
Emmeramsplatz 2,
8400 Regensburg, FRG

Prager, R.
Institut für Kardiologie
und Klinische Forschung,
Emmeramsplatz 2,
8400 Regensburg, FRG

Rüddel, H.
Psychosomatische Fachklinik,
St. Franziska-Stift,
Franziska-Puricelli-Straße 3,
6550 Bad Kreuznach, FRG

Schächinger, H.
Psychosomatische Fachklinik,
St. Franziska-Stift,
Franziska-Puricelli-Straße 3,
6550 Bad Kreuznach, FRG

Schlussel, Y. L.
The New York Hospital –
Cornell Medical Center,
525 East 68th Street, Starr-4,
New York, NY 10021, USA

Schmidt, T. F. H.
Präventiv- und Verhaltensmedizin,
Abteilung für Epidemiologie·
und Sozialmedizin,
Medizinische Hochschule Hannover,
Konstanty-Gutschow-Straße 8,
3000 Hannover 61, FRG

Schnall, P. L.
The New York Hospital –
Cornell Medical Center,
525 East 68th Street, Starr-4,
New York, NY 10021, USA

Schneiderman, N.
University of Miami, Behavioral
Medicine Research Center (D-110),
1500 N. W. 12th Avenue,
Jackson Medical Towers, 14th Floor,
Miami, FL 33136, USA

Schulte, W.
Medizinische Klinik,
Universität Bonn,
Sigmund-Freud-Straße 25,
5300 Bonn, FRG

Spitzer, S. B.
University of Miami, Behavioral
Medicine Research Center (D-110),
1500 N. W. 12th Avenue,
Jackson Medical Towers, 14th Floor,
Miami, FL 33136, USA

Sprangers, R. L. H.
TNO Biomedical Instrumentation,
Academic Medical Centre,
Suite 0-002, Mcibergdreef 15,
1105 AZ Amsterdam,
The Netherlands

Steinmetz, T.
Präventiv- und Verhaltensmedizin,
Abteilung für Epidemiologie
und Sozialmedizin,
Medizinische Hochschule Hannover,
Konstanty-Gutschow-Straße 8,
3000 Hannover 61, FRG

Steptoe, A.
Department of Psychology,
St George's Hospital Medical School,
Cranmer Terrace,
London SW17 ORE, UK

Stöhr, W.
Lehrstuhl Tierphysiologie,
Universität Bayreuth,
Postfach 101 251,
8580 Bayreuth, FRG

Talan, M. I.
National Institute on Aging,
Laboratory of Behavioral Sciences,
Gerontology Research Center,
Baltimore, MD 21224, USA

Tofler, G. H
Institute for Prevention of
Cardiovascular Disease, 1 Autumn St,
Boston, MA 02215, USA

Trazzi, S.
Ospedale Maggiore di Milano,
Centro di Fisiologia Clinica
e Ipertensione, Università di Milano,
Via Francesco Sforza 35,
20122 Milano, Italy

Vögele, C.
Department of Psychology,
St George's Hospital Medical School,
Cranmer Terrace,
London SW17 ORE, UK

Volmar, J.
Kardiologische Klinik,
Herzzentrum NRW,
Klinik der Ruhruniversität Bochum,
4970 Bad Oeynhausen, FRG

Wesseling, K. H.
TNO Biomedical Instrumentation,
Academic Medical Centre,
Suite 0-002, Meibergdreef 15,
1105 AZ Amsterdam,
The Netherlands

Wever, R. A.
Max-Planck-Institut für Psychiatrie,
Arbeitsgruppe Chronobiologie,
8138 Andechs, FRG

Wieling, W.
TNO Biomedical Instrumentation,
Academic Medical Centre,
Suite 0-002, Meibergdreef 15,
1105 AZ Amsterdam, The Netherlands

de Wit, B.
TNO Biomedical Instrumentation,
Academic Medical Centre,
Suite 0-002, Meibergdreef 15,
1105 AZ Amsterdam,
The Netherlands

Wittenhaus, J.
Präventiv- und Verhaltensmedizin,
Abteilung für Epidemiologie
und Sozialmedizin,
Medizinische Hochschule Hannover,
Konstanty-Gutschow-Straße 8,
3000 Hannover 61, FRG

Diurnal Variations –
Circadian Rhythms

Day-Night Variations in the Cardiovascular System. Historical and Other Notes by an Outsider

J. Aschoff

On the Physician's Pulse-Watch and the Proper Time for Getting Up

Among the earliest data-based documentations of diurnal variations in human physiological functions are those concerning heart rate and body temperature. In his famous textbook of 1801, Autenrieth states that "there occur within one minute in an adult human being in the morning 65 to 70, in the evening 75 to 80 pulsations" (my translation from German). In the same year, Gruner (1801) reported results from hourly measurements on two subjects; he found 65 pulses/min at 8 a.m, and 80 at 4 p.m. Similar observations had already been made by Reil (1796) who emphasizes that the acceleration of the pulse toward the evening does not occur in response to changes in conditions but is due to a "steady increase in irritability from morning to evening." However, one has to remember that almost 100 years earlier John Floyer (1707–1710) published his monograph "The Physicians Pulse-Watch" which according to Albrecht von Haller (1788) "broke the ice" in the measurement of pulse rate, and in which exact numbers are given on pulse rate under various conditions such as food intake, exercise and sleep. In the introduction, Floyer mentions that initially he had made use of a sea minute-glass, "but because that was not portable, I caused a pulse watch to be made which run 60 seconds." He approached Samuel Watson, Mathematician-in-Ordinary to King Charles II and one of the masters of horology at that time, to construct for him a watch carrying a seconds hand. "There is no doubt about the identity of Samuel Watson as the maker of Floyer's pulse watch" (Gibbs, 1971; for the only earlier watch with a seconds hand cf. Britten, 1911, and Kümmel, 1974).

Most of the authors of that time who were interested in diurnal variations also mention that body temperature decrease at night, but it took three more decades until the full temperature cycle was documented by Gierse (1842) (cf. Fig. 1 in Aschoff, 1955). On the other hand, the regularity and ubiquity of diurnal variations were obviously common knowledge at the turn of the century. In 1811, Burdach published his Dietetics for Healthy People in which he describes in what way bodily functions differ in their state at night from that seen during the daytime: "The digestion is slowed down, the breaths don't follow each other as quickly, the pulse is decelerated, and the heat of the body is lower by 0.5° Réaumur." In view of these rhythmic changes Burdach envisaged the possibility

Schmidt/Engel/Blümchen (Eds.)
Temporal Variations of the Cardiovascular System
© Springer-Verlag Berlin Heidelberg 1992

to shape, in analogy to Linné's "Flower-Clock", a "Man-Clock" (Menschenuhr) from which one could predict how a person will react to certain conditions in the morning and in the evening; this was written three years prior to Virey (1814) who coined the term "L'horloge vivante". Nowadays, Burdach will probably not get much approval for his claim that "five o'clock in the morning is the most becoming time to rise, and that those who abandon their pillow only at eight o'clock or later never reach that dispassionate self-consideration to which we are roused in the small hours." Ludwig (1861) who in his textbook introduced the graphic representation of pulse measurements (cf. Vol. 2, Fig. 32 and 33) summarizes the knowledge of his time in the plain sentence: "Heart rate changes with the time of day, independent of food intake and body movement." (All my translations from German).

At this point a brief digression seems permissible. Quite some time before the physicians began to record the pulse rate by means of precise watches, pulsations were used to determine time intervals, as did Galilei when studying the laws of the pendulum (cf. Viviani, 1654). Also at his time, the mathematician and philosopher Hieronymus Cardanus (1570) tried to illustrate the speed of the moon's movement by calculating the distance which it travels within one pulsation; in this context, Cardanus arrived at the astonishing correct number of 4000 pulsations per hour (= 67 pulses/minute) (cf. for this and further examples Kümmel, 1974). It was however up to the musicians to really introduce the pulse as a kind of metronom (Kümmel, 1977). In 1789, Johann Joachim Quantz, flutist and composer at the court of Frederic the Great, published his "Versuch einer Anweisung die flute traversière zu spielen" (Attempt of an introduction to play the German flute). In this remarkable document, Quantz recommends, in search of the right measure of time, to make use of the pulse because "it is as much convenient as it is inexpensive, and everybody has it always at hand." In discussing the pros and cons of such a procedure, he mentions as a possible objection that the pulse does not go at the same rate at each hour of the day: "One will argue that the pulse in the morning is slower than at noon, and still faster in the evening" (all my translations). For these reasons, and in view of effects of mood on the pulse, Quantz suggests that the pulse measured between lunch and evening in a gay and cheerful person might offer the right tempo.

Interests in diurnal variationed became renewed after methods had become available to measure blood pressure. From measurements made at the hand, Zadek (1881) concluded that the blood pressure is "submit to a daily variation, that it rises in the course of the afternoon independent of lunch, and that it starts to decline already towards late evening." In a few of the following studies a fall in pressure at night was indicated (Hill, 1898; Weiss, 1900), but not so in others (Hensen, 1900; Jellinek, 1900). The rather large variations reported by Colombo (1899) are of interest because this author tried to eliminate those factors which according to our present terminology "mask" the rhythm (cf. Aschoff, 1988; Wever, 1985): "Nous avons cherché à éliminer toutes les causes d'erreur ... que la température ambiente, le mouvement et les repas pouvaient exercer sur la pression." Obviously, sleep was not prevented in Colombo's studies. Erlanger and Hooker (1904) gave much weight to the effects of food, but also noticed a meal-independent variation: "We therefore can distinguish a gradual increase of pulse pressure throughout the day upon which is built up the wave-like increase that follows upon the ingestion of meals." Similar data were published by Weysse and Lutz (1915), indicating an almost parallel oscillation over the day in pulse rate and blood pressure, with a somewhat larger amplitude in systolic than in diastolic pressure. Eyster and Middleton (1924) point out that "a diurnal variation exists, the pressure tending to rise throughout the day and reaching its lowest level before getting out of bed."

Finally, specific attention was payed to the effects of sleep: "During sleep the blood pressure falls during the first few hours and then gradually rises up to the time of awakening" (Brush and Fayerweather, 1901). In a more detailed study, Brooks and Carroll (1912) arrived at the conclusion "that the preliminary drop after sleep is a very rapid one and that the rise thereafter begins during sleep, very soon after the point of minimum pressure and extends gradually throughout the reminder of the sleep period, to slowly rise during the day until the maximum pressure of the afternoon is reached." These authors also tried to separate the "masking" effects of sleep from a more basic oscillation by shifting sleep times: "It seems that the fall in pressure is much more pronounced after the customary regular or rhythmic sleep . . . . . while the drop which occurs as a result of the sleep taken at irregular intervals is usually less in degree and less abrupt in appearance." Similarily, in pulse rate a larger drop was found during night sleep than during day sleep (Klewitz, 1913).

In only a few of the studies mentioned so far attempts had been made to document a "basic" 24-h rhythm in the circulatory system by excluding simultaneously several of the masking factors (cf. Colombo, 1899). One way of doing this was to keep the subjects at strict bedrest. It is not surprising that under those conditions a diurnal rhythm still remained as long as the subjects were allowed to sleep at night (e.g. Reinberg et al., 1970; Halberg et al., 1970; Wertheimer et al., 1974). In an experiment in which 8 subjects were kept in bed for 56 days "the heart rate rhythm remained more stable .. than the other rhythms studied" (Winget et al., 1972). However, a diurnal rhythm has also been described in bedrest-studies in which the subjects presumably have been kept awake by frequent measurements. Morimoto and Shiraki (1970) who measured in 3-hourly intervals just prior to the ingestion of standarized meals found that at midnight the circulating blood volume was lowered by about 6%. One year previously, clinicians of the Klinikum Steglitz at Berlin had published data from 15 subjects who had been kept at strict bedrest (Schroeder et al., 1969). Sleep conditions are not mentioned but since measurements were made in 2-h intervals, each lasting for 30 minutes, it seems unlikely that the subjects had a solid sleep time. From the curves reproduced in the paper the following maxima and minima can be derived: heart rate (strokes/min) 61.4 ± 6.4 at 10 a.m. (with a 2nd maximum at 6 p.m.), 50.7 ± 6.4 at 4 a.m.; rate of pressure development (msec) 47.0 ± 10.4 at 6 a.m., 32.5 ± 5.7 at 6 p.m.

Experiments with rigorous sleep deprivation gave controversial results: Ahnve and coworkers (1981) failed to see a rhythm in heart rate and blood pressure during a 64-h vigilance (while a rhythm persisted in urinary excretion), in contrast to Rudolf and Tölle (1977) who did find a rhythm though of reduced amplitude in comparison to conditions with sleep. It was 80 years earlier that Johansson (1897)

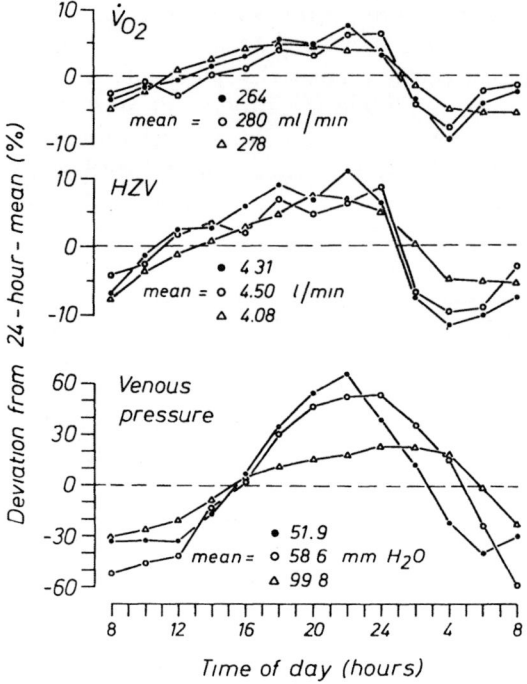

Fig. 1. Oxygen uptake ($\dot{V}_{O_1}$), cardiac output (HZV), and venous pressure recorded in 2-h intervals in 3 subjects at bedrest. Standarized meals were given every 4 h. (Adapted from Kroetz, 1940)

published data on body temperature, taken from subjects who had been fasting for 12 h, were kept awake, and avoided muscular movements as much as possible while resting in bed; the results reveal a clear rhythm, with a maximum of 36.5°C at 6 p.m., and a minimum of 35.8°C at 4 a.m. In this context, the experiments of Kroetz (1940) are to be mentioned. The "well-trained" (as Kroetz mentions) subjects rested in bed for 48 h, received a standardized meal every 4 h, and were kept awake. The results reproduced in Fig. 1 show a clear 24-h rhythm in oxygen consumption, cardiac output, and venous pressure. Unfortunately, in these experiments effects of sleep were not excluded with certainty; Kroetz admits that sometimes a subject had to be woken up for measurements.

The last step in the efforts to exclude masking is represented by a protocol which has become known as "constant routine" (Mills et al., 1978), and which attempts "to minimize or remove masking effects and so to uncover the internal clock" (Minors and Waterhouse, 1987). The constant routine as used at Manchester includes continuous lighting, hourly equal meals, sedentary position, and continuous wakefulness. In experiments, presently ongoing in the Psychiatric Clinic at Basel, distinct rhythms in heart rate have been demonstrated. The example provided in Fig. 2 is typical for 12 out of 15 subjects studied so far; in 3 subjects no rhythm was left in heart rate though the rhythm in rectal temperature was as clearly expressed as in Fig. 2 (unpublished data from Kräuchi and Wirz-

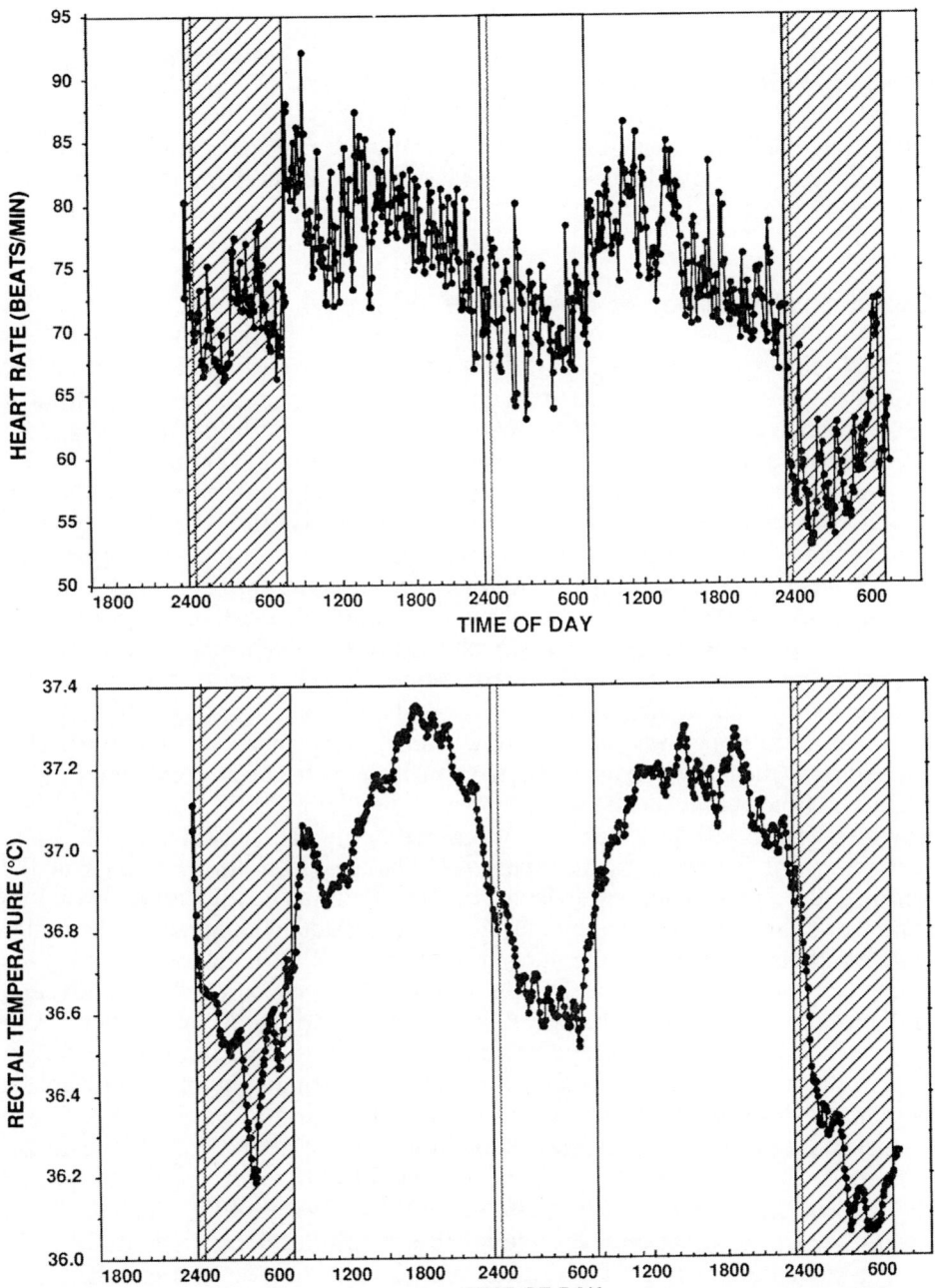

Fig. 2. Diurnal rhythms in heart rate and rectal temperature recorded in a male subject during constant routine. Shaded areas: sleep in darkness. (Courtesy of Kurt Kräuchi and Anna Wirz-Justice; unpublished data)

Justice). In slight deviation from the Manchester protocol the conditions at Basel were: continuous bedrest in a constantly illuminated, sound-attenuated room, standardized meals at 2-h intervals, and measurements of oxygen uptake every hour for 30 minutes. There is no doubt that the subjects studied at Basel did not fall asleep. Unfortunately, in none of the laboratories using constant routine enough data are available to support the likely hypothesis that a diurnal rhythm also persists in blood pressure.

On the Redistribution of Blood Flow Within 24 Hours

It is not surprising to notice that in studies on diurnal variations within the circulatory system data on heart rate and blood pressure outnumber by far all of the measurements one can think of. In an extensive review article (Smolensky et al., 1976) several Tables are given which cover the literature from about 1950 to 1975; they list 17 publications on blood pressure and 14 on heart rate, but only 4 on cardiac output or stroke volume, and 3 on blood flow. Without doubt, variations in heart rate and blood pressure are of relevance in medical theory and practice, but one wonders why not more attention is payed to that function which is served by the work of the heart, i.e. to the blood supply to various tissues. In the following, an attempt is made to briefly illustrate the problem with a few examples.

The diurnal variation in body temperature is partly due to changes in heat production, but also results from a diurnal rhythm in heat loss (Aschoff, 1947). In Fig. 3 the two uppermost curves show the rhythms in rectal and mean skin temperature (the latter one averaged from measurements at 11 points on the skin surface). The lower most two curves represent the rhythms in heat production and heat loss. The variations in heat loss are caused by changes in skin blood flow and the consequent changes in skin temperature. The conditions for heat loss from the body to the environment are described by "thermal conductance" which is expressed as heat flow divided by the temperature gradient along which the heat is lost; the dimension of conductance is $watt/m^2 \times {}^\circ C$. "Total conductance" is defined as heat flow devided by the gradient between core of the body and environment, "internal conductance" as heat flow divided by the gradient from core to skin. Variations in *internal* conductance reflect almost exclusively changes in skin blood flow. As can be seen from Fig. 3, internal conductance reaches a minimum of about 20.2 $(watt/m^2 \times {}^\circ C)$ at noon, and a maximum of 23.7 at 2 o'clock in the morning. Hence, skin blood flow varies by about $\pm 15\%$ from its 24-h mean; it reflects drastic changes in the distribution of blood between the core and the shell of the body (Aschoff, 1956; Aschoff and Wever, 1958). This order of magnitude in changes of skin blood flow can certainly not be considered irrelevant for the circulation at large if one takes into account that, on average, the blood vessels of the skin participate with 25% in the total blood volume and with 4.5% in the flow resistance which itself is in the skin even more variable than in the muscles (Aschoff, 1954). (It should be noticed that the rhythm in heat production phase-leads the rhythm in heat loss by 1.2 h; the rhythm of rectal temperature begins to decline when the curve of decreasing heat production crosses the still increasing curve of heat loss; cf. Fig. 8.7 in Aschoff et al., 1974; for the interaction

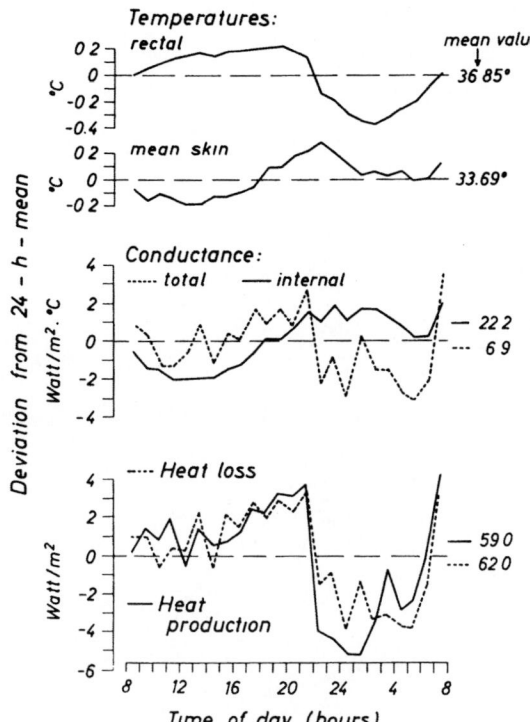

Fig. 3. Hourly averages of heat balance in 8 female subjects, each recorded twice throughout 24 h during bedrest at an ambient temperature of 28 °C. Sleep from 21:30 to 07:30. (Adapted from Schmidt, 1972)

between these three rhythms and that of conductance cf. Fig. 13.8 in Aschoff, 1982).

Impressive as the 24-h variations are in the values of heat transfer from the core of the body to its surface as a whole, they are outweighed by the 24-h redistribution of blood flow which occurs within the shell of the body. During the forenoon conductance in the extremities is far below that measured at the trunk, but in the afternoon this relationship becomes reversed: conductance at hands and feet reaches values which are about twice as large as those measured at the trunk. An example is given in Fig. 4 by the data from one female subject, measured in the nude and in a reclining position at an ambient temperature of 24 °C. It is obvious that the steep increase in conductance (i.e. in blood flow) is confined to the distal parts of the extremities; at the chest, conductance even slightly decreases. In comparing the data from various parts of the body's shell, one has to keep in mind that conductance when measured at the trunk gives only a qualitative estimate of blood flow. On the fingers, however, a proportional relationship has been demonstrated between conductance and blood flow as measured by plethysmographic techniques (cf. Fig. 3 in Aschoff and Wever, 1957). Hence it can be estimated that there is an about 30 fold increase in finger blood flow between 8 and 10 p.m.

The abrupt increases in blood flow which occur in the distal parts of the extremities toward the evening could be considered to be caused by the onset of sleep. However, a closer inspection of such curves reveals that conductance which

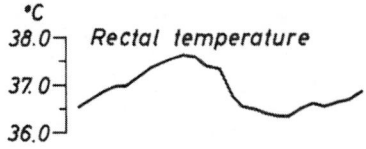

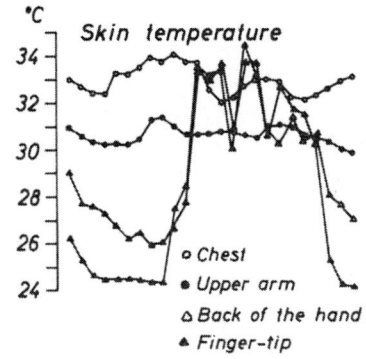

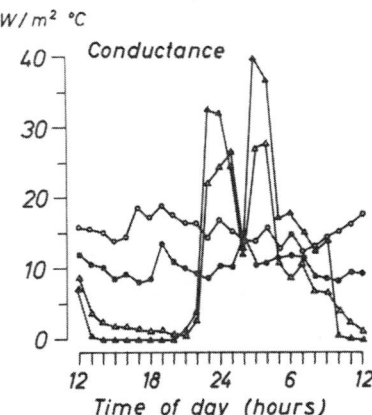

Fig. 4. Hourly values of rectal and skin temperature, and of internal conductance, recorded in a male subject at an ambient temperature of 24 °C. (Adapted from Heise, 1969, in Aschoff and Heise, 1972)

falls throughout the afternoon, begins to rise 2.5 h before the subject falls asleep, in contrast to other parts of the shell where conductance begins to decrease with the onset of sleep. For four sites, this is shown in Fig. 5 by data averaged from the records of 8 female subjects. The daily turning-point in the dynamics of the circulatory system in late afternoon (when one's shoes become tight) does neither depend on a change in position nor on sleep. If sleep is prevented, the patterns of curves describing changes in skin blood flow are similar to those presented in Fig. 5, though the ranges of oscillation are distinctly smaller (Damm et al., 1974). In summary: there is a basic, meal- and sleep-independent 24-h rhythm in the redistribution of blood flow.

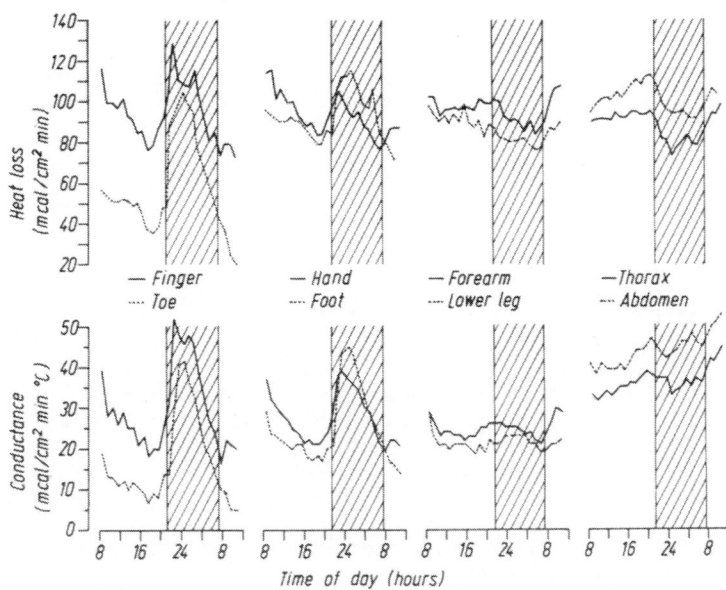

Fig. 5. Heat loss from 8 areas of the skin surface, as well as internal conductance, drawn as a function of time of day. Mean values from 8 female subjects, measured twice during bedrest at an ambient temperature of 28 °C. Shaded area: sleep in darkness. (Adapted from Schmidt, 1972, in Aschoff et al., 1974)

Concluding Remark: On the Proper Time to Retire

So far, the Patron Saint of chronobiology, Hufeland, has not been mentioned; the reason is that, despite of his interest in the 24-h period as the unit of natural chronology, he has nowhere given detailed figures on rhythmic functions. Reference to him is now made because of a literary speciality: The first edition of his bestseller "Die Kunst das menschliche Leben zu verlängern" (The art for prolonging human life; Hufeland, 1797) carries the following dedication: "Dem Herrn Georg Christoph Lichtenberg, Königl. Großbrittan. Hofrath und Professor zu Göttingen, seinem verehrtesten Lehrer und Freund, zum öffentlichen Zeichen der aufrichtigsten Hochachtung und Dankbarkeit gewidmet vom Verfasser." Lichtenberg was primarily physicist, but interested in all aspects of life. One possibly doesn't go wrong in supposing that he himself has been aware of the 24-h periodicity and its internal routes. And indeed: in one of his popular articles published in the "Göttinger Taschen-Kalender" of 1773, Lichtenberg writes: "Die sogenannten Leute nach der Uhr werden gewöhnlich alt. Das Handeln nach der Uhr aber setzt innere uhrmäßige Anlage voraus...." (The so-called people-by-the-clock usually grow old. But to act up to the clock presupposes an internal clock-like disposition). If one tries to live in accordance with one's clock-like disposition one needs to have a feeling for the course of the internal clock. What comes to mind is the stomach. A latin saying runs: "Venter optimum est horologium" (the stomach is the best clock). But circulation may as well be suitable for use, especially in the evening when we attempt to time our sleep in such a way that its masking effects don't conteract but enforce what the internal clock demands. Not long after the turning-point in peripheral blood flow, when heat loss reaches its maximum and rectal temperature begins to decline, onset of sleep seems to be most appropriate. As a true poet who apparently has a deep insight into the human circadian machinery, Elias Canetti (1935) recommends: "A respectable man retires at nine o'clock."

References

Ahnve S, Theorell T, Akerstedt T, Fröberg JE, Halberg F (1981) Circadian variations in cardiovascular parameters during sleep deprivation. Europ J Appl Physiol 46:9–19

Aschoff J (1947) Einige allgemeine Gesetzmässigkeiten physikalischer Temperaturregulation. Pflügers Arch 249:125–136

Aschoff J (1954) Regelgrössen des Kreislaufes. Nauheimer Fortbildung Lehrg 20:2–17

Aschoff J (1955) Der Tagesgang der Körpertemperatur beim Menschen. Klin. Wochenschr. 33:545–551.

Aschoff J (1956) Wechselwirkungen zwischen Kern und Schale im Wärmehaushalt. Arch Physikal Therapie 8:112–133.

Aschoff J (1982) The circadian rhythm of body temperature as a function of body size. In: Taylor CR, Johansen K, Bolis L (Eds): A Companion to Animal Physiology Cambridge University Press, Cambridge, pp. 173–188.

Aschoff J (1988) Masking of circadian rhythms by zeitgebers as opposed to entrainment. In: Hekkens WThJM, Kerkhof GA, Rietveld WJ (Eds): Trends in Chronobiology. Pergamon Press, Oxford-New York, pp. 149–161.

Aschoff J, Biebach H, Heise A and Schmidt T (1974) Day-night variation in heat balance. In: Monteith JL, Mount LE (Eds): Heat Loss from Animals and Man. Butterworth, London, pp. 147–172.

Aschoff J and Heise A (1972) Thermal conductance in man, its dependence on time of day and on ambient temperature. In: Ito S, Ogata K, Yoshimura H (Eds): Advances in Climatic Physiology, Igaku Shoin Ltd., Tokyo, pp. 334–348.

Aschoff J and Wever R (1957) Durchblutungsmessung an der menschlichen Extremität. Verhandl Dtsch Ges Kreislaufforsch 23: pp. 375–380.

Aschoff J and Wever R (1958) Kern und Schale im Wärmehaushalt des Menschen. Klin Wochenschr 45:477–485.

Autenrieth JHF Handbuch der Empirischen Menschlichen Physiologie, Band 1, Tübingen 1801/02.

Britten FJ (1911) Old Clocks and Watches and their Makers. Batsford, London, 1911.

Brooks H and Carroll JH (1912) A clinical study of the effects of sleep and rest on blood-pressure. Arch Int Med 10:97–102.

Brush CE and Fayerweather R (1901) Observations on the changes in blood-pressure during normal sleep. Am J Physiol 5:199–210.

Burdach KF (1811) Die Diaetetik für Gesunde. Heinrich IC, Leipzig

Canetti E (1935) Die Blendung. Fischer, Frankfurt.

Cardanus H (1570) Opus novum de proportionibus numerorum, motuum, ponderum, sonorum aliarumque rerum mensurandum... Basel.

Colombo C (1899) Recherches sur la pression du sang chez l'homme. Arch Ital Biol 31:345–368.

Damm F, Döring G and Hildebrandt G (1974) Untersuchungen über den Tagesgang von Hautdurchblutung und Hauttemperatur unter besonderer Berücksichtigung der physikalischen Temperaturregulation. Physikal Medizin Rehabilitat 15:1–6.

Erlanger J and Hooker DR (1904) An experimental study of blood-pressure and of pulse pressure in man. John Hopkins Hospital Reports 12:145–378.

Eyster JAE and Middleton WS (1924) Clinical studies on venous pressure. Arch internal Med 34:228–242.

Floyer J (1707–1610) The Physician's Pulse-Watch; or, am Essay to Explain the Old Art of Feeling the Pulse and to Improve it by the Help of a Pulse-Watch. Smith S and Walford B, London, Vol. 1 and 2.

Gibbs DD (1971) The physicians pulse watch. Medical History 15:187–190.

Gierse A (1842) Quoniam sit ratio caloris organici ... Med. Thesis, Halle.

Gruner ChG (1801) Physiologische und Pathologische Zeichenlehre zum Gebrauch Akademischer Vorlesungen. Akademische Buchhandlung, Jena.

Halberg F, Vallbona C, Dietlein LF, Rummel JA, Bewy ChA, Pitts GC and Nunneley SA (1970) Human circadian circulatory rhythms during weightlesness in extraterrestrial flight or bedrest with and without exercise. Space Life Sci 2:18–32.

Haller A von (1776–1788) Bibliotheca medicinae practicae. Bern und Basel, Vol 1–4.

Heise A (1969) Der Einfluss der Umgebungstemperatur auf verschiedene temperaturregulatorische Grössen beim Menschen mit besonderer Berücksichtigung der Tagesperiodik. Med Thesis, München.

Hensen H (1900) Beiträge zur Physiologie und Pathologie des Blutdruckes. Dtsch Arch Klin Med 67:436–530.

Hill L (1898) On rest, sleep, and work and the concomitant changes in the circulation of the blood. The Lancet 1898, I:282–285.

Hufeland ChW (1797) Die Kunst das menschliche Leben zu verlängern. 1. Aufl., Thad Edl v Schmidball, Wien.

Jellinek S (1900) Über den Blutdruck des gesunden Menschen. Z Klin Med 39:447–472.

Johansson JE (1897) Über das Verhalten der Kohlensäure und der Körpertemperatur bei möglichst vollständiger Ausschliessung der Muskeltätigkeit. Nordiskt med Ark 30, Nr. 22.

Klewitz F (1913) Der Puls im Schlaf. Dtsch Arch klin med 112:38–47.

Kroetz Ch (1940) Ein biologischer 24-Stunden-Rhythmus des Blutkreislaufs bei Gesundheit und bei Herzschwäche. Münch Med Wschr 87:284–288 and 314–317.

Kümmel WF (1974) Der Puls und das Problem der Zeitmessung in der Medizin. Medizinhist Journal 9:1–23.

Kümmel WK (1977) Musik und Medizin. Freiburger Beitr. zur Wissenschafts- und Universitätsgeschichte. Karl Alber, Freiburg/München.

Lichtenberg GCh (1793) Hupazoli und Cornaro, oder: Thue es ihnen nach wer kann. Göttinger Taschen-Kalender 1793:137–143

Ludwig C (1861) Lehrbuch der Physiologie des Menschen. 2. Aufl. C. F. Wintersche Verlagsbuchhandlung, Leipzig und Heidelberg.

Mills JN, Minors DS and Waterhouse JM (1978) Adaptation to abrupt time shifts of the oscillators controlling human circadian rhythms. J Physiol 285:455–470.

Minors DS and Waterhouse JM (1987) The problem of masking and some ways to deal with it. In: Hildebrandt G, Moog R, Rascke F (Eds): Chronobiology and Chronomedicine. Verlag Peter Lang, Frankfurt, pp. 119–135.

Morimoto T and Shiraki K (1970) Circadian variation in circulating blood volume. Jap J Physiol 20:550–559.

Quantz JJ (1789) Versuch einer Anweisung die flute traversière zu spielen. Berlin, 3. Aufl. Nachdruck im Bärenreiter-Verlag, Kassel und Basel, 1953.

Reil JCh, Von der Lebenskraft. Arch für die Physiol 1:8–162.

Reinberg A, Ghata J, Halberg F, Gervais P, Abulkev Ch, Dupont J and Gaudeau Cl (1970) Rythmes circadiens du pouls, de la pression artérielle, des excrétions urinaires en 17-hydroxycorticosteroides, catécholamines et potassium. Ann d'Endocrinol 31:277–287.

Rudolf GAE and Tölle R (1977) Circadian rhythm of circulatory functions in depressives and in sleep deprivation. Int Pharmacopsychiat 12:174–183.

Schmidt TH (1972) Thermoregulatorische Grössen in Abhängigkeit von Tageszeit und Menstrualzyklus. Med Thesis, München.

Schröder R, Dennert J, Neumann H, Prokein E, Ramdohr B, Schachinger H and Schüren KP (1969) 24-Stunden-Rhythmus im Inotropiezustand des Herzmuskels bei gesunden jungen Männern. Verhandlg Dtsch Ges Kreislaufforschg 35:370–375.

Smolensky MH, Tatar ShE, Bergman SA, Losman J, Barnard ChN, Dacso CC and Kraft IA (1976) Circadian rhythmic aspects of human cardiovascular function: a review by chronobiologic statistical methods. Chronobiologia 3:337–371.

Virey JJ (1814) Ephémérides de la vie humaine ou recherches sur ala révolution journalière, et la périodicité de ses phénomènes dans la santé et les maladies. Med Thesis, Paris.

Viviani V (1966) Lettere di Vincenzo viviani al Principe Leopoldo de' Medici intorno all' applicazione del pendolo all' orologio. In: Le Opere di Galileo Galilei. Nuova Ristampa della Edizione Nazionale, Firence, Vol. 19, pp. 647–659.

Weiss H (1900) Blutdruckmessung mit Gärtler's Tonometer. Münchn Med Wschr 47:79–74.

Wertheimer L, Hassen A, Delman A and Yaseen A (1974) Cardiovascular circadian rhythm in man. In: Scheving LE, Halberg F, Pauly JE (Eds): Chronobiology Georg Thieme Publ., Stuttgart, pp. 742–747.

Wever RA (1985) Internal interactions within the human circadian system: the masking effect. Experientia 41:332–342.

Weysse AW and Lutz BR (1915) Diurnal variations in arterial blood pressure. Am J Physiol 37:330–347.

Winget CM, Vernikos-Danellis J, Cronin SE, Leach CS, Rambaut PS and Mack PB (1972) Circadian rhythm asynchrony in many during hypokinesis. J Appl Physiol 33:640–643.

Zadek I (1881) Die Messung des Blutdrucks am Menschen mittels des Basch'schen Apparates. Z Klin Med 2:509–551.

Basic Principles of Human Circadian Rhythms

R. A. Wever

Introduction

24-Hour Rhythms

Virtually all variables that can be measured in living organisms, both physiological and psychical, undergo daily rhythms, that is, they show one maximum value and one minimum value over a 24-h period; only in rare cases may a variable show two nearly equivalent extreme values per day.

To elucidate this rhythmicitiy, Fig. 1 presents the courses of a number of variables that were measured continuously for 10 days in a healthy young man who lived under a strict 24-h routine. All these variables show regular daily rhythms with a high reliability; on the right side of the figure cycles are shown as averages over the 10 successive days (in this case it is clear without additional analysis that the averaging period must be 24 h). As another example, Fig. 2 shows educed cycles of blood pressure (systolic and diastolic) and heart rate measured over the natural 24-h day in a healthy young man for 14 successive days; while continuing his normal routine and performing his normal activities, he measured the variables in hourly intervals (with only very few missing data). Both figures show the standard deviations over all successive cycles to give an impression of the intraindividual variability of the data. These standard deviations, however, cannot be used for statistical purposes because of the interdependence of successive events in biological time series. Thus, the calculation of intraindividual statistics is not possible in the conventional manner but requires special time series analyses. Interindividual statistics, on the other hand, can be calculated without restriction (Wever 1979), for example, summarizing the values of rhythm parameters obtained in independent experiments or correlating the values of different parameters from subjects tested in independent experiments.

Circadian Rhythms

Apparently, the daily rhythms of all variables are based on the 24-h periodicity of nearly all environmental parameters. Since light intensity, ambient temperature, air pressure, ambient noise level, most electromagnetic phenomena, and many

Schmidt/Engel/Blümchen (Eds.)
Temporal Variations of the Cardiovascular System
© Springer-Verlag Berlin Heidelberg 1992

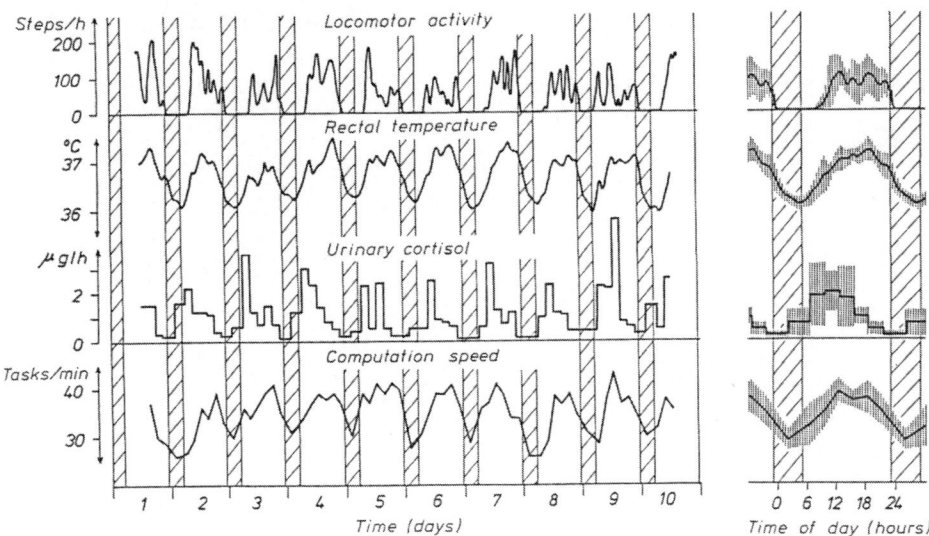

Fig. 1. Courses of several variables in a 26-year-old man living for 10 days under a carefully controlled 24-h routine (*hatched areas*, dark time). *From top to bottom:* locomotor activity (measured by contact plates under the carpet), rectal temperature (measured continuously), urinary excretion of free cortisol (urine samples were requested at 3-h intervals during day time and at 4.5-h intervals during night time), and the highest possible computation speed (adding and substracting of random digits for 3 min each at the time of micturitions). *Right*, educed cycles of the variables over the 10 days presented (with standard deviations)

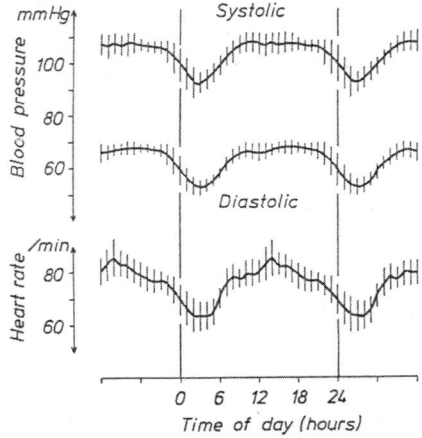

Fig. 2. Educed cycles of blood pressure (systolic and diastolic) and heart rate, measured at about hourly intervals in a 30-year-old man over 14 days while he lived a normal 24-h day and performed his normal activities (with standard deviations)

more meteorological variables show strong 24-h periodicity (based on the day-night cycle and hence the earth's rotation), it seems plausible that biological 24-h rhythms are merely reactions to the environmental 24-h period. However, this simple assumption can easily be shown to be incorrect. After having been detached from the time cues of the day-night cycle (under experimental conditions held constant for many days), all variables continue to show rhythmic courses. The efficacy of the detaching can then be seen in the resulting deviation of the period of such "free-running" or "autonomous" rhythms from 24 h. In humans this period is always close to 25 h; in some animal species (e.g., in many birds) this period may also be consistently shorter than 24 h. Since our environment does not include corresponding rhythms, the deviation of free-running periods from 24 h confirms the endogenous origin of the rhythms, i.e., the generation of the rhythm within the organism. Due to this deviation from 24 h, moreover, one should speak not of 24-h rhythms but of circadian ("about daily") rhythms (Wever 1979).

Since all biological variables in the normal environment show rhythms with a period of precisely 24.0 h, the endogenous origin of these rhythms means that the rhythms are commonly synchronized to the day-night cycle by periodic external stimuli (Zeitgeber). The day-night cycle is therefore not necessary for generating the rhythms, but it is inevitable in synchronizing the "heteronomous" rhythms to the periodically changing environment. Fortunately, such a synchronization is possible not only by natural zeitgebers connected to the day-night cycle but also, under laboratory conditions, by artificial zeitgebers of various features. This allows us to measure characteristics of circadian rhythms not only under constant conditions (and hence the mere biological regularities) but also under periodically varying conditions which correspond closer to natural conditions. Both types of experiments can be performed only under temporal isolation of the subjects, and both demand long-term experiments (Wever 1979).

Performance of the Experiments

The results discussed below derive from a series of over 450 long-term experiments, performed over 25 years in a special underground station constructed particularly for such experiments; it is worth mentioning that all these experiments proceeded without a hitch. Only volunteers participated in the experiments, lasting 1–3 months; the great majority of these subjects lived alone during the experiment, but 28 were isolated in groups of two each and 12 in groups of four each. While it may perhaps sound strange to require such long-term isolation, it has been our experience that the very great majority of volunteers felt very well during the experiment. Subjects were free to terminate the experiment at any time; they were also informed that it would be meaningless or perhaps injurious, also to the experimenter, to continue an experiment past one's endurance – "to play the hero" would substantially reduce the objective utility of the rhythm measurements. The experimental rooms were not locked, and subjects were free to leave even without informing the experimenter (but, of course, not without being seen by the experimenter). Only nine subjects terminated the experiment early, some of whom for reasons that were independent of the experimental conditions. On the other hand, the great majority of the subjects

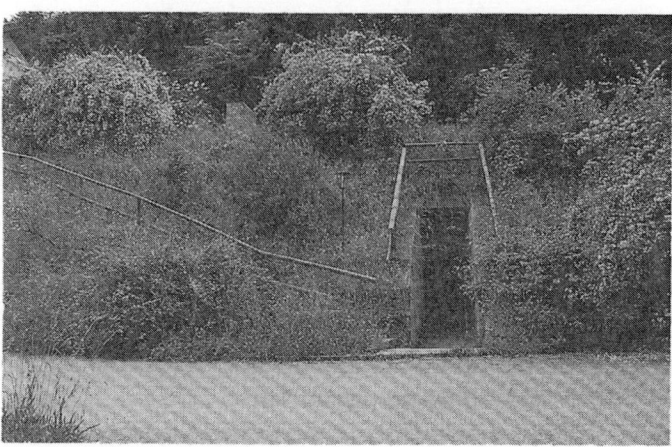

Fig. 3. Entrance to the station constructed specifically for performing experiments under temporal isolation

(over 80 %) asked, upon terminating the experiment, for a chance to participate in an additional experiment; 52 subjects, in fact, participated in two, three or even four successive experiments, with intervals between the experiments from 1 month to 19 years (the majority of subjects requesting another experiment ultimately did not find the time for such an experiment).

The very good condition of the volunteers is evident when one examines their performance in the experiments. The subjects did not live in a laboratory but in a rather comfortable apartment, consisting of a living room, bathroom, and kitchen. Figure 3 shows the entrance to the station, which includes two separate apartments (insulated independently with glass wool without any fixed connection to the outer concrete building); for special group experiments the two apartments could be connected. Figure 4 gives a view of one of the experimental units. During the experiment the subject was free in his activities for about 95 % of his time. Many subjects were students preparing for an examination or writing a thesis; many of these upon terminating an experiment applied immediately for another in advance of the next examination. Other subjects were drawn from nearly all strata and occupations, including artists preparing new works, school pupils (from 17 years of age) working for school, and elderly persons (up to 81 years of age) writing their memories or knitting for their grandchildren. Great attention was paid to the well-being of subjects; if possible, special wishes were fulfilled (contacts between subject and experimenter were possible only by written messages; Wever 1979).

It is possible that the participation exclusively of volunteers in these experiments leads to a bias in the sample. The generalization of quantitative results is therefore not necessarily possible. However, all subjects were tested psychologically before and after the experiment; on each tested item (e.g., neuroticism or introvertism) the mean among our subjects coincided with that among the total population. Nevertheless, experiments were performed in such a manner that the main weight of the results related to yes/no answers and not to quantitative data. Comparison

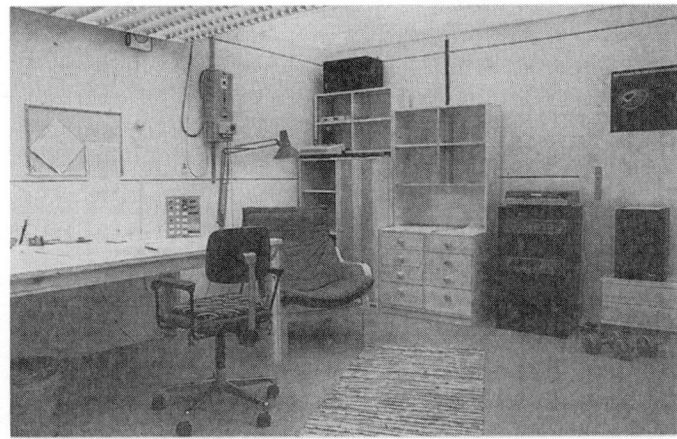

Fig. 4. One of the two experimental units (each unit included its own kitchen and bathroom)

of test scores before and those after experiments showed no systematic change in any item; hence the participation in an isolation experiment did not appear to change the personality data of subjects (for example, subjects did not become neurotic or depressive during experiments).

Experiments were conducted only with healthy subjects. However, in six cases subjects became ill during an experiment, as indicated by an increase in rectal temperature (up to 39.5 °C) or reactions in the immune system (increases in neo- and monapterin up to about five times the original levels). In each of these cases the subject insisted upon continuing the experiment, and each recovered from the illness within a few days (see Fig. 16). The results of these experiments deviated from those conducted with healthy subjects; hence, the consideration of these unintended modifications in the experimental design provides the unexpected opportunity to evaluate rhythm disorders in ill patients. Moreover, subjects aged up to 81 years were tested, and the results of experiments with elderly subjects (older than about 70 years) deviated from those of experiments with younger subjects in the same direction as those of the ill patients (see Fig. 25). Despite the small number of experiments with ill or elderly subjects, therefore, these results suggest possible relationships between disorders in circadian rhythms and health disorders, in particular mental disorders (Wever 1988).

Autonomous Rhythms

Internally Synchronized Rhythms

Examples of Experiments

When humans live under constant conditions without environmental time cues, their rhythms persist but with a period deviating slightly from 24 h. This can be

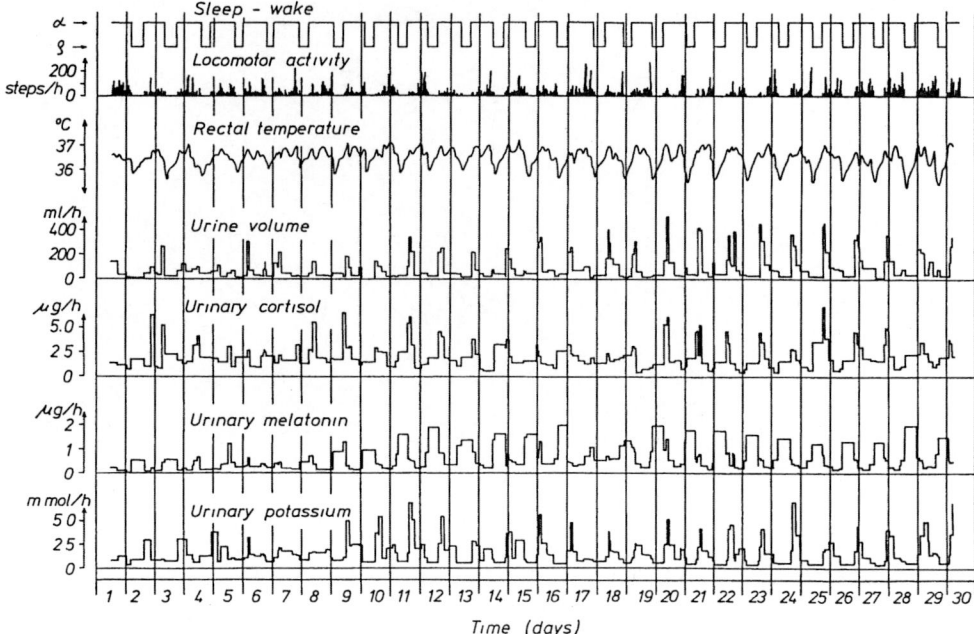

Fig. 5. Course of an experiment in which a 24-year-old woman lived for 1 month under carefully controlled constant conditions (light intensity 3000 lux) and without external time cues. *From top to bottom*, the alternation between sleep and wake, the course of locomotor activity, rectal temperature, and four urine constituents (in the constant-condition experiments micturitions could be performed only at intervals that were determined by the subject)

seen in the example of a healthy young woman shown in Fig. 5; the courses of all variables remained rhythmical (including some not shown). The slight shifts from the vertical lines (midnight in local time) demonstrate the deviations of the free-running period from 24 h. The figure also shows the remaining internal phase relationships between the rhythms of different variables; for instance, despite the deviation of the period from 24 h, the maximum values of body temperature always occurred in the wake state, and the maximum values of melatonin excretion always occurred during sleep (i.e., when the eyes were closed, and it was hence subjectively dark). This also means that in the free-run the rhythms of all variables were synchronous with one another, as in the 24-h day. As is shown below, such internal synchronization does not occur in all subjects and under all conditions (Wever 1979).

Longitudinal presentation of the data as in Fig. 5, permits the comparison between the courses of several variables and recognition of the persistence of the rhythms. The assessment of the period, on the other hand, is possible only in further analyses, as in Fig. 6; on the left are the results of periodogram analysis of the data presented directly in Fig. 5. The ordinates show normalized reliabilities of the rhythms, i.e., the portion of the total variability of the time series that is due to a rhythm, with the period indicated at the abscissa, supplementing that portion of the total variability due to random fluctuations (normalized to a standard

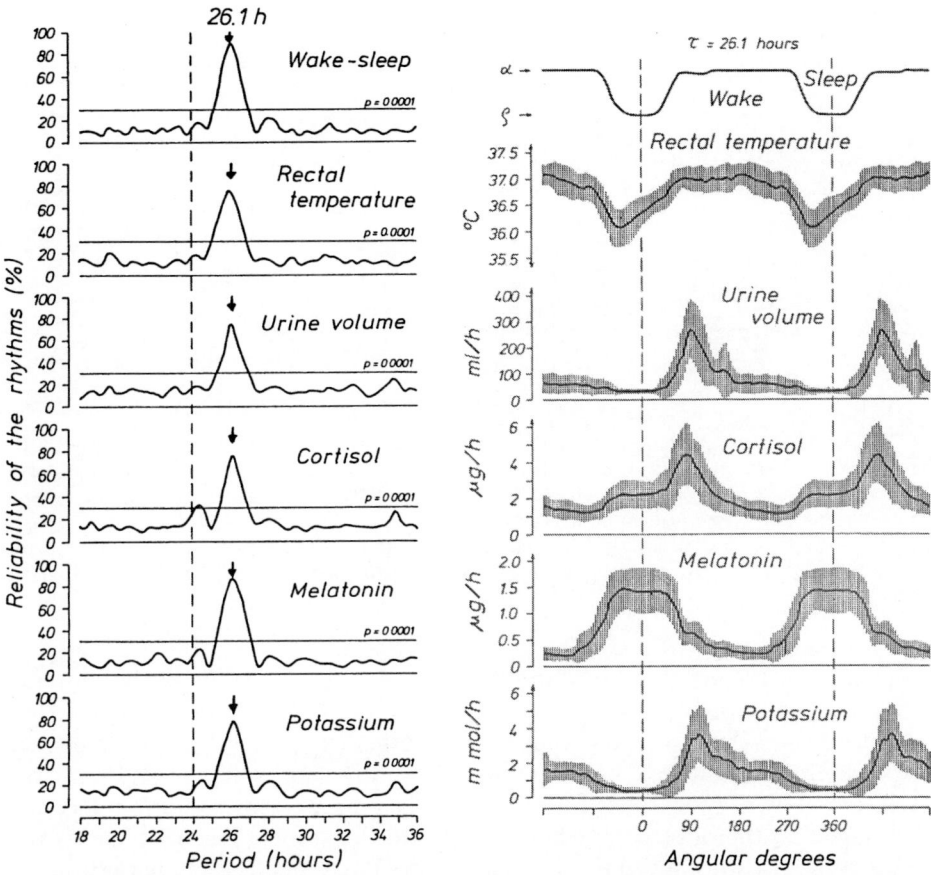

Fig. 6. Computer analysis of the experiment in Fig. 5. *Left*, periodogram analysis. All variables show highly reliable free-running rhythms with identical periods deviating from 24 h. In this experiment the free-running period was especially long due to the particularly bright illumination. *Right*, educed cycles of the same variables, averaged with the single coinciding prominent period from the periodogram analysis, indicating the high reliabilities of all rhythms; this presentation shows the internal phase relationships among the rhythms of the presented variables

circadian time series of 25 successive cycles and 24 measuring points per cycle). A normalized reliability of 30% means (independently of the actual length of the time series) a chance probability of $p = 0.0001$ of the time series being rhythmic with the indicated period. In the following, this value is taken as the threshold for rhythmicity (Wever 1979). The data show all variables to have peak periods at 26.1 h and to be remarkably reliable. This free-running period is clearly longer than usual due to the comparatively bright light to which this subject was continuously exposed (see "External Modifications of Autonomous Rhythms"). On the right of Fig. 6 educed cycles are shown, again of the same variables (averaged with the only prominent period of 26.1 h). These data show again the very high reliabilities of all rhythms and, in addition, they show the mean wave shapes, and they give obvious insight into the structure of the system as

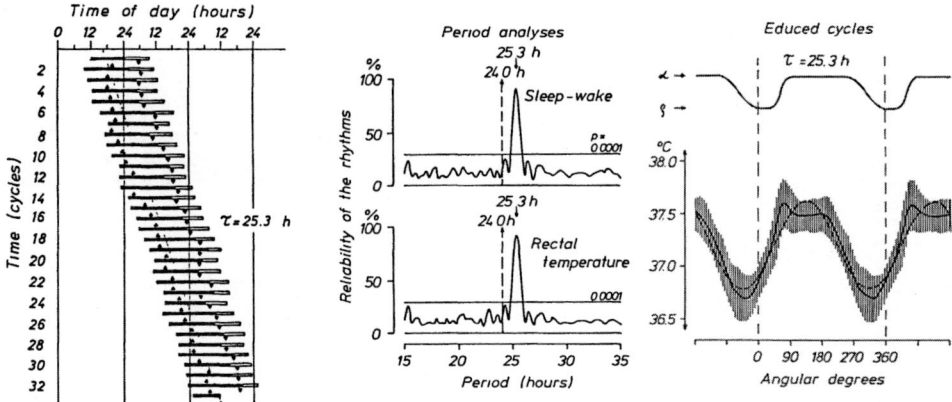

Fig. 7. Results of an experiment in which a 26-year-old man lived under constant conditions (light intensity 300 lux) without external time cues. *Left*, course of the experiment. Successive cycles of sleep-wake (*bars*) and body temperature (*triangles*, temporal positions of extreme values) are drawn beneath one another as a function of local time (*abscissa*). *Middle*, periodogram analysis of the two time series, with indication of the (coinciding) prominent periods. *Right*, educed cycles of the two time series, averaged with the prominent period from the periodogram analysis

represented by the internal (or mutual) phase relationships between the rhythms of the different variables.

Figure 7 shows the (similar) outcome of another experiment of the same type, but presenting the course of the experiment in another way. On the left, successive cycles are drawn beneath one another. This type of representation has the advantage that the slope in the data (relative to the vertical lines) highlights the period of the rhythms; it can be seen that this period is identical in the rhythms of all variables (i.e., that all rhythms are mutually synchronous). In particular, it shows that this period is maintained from the 1st day throughout the entire experiment without temporal trend or long-term fluctuations. This presention of the data thus demonstrates clearly the long-term stability of free-running rhythms. The disadvantage, on the other hand, is that it allows the simultaneous presentation of only a few rhythms. However, this is not a serious limitation since, as we have shown, either the rhythms of all variables are mutually synchronous (internal synchronization), and the presentation of others would not improve understanding of the system properties, or, in case of internally desynchronized rhythms (see "Internally Desynchronized Rhythms"), the great variety of overt rhythms can be represented by only two different rhythms (commonly, sleep-wake and body temperature) since all other rhythms are synchronous with one of these rhythms; in only a few special cases is it necessary to take three (or even four) separate rhythms. In case of the latter example (Fig. 7) computer analyses are also added. However, in contrast to the former example (Fig. 5) these analyses do not contribute essentially to the understanding of the course of this experiment (they show, for instance, the wave shape of the body temperature rhythm and the internal phase relationship between the rhythms of sleep-wake and body temperature); these are added mainly for completeness.

Internal Phase Relationships

We have seen in Figs. 6 and 7 that the internal phase relationship between the rhythms of sleep-wake and body temperature during the free-run deviates from that of the 24-h day. While the maximum of body temperature is normally reached in the late afternoon, in the free-run it is always in the first half of the activity period (i.e., in the subjective late morning), and while the temperature minimum in the 24-h day is generally close to the end of sleep, in the free-run it is always close to sleep onset (frequently even in the last part of the wake episode). Due to this internal phase shift one sleeps in the 24-h day with decreasing body temperature; in the free-run, however, one sleeps with increasing body temperature. Other variables show similar but not identical internal phase shifts; this means that the internal organization of the circadian system changes completely with the transition from the 24-h day to a free-run (Wever 1979). It could be argued that this internal change is due to the complete change of all living circumstances with the transition from the "normal world" to temporal isolation. However, some experiments have included examination of the transition from 24-h synchroniza-tion to free-run (or vice versa) without perceptible change in the environment and these show the same internal phase shifts (Wever 1982). Consequently, these shifts are due only to the forced change in the state of the rhythm and its period and not to the change in any behavioral parameter of the subjects.

The reversal in the course of body temperature during sleep has consequences for the pattern of sleep. While in the 24-h day the amount of REM sleep increases during the night, in the free-run the first REM episode of every sleep episode is the longest, and the following REM episodes shorten with advancing sleep episode. There is thus a correlation between body temperature and the amount of REM sleep: the lower the temperature at a specific time the longer are the REM episodes at this time. On the other hand, the structure of deep (or slow-wave) sleep is the same in the 24-h day and the free-run; slow-wave sleep is always concentrated at the beginning of each sleep episode, independently of the position of the temperature minimum. REM and slow-wave sleep are clearly controlled by different rhythms; REM sleep tends to be synchronous with the rhythm of body temperature, and slow-wave sleep tends to be synchronous with the sleep-wake rhythm. Finally, the percentages of REM and of slow-wave sleep are about the same in the 24-h day and in the free-run (Wever 1985b).

The change in the internal phase relationship between the rhythms of sleep-wake and body temperature, in addition, has consequences for the performance of experiments. The internal phase shift is, in fact, completed in some experiments within a few days (see Fig. 7); in other experiments, however, it lasts up to about 1 week; and during these transient states the two rhythms apparently run with different periods. If such an experiment were terminated after this week, inspection of its course and also of period analysis would lead to a misleading interpretation: different prominent periods for the rhythms of sleep-wake and body temperature would seem to indicate internal desynchronization. Moreover, during the transient state the period of the temperature rhythm is generally shorter than that of the sleep-wake rhythm and, by chance, is often close to 24.0 h; it could be concluded, therefore, to a free-run only of the sleep-wake rhythm with the temperature rhythm remaining synchronous with some 24-h zeitgeber that was overlooked or could not be eliminated (e.g., air pressure or cosmic rays). Continuation of such experiments clearly would demonstrate the incorrectness of these interpretations.

During transient states it is not meaningful to evaluate rhythm parameters (for instance, the term "period" is defined only in the steady state). Consequently, circadian experiments must last long enough, i.e., until the transients have faded away and the final steady state is maintained for a sufficiently long span of time to evaluate rhythm parameters; during transients it cannot even be decided in all experiments what the final steady state will be (i.e., internal synchronization or desynchronization). On the other hand, the transient state is of interest in itself because it gives insight into the dynamics of the circadian system; for instance, the maximum value of body temperature generally advances (relative to sleep-wake) more and faster than the minimum, indicating a change in the shape of the temperature cycle with the transition from the 24-h day to free-run.

Reliabilities of Rhythm Parameters

Before quantitative analyses between rhythm parameters from different subjects are possible, it must be certain that the values obtained in the experiment are individual constants and not accidental measurements. The parameters may depend on the experimental conditions, and they may vary from subject to subject; extensive analyses, however, are meaningless if the values obtained in different experiments also vary when the experimental conditions and the subject remain the same. Fortunately, a large number of experiments have been repeated with the same subjects (see "Performance of the Experiments") under identical experimental conditions. Considering all repetition experiments together, one can observe that the differences between all rhythm parameters in different experiments with the same subject (and identical experimental conditions) are significantly smaller than in experiments with different subjects (and also identical conditions; Wever 1983b). In other types of experiments (of longer duration) the experimental conditions were altered several times between exposure to a zeitgeber of various periods and exposure to (each identical) constant conditions; the aim of these experiments was to examine the influence of the previous zeitgeber period (for instance, of zeitgebers with periods shorter or longer than the free-running period) on the subsequent free-run. The result of these experiments was that there is not such an influence, or after-effect; i.e., the free-running period and the other rhythm parameters are independent of the previous zeitgeber period (or any other experimental condition).

Figure 8 demonstrates two examples of the coincidence between data obtained in repetition experiments. Data presented on the left are from an elderly woman who repeated the experiment after 1 year (in the meantime she had retired, moved from a big city to a little village, and completely changed her lifestyle); data on the right are from a young man who repeated the experiment after 5 years. Both subjects showed free-running periods that deviate substantially from the interindividual mean but are very similar in both experiments each, as can be seen in the upper panels of Fig. 8. The subject on the left showed the shortest free-running

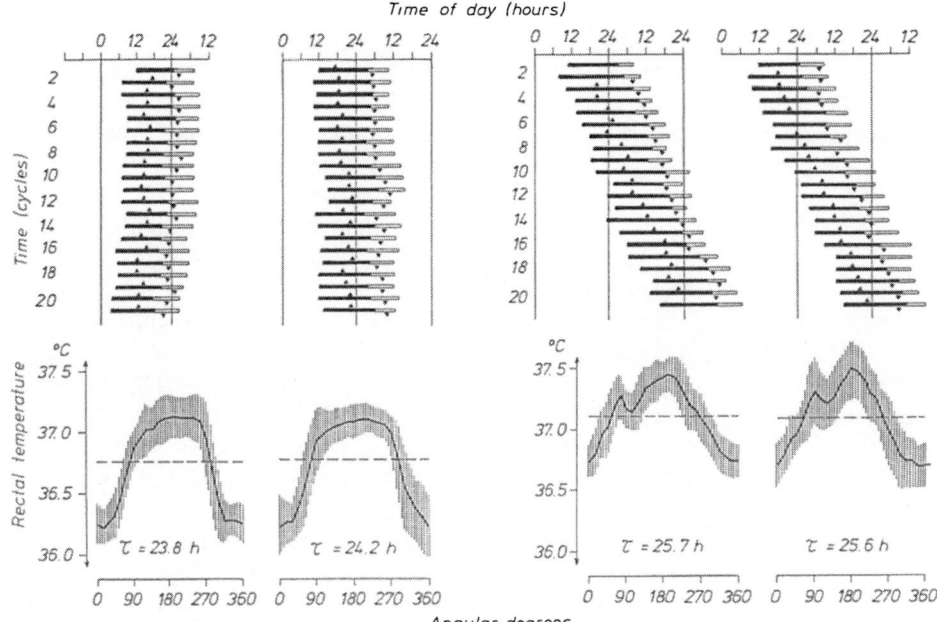

Fig. 8. Results of experiments with two subjects who lived under identical constant conditions in two successive experiments each. *Left,* 61–62-year-old woman with repetition after 1 year; *right,* 21–26-year-old man with repetition after 5 years. *Above,* courses of the experiments (in the same manner as in Fig. 7, left); *below,* educed cycles of body temperature rhythms, averaged with the prominent period as indicated (calculated previously by means of periodogram analysis)

period observed in any of the experiments, and the subject on the right showed free-running rhythms with about the longest periods, which did not show an immediate switch to internal desynchronization (see "Spontaneous Occurrence of Internal Desynchronization"). Similarities in the period can also be clearly seen in subjects with the most probable period close to 25.0 h; however, in this range similarity of the period in the repetition experiment should be expected even when there is no inherent consistency. The lower panels present educed cycles in the rhythms of body temperature; these show coinciding mean values and amplitudes and remarkably coinciding individual patterns in each subject (as "finger-prints"). While individual patterns can be distinguished from each other, the experimenter is not able to distinguish between patterns deriving from different experiments performed with the same subject. Hence, the precondition is fulfilled for analyzing the outcomes of all experiments statistically under comparable experimental conditions (Wever 1979).

Internal Stabilization of Autonomous Rhythms

As we noted in considering Fig. 7, the long-term stability of a free-running rhythm is striking; the actual cycle-to-cycle variability should lead to a much less consistent period in the long run. The basis for such stabilization of the period is a highly consistent negative serial correlation among successive cycles. This means that every cycle (sleep-wake cycle measured, for instance, from one wake onset to the next; or temperature cycle measured, for instance, from one temperature minimum to the next) which is, for any reason, longer than the long-term average in this subject, is generally followed by a cycle which is shorter than average (and even the second following cycle is shorter than average); and, vice versa, every cycle which is shorter than the intraindividual average is followed by cycles that are longer than average. Hence, every disorder in the rhythm's period is immediately corrected. The coefficients of these serial correlations are very consistent: the first-order serial correlation (i.e., between neighboring cycles) is -0.402 ± 0.132 and the second-order (i.e., between every second cycle) is -0.101 ± 0.125. In addition, there is a significant negative interindividual correlation between coefficients of first and second orders ($r = -0.673$), so that the sum of these coefficients (the coefficient of the third-order serial correlation and those of higher orders cannot be differentiated from zero) characterizes a very highly significant "internal stabilization capacity" (($r_s = -0.503 \pm 0.104$; Wever 1984 b).

Apart from the negative serial correlations between successive cycles indicating an inherent stabilization mechanism, there are those between adjacent wake and sleep episodes. Every wake episode which is, for any reason, longer than the long-term average in a subject is generally followed by a sleep episode that is shorter than average; and, vice versa, every wake episode that is shorter than the intraindividual average is followed by a sleep episode that is longer than average ($r_s = -0.527 \pm 0.221$). Moreover, every wake episode that is longer than the long-term average in a subject is followed, with lower but still significant probability, by a wake episode that is shorter than average, and vice versa ($r_s = -0.119 \pm 0.214$). These serial correlations between adjacent episodes supplement each other; in spite of the different levels of significance, therefore, they are of equal importance for the dynamics of the circadian system (Wever 1984 b). For instance, they indicate that the stabilization mechanism described above aims exclusively at the length of the total cycle and not at the length of specific episodes.

Age and Sex Dependence of Rhythm Parameters

Several parameters of free-running rhythms depend on the age and sex of the subject, but in different ways. Figure 9 illustrates three different types of age and sex dependence which have been observed among healthy volunteers. In all three cases the assessment of age dependence suffers from a lack of data from subjects aged between about 30 and 60 years; those in these age cohorts do not commonly have the time to participate in such long-term experiments. The lower panel shows the dependence of the internal stabilization capacity as just discussed. Despite the lack of data in the middle aged patients, there are highly significant correlations with the age of the subject in both women and men ($r = 0.891$), but there is no recognizable difference between the data of the sexes. This means that the mechanism stabilizing the rhythm can be disturbed (as it is in elderly subjects) without the mechanism generating the rhythm being in disorder; in elderly women the amplitude of the rhythm, as an indicator of the efficacy of this mechanism, is

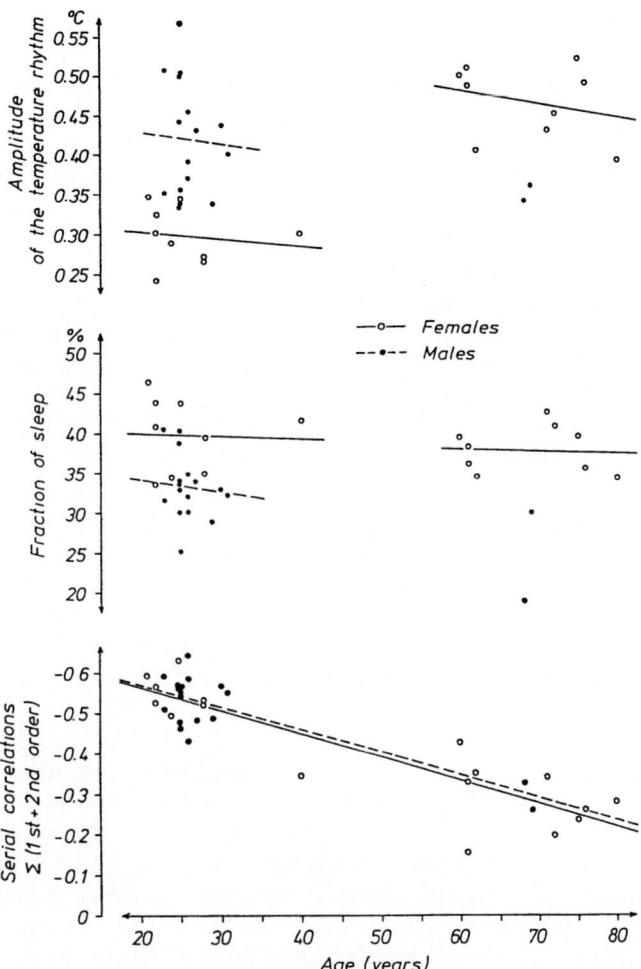

Fig. 9. Three different types of age and sex dependence in parameters of free-running circadian rhythms. *Below,* coefficients of serial correlations between successive sleep-wake cycles (index of long-term stability); consistent age dependence, no sex difference. *Middle,* fraction of sleep in the sleep-wake cycle: no age dependence, consistent sex difference. *Above,* amplitude of the rhythm of body temperature; threshold age in women (significantly higher amplitudes in elderly than in young women) but no age dependence within the groups of the young or elderly women; no age dependence in men; sex difference only between young women and men (of any age) but no sex difference between elderly women and men

even higher than in young women, and in men it is independent of age (see upper panel of Fig. 9). The same disorder in stabilization as in elderly occurs in ill patients (the coefficients of serial correlation as measured in the few subjects becoming ill during the experiment were, in fact, distinctly lower than those of healthy subjects of the same age). This means that a rhythm which is obviously intact can be disturbed in its stabilization ability (which can be measured only by extensive analyses) and hence indicates a rhythm disorder as a symptom of a health disorder (Wever 1988).

The middle panel of Fig. 9 shows the mean fraction of sleep in the sleep-wake cycle. This fraction is generally higher in women than in men (normalized to the 24-h day, women slept longer than men by 93.6 min $\pm$ 65.5 min per cycle). Since subjects in these experiments had no knowledge (and no subjective feeling) of the exact duration of their sleep episodes, this difference can be regarded as a biological necessity (in normal life the duration of sleep is frequently affected by real or imagined social constraints and hence does not necessarily reflect the biological need for sleep). The measured fraction of sleep (or even the need for sleep; see above) does not depend on the age of the subjects, either in women or in men; this is true at least when the subjects do not know the duration of the sleep, and if the naps, which may increase with age, are included in the sleep (Wever 1989 b).

The upper panel of Fig. 9 shows the amplitude of the rhythm of body temperature. In young subjects it is very significantly lower in women than in men (on average, by $34\% \pm 17\%$); in contrast, in elderly subjects there is no recognizable sex difference. On the other hand, while the amplitudes are similar in young and in elderly men, there is a distinct age dependence in women; elderly women show very significantly larger amplitudes than young women (on average, by $51\% \pm 10\%$). Since within the groups of young and elderly women no correlations with age can be established when considered separately, this result means that there is a threshold age in women (but not in men) above which the amplitude is distinctly larger than below it. Due to the lack of data in subjects in middle age, the position of this threshold cannot be determined precisely; since it is in the range of 50–60 years, it is plausible to combine this age with the menopause (Wever 1986).

Apart from the three parameters presented in Fig. 9, several other parameters of free-running rhythms show dependence on the age and/or the sex of the subject. These include the period of these rhythms, which is significantly shorter in women than in men (on average by 22.2 min $\pm$ 34.8 min; Wever 1984c). A dependence of the period on the age of the subject is not recognizable. Hence, the dependence of this parameter is equivalent to that of the sleep fraction shown in Fig. 9 (middle panel) which is clearly a property of the sleep-wake rhythm. As is shown below, the sex difference in the period of free-running rhythms is exclusively a property of the sleep-wake rhythm and not of the rhythm of body temperature. It is suggested, therefore, that the type of age and sex dependence as illustrated in the middle panel of Fig. 9, is a characteristic of the sleep-wake rhythm (Wever 1984c).

Further age and sex dependence can be observed in parameters of the rhythm of body temperature, but only regarding data on young subjects. For instance, the mean value of body temperature is significantly higher (on average by $0.176\,°C \pm 0.078\,°C$) in (young) women than in men (of any age); the data on elderly women are not distinguishable from those on men (of any age). Only in this parameter can the sex difference be deduced from well-known hormonal control mechanism. In young women the body temperature alternates in a monthly rhythm (with a period similar to the usual duration of an experiment) between lower preovulatory values (which are similar to body temperature values of men) and higher postovulatory values; in elderly women this rhythm ceases, and body temperature is consistently similar to that of men. Moreover, even the wave shape shows a significant sex difference: the increasing slope of the temperature cycle (relative to the decreasing slope) is steeper in women than in men. Finally, the intra-individual variabilities on all of these parameters are higher in (young) women than in men (of any age). On none of these parameters do the data from elderly subjects show any sex difference. Thus the data from young and from elderly women differ significantly from each other, with a threshold age around the menopause. In summary, all parameters of the rhythm of body temperature behave, with respect to the dependence on age and sex, as the parameter illustrated in the upper panel of Fig. 9. This type of dependence, with a (hormonally conditioned) threshold age in women but not in men therefore appears to be a characteristic of the rhythm of body temperature.

Intercorrelations Among Rhythm Parameters

Most of the parameters mentioned, of the sleep-wake rhythm and the rhythm of body temperature, are correlated with one another interindividually (and intraindividually). This means, for instance (at least, within a sex; see above section), that the higher a subject's mean amplitude of the temperature rhythm (within the range of the interindividual variabilities), the shorter the period of his rhythms, the larger the fraction of sleep in the sleep-wake cycle, the higher the mean value of his temperature rhythm, the steeper the increasing slope of the temperature cycle relative to the decreasing slope, the later the temperature rhythm relative to the sleep-wake rhythm, and the less the variabilities among all these parameters (i.e., the greater is the overall reliability of his rhythm); all these correlations are statistically significant. The reference of all other rhythm parameters to the amplitude of the temperature rhythm is of course arbitrary; correlations of the same quality would be obtained with reference, for instance, to the period or any other rhythm parameter.

Of special interest is the correlation between the amplitude of the temperature rhythm and the sleep fraction in the sleep-wake cycle. This correlation combines parameters of the two rhythms which show different types of age and sex dependence (see above section), and which can be separated completely from each other so that they run with different periods (see "Internally Desynchronized Rhythms"). Nevertheless, there are highly significant correlations between these two parameters, but only when the data from (young) women ($R = 0.90$) and men ($R = 0.88$) are considered separately (the data on elderly women fit the regression line of the men). When the data of both sexes are considered together, there is no correlation ($R = 0.04$). The strong correlation between temperature amplitude and sleep fraction clearly shows that the two rhythms are generally very closely related to each other, and in particular that changes in one of the rhythms are followed systematically by changes in the other. Moreover, this correlation is of practical interest because it allows to predict, in every individual subject, the specific biological need for sleep, and that by measuring the amplitude of the temperature rhythm of this subject; the practical importance of this correlation is

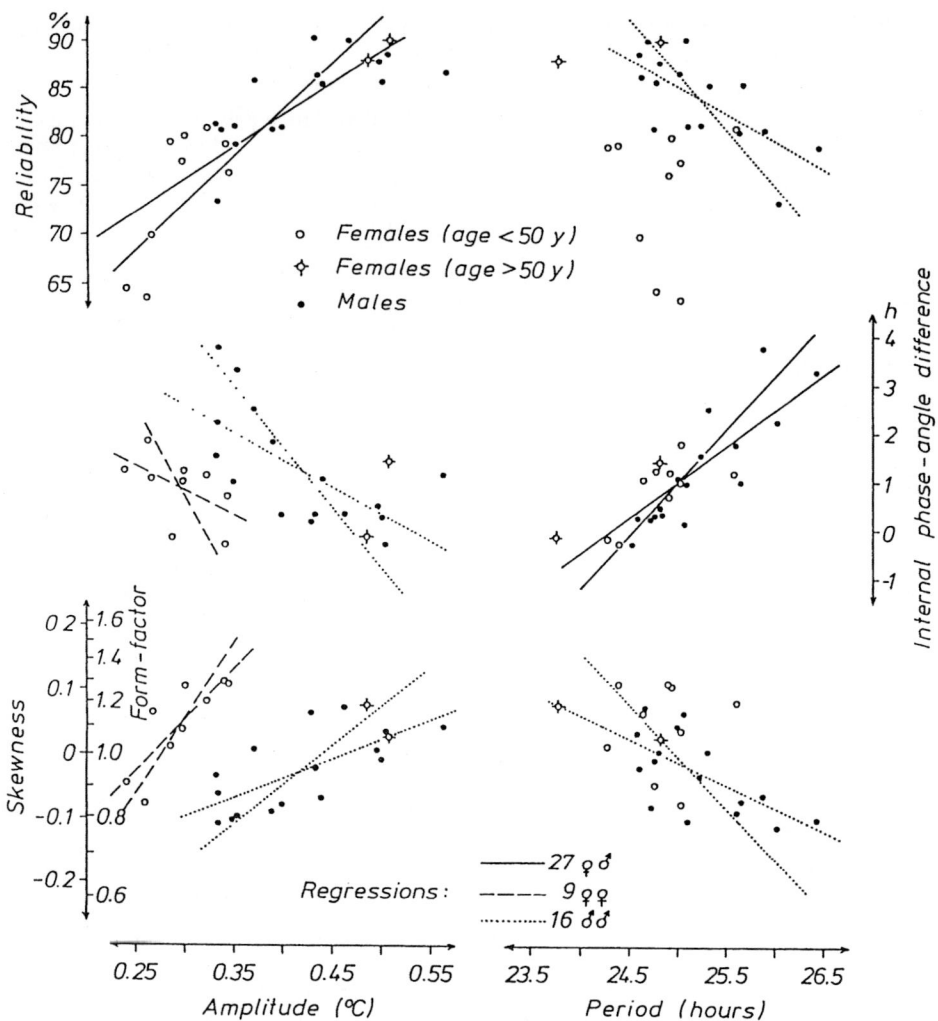

Fig. 10. Intercorrelations between various parameters of free-running circadian rhythms of different subjects. The interindividual correlations are drawn between amplitude of the body temperature rhythm and period (*abscissa*) and total reliability of the temperature rhythm, internal phase relationship between the rhythms of sleep-wake and body temperature, and skewness of the temperature cycle (*ordinate*). Regression lines are drawn (in both directions each) only in significant correlations. Several correlations are significant if all data are considered together (in these cases, the correlations are also significant if the data of the two sexes are considered separately); other correlations are significant only if the data on women and men are considered separately

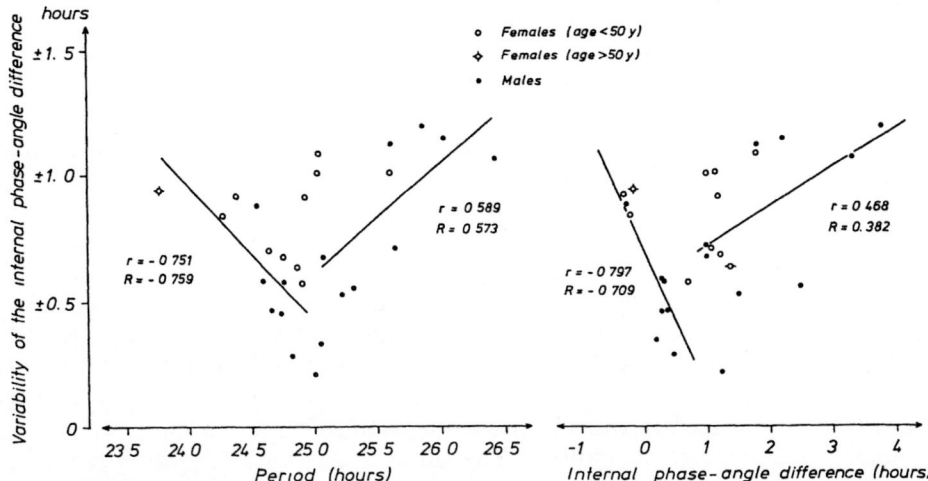

Fig. 11. Intercorrelations between the variability of the internal phase relationship between the rhythms of body temperature and sleep-wake (reciprocal of internal stability; *ordinate*) and the period (*left*) and the internal phase relationship itself (*right; positive values*, advance; *negative values*, delay of the temperature rhythm relative to the sleep-wake rhythm), taken from the same sample of subjects as in Fig. 10. Correlations are calculated separately from all data with shorter and longer periods than the optimum period, and separately from all data with internal phase relationships earlier and later than the optimum phase relationship

the greater since its validity had been shown not only in free-running rhythms but also in the 24-h day (Wever 1981).

Some of the intercorrelations are illustrated in Fig. 10; here regression lines (in both directions) are drawn only in the case of significant correlations. The figure shows that the correlations between some parameters are significant only when the data on women and men are considered separately (these follow different regression lines). Correlations between other parameters are also significant when the data on all subjects are considered together; in these cases, of course, the separate consideration on data from women or men also lead to significant correlations (they follow the same regression lines).

Another type of correlation between different rhythm parameters can be observed when not the internal phase relationship itself is considered (as in Fig. 10) but the intraindividual variability of this relationship, i.e., the internal stability of the rhythmic system. Correlations of this stability with the period and the internal phase relationship itself are shown in Fig. 11. There is not, as in all other correlations (see Fig. 10), a unidirectional relationship but an optimum function. At a specific period and at a specific phase relationship the internal variability is smallest (and hence the internal stability is greatest), and with increasing as well as decreasing periods, and also with increasing as well as decreasing internal phase relationships, the internal variability increases. The correlations with both sides of the optimum have been calculated for arbitrarily assumed optimum values for periods between 24 and 26 h and for internal phase relationships between 0 and 2 h (at intervals of 0.1 h each). All correlations were strongest with the optimum at a period of 25.0 h and an internal phase relationship of 1.0 h (advance of the temperature rhythm relative to the sleep-wake rhythm). It is striking that these optimum values coincide with the means of the parameters in the whole sample of experiments. This means, on the one hand, that there is a strong tendency to accept values that assure the highest internal stability of the system. This means, on the other hand, that a free-running period of 25.0 h assures higher internal stability than one of 24.0 h, which could be – as it turns out now, erroneously – assumed to be more reasonable.

It should be emphasized that these correlations between rhythm parameters are not merely empirical but also derived from predictions of a simple mathematical model of circadian rhythms that was developed nearly 30 years ago (before experiments with human subjects had started; Wever 1984a, 1987). All model predictions have indeed been confirmed experimentally, even quantitatively. This means that the correlations are not based on specific biological peculiarities but on general regularities of oscillations. The same is true with regard to the serial correlations discussed above (see "Internal Stabilization of Autonomous Rhythms"); these features were also predicted originally by the mathematical model. The serial correlations which establish a very powerful internal stabilization mechanism are therefore based on general rhythm properties and not on specific biological peculiarities. To be sure, the mathematically defined rhythm properties which seem to reflect biological peculiarities, are in these (and in other comparable) cases due to specific and well-known nonlinearities in the oscillation equation (Wever 1984a, 1987).

Internally Desynchronized Rhythms

Up to now we have considered results only of experiments involving constant conditions in which the rhythms of all variables are synchronous (internally synchronized rhythms). This state of free-running rhythms was, in fact, reached in most subjects. In a minority of subjects (up to the present in 52), however, we observed internal desynchronization, i.e., a state in which the rhythms of different variables run in the steady state with different periods. In most of these cases, the rhythms of body temperature and sleep-wake can be taken as representative, and the rhythms of all other variables run either with the period of the temperature rhythm or with the (considerably deviating) period of the sleep-wake rhythm. In the state of internal desynchronization, the rhythm of body temperature almost maintains its period (the mean period of the separate temperature rhythm of all 52 subjects was 24.86 ± 0.21 h) while the rhythm of sleep-wake showed periods (in the steady state and not only a short-term transient state) between (up to the present) 12 and 65 h.

Examples of Experiments

Figure 12 gives an example of the state of internal desynchronization. The left panel shows the course of this experiment; for the sake of clarity, it is not drawn in the common double-plot manner but in a triple-plot manner. This diagram shows that the rhythm of body temperature takes a similar course as in the examples

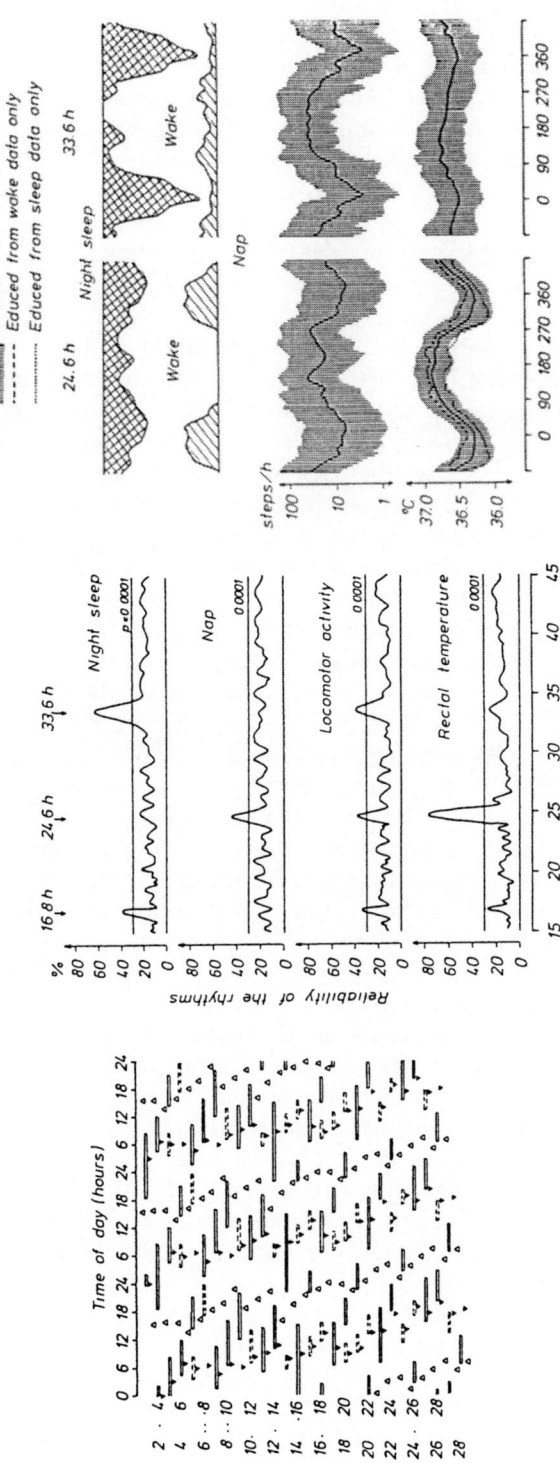

Fig. 12. Results of an experiment in which a 23-year-old man lived under constant conditions (light intensity 300 lux) without external time cues. *Left*, course of the experiment. The sleep-wake rhythm is represented by the sleep episodes (*bars*; *dotted bars*, sleep episodes scored subjectively as naps) and the rhythm of body temperature by the temporal positions of extreme values (*triangles*); data of successive days are drawn beneath one another (for clarity, in addition, data of three successive days each are drawn side by side). *Middle*, periodogram analysis, calculated separately for sleep episodes scored subjectively as night sleeps and as naps, and for locomotor activity and rectal temperature (each measured continuously). The prominent periods are indicated (the period of 16.8 h does not indicate an independent rhythm but indicates, as the second harmonic, the rectangular wave shape of the sleep-wake alternation). *Right*, educed cycles of the rhythms of the periodogram analysis. Due to the two prominent periods the averaging procedure was been calculated twice for each variable

shown above; its slope again indicates a period close to 25 h. The slope of the sleep episodes, on the other hand, indicates a much longer period. To be sure, there are several naps between these, and the naps seem to indicate, when combined with the night sleep episodes, a weakly marked component of the sleep-wake period similar to that of body temperature (i.e., indicating internal synchronization and not desynchronization). An explanation can be provided only by computer analysis. The overall periodogram analysis from the sleep-wake data (independently of whether the subject had scored the sleep subjectively as a night sleep or a nap) shows, in fact, a dominant peak at the period of 33.6 h and, in addition, a secondary (clearly smaller) peak at 24.6 h.

More explanatory is the separate analysis of night sleeps and naps. (In this experiment, and in virtually all others, there was never any doubt for the subject whether a sleep was a real night sleep or only a nap, even when a nap lasted longer than a night sleep). Separate periodograms are shown in the middle panel of Fig. 12. The analysis of the sleep episodes which were scored subjectively as night sleeps shows only one period at 33.6 h (the secondary period at 16.8 h does not represent an independent rhythm but the second harmonic of the dominant period indicating the rectangular wave shape of the sleep-wake alternation), and the analysis of the subjective naps results in only one period at 24.6 h (again, there is a secondary period at precisely half this period which, however, is not included in the diagram). This means that the rhythms of night sleeps and naps run with different periods (where the period of the naps coincides with that of body temperature; Wever 1986). The periodogram analysis of the locomotor activity of this subject again results in two periods, at 24.6 and at 33.6 h (a small peak at 16.8 h, again, describes only the rectangular shape of the rest-activity cycle). In contrast to the sleep analyses, here the two periods are nearly equivalent; this is due to the fact that in the locomotor activity not only the naps contribute to the shorter period but also the corresponding dips in activity on the days without naps. Finally, the middle panel of Fig. 12 includes the periodogram of the rhythm of body temperature; here there is only one very clear period at 24.6 h.

The right panel of Fig. 12 shows educed cycles of the different time series; in contrast to the corresponding calculations with internally synchronized rhythms, in internally desynchronized rhythms the calculation is meaningful (at least) twice, i.e., with the dominant periods of the rhythms of the different variables. With the period of 24.6 h (i.e., with the period as characteristic of the body temperature rhythm) the naps show highly reliable rhythms; more than half of the cycle is free of any naps. In contrast, all phases of this 24.6-h cycle show virtually even probabilities for a night sleep. On the other hand, with the 33.4-h cycle, there is an almost even distribution of the probability for naps, indicating the absence of any rhythmicity; however, there is a clear indication of a reliable rhythm in the night sleep with this period. The educed cycles of locomotor activity with the two periods show cycles of similar clarity but typically different wave shapes. The educed cycles of body temperature show a highly pronounced rhythm with 24.6 h, but a rhythm that cannot be differentiated from the noise level with 33.4 h.

In summary, this rhythm shows different prominent periods in body temperature and sleep-wake (even with equal consideration of the naps), and it shows different prominent periods in the night sleep episodes and the naps (according to the subjective scoring). The rating of a rhythm to be internally synchronized or desynchronized is therefore independent of the presence of naps (naps were expressly allowed in nearly all experiments, but in about half the experiments, including those showing internal desynchronization, the subjects never took a nap). Hence, the state of internal desynchronization is real, and it can be utilized for further analysis of the circadian system which is not possible with internally synchronized rhythms. There is, for instance, the interaction between the rhythms of different variables (mainly between the rhythms of body temperature and sleep-wake). This interaction leads to full mutual synchronization in internally synchronized rhythms, so that they appear outwardly as controlled by only one single rhythm. In internally desynchronized rhythms, on the other hand, the residual interaction between the different rhythms can clearly be seen in the scalloped pattern of the phases of the different rhythms, indicating internal relative coordination (see the left panel of Fig. 12).

Spontaneous Occurrence of Internal Desynchronization

In about one-third of experiments in which internal desynchronization occurred, this state was present from the beginning of the experiment (as in the case in Fig. 12). In the majority of experiments this occurred spontaneously during the experiment (in the more than 50 experiments, a spontaneous termination of the state of internal desynchronization was never observed). This allows us to compare, in the same experiment, sections with internally synchronized and desynchronized rhythms (Wever 1979). Figure 13 illustrates this spontaneous occurrence with two examples. In both experiments the rhythms were originally

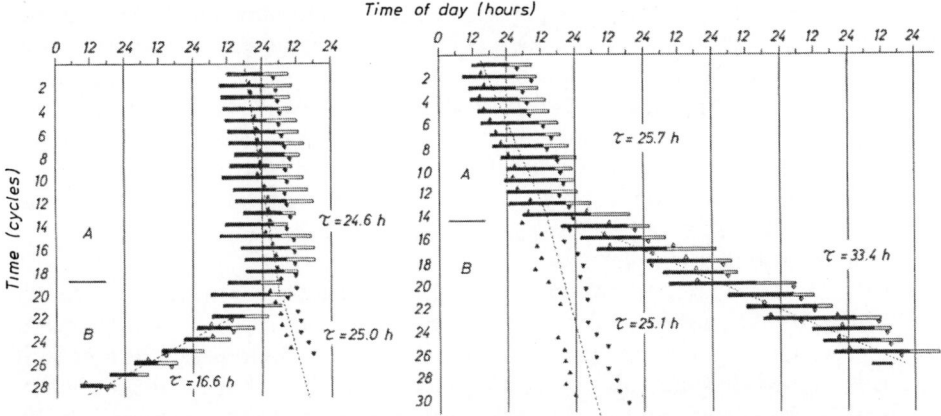

Fig. 13. Results of two experiments in which subjects (*left*, 24-year-old man; *right*, 25-year-old woman) lived under constant conditions without external time cues. The courses are as shown in Fig. 7, left (*open triangles*, temporally correct repetitions of already drawn triangles). In both experiments the rhythms initially ran internally synchronized (*A*); during the experiments, spontaneously (i.e., without any change in the experimental conditions) internal desynchronization occurred in each (*B*). (The separation into two sections was taken subsequently, to perform separate analyses)

internally synchronized; after 18 cycles (left) or 14 cycles (right) internal desynchronization occurred spontaneously, either with a dramatic shortening (left) or a dramatic lengthening (right) of the sleep-wake period. In both experiments, therefore, properties of internally desynchronized rhythms (and that with desynchronization in both directions) can be compared with properties of internally synchronized rhythms in the same subject.

The examples shown in Fig. 13 represent an initial description of 33 experiments during which internal desynchronization occurred spontaneously (13 with desynchronization by shortening, see Fig. 13, left panel; and 20 with desynchronization by lengthening, right panel). The fraction of sleep in the sleep-wake cycle was significantly shorter during internal desynchronization (independently of its direction) than during synchronization (Wever 1979). This means that with the transition to internal desynchronization by shortening, when the whole sleep-wake cycle shortened considerably, the sleep episode shortened relatively more than the whole cycle; with the transition to internal desynchronization by lengthening, on the other hand, when the whole sleep-wake cycle lengthened considerably, the sleep episode lengthened relatively less than the whole cycle. The amount of the relative reduction in sleep with the transition to internal desynchronization was significantly greater in women than in men; thus, the sex difference in the fraction of sleep (more sleep in women than in men; see Fig. 9, middle panel) is smaller during the state of internal desynchronization than that of synchronization.

In addition, each (always considerable) alteration in the sleep-wake period was accompanied by an (always slight but significant) alteration in the temperature period in the opposite direction (see Fig. 13). The proportion of alterations in the periods of the two rhythms was always close to 1:12; this means that every (very obvious) alteration of the sleep-wake period was accompanied by an alteration about 12 times smaller in the temperature period in the opposite direction. The fact of the transition to internal desynchronization and the direction of this desynchronization can therefore be deduced from inspection of the body temperature rhythm, without the need to score the sleep-wake rhythm, which may raise problems such as the subjective scoring of naps. Since the period of temperature rhythms after the separation was independent of the direction of internal desynchronization, the periods of the combined rhythms during the state of internal synchronization were significantly different depending on the direction of the later desynchronization (Wever 1979). From this result, predictions can be deduced concerning the probability of a later desynchronization. If an internally synchronized rhythm shows a free-running period of about 24.9 h $\pm$ 0.4 h, there is a high probability that this rhythm will not desynchronize internally in the long run. If the combined rhythms show a period of about 24.5 h or shorter, they will very probably desynchronize internally by accelerating the sleep-wake rhythm. If the combined rhythms show a period of about 25.4 h or longer, they will very probably desynchronize internally in the long run by retarding the sleep-wake rhythm.

The periods of the separate rhythms of body temperature (i.e., after they have been detached from the sleep-wake rhythms in the state of internal desynchronization) show a remarkably small interindividual variability (24.86 h $\pm$ 0.21 h). This value is independent of the direction of internal desynchronization (i.e., whether this period is accompanied by an extremely short or an extremely long sleep-wake period). In addition, it is independent of the sex of the subject; the free-running period of separate temperature rhythms was 24.85 h ± 0.24 h in women and 24.87 h ± 0.19 h in men (Wever 1984c). Since, in the state of internal synchronization, women showed a significantly shorter period of the combined rhythms than men (i.e., the period of the temperature rhythm was also shorter in women than men; see "Age and Sex Dependences"), this sex difference must be exclusively a property of the sleep-wake rhythm; this is, in fact, the case. Since women tend significantly more frequently to desynchronization by shortening than men, and men more frequently than women to desynchronization by lengthening, the mean of the separate sleep-wake periods is clearly shorter in women than in men (on average, by about 4 h).

The Multioscillator Concept

The above results force us to accept a multioscillator concept instead of the simple one-oscillator concept. The assumption of only one internal clock is insufficient; we need at least two internal clocks with slightly different properties, which are, to be sure, in interaction with one another. For simplicity, these two clocks can be seen as represented by the rhythms of body temperature and sleep-wake. These internal clocks do not usually show coinciding component periods. If these periods are close enough together, and the interaction between the two clocks is strong enough, the different clocks synchronize each other by adopting a compromise period. Since the experimentally determined compromise period is not precisely in the middle between the two separate periods but closer to the period of the temperature clock, the two clocks cannot be equally strong (rather, the temperature clock is about 12 times stronger than the sleep-wake clock; see "Spontaneous Occurrence of Internal Desynchronization"). If, on the other hand, the component periods of the two clocks are too far apart, or if the interaction between the clocks is not strong enough, the two clocks are outside the range of mutual entrainment, and hence they run separately from each other with their own inherent periods (and hence showing internal desynchronization). Also in this state, the interaction does not cease (but is only too weak for mutual synchronization), as can be seen by the consistent presence of relative coordination (seen in Figs. 12 and 13 in the scalloped patterns of the phases of both rhythms).

The probability of spontaneous internal desynchronization is significantly increased in elderly subjects and in those with high neuroticism scores (as measured with standard questionnaires) (Wever 1979). Dependence of the free-running period on the age of the subject or on the state of his health could not be found (see above); we can only assume, therefore, that in these groups the mutual coupling of different internal clocks is less than in young and healthy subjects, and hence that the weakening of interaction between the different rhythms causes the increased tendency toward internal desynchronization. At least in elderly subjects, evidence for such a weakening has been shown independently (see "Peculiarities in an Elderly Subject").

Internal Interactions: The Masking Effect

The state of internal desynchronization can be used to examine properties of the interaction between the different clocks; a complete knowledge of the circadian system presupposes a knowledge not only of the properties of the single rhythms but also of the regularities of the interaction among these rhythms (Wever 1983 b). It is a complication in the evaluation of this interaction that there are several (at least two) different modes of such an interaction, and these may obscure each other. Most importantly, not only do the basic oscillators, or clocks, or pacemakers, controlling the rhythms of different variables interact with one another but also the overt rhythms themselves. This latter direct or reactive influence of one variable on another is called the "masking effect." It can be observed, for instance, in increased body temperature, blood pressure or excretion of a hormone during the state of activity in comparison to rest, almost independently of the circadian phase and nearly additively with the circadian variation. Since the alternation between activity and rest may be due not only to circadian rhythmicity but also to forced behavior, it may via the masking effect cause changes in physiological variables that are not basically controlled by biological impulses. It is therefore of great importance to evaluate the influence of the masking effect on the observed variations in a physiological variable. In the following, the meaning of the masking effects is discussed in the reaction of body temperature to sleep-wake alternations (Wever 1985 a).

In internally synchronized rhythms, the rhythms of body temperature and sleep-wake, and hence also the masking effect of sleep-wake on body temperature, are synchronous with each other. Consequently, the masking effect makes itself felt only in an enlarging of the amplitude of the temperature rhythm, the extent of which, however, is unknown. This means that the portions of a (hypothetical) pure circadian component and a masking component of an observed rhythm cannot be evaluated in internally synchronized rhythms. Such evaluation seems to be possible during continuous bedrest for several days (where a masking effect should be lacking) or during continuous activity for several days without any rest (where the masking effect should be present but temporally constant); however, both these unnatural states may cause rhythm disorders which prevent the measurement of parameters of undisturbed rhythms (a phase delaying effect of sleep deprivation, for instance, is well known). In internally desynchronized rhythms, on the other hand, the rhythms of body temperature and sleep-wake, and hence the hypothetical components of the temperature rhythm, circadian and masking, run with different periods; consequently, they may be separated from each other (Wever 1985 a).

As an example, Fig. 14 shows data from an experiment performed under constant conditions where the rhythms were internally desynchronized during the whole experiment (29 days); the period of the temperature rhythm was 25.0 h, and that of the sleep-wake rhythm was 30.2 h (the subject never took a nap). Figure 14 presents the cycles of the temperature rhythm; the measurements use all corresponding data (dotted line), as in all examples up to here (see Figs. 1, 2, 6, 7, 12) and data obtained exclusively during the wake episodes (upper solid line) or the sleep episodes (lower solid line). It has previously been shown that

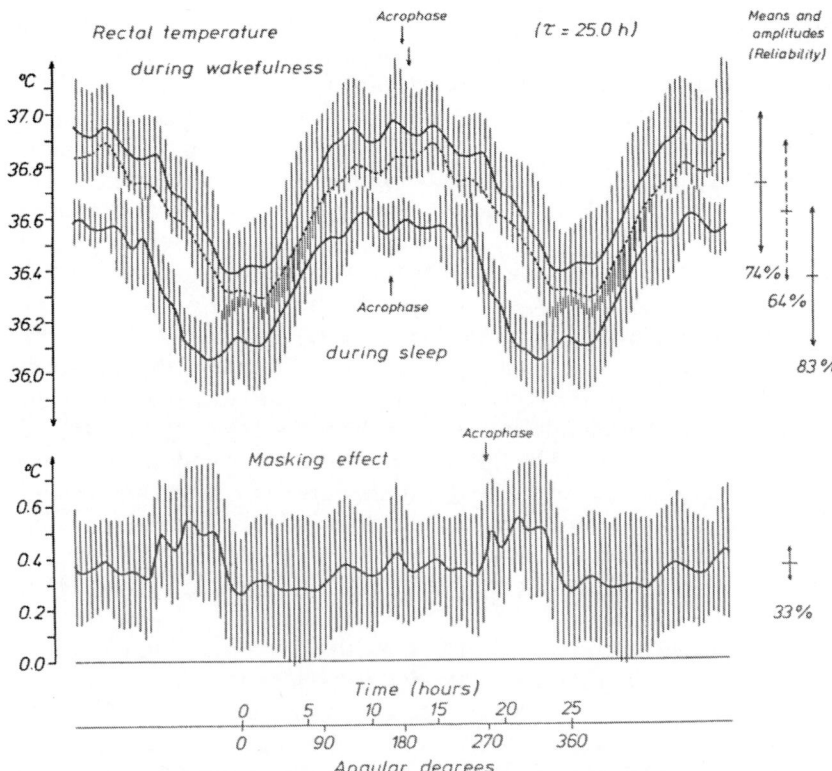

Fig. 14. Results of an experiment in which a 24-year-old man lived under constant conditions without external time cues; the rhythms were internally desynchronized during the entire experiment. *Above*, educed cycles of the body temperature rhythm, using all data (*dotted line*) and data obtained only during the wake episodes (*upper solid line*) and only during the sleep episodes (*lower solid line*), each averaged with the prominent period of the temperature rhythm of 25.0 h; standard deviations are drawn from the separate wake and sleep cycles. *Below*, extent of the masking effect (difference between wake and sleep cycle, with standard deviations). *Right border*, mean values, amplitudes, and reliabilities of the different educed cycles and the masking effect; acrophases are also indicated

periodogram analysis from separate wake and sleep data also result in a dominant 25.0-h period, as does the analysis of all data (Wever 1985a). Since due to the difference in the periods there is a manyfold overlap between the rhythms of body temperature and sleep-wake, the latter measurements also result in closed average cycles. For clarity only in the latter are standard deviations drawn around the mean cycles (there is almost no overlap in the standard deviations, indicating the high consistency of the masking effect). Figure 14 shows clearly that the mean wake temperature cycle and the mean sleep temperature cycle run parallel to each other, also in individual details such as the splitted minimum and the fourfold maximum (with the last maximum as the smallest). The two cycles are separated by the mean masking effect which in this case is 0.36 °C. A closer inspection suggests a phase delay of the wake cycle relative to the sleep cycle, which is expressed in all individual details mentioned, by about 1 h (this phase delay is in agreement with the phase delay during continuous wakefulness in internally synchronized rhythms, which also amounts to about 1 h per cycle; Wever 1979). As a consequence of this internal phase shift, the masking effect is smaller during the ascending section of the temperature cycle than during the descending section. In summary, the masking effect is, albeit only to a small extent, phase dependent. This becomes obvious in the lower panel of Fig. 14, which presents the course of the masking effect, i.e., the differences between the wake and the sleep temperature cycles, together again with the standard deviations of these differences.

At the right border of Fig. 14, mean values and amplitudes of the different educed cycles and the masking effect are indicated; the numbers indicate reliabilities. The educed cycles of the separate wake and sleep data show higher reliabilities (and larger amplitudes) than the educed cycle of all data; the reason is that they are not obscured by the masking effect, as the educed cycle for all data is. Also, the sleep cycle shows a higher reliability (and larger amplitude) than the wake cycle; this is because the activity (which induces the masking effect) is more consistent during sleep than wake. The masking effect itself (lower panel) shows a reliability which indicates the significance (though close to the border) of its phase dependence.

In the experiment presented in Fig. 14, the mean masking effect was 0.36 °C. This value is clearly larger than the average, which in a large sample of experiments is 0.28 °C $\pm$ 0.06 °C. The extent of the masking effect is obviously larger the more subjects are subjectively under behavioral stress; this is the case, for instance, in elderly subjects and in young subjects under complicating experimental conditions (from the subject in Fig. 14, complete EEG sleep recordings were taken which irritated the subject, according to his statements). Hence, the extent of the masking effect can be taken as a measure of stress. On the other hand, the amount of the phase delay of the wake cycle relative to the sleep cycle (mean: 52 min $\pm$ 15 min) does not show a recognizable relationship to any other parameter.

A masking effect from sleep-wake (resulting in higher values during wake than sleep) is present not only in body temperature but also in many other physiological variables. Its extent (relative to the circadian range of this variable) which is roughly one-third in body temperature, varies considerably from variable to variable. In the urinary excretion of several electrolytes and of cortisol and also in psychomotor performances it is frequently close to 50%; the phase delay of the wake cycle relative to the sleep cycle is close to 1 h also in these variables. In the excretion of melatonin almost no masking effect is recognizable; i.e., its amount is close to 0%. On the other hand, blood pressure (and heart rate) seem to be controlled overwhelmingly by masking (see Fig. 2); its effect can be close to 100%. Nevertheless, also here knowledge of the composition of the observed rhythms from two components, a true circadian and a masking component, is necessary for understanding the regularities of the overt rhythmicity. In contrast to the examples of the masking effect discussed hitherto, sleep-wake also undergoes direct (masking) influences of body temperature and other physiological variables; for instance, the higher the body temperature, the greater the probability for wake is, again almost independently of the circadian phase and almost additively to the circadian variation of sleep-wake.

Many parameters of the rhythm of a variable may be influenced by the masking effect (e.g., amplitude, phase, wave shape), but not the period. Thus the influence by the masking effect can never result in a mutual synchronization (at most, if the masking effect is close to 100%, it can simulate synchronization). Mutual synchronization can be affected only by another type of internal interaction, oscillatory interaction, in which one oscillator affects another in the same way as an external zeitgeber (see "Heteronomous Rhythms"). Since in most free-running rhythms all overt rhythms are generally mutually synchronous, this oscillatory interaction is the most common type of internal interaction (Wever 1983 b).

The way in which the different types of internal interaction have been discussed may suggest completely different pathways of the effects; the oscillatory interaction should be active immediately between the different oscillators while the masking effect should be active, by-passing the "clocks," independently of the oscillators. This picture, however, cannot be correct, as can be shown by model considerations. Rather, the masking effect must also be an integral part of the oscillatory mechanism. The original model equation was established by adding successively alternative terms (i.e., nonlinearities) to a simple oscillation equation and comparing the resulting modifications with biological results, i.e., by "trial and error." In this way a simpler version that included the masking effect inherently was compared with a more complicated version not including the masking effect but in which this effect was subsequently added by a separate equation. Both versions, of course, produce equivalent predictions concerning the masking effect (otherwise a calculation error would be included); however, they differ from each other in various predictions unrelated to the masking effect but involving apparently completely deviating properties. In all these respects only the original, simpler version including the masking effect leads to full agreement with biological results, while the combined version which separates the masking effect from other properties of the oscillator leads to predictions not in agreement with the biological results (Wever 1984 a). Since the original model equation fits the results obtained in the measurements of human circadian rhythms in all hitherto known respects, even quantitatively, it seems plausible that the model equation leads to meaningful interpretations also with regard to the masking effect (to be included in the oscillatory mechanism). This means that a separation of the masking effect from the oscillatory interaction may be of some pragmatic value in practical respects, but that this separation cannot contribute to a theoretical understanding of circadian rhythms.

Apparent Internal Desynchronization

Apart from the type of internal desynchronization as discussed above, with different free-running periods in rhythms of different variables and a constantly changing internal phase relationships between the involved rhythms, there is another type which, in fact, meets the first definition given above but not the second. The internal phase relationship between the rhythms of sleep-wake and body temperature is temporally constant, in spite of different periods of the two rhythms. Here, the periods of the two rhythms are integrally related. This means, for instance, that a temperature rhythm with a period of about 25 h is combined with a sleep-wake rhythm with a period of about 50 h, i.e., one sleep-wake cycle covers precisely two temperature cycles ("circabidian" sleep-wake rhythm). Or a temperature rhythm with a period of about 25 h is combined with a sleep-wake rhythm with a period of about 12.5 h, i.e., two sleep-wake cycles cover precisely one temperature cycle ("circasemidian" sleep-wake rhythm). In these cases (up to the present, 14 experiments of this type have been observed), there is an internal synchronization, not in the common 1:1 manner but 1:2 or 2:1. Since the obvious criterion of the different period values dominates, in a rough inspection of the course of an experiment, that of the internal phase relationship, this type had been called "apparent internal desynchronization" (Wever 1979).

In particular, the case of circabidian sleep-wake rhythms deserves attention; it has been observed in 12 (overwhelmingly male) subjects (circasemidian rhythms in only two female subjects). Wake and sleep episodes are each about twice as long as usual, i.e., 30–35 h of wake (in about half the experiments without any nap) alternate with 15–20 h of sleep (partly with full EEG records of all sleep episodes, showing 10–12 normally structurized REM-non-REM cycles per sleep episode instead of usually about 5 cycles), with a small variability in the duration of the total cycle and distinctly larger variabilities in the durations of the episodes, as is common in internally synchronized rhythms. It is worth mentioning again that no subject showing this state of the rhythm, consciously realized a change in the duration of his subjective day; each refused to believe, after terminating the experiment, that he could be out of real time for several weeks. It is also worth mentioning that all subjects showing this state had, after a wake episode twice as long as normal, a sleep episode which was normally structured but twice as long as usual, and not a typical "recovery sleep" (showing deep sleep and REM rebounds, and being only about 20% longer than usual) as they would have shown after a forced sleep deprivation of the same length (Wever 1985b).

External Modifications of Autonomous Rhythms

Although circadian rhythms are of endogenous origin and hence capable of free-running autonomously (with periods usually deviating from the day-night cycle), they are not independent of external stimuli. Rather, the biological significance of these rhythms is based on the observation that they usually run synchronously to the day-night cycle. The temporal fit of the internal rhythm to the earth's rotation is possible only by reactive modifications in the rhythms by external stimuli which are connected to the day-night cycle. This means that these external stimuli, when operating periodically, can be effective as zeitgebers synchronizing the endogenously generated rhythms (compare next section). The same stimuli, when operating continuously, are able to modify all parameters of free-running rhythms, including the tendency to internal desynchronization (Wever 1979).

The first external stimulus to be evaluated, was that of light. The experiments were performed so that the intensity of light to which a subject was continuously exposed altered once or twice during a long-term experiment, at intervals of 10–14 days; the temporal sequences of the different light intensities changed from experiment to experiment. An unexpected result was that no rhythm parameter depended, at least on average, in any way on the intensity of light. This was true with light intensities ranging from continuous total darkness up to the highest intensities originally attainable, i.e., up to 1500 lux (artificial indoor light is commonly not higher than 1000 lux, and even this intensity is only in use in specific cases). The results of experiments under total darkness have been confirmed by those of an experimental series with blind subjects; the rhythms in the blind were indistinguishable from those in the sighted (only the interindividual differences of rhythms in the blinds were larger than those in the sighted). There were a few experiments in which the period (and other rhythm parameters) changed on the day of alternation in light intensity; however, there was not a consistent direction of the correlation between light intensity and period, so that the results of these experiments have not influenced our view regarding the ineffectiveness of light in the control of human circadian rhythmicity (in most animal experiments, light intensity shows a strong influence on circadian rhythms; Wever 1979).

The picture changed dramatically after it was possible to use considerably higher light intensities. When subjects were exposed continuously to light of 3000–5000 lux in the total room (for details, see "Bright Light as a Zeitgeber"), the period was significantly longer, and the tendency to internal desynchronization was stronger than under light of normal intensity or under total darkness. Thus, after exceeding a threshold of light intensity known for the suppression of melatonin (Lewy et al. 1980), light gains another quality in the control of human circadian rhythms, one that is similar to that in animal experiments. The previous statement concerning the ineffectiveness of light must therefore be revised, i.e., restricted to light intensities within the range of common artificial illumination; it is not true for natural outdoor illumination (on not overly cloudy days) and for special types of very bright artificial light (which are possible to verify, but very expensive and not in use to-day; Wever 1985d, 1989a).

Another constant stimulus to the subjects was that resulting from their being isolated not alone but in a group. In such a group they enjoy social contacts which are lacking when they live singly. In group experiments the rhythms of the different subjects became synchronized with one another; this mutual synchronization did not concern only the sleep-wake rhythms but also the rhythms of physiological variables (e.g., body temperature), even when they are separated from sleep-wake in the course of internal desynchronization and hence run independently from sleep-wake. In particular the periods were significantly longer and the tendency to internal desynchronization stronger in groups than in singly isolated subjects. This means, apart from bright light, social contacts affect free-running circadian rhythms. Results from group experiments also refute the view that social deprivation during isolation accounts for the deviation of free-running periods from 24 h, as here the deviation is greater than in the single experiments, although the subjects are certainly less deprived socially than in the single experiments (Wever 1979).

A further stimulus that was considered was physical workload. During one section in the respective experiments subjects had to exercise on a bicycle ergometer about seven times per wake episode. The workload of 100–200 W for about 20 min was such that every work episode resulted in an increase in body temperature of about 1 °C. During another section of the same experiment (again, in changing temporal sequences), subjects were asked to avoid any physical workload including, for instance, gymnastics (the realization of this request could be controlled by the inspection of the course of body temperature). There was no difference in any respect between the sections with and those without the workload (apart from the steep temperature increases during the exercising episodes). This result demonstrates that the lack of physical activity during an isolation experiment is not responsible for the deviation of the free-running periods from a period of 24 h (Wever 1979).

We also investigated the influence of nutrition on circadian rhythms. Among the hundreds of volunteers participating in the experiments, many asked for special diets during the experiment; these requests were granted on the condition that the subjects maintained the special diet consistently. There were, for instance, subjects who were vegetarians, others who asked for nutrition very rich in proteins, or subjects requesting for nutrition very low in proteins and rich in carbohydrates, or even very low in carbohydrates, and so on. There was not any systematical dependence of rhythm parameters such as period on diet; hence, the kind of the nutrition did not have any influence on circadian rhythms. Finally, a few subjects asked for a complete fast during the experiment. Even this request was granted, on the precondition that they ate normally during half the experiment (so that the influence of fasting could be investigated with the subject as his own control). Fasting also showed no effect on the rhythms, either under continuous bright light, continuous normal light, constant total darkness, or the influence of a 24-h zeitgeber. In summary, even complete fasting is without any effect on the parameters of human circadian rhythms.

Heteronomous Rhythms

Although they are of endogenous origin, circadian rhythms in our natural environment are meaningful only after being synchronized by external zeitgebers to the 24-h period of the environment. The temporal fit of internal rhythms to this environment (and the temporal fit of the different rhythms to one another) is the ultimate goal of the circadian system. Two questions arise here: What are the external periodic stimuli that serve as zeitgebers; and what are the regularities of the control by an effective zeitgeber (for instance, in what ranges of periods can a zeitgeber synchronize the endogenously generated rhythms)?

Relative Light-Dark Alternations

Pure Light-Dark Alternations

The most important stimulus in our environment is light; consequently, the light-dark cycle as an integral component of the day-night cycle is the most important external zeitgeber in nearly all organisms, both animals and plants. In humans a light-dark cycle originally seemed ineffective. Figure 15 shows the course of two

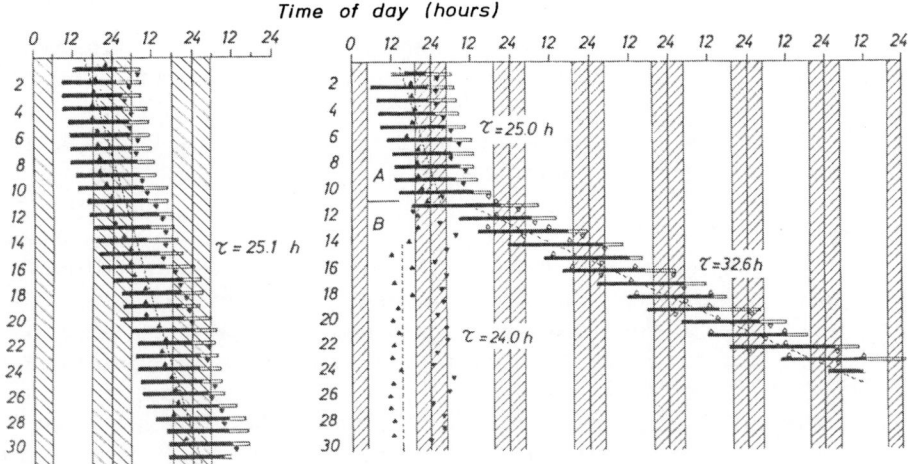

Fig. 15. Courses of two experiments in which a 29-year-old man (*left*) and a 25-year-old man (*right*) lived without environmental time cues but under the influence of artificial light-dark alternation (300:0.03 lux), with the option of switching on small auxiliary lamps during dark (relative light-dark); the zeitgeber period in both experiments was continuously 24.0 h. The courses of the rhythms of sleep-wake and body temperature are shown with the same designations as in Fig. 13 (*shaded areas*, dark time of the zeitgeber). *Left*, the rhythms ran freely internally synchronized throughout, with slight indications of relative coordination. *Right*, the rhythms ran freely initially internally synchronized (*A*); during the experiment, spontaneously (i.e., without any change in the experimental conditions) internal desynchronization occurred (*B*); in the latter, the rhythm of body temperature did not run freely but was synchronized to the light-dark alternation

experiments in which subjects were exposed to an artificial 24-h light-dark cycle. During the dark phase subjects could switch on small auxiliary lamps that allowed reading and other activities; such a relative light-dark alternation corresponds to the natural conditions in which sunset means rather a need to switch on artificial lamps than a compulsion to go to bed. In about half the experiments of this series the subjects were informed of the conditions before starting the experiment (Wever 1979). None of the subjects became fully synchronized to the zeitgeber. In 70% of experiments the rhythms ran internally synchronized, as presented in the left panel of Fig. 15, i.e., they showed subjective days with a duration close to 25 h coinciding in all variables. In 30% of experiments the rhythms ran internally desynchronized during part of the experiment, as in the right panel of Fig. 15 (these percentages were similar to those in experiments under constant conditions; see Figs. 12, 13). In all these experiments the sleep-wake cycles (which only could be perceived consciously) were considerably longer than the temperature cycles (between 32 and 38 h). In the experiments in which subjects were informed previously about their exposure to a 24-h day, they did not believe this after the experiment; what they felt subjectively was a clear deviation of the light-dark alternation from their days (which were always experienced as 24-h days).

The initial inspection of Fig. 15 might lead to the – rash – impression that the light-dark cycle was completely ineffective. In all cases with internally synchronized rhythms (left panel), however, relative coordination was recognizable; the phase of the rhythm shifted more slowly against the zeitgeber when the external phase relationship was "right" (sleep and temperature minimum during dark, wake and temperature maximum during light) than when the phase relationship was "wrong" (sleep and temperature minimum during light, wake and temperature maximum during dark). Such a relative coordination indicates the presence of a zeitgeber which in principle is effective but is too weak for full entrainment. Moreover, in all cases with internally desynchronized rhythms (right panel of Fig. 15), the rhythms of body temperature show, after the separation from sleep-wake, periods that are considerably shorter than those of the sleep-wake rhythms and also shorter than the temperature periods before the separation (as is common in desynchronized rhythms under constant conditions; see Fig. 13). In all these cases, however, the periods of the temperature rhythm were precisely 24.0 h, at least temporarily, i.e., for a section of not less than 10 days (which was never the case under constant conditions). It could be argued that in all these cases the temperature rhythms ran freely with periods which were, by chance, coincidingly very close to 24.0 h. There are, however, several independent arguments that the temperature rhythms did not run freely but were synchronized to the light-dark alternation. The main argument is the external phase relationship to the zeitgeber, which coincided in all these cases with that as measured under the influence of effective light-dark zeitgebers (see below). Observations both in internally synchronized and in internally desynchronized rhythms clearly show a residual zeitgeber effectiveness of the light-dark alternation (although it is too weak for full entrainment). In other words, relative light-dark alternation is in principle a (weak zeitgeber, but the range of entrainment of this zeitgeber is so small that it does not cover the period of 24.0 h (Wever 1979).

Peculiarities in an Ill Patient

This series included one experiment with a slightly different intention; in addition, this experiment was modified by unintended conditions, and it took an unexpected course. Figure 16 shows the outcome of this experiment. The (female) subject was exposed continuously to a relative light-dark alternation with a period of 25.25 h (left panel) which was expected to be very close to the free-running period, so that this period was intended to be inside of the (albeit small) range of entrainment; in addition, the subject was asked to follow the zeitgeber if possible. During the first few days of the experiment the rhythm was clearly synchronized externally and internally. However, after about 1 week the subject became ill (German measles with fever of 39 °C; see right border of the left panel of Fig. 16), but she insisted to continue the experiment according to the original protocol. Thereafter the rhythm of body temperature became detached from the zeitgeber and started to run freely; the sleep-wake cycle, on the other hand, remained synchronized to the zeitgeber although with considerably increasing variability, so that the rhythm desynchronized internally (i.e., partial external synchronization occurred, opposite to that as observed in Fig. 15, right). After recovery from the illness, the rhythm did not return to its original state but continued to run internally desynchronized. The special quality of this course is the state of internal

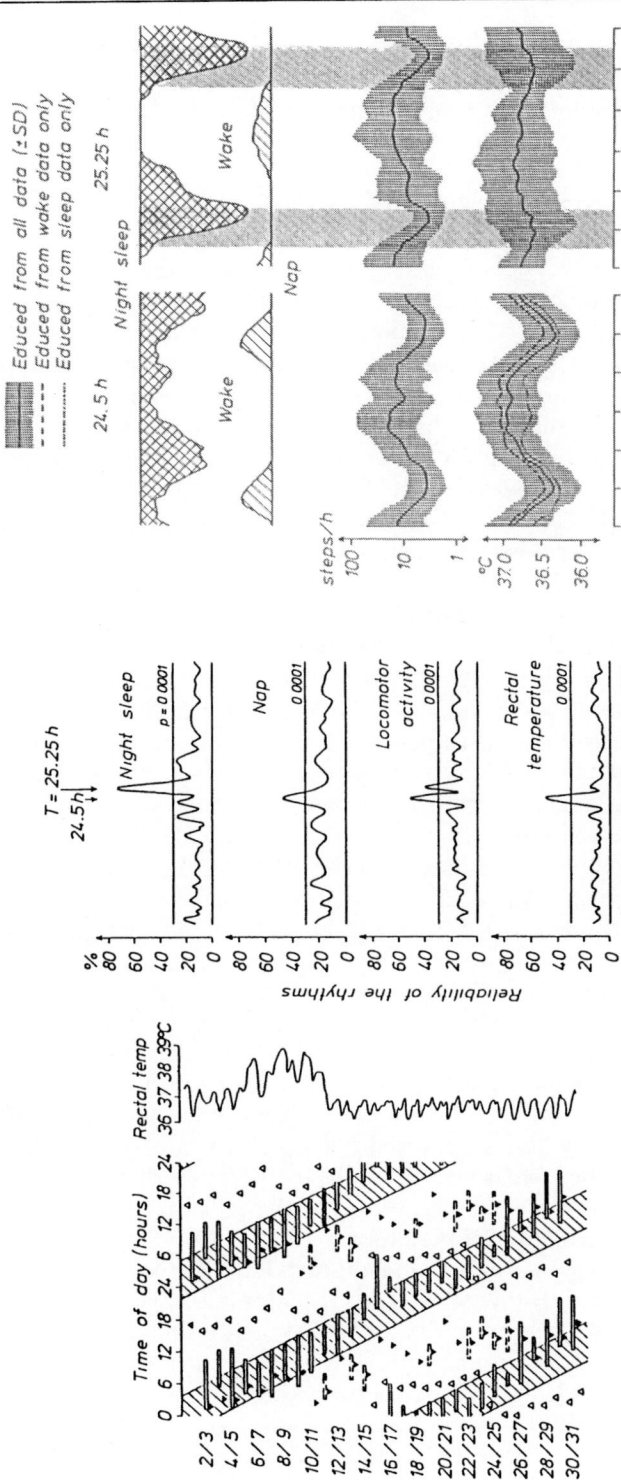

Fig. 16. Results of an experiment in which a 23-year-old woman lived without environmental time cues but under the continuous influence of artificial light-dark alternation (relative light-dark; 300:0.03 lux) with a period of 25.25 h. *Left,* course of the experiment; presented are the courses of the rhythms of sleep-wake and body temperature, with the same designations as in Fig. 12 (*shaded areas,* dark phase of the zeitgeber); *right border,* course of body temperature, with high fever from about day 6 to day 11. *Middle,* periodogram analysis. *Right,* educed cycles (as in Fig. 12)

desynchronization with the periods of the separated rhythms being so close together; the interval between the two rhythms (or between the zeitgeber period and the free-running period of the temperature rhythm) was not more than 45 min, i.e., rather smaller than the common interval between the 24-h day and the free-running period.

Prior to the experiment the subject stated that she normally never took a nap and expected during the experiment also not to do so. After about 10 days she wrote that a nap would now be inavoidable, obviously due to her illness. After her recovery, however, she continued to take naps frequently. All her naps occurred around the minimum in body temperature; thus, the naps in the first part of the experiment were close to the end of the wake episode (after lunch) and in the second part of the experiment close to the onset of the wake episode (before lunch), without the subject realizing this internal phase shift.

The middle panel of Fig. 16 shows a periodogram analysis, again calculated separately for sleep episodes that had been scored subjectively for night sleeps and naps, as in Fig. 12. Both night sleeps and naps show a reliable rhythm but at slightly different periods; the night sleeps show a period coinciding with the zeitgeber period (25.25 h), and the naps show a period coinciding with the free-running period of the temperature rhythm (24.5 h). The analysis of locomotor activity demonstrated two closely neighboring periods, coinciding with the two (separate) periods of the two types of sleep; analysis of body temperature revealed a single free-running period at 24.5 h. This analysis confirms the existence of two separate rhythms within one subject, with periods closer to one another than was observed in any healthy subject; this was obviously due to the illness of the subject. The analysis also confirms the control of night sleeps and naps by different oscillators in the human multioscillator system (see Fig. 12).

The right panel of Fig. 16 shows educed cycles of the same variables as shown in the middle panel; as usual in internally desynchronized rhythms, the measurements were each made twice, with the two prominent periods included in the analysis (see Fig. 12). Night sleep showed a pattern clearly with the zeitgeber period, and the naps showed a pattern clearly with the free-running period. With the other period in each case the distributions were not really even because there was in internal phase shift between the two rhythms of less than 360° (i.e., only about 240°) due to the small interval between the periods (in Fig. 12 the two rhythms shifted more than 7 times 360° against each other). Measurement of the rhythm of locomotor activity showed two cycles of similar reliability but having different wave shapes. Measurement of the temperature rhythm revealed a reliable rhythm only with the free-running period; with the zeitgeber period it could not be differentiated from random fluctuations.

These results suggest that a similar partial synchronization combined with internal desynchronization can also occur under natural conditions, at least in ill patients and possibly also in the elderly. The interaction between the rhythms of body temperature and sleep-wake was so weak that it led to internal desynchronization even with periods that were closer together than in all experiments in which internal desynchronization occurred in healthy subjects. It must therefore be considered that such a disorder (partial external synchronization combined with internal desynchronization) is also more frequent under natural conditions, in particular in the ill and the elderly (see "Peculiarities in an Elderly Subject") than is commonly assumed. This means that an obviously 24-h sleep-wake cycle does not guarantee a 24-h rhythm in physiological rhythms; these rhythms, rather, can possibly run freely with a period longer than 24 h. The problem is that such a free-run, in contrast to the 24-h rhythm in sleep-wake, would be recognizable only after laborious long-term investigations which would be difficult to perform particularly in the groups of subjects in whom it would be most desirable. Consequently, long-term measurements of physiological variables which could answer this question, are very rare.

Relative Light-Dark Supplemented by Regular Request Cues

In another experimental series the light-dark cycle was supplemented by regular signals (transmitted acoustically by a gong) requesting of the subjects mictions and the performance of several tests (in all experiments discussed hitherto, mictions and tests were performed only at self-selected and hence varying intervals, generally with a large night gap in the data). The signals were given in a 24-h day at regular intervals of 3 h during the light phase and 4.5 h during the dark phase; on days of varying durations, the intervals were altered proportionally. This means that there were consistently seven signals per cycle, independently of the cycle duration. Results deviated clearly from those of experiments without request cues. The rhythms were entrained to such a combined zeitgeber within a range of periods between about 23 and 27 h. An example of such an experiment is shown in Fig. 17. Here the subject was exposed to a relative light-dark alternation, supplemented by seven request cues per cycle, with periods of 26:40, 25:20 and 24:00 h for about 10 days each. An initial result of this experiment was that the subject's rhythm was synchronized to all these zeitgeber periods. In addition, the phase relationships altered systematically; the shorter the period, the later were the rhythms relative to the zeitgeber (i.e., the external phase relationship) and the later the temperature rhythm relative to the sleep-wake rhythm (i.e., the internal phase relationship; Fig. 17, right). Finally, it was demonstrated that the fraction of sleep increased with shortening zeitgeber period to such an extent that the absolute length of the sleep episodes remained constant with changing zeitgeber period (Wever 1979).

Of special interest in this experiment was the variability of the phase relationships; in particular, this concerned the temporal position of the temperature minimum as the sharpest marked phase of the temperature rhythm. In the 26:40-h day this minimum was close to the beginning of sleep and was rather stable; in the 24:00-h day it was close to the end of sleep and was also rather stable. In the 25:20-hour day, however, the minimum was not in the middle of the sleep episode as would be expected, but a split temperature minimum was recognizable that needed further attention. An inspection of all single nights in this experiment showed that in the 26:40- and the 24:00-h days the temporal positions of the temperature minimum were consistently at the beginning or at the end of sleep; in the 25:20-h day, on the other hand, the minimum was in some nights at the beginning (as in the 26:40-h day) and in others at the end of sleep (as in the 24:00-h day). In about half the nights it was hard to determine a position of the minimum

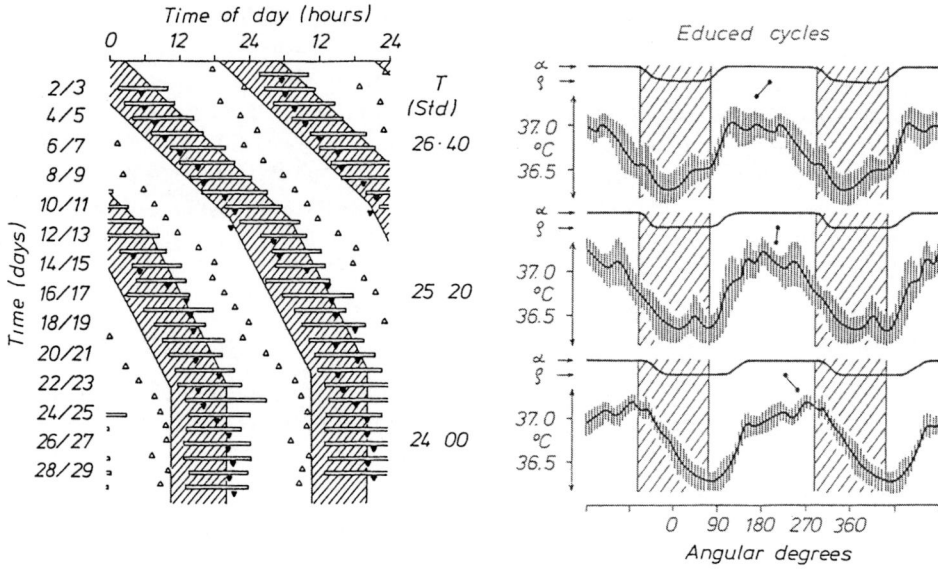

Fig. 17. Results of an experiment in which a 24-year-old man lived without environmental time cues but under the influence of a combined zeitgeber consisting of an artificial light-dark alternation (relative light-dark; 300:0.03 lux) and seven signals per cycle in regular intervals requesting the subject for mictions and the performance of several tests, with two changes in the zeitgeber period. *Left*, course of the experiment, with the same designations as in Fig. 16. The rhythm was fully synchronized externally and internally during the entire experiment, i.e., with all zeitgeber periods. *Right*, educed cycles of the rhythms of sleep-wake and body temperature, calculated separately for the three sections; the acrophases of the two rhythms are connected by lines

within the sleep episode at all (a split minimum as in the average cycle was not observable in any night). In summary, in contrast to the stable positions in the 26:40- and the 24:00-h days, the phase relationship in the 25:20-h day was rather unstable. This is remarkable as the 25:20-h day corresponds closest to the free-running period. Thus, the phase relationship under the influence of a zeitgeber was more stable when the zeitgeber period deviated (in either direction) from the free-running period than when it coincided with the free-running period. In other words, the system was more stable when it was under constant temporal pressure than when it was in an indifferent equilibrium (this result, again, is in agreement with model predictions).

This result refutes the often heard view that the deviation of the free-running period from the period of the day-night cycle can only be based on insufficient evolution in controlling the free-running period. Rather, this deviation is of evolutionary advantage, for it assists in stabilizing the circadian system. The evolutionary pressure to keep the free-running period at variance from the day-night cycle can also be deduced in another way. The earth's rotation is now slower than in earlier times; it is continuously retarded by the friction of the tides. Several million years ago when the period of the earth's rotation was 23 h or shorter, organisms with a free-running period of 25 h (as we now have) could not survive because their free-running period would have been out of the range of entrainment (the range of entrainment of the natural zeitgeber is similar to that of the artificial zeitgeber just discussed, i.e., about 2 h to either side of the free-running period; see next section); this means that our ancestors had a free-running period that was shorter than 25 h (e.g., 24 h); if there were no pressure of evolution to retard the free-running period to keep a distance to the retarding actual day-night period, today we would have a 24-h period rather than a 25-h period. In other words, the present 25-h period is clear proof of evolutionary pressure to keep a distinct difference between the periods of the day-night cycle and the free-running rhythms.

The experimental series with the combined zeitgeber (relative light-dark alternation and regular request cues) included 17 experiments with one to three alterations in the zeitgeber period. These experiments confirm in all respects the results obtained from the experiment discussed above. On the basis of these results we can make a number of generalizations. First, the rhythms are entrained to the zeitgeber within a limited range of entrainment (between about 23 and 27 h); outside this range they run freely. Second, inside this range the rhythms of all variables delay, relative to the zeitgeber, with shortening zeitgeber period, but the rhythms of different variables to different extents, so that with changing period the total temporal organization of the circadian system changes (in particular, the rhythm of body temperature delays relative to the sleep-wake cycle with shortening zeitgeber period). Third, the fraction of sleep within the sleep-wake cycle is greater the shorter the period is; the absolute duration of the sleep episodes is in fact different from subject to subject but is the same with all zeitgeber periods in any given subject. Fourth, the variability of the internal phase relationship is smallest, and hence the internal stability is greatest, with a free-running period of about 25 h, i.e., with a period which is precisely the mean of the free-running periods in all experiments. Finally, outside the range of entrainment relative coordination occurs, and this coordination is the more marked the closer the rhythm to the limit of entrainment is. All these relationships are statistically significant (Wever 1979).

Comparison of the results of experiments in which subjects lived under relative light-dark alternation with and without additional request cues suggests an overwhelming zeitgeber effectiveness, not of the light-dark alternation but of the request cues. When subjects were asked after both types of experiments for their subjective experiences, they considered the light-dark alternation to be controlled by a switch clock (as was, in fact, the case); the gong signals, however, most subjects thought to be released personally by the experimenter, i.e., as a direct social contact (which it was not). Only after drawing the subject's attention to the switch clock (which they had postulated themselves previously, in connection with the light-dark alternation) which also released the gong signals, they regretted finding that the request cues were also a mechanical operation; frequently, the subjects added "what a pity." This turned out to be a key: the subjects believed in a social contact while knowing that it existed only in their imagination. Finally, experiments were also performed (complementing the experiments with the sole exposure to the relative light-dark alternation) with the sole exposure to the regular request cues under constant light intensity. These experiments showed an entrainment of the rhythms in similar limits as with the combined zeitgeber. Thus, these experiments also indicated the dominant role of social contacts in effective zeitgebers (Wever 1985 d).

Phase Shifts of the Zeitgeber: Jet Lag Simulation

When the combined zeitgeber is able to entrain circadian rhythms within a reasonable range of entrainment, it should also be able to shift the phase of the rhythm and hence simulate the jet lag phenomenon. Consequently, several experiments were performed in which subjects lived under an artificial 24-h zeitgeber with the phase shifted successively 6 h each in opposite directions, simulating first an eastward flight over six time zones and thereafter (10–14 days later) a westward flight also over six time zones (Wever 1980). Figure 18 shows the results of an experiment of this series. The left panel shows the course of the experiment; it can be seen that both rhythms adjust, or reentrain, to the shifted zeitgeber within a few days, with the sleep-wake rhythm adjusting much faster than the temperature rhythm. The middle panel shows the educed cycles, calculated separately for the three sections (after deleting the first 2 days of each section); it shows, in fact, that the rhythm adjusts completely to the zeitgeber in every section. The right panel shows smoothed courses of several variables and their amplitudes. One sees primarily a considerable reduction in the amplitude of the temperature rhythm immediately following the "eastward" shift and simultaneously a considerable dip in performance level, interrupting the steady increase in practice, indicating the jet lag syndrome.

The outcomes of all experiments in this series were similar, so that a number of statistically significant generalization can be made. These generalizations are particularly valid since the strength of the artificial zeitgeber used in these experiments can be shown to be similar to the strength of the natural zeitgeber. Apart from the size of the range of entrainment, the rate of reentrainment after a phase shift of a zeitgeber is a direct measure of the strength of the controlling zeitgeber; in these simulation experiments this rate is about the same as the mean rate in a large number of real flight experiments, i.e., in experiments in which numerous subjects were transported over many time zones (Aschoff et al. 1975). The generalizations can thus be taken as valid not only in the simulation experiments as discussed here but also under natural conditions, i.e., after long-distance transmeridian flights.

First, the rate of reentrainment differs for the rhythms of different variables; immediately after each shift there is therefore a transient state during which the temporal organization of the circadian system differs considerably from that in the steady state. Second, during the transient state the rate of reentrainment is greater for onset than end of sleep, and it is greater for the minimum than for the maximum of the rhythm of body temperature. Third, the rate of reentrainment is greater after an "eastward" than after a "westward" shift. Fourth, the amplitude of the rhythm of body temperature is considerably reduced after a phase shift, at least after an "eastward" shift. Fifth, the "direction asymmetry" in the reentrainment rates is the stronger the more the rhythm's amplitude is reduced after the "eastward" shift. Extrapolating this correlation to an amplitude

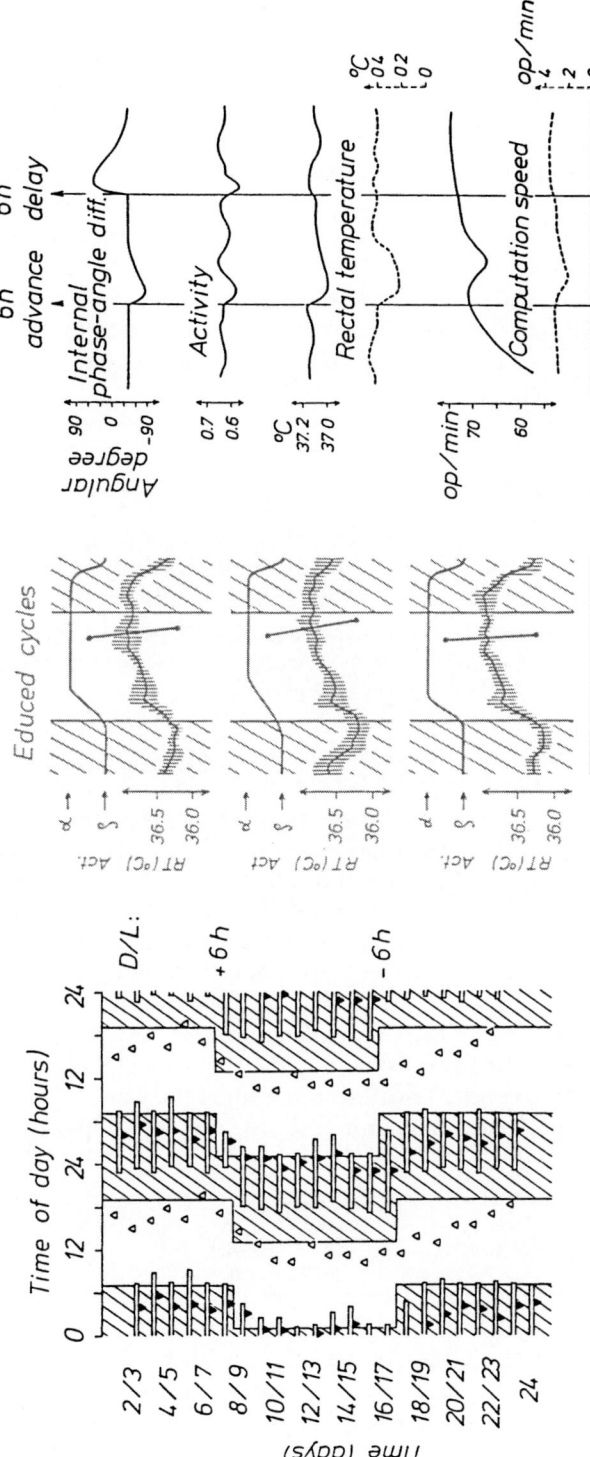

Fig. 18. Results of an experiment in which a 26-year-old man lived without environmental time cues but under the influence of the same combined zeitgeber as in Fig. 17 (relative light-dark plus regular request cues), with a period of 24.0 h and two opposite phase shifts of the zeitgeber for 6 h each. *Left,* course of the experiment, with the same designations as in Fig. 17. The rhythm followed the zeitgeber shifts but with different reentrainment rates for the rhythms of sleep-wake and body temperature. *Middle,* educed cycles of the rhythms of sleep-wake and body temperature, calculated separately for the three sections (after deletion of the first two cycles of every section); consistent entrainment patterns in all sections. *Right,* smoothed courses of several variables and their circadian amplitudes (dotted lines). Of particular interest is the reduction in the rhythm's amplitude immediately following the first "eastward" shift and the simultaneous dip in the level of performance

remaining constant, the direction asymmetry would be reversed, i.e., the reentrainment rate after the "westward" shift would be greater than after the "eastward" shift (which is often considered for reasonable due to the free-running period being longer than 24 h). Sixth, the reentrainment rate in both directions is greater the smaller the amplitude of the rhythm of body temperature is; since there is a strong correlation between the rhythm's amplitude and the length of sleep (see "Intercorrelations Among Rhythm Parameters"), this means that "short-sleepers" reentrain faster to a shifted zeitgeber than do "long-sleepers." Seventh, the impairment of subjectively scored well-being and the reduction in objectively measured efficiency (i.e., the jet lag syndrome) is greater after "eastward" than after "westward" shifts. Finally, both these impairments are stronger in subjects with an early temperature maximum ("morning types") than in those with a late temperature maximum ("evening types;" Wever 1980).

Absolute Light-Dark Alternations

In another series of experiments the possibility of switching on auxiliary lamps during the dark phase, was eliminated (absolute light-dark alternation), and subjects were more or less forced to go to bed at "sunset" (subjectively, almost no subject consciously realized alterations in the zeitgeber period, even when these alterations were dramatic, so that the term "forced" by no means reflects the subjective situation; Wever 1979). As a general result, the range of entrainment was about the same as that with the previously discussed zeitgeber (relative light-dark plus regular request cues), but only with regard to the physiological rhythms. The sleep-wake cycle, on the other hand, was synchronized to an absolute light-dark alternation within a wide (or even unlimited) range. Supplementation by the regular request cues did not influence the strength of this zeitgeber; the range of entrainment was about the same with and without these signals. The request cues, however, were very useful in another respect, for they give us the chance to obtain urine data and, in particular, performance data, not only at equidistant intervals but, more importantly, also during the sleep episodes (by waking the subjects). Thus test data were available "around the clock;" this was also true in internally desynchronized rhythms, so that these experiments also provided performance data in free-running physiological and psychological (but, of course, not in free-running sleep-wake) rhythms (under constant conditions the generally unavoidable night gap in the data prevented a meaningful measurement of parameters of those rhythms).

Absolute Light-Dark with Constant Zeitgeber Periods

Figure 19 presents results from an experiment of this series. The subject was exposed successively to a zeitgeber (absolute light-dark plus regular request cues) with periods of 24.0, 28.0, and 32.0 h. As the left panel shows, sleep-wake was synchronized to this zeitgeber during the entire experiment; the rhythm of body temperature, on the other hand, was so only during the first section (24-h day) while it ran freely during the second and third sections (28- and 32-h days, without

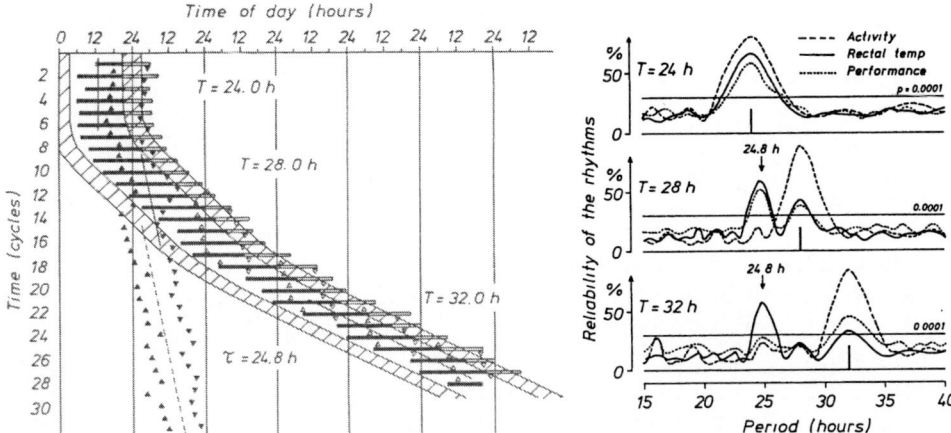

Fig. 19. Results of an experiment in which a 31-year-old man lived without environmental time cues but under the influence of a combined zeitgeber, consisting of an artificial light-dark alternation (absolute light-dark, i.e., without the option of switching on any lamps during dark; 300:0.03 lux) and seven regular request cues per cycle, with two changes in the zeitgeber period. *Left*, course of the experiment, with the same designations as in Fig. 15 (*solid lines*, schematic courses of the acrophases of the performance rhythm); the sleep-wake rhythm was snychronized to the zeitgeber during the entire experiment, while the rhythm of body temperature was synchronized only during the first section (with coinciding free-running periods during the second and third sections), and the performance rhythm was synchronized to the zeitgeber (and sleep-wake) during the first and third sections but not during the second (here, it was snychronous with the temperature rhythm). *Right*, periodogram analysis of the three rhythms, computed separately for the three sections of the experiment; the prominent periods are indicated and the zeitgeber periods are marked

difference in the free-running periods). In addition, the schematic course of the acrophases of a performance rhythm (maximal possible computation speed) is presented. During the first section, this rhythm was also synchronized to the zeitgeber and to all other rhythms; during the second section it run freely, i.e., it ran synchronously with the temperature rhythm but not to the zeitgeber or the sleep-wake rhythm; and during the third section it was synchronized by the zeitgeber and the sleep-wake rhythm and was hence desynchronized from the temperature rhythm. The right panel of Fig. 19 shows a periodogram analysis, computed separately for the three sections and the rhythms of the three variables. The analysis of sleep-wake and body temperature confirms the interpretation of the courses (left panel) of a limited range of entrainment for body temperature but not for sleep-wake. During the state of internal desynchronization (second and third sections), the analysis shows secondary periods at values where the other rhythms show their primary periods. Analysis of the performance rhythm establishes a rule which is valid generally: while the performance rhythms (particularly that of computation speed) during internal desynchronization tend to follow body temperature in short term, they tend to follow sleep-wake in the long run; this is the only indication of a temporal trend in human circadian rhythmicity known so far (Wever 1979, 1985d).

It was the general result of all experiments with an absolute light-dark alternation that the state of internal desynchronization, which gives us special insight in the circadian system which cannot be gained in internally synchronized rhythms, can be observed in every subject, not only in the elderly or in subjects with high scores of neuroticism; this state does not occur spontaneously as under constant conditions (see "Internally Desynchronized Rhythms") but forced by a zeitgeber with a period shorter than 23 h or longer than 27 h (where again the term "forced" is inadequate for the description of the subjective situation because nearly no subject had realized consciously the exposure to such a zeitgeber). Like in internal desynchronization under constant conditions the rhythms of the different variables follow either the sleep-wake rhythm (which stays commonly synchronous to the zeitgeber) or the rhythm of body temperature (which commonly runs freely under this condition). It seems to be a characteristic exception that in the courses of the excretion of the different pterins any rhythmicity disappears completely after the transition to forced internal desynchronization, unlike the courses of other variables: this is true although also the pterins show highly reliable rhythms in the free-run and under the influence of a zeitgeber as long as the rhythms remain internally synchronized.

The state of internal desynchronization as forced in these experiments, allows us, for instance, again to examine masking effects. In contrast to experiments performed under constant conditions (see Fig. 14), here masking effects can also be assessed in performance rhythms. Figure 20 presents data of an experiment in which a subject lived for 25 days under the continuous influence of a 28.0-h zeitgeber (absolute light-dark plus regular request cues). In the left panel the courses of body temperature and computation speed are synchronized to wake and sleep onsets. Regarding body temperature, the figure shows the virtually rectangular course of the masking effect (high temperature values during wake and low values during sleep) with the about 50% overshoots immediately following wake and sleep onsets. In psychomotor performance the data show a similar pattern, indicating a masking effect of about three tasks per minute (the mean level was about 42 tasks/min). The overshoots are clearly smaller than with body temperature; however, this is due principally to the much less rigorous screening of the performance data (3 h versus 0.25 h) which is unavoidable because of the much smaller set of data, but which smoothes the overshoots to a considerable extent (Wever 1985 a).

The right panel of Fig. 20 shows the educed cycles of the two rhythms, computed with the previously determined coinciding period of 24.8 h; these are from all data and from data obtained only during the wake and during the sleep episodes. As under constant conditions (see Fig. 14), there are separate wake and sleep cycles which run parallel in individual details but are phase-advanced during sleep in comparison to wake for about 1 h. In body temperature the mean masking effect (0.22 °C) is clearly smaller than in the previous example under constant conditions (Fig. 14). One of the reasons is the generally increased score on neuroticism in constant-condition experiments with internally desynchronized rhythms (with low scores internal desynchronization would not occur; see "Spontaneous Occurrence of Internal Desynchronization"), which was shown to increase the mean masking effect, while in zeitgeber experiments internal

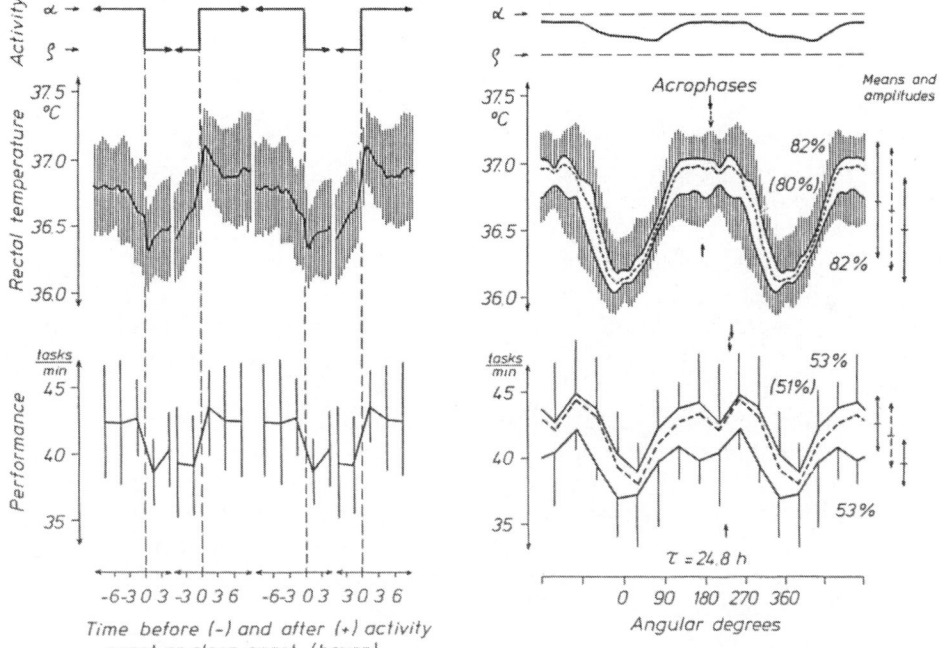

Fig. 20. Results of an experiment in which a 26-year-old man lived without environmental time cues but under the influence of a 28.0-h zeitgeber of the same modality as in Fig. 19 (absolute light-dark plus regular request cues) for 25 days. Presented are educed cycles of the rhythm of body temperature and performance (computation speed; with standard deviations). *Left*, synchronization to the times of wake and sleep onsets. *Right*, educed (by applying the previously determined period of the temperature rhythm of 24.8 h) using all data (*dotted lines*) and data obtained only during the wake episodes (*upper solid lines*) and only during the sleep episodes (*lower solid lines*); *right border*, mean values and amplitudes of the educed cycles (the reliabilities are marked)

desynchronization can be forced in every subject, independently of neuroticism score. Concerning the performance rhythm it may be surprising that the pure circadian variation (i.e., in the separate wake or sleep cycles) clearly dominates the masking-induced variation (i.e., the reduction in performance during sleep episodes immediately after wakings). Of particular interest is the "post-lunch dip" in performance, which is desynchronized from the zeitgeber and hence from the rhythm of sleep-wake and of meals. This means that the performance dip cannot be due to a previous meal or to the duration of the prior wakefulness; it is present even after waking from sleep in cycles in which sleep-wake and body temperature are virtually counterphased. Rather, the performance dips are bound to the temperature rhythm, and they always occur around the maximum in body temperature, independently of the phase relationship between the rhythms of body temperature and sleep-wake. Since the performance dips in several subjects led to naps (though not in the present subject, who never took a nap), this correlation between temperature rhythm and performance dip is another independent indication that the naps are controlled by the rhythm of body temperature and not by the sleep-wake rhythm (see Figs. 12, 16; Wever 1985 a).

Experiments of this series show also another consistent results that deserves attention: the subjectively scored well-being of subjects is better and the objectively measured level of psychomotor performance is higher during the (forced) state of internal desynchronization than during synchronization. This apparently paradoxical result can hardly be distinguished from a temporal trend (which would be more plausible) in the experiments underlying Figs. 19 and 20; the increase, at least in performance, due to the common practice effect is superimposed in an unsystematic manner upon the effect to be examined. To secure this result numerous additional experiments of this type were performed in such a way that more than two sections with different rhythm states alternated with one another and that the temporal sequence of the sections with internally synchronized and desynchronized rhythms (i.e., with zeitgeber periods close to 24 h, on the one hand, and with periods of 28 h and longer or 20 h and shorter, on the other hand) were varied again and again. To give an example, in an experiment a section with internally synchronized rhythms was in the middle and hence was preceded and followed by sections with internally desynchronized rhythms; then, in the next experiment a section with internally desynchronized rhythms was in the middle and hence was surrounded by sections with internally synchronized rhythms (Wever 1979).

The smoothed courses of performance variables in all these experiments showed, primarily, the well-known practice effect, with a steady increase during the first one or two weeks. Secondarily, however, they all showed clearly recognizable superimpositions of modifications which depend on the internal organization of the rhythmic system. All these variables showed higher values during the sections with internally desynchronized rhythms than internally synchronized rhythms; and in the sections first mentioned they showed maximum values at days when the internal phase relationship between the rhythms of sleep-wake and body temperature was exactly the opposite of the normal phase relationship (with the temperature maximum during wake and the temperature minimum during sleep). In other words, the psychical efficiency of the subjects was, paradoxically enough, the higher the farther away the rhythmic system was from its steady state, the maintenance of which is the basic function of the circadian system. Also the fractions of wake within the sleep-wake cycle showed rather higher levels during internal desynchronization than synchronization (this is in agreement with results obtained under constant conditions; see Fig. 13); this means that the subjects slept less during the sections with internally desynchronized than synchronized rhythms, in spite of the fact that they are more efficient during these sections.

While the objectively measurable psychomotor performances (e.g., maximal possible computation speed, or reaction time) normally show practice effects (or learning increases) which may slightly obscure the dependence of the obtained data on the internal organization of the rhythmic system, this is not the case with subjectively scored mood data. When a subject, for instance, has to indicate subjectively in regular intervals (as indicated above, according to seven signals per cycle, including awakenings during the sleep episodes) his feeling of "contentment" (and of other items) on a visual analog scale, the results are higher levels during the sections with internally desynchronized than during sections with internally synchronized rhythms; and the mood levels are higher at days with internal phase relationships between the rhythms of sleep-wake and body temperature being just opposite to the "right" relationship (temperature maximum during wake and temperature minimum during sleep) than at days with phase relationships according to the normal order. Moreover, the absence of an obscuring practice effect allows, in these variables, the demonstration of the rhythmic courses. Amplitudes of the mood rhythms remain nearly unchanged when the state of the rhythm changes (with a pattern of the rhythms remaining also nearly unchanged), so that all phases of the mood rhythms (e.g., the wake values as well as the sleep values) change about equivalently with the state of the rhythm. The phases of the mood rhythms (measured in comparison to the phases of the zeitgeber or the sleep-wake cycles), on the other hand, change regularly with the zeitgeber period: the longer the zeitgeber period, the earlier are the mood rhythms.

The significant result of the objective and subjective improvement of the subjects by the unphysiological state of internal desynchronization is paradoxical and in contradiction to all expectations. On the one hand, this result has the advantage – independent of its theoretical meaning – that it justifies the performance of isolation experiments with human subjects, even when there is the possibility of the occurrence of internal desynchronization (if such experiments had adverse effects, their performance could not be justified). On the other hand, an interpretation of these results is difficult. It may be speculated that this result is due to a short-term (i.e., lasting for not more than a few weeks) euphoria, which may reverse in the long run. Another hypothesis is based on the fact that the input of too few stimuli (sensory deprivation) leads to stress as does the input of too many stimuli; this means that an optimum of stimulation exists where the well-being of the subjects and their psychical efficiency is at its maximum. It is plausible that during the isolation the stimulus input is smaller than usual (i.e., below the optimum), and that the additional internal stimulus of the internal desynchronization raises the total stimulation and hence the well-being of the subjects closer to its optimum (in the normal situation where the stimulation of most persons is certainly not below the optimum, an additional internal stimulus would shift the total stimulation further away from the optimum, i.e., to more stress, and hence it would rather impair the well-being). Independent of the mechanism underlying the paradoxical effect indicating an psychical improvement of the subjects by the state of internal desynchronization, the exposure to internal desynchronization may be of value as a stimulation therapy in specific patients.

Absolute Light-Dark Supplemented by External Modifications

Apart from an independent evaluation of the effects of an absolute light-dark alternation, forcing internal desynchronization can be used as a tool to examine other aspects not directly related to this specific type of zeitgeber, for instance the influence of behavioral stress on human circadian rhythms. There are a number of vague indications of a lengthening effect on free-running rhythms; these come

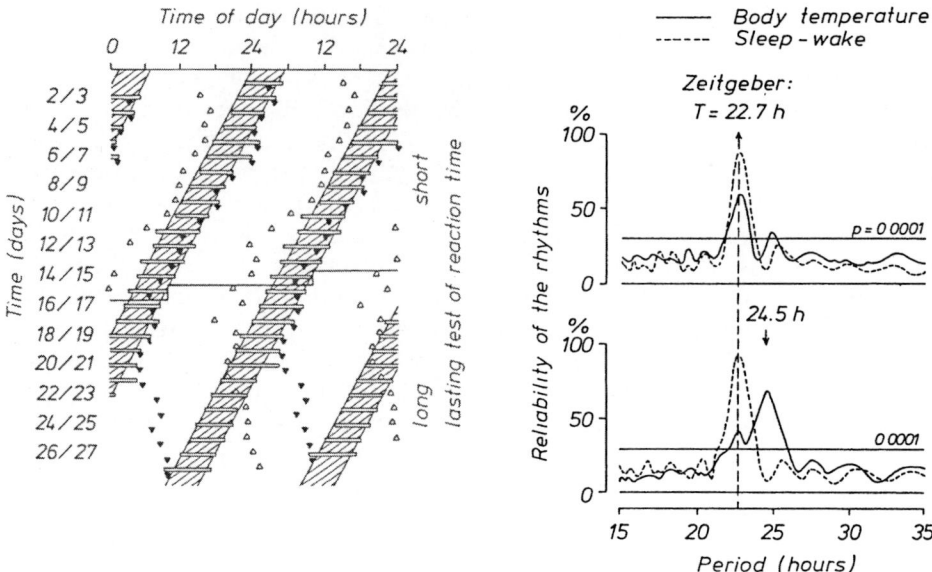

Fig. 21. Results of an experiment in which a 26-year-old man lived without environmental time cues but under the influence of an artificial zeitgeber of the same modality as in Fig. 19, with a constant period of 22:40 h. In the first section the subject performed a short-term (5-min) reaction time test (which he performed happily); in the second the duration of the test sessions was increased to 20 min (which obviously "stressed" the subject). *Left*, course of the experiment; designations as in Fig. 16, left. Internal (and external) synchronization during the first section but forced internal desynchronization during the second. *Right*, periodogram analysis of the two rhythms, computed separately for the two sections of the experiment

from the comparison of results obtained over the years during which various psychomotor tests were performed (involving different levels of behavioral stress); and during these years the free-running periods and other rhythm parameters varied systematically (see "External Modifications of Autonomous Rhythms"). However, the lengthening effect was only in the range of about 0.2 h and hence too small for drawing realistic conclusions; in particular, it was too small for performing measurements in single experiments in which subjects are exposed to behavioral stress in one section and protected from stress in another section so that they can serve as their own controls. To answer the question for a possible effect of stress, therefore, we attempted to use instability close to the limit of entrainment for an amplification process (Wever 1979).

In the experiment described in Fig. 21, the subject was exposed continuously to a zeitgeber (absolute light-dark plus request cues) with a period of 22:40 h (which was known from previous experiments to be very close to the lower limit of entrainment of the physiological rhythms). For the first 2 weeks the subject performed a reaction time test (lasting 5 min at every test session) which he considered a welcome diversion from his studies (see left panel). In this first section not only the rhythm of sleep-wake but also that of body temperature was synchronized to the zeitgeber (right panel). After 2 weeks the duration of the test sessions was lengthened to 20 min (without informing the subject). After a few days the subject wrote a strongly worded message that he was beginning to hate the test (without realizing the objective reason), and he urgently requested that it be cancelled. It was possible to convince him, however, that in this specific experiment performance on the test was of particular importance, and he continued to perform it despite his reluctance. Also in the diary which he submitted upon going to bed each time he indicated that he felt stressed during the second section of the experiment (as was intended). In this second section, the rhythm of body temperature started to run freely and hence to desynchronize internally; the periodogram analysis (right panel of Fig. 21) confirms this result. Other experiments of this series showed similar results, and it was concluded that under these conditions behavioral stress leads to internal desynchronization.

The introduction of behavioral stress thus led to a lengthening of the inherent period of the temperature rhythm to only a small degree. This alteration in the period would be too small to be recognizable directly but it was sufficient barely to exceed the limit of entrainment so that the temperature rhythm could no longer be synchronized to the zeitgeber (and the sleep-wake rhythm) but ran freely. Consequently, the overt period altered for not less than about 2 h (from synchronization to 22:40 h to a free-run with a period of 24.5 h) which was easily recognizable. Therefore the experiment confirms, due to its amplification capacity, the lengthening effect of behavioral stress, which would be hard to establish without this procedure.

Another problem concerns the influence of social contacts within a group of collectively isolated subjects. Preliminary answer to this question came from those four group experiments under constant conditions in which the rhythms desynchronized internally during the experiment (see "External Modifications of Autonomous Rhythms"); in these experiments not only the sleep-wake rhythms of the different subjects were synchronous with one another but the rhythms of body temperature, which were independent of the sleep-wake rhythms, also. However, the sections showing the state of internal desynchronization were too short to decide finally whether this synchronization was due to an accidental coincidence in the free-running periods of the different subjects or to mutual entrainment (which then could be effected only by the social contacts among the subjects). To examine the problem of the mutual synchronization more precisely, a group of four subjects were exposed to a 30-h day (absolute light-dark plus request cues) which was known from previous experiments to be outside of the range of entrainment of the physiological rhythms. As was expected, the sleep-wake rhythms of all subjects became synchronized to the zeitgeber and therefore also to one another; they ate together, learned together, and went to bed at the same time. It was, however, surprising that their rhythms of body temperature (and other physiological and psychological rhythms) also became synchronous with one another during the entire experiment, independently of the perceivable sleep-wake rhythms. Here the long-term course of internal desynchronization (29 objective days including 28 temperature cycles) allowed a clear decision concerning the origin of the synchronization. Particularly the constantly changing temporal sequence of phase positions of the temperature rhythms of different subjects demonstrated that the synchrony in the periods was not due to an accidental coincidence of independently free-running rhythms but to a mutual entrainment.

The modality of this mutual entrainment (possibly olfactory pathways?) is still unknown; it is unsatisfactory to speak of social contacts as the zeitgeber. Nevertheless, this mutual synchronization of imperceptible rhythms is of practical significance. It prevents investigation of rhythms in patients who cannot stay alone (e.g., in depressives). In fact, it has been proposed (and even shown in a few experiments) that such patients live in isolation but under the constant control of physicians and nurses in randomly changing schedules and sequences. In this way, a transfer of the (differing) sleep-wake rhythms of the observers to the patient can be avoided, according to the present results, but not, however, a synchronization by their (coinciding) rhythms of body temperature (which in all observers have the same 24-h period and about the same phase, independently of the individual sleep-wake schedules). Consequently, an independent free-running rhythm of the patient cannot necessarily be expected. In fact, in the few experiments with depressives under intentionally constant conditions, the periods were so close to 24.0 h – and the experiments so short – that they could not be clearly coordinated to free-running rhythms. This means that it is hard to study rhythm parameters in such patients (Wever 1979).

Absolute Light-Dark with Constantly Changing Zeitgeber Period: Fractional Desynchronization

Several problems – in particular those of practical interest – require precise knowledge of the limits of entrainment. In the experiments discussed hitherto, the zeitgeber period was altered in steps of several hours each so that entrainment limits could be determined only at intervals of several hours. To obtain more precise values for these limits, an experimental design was used involving exposure to a zeitgeber whose period changed slowly and constantly. Since experiments have shown the entrainment limits of the rhythms of different variables to be slightly different such that the rhythms detach from the zeitgeber successively on different days, this experimental technique has been called "fractional desynchronization" (Wever 1983a). Figure 22 illustrates this technique. In the upper panel a subject was exposed to a zeitgeber (absolute light-dark plus regular request cues) with a length of 24.0 h in the first cycle and 5 min shorter in each following cycle than in the previous one. Due to the zeitgeber modality (see "Absolute Light-Dark with Constant Zeitgeber Period") sleep-wake followed the zeitgeber during the entire experiment, but not the rhythm of body temperature. The latter was clearly synchronous with the zeitgeber down to a period of 22:30 h; in the next cycle (with a length of 22:25 h), it detached from the zeitgeber and started to run freely (with the characteristic free-running period of 24.8 h and with clear indication of relative coordination due to the remaining zeitgeber effectiveness). In the lower panel another subject was exposed to a zeitgeber of the same modality, starting with a period of 26:00 h and maintaining this for four cycles (to obtain a steady state); thereafter each cycle was 10 min longer than the previous one. Sleep-wake was again synchronized to the zeitgeber during the entire experiment, the rhythm of body temperature, however, only up to a period of 26:50 h; beginning with the next cycle (with a length of 27:00 h) it ran freely (again with clear indication of relative coordination) with a period of 24.6 h. In

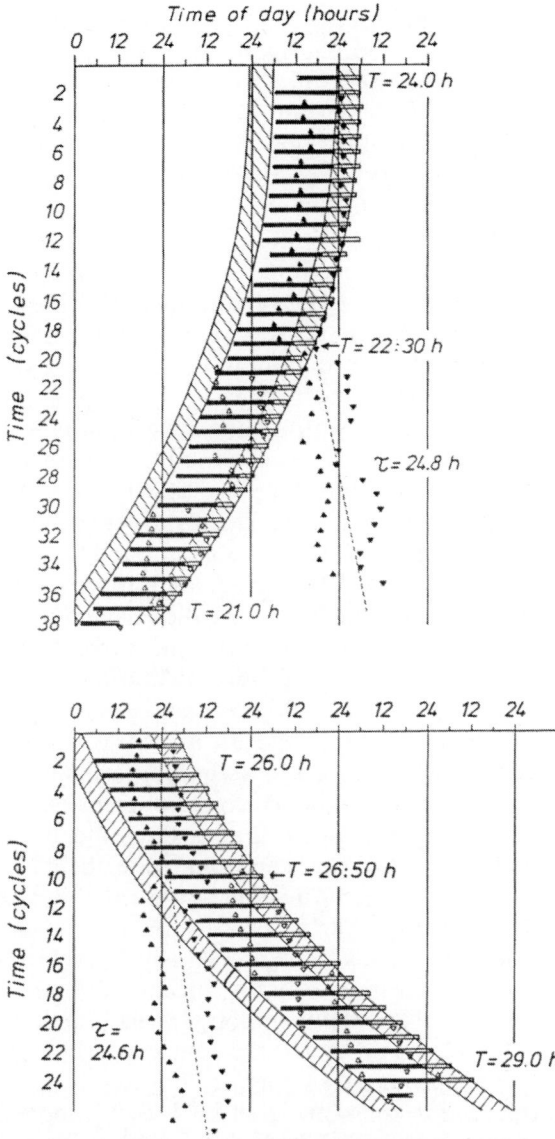

Fig. 22. Courses of two experiments in which a 24-year-old man (*above*) and a 22-year-old man (*below*) lived without environmental time cues but under the influence of artificial zeitgebers of the same modality as in Fig. 19 (absolute light-dark plus seven regular request cues per cycle), with slowly and constantly changing period. *Above*, beginning with a cycle duration of 24.0 h, every subsequent cycle was 5 min shorter than the previous one; *below*, beginning with four cycles with a duration of 26.0 h, every subsequent cycle was 10 min longer than the previous one. In both experiments, the sleep-wake rhythms were synchronized to the zeitgeber during the entire experiments. *Above*, the rhythm of body temperature was synchronized only down to a period of 22:30 h; in the next cycle (with a duration of 22:25 h) it detached from the zeitgeber and began to run freely (with a period of 24.8 h). *Below*, the rhythm of body temperature was synchronized only up to a period of 26:50 h; in the next cycle (with a duration of 27:00 h) it detached from the zeitgeber and began to run freely (with a period of 24.6 h)

these experiments, the limits of entrainment of the rhythm of body temperature could therefore be determined with a precision of 5 min (upper panel), or 10 min (lower panel). The smaller the changing rate, the more precise is the determination of entrainment limit, but the smaller the range of periods is that can be covered within a reasonable span of experimental time.

In all there are 12 experiments with fractional desynchronization by shortening (performed with young and healthy subjects), with changing rates of 5 min/cycle (Fig. 22, upper panel) and changing rates of 10 min/cycle. The (lower) entrainment limits of the rhythms of body temperature to be obtained with both these rates coincided, so that even the changing rate of 10 min/cycle is small enough to guarantee a continuous steady state; the mean entrainment limit of the temperature rhythm obtained with both rates was 22.41 ± 0.17 h. The seven experiments with fractional desynchronization by lengthening (again considering only experiments performed with young and healthy subjects), with changing rates of 10 min/cycle (Fig. 22, lower panel) resulted in an (upper) entrainment limit of the temperature rhythm of 26.91 ± 0.24 h. These data show that the entrainment limits vary only very little from subject to subject; nevertheless, even this small variability depends systematically on the free-running period of the temperature rhythms which had been measured after the detaching from the zeitgeber: the shorter the free-running period, the smaller the range of entrainment ($r = 0.93$). In subjects with an extraordinarily short free-running period, the range of entrainment is small in terms of the correlation mentioned, but it is sufficient to entrain the rhythm to the 24-h day because such a period is necessarily close to 24 h. On the other hand, subjects with an extraordinarily long free-running period (in extreme cases up to 28 h) also become synchronized to the 24-h day because they have, in terms of the correlation mentioned, a particularly wide range of entrainment (extrapolating the data mentioned, rhythms with free-running periods up to 28.3 h are entrainable to the 24-h day) (Wever 1983a).

Considering Fig. 22 it could be argued that the establishment of an entrainment limit is more or less arbitrary because, for instance, the masking effect (see above) can obscure the determination of single cycles. Fortunately, however, there is a physiological variable that is virtually free of masking effects or other rhythm distortions; this is the excretion of melatonin in the urine (Wever 1986). Figure 23 shows (in the right panel) the course of urinary melatonin in an experiment with the same protocol as that in Fig. 22, lower panel. Each zeitgeber cycle is normalized to the same length ($0° - 360°$), independently of its actual increasing length (as indicated at the right border). Here, even consideration of the raw data shows, without any doubt, external synchronization up to a period of 27:10 h and thereafter a free-run (with a period shorter than the actual zeitgeber periods). By comparison, the left panel of Fig. 23 shows the course of urinary cortisol, which is often taken as a good indicator of a physiological rhythm. In contrast to the right panel, the one on the left shows a course that is hard to interpret without detailed computer analysis. During the first part of the experiment, cortisol excretion was concentrated principally shortly after "sunrise", or wake onset, as usual; however, in the second part of the experiment, where the melatonin rhythm clearly ran freely, a cortisol concentration after "sunrise", or wake onset was also recognizable (here it represents a considerable masking effect). One needs some

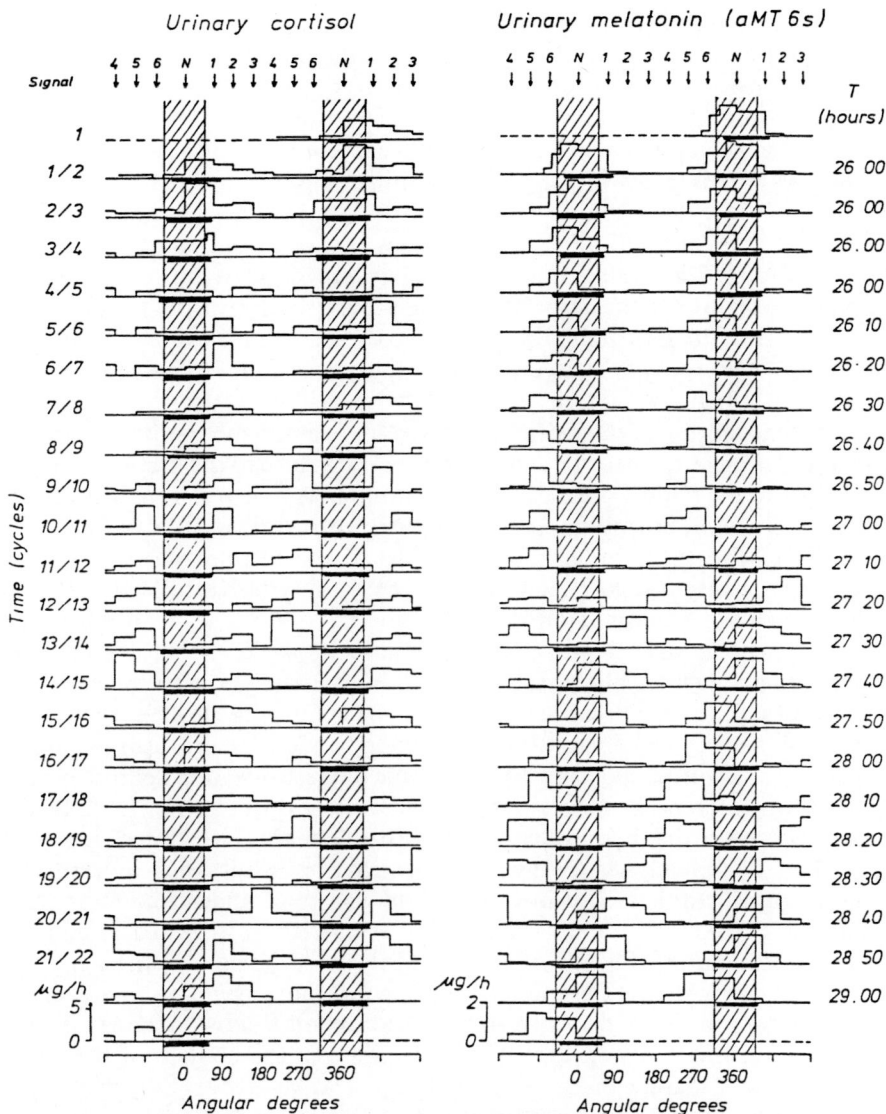

Fig. 23. Results of an experiment in which a 30-year-old man lived without environmental time cues but under the influence of the same artificial zeitgeber as in Fig. 22, below. Presented are the courses of the sleep episodes (*bars;* identical in both diagrams), of urinary cortisol (*left*) and urinary melatonin (measured as aMT6s; *right*). The data of successive cycles are drawn beneath one another (for clarity, in addition, data of two successive cycles each are drawn side by side); every zeitgeber cycle is normalized to 360°, independently of its (constantly lengthening) actual duration (*right border*). The rhythm of melatonin was clearly synchronized to the zeitgeber (and sleep-wake) up to a period of 27:10 h and thereafter ran freely, with the same clarity (i.e., showed forced internal desynchronization). The course of the cortisol rhythm may be similar but is much less obvious

imagination to perceive a free-running component here (parallel to the free-run of melatonin) by simple optical inspection (specific period analysis also leads to a coinciding free-running component in urinary cortisol). The precise determination of entrainment limits by simple eye inspection can therefore be supported by a number of variables such as melatonin excretion. Verification of this concept in most variables, however, requires specific computer analysis.

With regard to melatonin excretion itself, Fig. 23 shows an additional result. From its initial normal value this declines to about one-third of the normal excretion rate with lengthening zeitgeber period, i.e., with approximation of the entrainment limit. On the day when the melatonin rhythm begins to run freely, the excretion rises to its original value. It is the clear impression (which is also supported by the results of several other experiments) that melatonin secretion is suppressed when its rhythm is forced by a zeitgeber operating close to its entrainment limit; as long as the rhythm is not under such pressure, i.e., if it is either under the influence of a zeitgeber operating close to the free-running period (i.e., close to the middle of its range of entrainment) or is free-running, melatonin excretion shows its normal value. The suppression mentioned (down to about one-third) is of the same order of magnitude as the well-known suppression of melatonin by bright light (Lewy et al. 1980). It may be speculated that the two types of melatonin suppression are related to each other. The melatonin excretion peak, in fact, is shifted into the light phase (and the wake episode) by the lengthening zeitgeber; this phase position, however, cannot be the cause of the melatonin suppression because the melatonin peak during the later free-run is also frequently in the light phase (and the wake episode) without being suppressed.

The original purpose of using the technique of fractional desynchronization was to look for differences in the entrainment limits of different rhythms. If there is such a difference, the rhythms of the variables under consideration run, at least for a few days, completely separately: while one rhythm is still synchronized, another is already free-running. This means that the variables underlying these rhythms cannot be related functionally to one another or even be in a causal relationship. Figure 24 illustrates this use of fractional desynchronization; the results (only from analysis of the rhythms of body temperature and psychomotor performance, i.e., computation speed) derive from two experiments following the same protocol as in Fig. 22, lower panel. The upper panel shows the courses of the temporal positions (acrophases) of the two rhythms relative to the zeitgeber. The left diagram demonstrates a detaching of the performance rhythm 2 days later than that of the temperature rhythm; during the later free-run, the phases of the performance rhythm cross the zeitgeber, in the course of relative coordination, consistently 2 days later than the temperature rhythm. Thus the (upper) entrainment limit of the performance rhythm is passed 2 days later, and the period is 20 min longer than that of the temperature rhythm. This difference is confirmed by the course of the circadian amplitudes of the two rhythms (middle panel); the minimum values of the amplitudes which are combined systematically with the zeitgeber crossings, occur consistently 2 days later in the performance than in the temperature rhythm.

In the experiment on the right the performance rhythm detached from the zeitgeber not later, as in the left panel, but 3 days earlier than the temperature

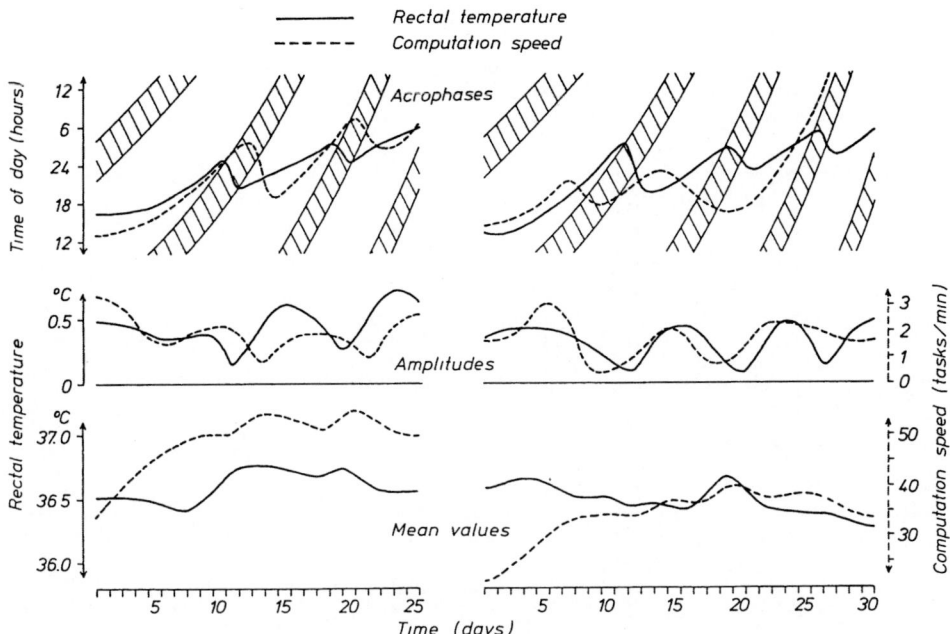

Fig. 24. Results of two experiments in which a 25-year-old man and a 20-year-old woman lived without environmental time cues but under the influence of same artificial zeitgebers as in Fig. 22, below. Presented are, from the rhythms of body temperature and performance (computation speed), the courses of the temporal positions of the acrophases (*above; shaded areas,* dark phases of the zeitgebers), circadian amplitudes (*middle*), and the smoothed levels (mean values; *below*)

rhythm; here the (opposite) difference in the entrainment limits of 30 min is also confirmed by the inspection of the rhythm's amplitudes. Analysis of entrainment limits in the other experiments of this series leads to similar results. We can therefore conclude that the ranges of entrainment of the rhythms of body temperature and psychomotor performance differ from each other in their widths in each subject but in different directions and to different extents (so that the two means of the ranges of entrainment are very similar). This obviously means that there cannot be a functional dependence, or a causal relationship between body temperature and psychomotor performance. Similar differences between rhythms have been observed in other variables, for instance, between sodium and potassium excretion, cortisol excretion and body temperature, and even between different types of performances (with and without the participation of memory) (Wever 1983a).

Peculiarities in an Elderly Subject

Another experiment with this protocol (Fig. 22, lower panel) was performed with a 81-year old woman; this was the third experiment with this subject. This one differed from experiments conducted with younger subjects. The rhythms of physiological variables ran freely during the entire experiment, i.e., the upper

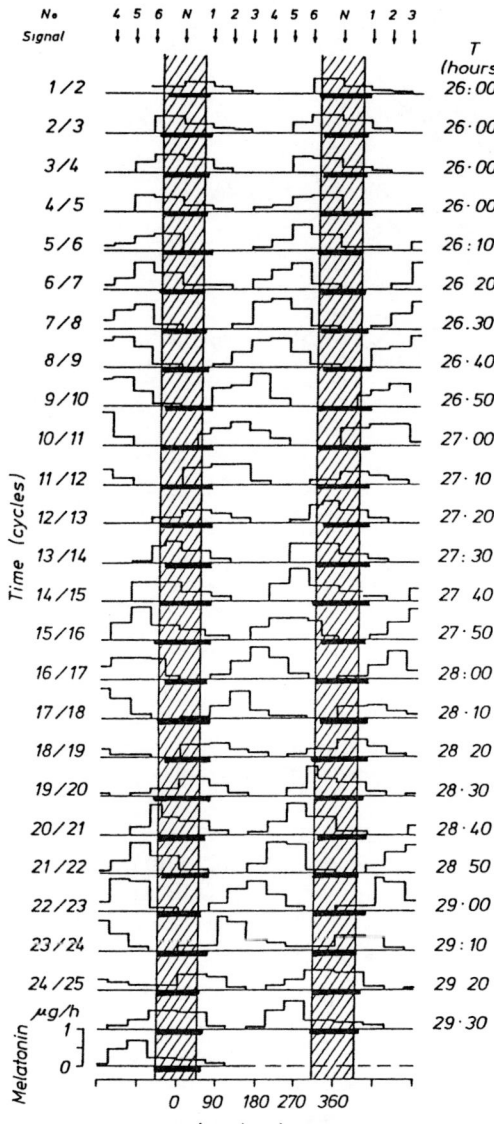

Fig. 25. Results of an experiment in which an 81-year-old woman lived without environmental time cues but under the influence of the same artificial zeitgeber as in Fig. 22, below. Presented are the courses of the sleep episodes and urinary melatonin in the same way as in Fig. 23. The rhythm of melatonin ran freely and hence was desynchronized externally from the zeitgeber and internally from sleep-wake during the entire experiment

limits of entrainment were – unexpectedly (otherwise the experiment had been started with a shorter period) – at periods shorter than 26.0 h. Figure 25 shows the courses of sleep-wake and urinary melatonin (the courses of other rhythms are more or less obscured by the masking effect, which is larger than normal in this subject because of her age; see "Internal Interactions: The Masking Effect"). From the beginning (with a period of 26.0 h) the excretion peak shifted to earlier phases of the zeitgeber (and the sleep-wake cycle); during the overall experiment the melatonin rhythm crossed the zeitgeber and sleep-wake rhythm more than three times. In addition, Fig. 25 shows a peculiarity of melatonin excretion in elderly subjects: when melatonin excretion occurs in a light phase and hence a wake episode (where it never occurs under natural conditions), it is twice as large as when it occurs at its normal time, namely in a dark phase and hence a sleep episode. As is well-known in the elderly, this subject's melatonin excretion was only about half that of young subjects. This holds, however, only when melatonin excretion occurs at its normal temporal position, i.e., during the dark phase and hence a sleep episode; melatonin excretion in this elderly subject was similar to that in young subjects when this occurred during the light phase and hence a wake episode (Wever 1989 a).

Information as a Zeitgeber

After discussing many different types of experiments using absolute light-dark alternation and constantly changing zeitgeber period, the actual synchronizing stimulus is still unclear. Absolute light-dark alternation has two very different aspects. First, it includes a physical stimulus which may exert direct physiological effects; such a direct light effect is the basis for the very effective light-dark zeitgebers in nearly all animal experiments. On the other hand, the transition from light to dark operates, independently of a possible direct effect of light, as a cue to go to bed, and the transition from dark to light makes it possible for the subject to resume his activities. Hence, the absolute light-dark alternation includes a behavioral component, and the zeitgeber effectiveness of this must be distinguished from that of the light per se.

Investigation of the direct light effect alone – with relative light-dark alternation and without request cues to the subject – have shown only residual effects of light. Investigation specifically of the effectiveness of the behavioral component is possible when the request cues (constituted by light transitions in absolute light-dark alternation) are given in the form of acoustically transmitted signals under constant light intensity (or even constant darkness). Experiments were thus performed under a constant light intensity of about 300 lux (and in one case under constant absolute darkness), and the subjects received two acoustic signals per cycle for getting up and going to bed (Wever 1983 b). Figure 26 shows the course of two different types of experiments following this concept. In the left panel the cues were given with a constant period of 23.5 h. This period was sufficiently far outside the range within which free-running rhythms could be expected and was close enough to the common free-running periods to allow synchronization even by a weak zeitgeber with a correspondingly small range of entrainment. This experiment (and several others with the same protocol) showed a clear synchronization to this purely information zeitgeber, not only regarding the rhythms of sleep-wake and body temperature but also all other rhythms that were measured. In the right panel the cues followed a constantly lengthening period, starting with 24.0 h and lengthening by 10 min in each succeeding cycle. Synchronization of the sleep-wake rhythm remained during the entire experiment (indicating the high motivation of the subject) and that of the rhythm of body temperature up to a period close to 27 h, with a subsequent free-run; the entrainment limit was here expected at a shorter period, otherwise the experiment had started with a longer period. The

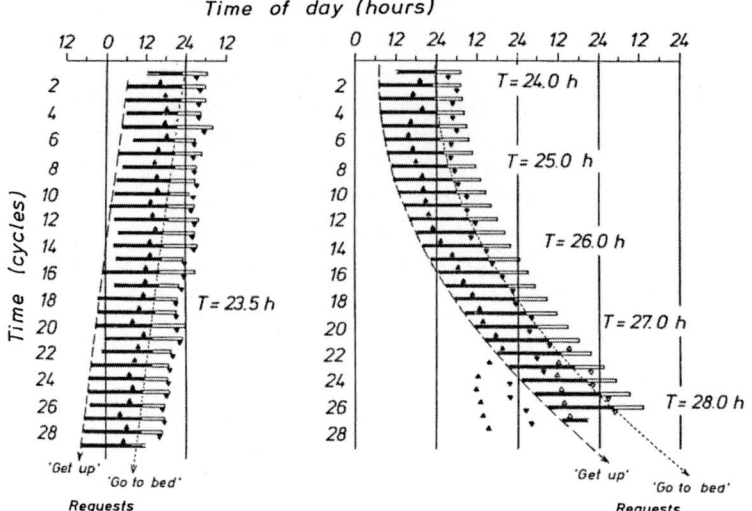

Fig. 26. Courses of two experiments in which a 26-year-old man (*left*) and a 47-year-old woman (*right*) lived under constant light (300 lux) and without environmental time cues but under the influence of information zeitgebers consisting of two acoustically transmitted requests per cycle. The courses of the rhythms of sleep-wake and body temperature are presented with the same designations as in Fig. 7, left. *Left*, the zeitgeber had a constant period of 23.5 h; the rhythms of sleep-wake and body temperature (and of all other variables measured but not presented) were synchronized to the zeitgeber during the entire experiment. *Right*, the zeitgeber had a constantly lengthening period (beginning with a cycle duration of 24.0 h, every subsequent cycle was 10 min longer than the previous one); synchronization of sleep-wake during the entire experiment and synchronization of the rhythm of body temperature up to a period of 27:10 h (thereafter ran the rhythm freely with a the period that cannot be determined because of the shortness of the section with the free-running rhythm)

same result was obtained in several more experiments of the same type and also in the experiment performed under total darkness, which excluded a role of the subjective light-dark alternation due to the opening and closing of the eyes. Furthermore, this was the same result as with absolute light-dark alternation, which should include, apart from the behavioral requests, direct effects of light. This means that there could be no such direct light effect; in other words, absolute light-dark alternation also operates overwhelmingly due to its behavioral cues and with only a negligible direct effect of light. This result is in agreement with that of the experiments using relative light-dark alternation, which can operate only due to a direct effect of light (i.e., there is no behavioral zeitgeber component) and which shows only a residual zeitgeber effectiveness (see "Pure Light-Dark Alternation;" Wever 1989a).

Other experiments were performed to compare the effects of two very different zeitgeber modalities but the same temporal protocol. These experiments make use of a constantly shortening zeitgeber (starting with 24.0 h), shortening by 5 min per cycle). The compared modalities were absolute light-dark alternation supplemented by seven request cues per cycle (the strongest zeitgeber known at that time) and only the two information cues under constant light intensity (information zeitgeber). The respective outcomes of these experiments are indistinguishable; independently of the zeitgeber modality they show synchronization of sleep-wake during the entire experiments and synchronization of the rhythm of body temperature down to periods of about 22:30 h, with a subsequent free-run. Consequently, the same results in these two types of experiment, in particular the same entrainment limits, indicate clearly the influence of zeitgebers of identical strengths. This again demonstrates that only the behavioral component influences the rhythms, not (or only negligibly) the direct effects of light (Wever 1989 a).

Bright Light as a Zeitgeber

Absolute Light-Dark Alternations with Bright Light

All experiments discussed so far were performed under light intensities between 0 and 1500 lux. Within this range light has been shown to exert only marginal effects on human circadian rhythms; in particular, light-dark alternations using intensities within this range are virtually ineffective. This picture alters dramatically with light intensities over 2500 lux. In the following, the zeitgeber effect of light-dark alternations is considered where the light intensity during the light phase is 3000– 5000 lux in the whole experimental room (Wever et al. 1983).

In the initial experimental series absolute light-dark alternation with the seven request cues per cycle was used (as in the experiments in Fig. 22). Figure 27 shows the course of two experiments with protocols similar to those in Fig. 22 but with a light intensity during the light phases ten times higher and changing rates of the zeitgeber period 5 min longer than in Fig. 22 (due to stronger zeitgeber effectiveness to be expected). The results were very different, however, to those in the previous experiments. Not only the sleep-wake rhythm but also the body temperature rhythm was synchronized to the zeitgeber throughout experiments, i.e., they showed entrainment limits lower than 18:30 h (upper panel) and higher than 31:30 h (lower panel). In fact, not only the rhythm of body temperature showed such a broad range of entrainment but also the rhythms of other physiological variables. Other experiments of this series showed similar results; in only a few of these experiments were the entrainment limits of the physiological rhythms exceeded (originally, the range of entrainment had not been expected to be so broad), and these were in fact only slightly outside of the periods in Fig. 27. In any case, the range of entrainment using a bright-light zeitgeber is considerably (i.e., about three times) broader than the zeitgeber with light of common intensities (compare Fig. 27 with Fig. 22); this means that the bright-light zeitgeber is about three times stronger than the normal-light zeitgeber (which is effective mainly due to its behavioral component; Wever 1985 d).

To perform the experiments shown in Fig. 27, one of the two experimental units had been equipped with additional lamps. In initially considering whether it would be worthwhile to perform experiments with bright light, mercury vapor lamps (which were at hand) were installed which produce bright light but of a spectral distribution which deviates considerably from that of natural light (after a few hours of adaptation, the subjects no longer perceived the strange spectral distribution; Wever et al. 1983). After these experiments had produced promising

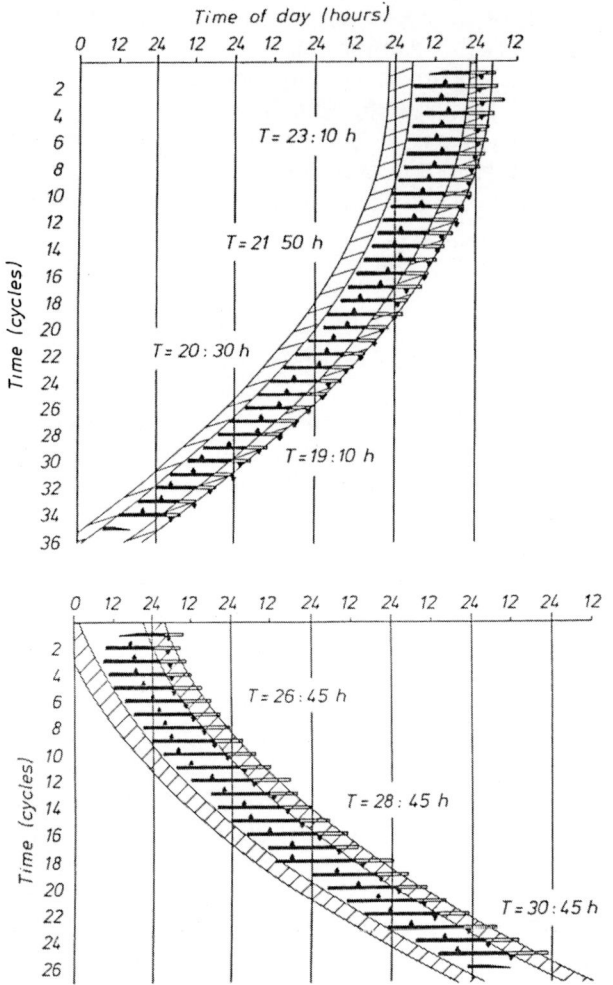

Fig. 27. Courses of two experiments in which a 21-year-old man (*above*) and a 19-year-old man (*below*) lived without environmental time cues but under the influence of artificial bright-light zeitgebers (absolute light-dark, 3000:0.03 lux, supplemented by seven regular request cues per cycle) with constantly changing period. *Above*, beginning with a cycle duration of 24.0 h, every subsequent cycle was 10 min shorter than the previous one; *below*, beginning with three cycles with a duration of 26.0 h each, every subsequent cycle was 15 min longer than the previous one. Presented are the rhythms of sleep-wake and body temperature with the same designations as in Fig. 19, left. In both experiments the rhythms of all variables were synchronized to the zeitgeber up to the end of the experiment

results, other lamps were installed that had a spectrum similar to that of natural sunlight and yet provided the needed intensity of light in the whole room (one of the greatest technical problems involved installing a cooling system adequate for a small temperature gradient in the room.) Subjects therefore did not have to sit in front of a relatively small light screen to be exposed to the bright light but were free to move around in the whole apartment without missing the exposure to the bright light. The results of the experiments with these two types of qualitatively different but quantitatively (i.e., when the intensity of illumination is measured in lux) similar illumination were indistinguishable; it must be concluded, therefore, that in humans mainly the intensity of light is relevant and not its spectral distribution (Wever 1985 d).

Relative Light-Dark Alternations with Bright Light

The experiments in Fig. 27 were performed using absolute light-dark alternation; consequently, a behavioral component is included in the overall zeitgeber effectiveness. It is plausible to assume that this component is not stronger with the bright-light than with the normal-light zeitgeber, and therefore that the considerably stronger effect of the bright-light zeitgeber is due to a powerful direct effect of light which is (nearly) lacking in the weaker effect of the normal-light zeitgeber. However, it cannot be completely excluded that the increased strength of the bright-light zeitgeber is nevertheless due to an increased strength of the behavioral component; this would mean that the bright-light zeitgeber also does not include (or only to a small degree) a direct effect of light. This question can be answered after exclusion of the behavioral component as in the case under relative light-dark alternation. To intensify discriminatory power, experiments were performed using light-dark alternation with a ratio between the light intensities of only 10:1 so that the subjects could also conduct all activities during the "dark" phase without any restrictions (and even without the necessity of switching on auxiliary lamps, as in the previous experiments under relative light-dark alternation with normal light; see "Relative Light-Dark Alternations"). The only precondition in these experiments was that the light intensities altered between values above and below the threshold of its effectiveness (at about 2500 lux; see above; Wever 1989 a).

Figure 28 shows the courses of three experiments in which subjects were exposed to such a relative light-dark alternation. In the right panel the light intensities were 3000:300 lux (i.e., alternatingly above and below the threshold of effectiveness) and in the left panel (with the same temporal protocol) 300:30 lux (i.e., for comparison, in both phases staying below the threshold); the middle panel (with likewise the higher light level but in a reversed temporal ratio) is discussed below (see "How Long Must Humans Be Exposed to Brigth Light"). In both light conditions of the right and left panel the subjects were free to pursue all activities during the "dark" phase as well as during the light phase (subjectively, all subjects experienced the contrast in the light intensities stronger under the lower light level than under the higher light level). The respective outcomes of the experiments were very different. Under the higher light level (right) the rhythm was fully synchronized to the zeitgeber down to a period of 20:30 h and then began to run

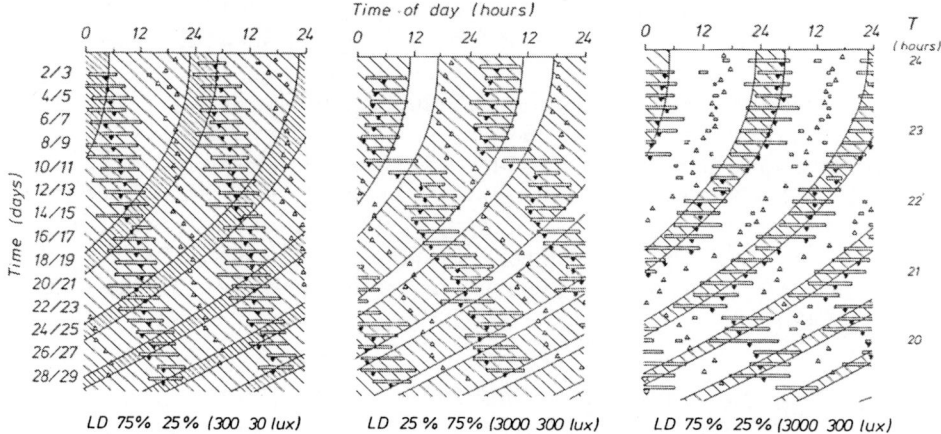

Fig. 28. Courses of three experiments in which subjects lived without environmental time cues but under the influence of artificial zeitgebers (relative light-dark with a ratio of light intensities of only 10:1), with constantly shortening periods (beginning with a cycle duration of 24.0 h, every subsequent cycle was 10 min shorter than the previous one). The courses of the rhythms of sleep-wake and body temperature are presented with the same designations as in Fig. 13, left. *Left*, light-dark 300:30 lux; no synchronization to the zeitgeber at all, i.e., free-run during the entire experiment. *Right*, light-dark 3000:300 lux; synchronization to the zeitgeber down to a period of 20:30 h and free-running thereafter. *Middle*, light-dark 3000:300 lux, as on the right, but with an inverse temporal ratio of 25%:75%; synchronization to the zeitgeber only down to a period of 23:00 h, and free-running thereafter

freely (while staying internally synchronized). Under the lower light level (but the subjectively stronger contrast; left) the rhythm ran freely during the entire experiment, i.e., it was not even synchronized to the zeitgeber with the initial period of 24.0 h (compare Fig. 15). The free-running also of the sleep-wake rhythms (during the entire experiment in the left panel and during the last section of the experiment in the right panel) indicates the absence of any behavioral component (as was present under the bright-light zeitgeber in Fig. 27). Hence, the great difference in the zeitgeber strengths depending on the light level can be due only to a powerful direct effect of light under the higher light level which is lacking under the lower light level. Six more experiments of the same type (with constantly shortening zeitgeber period) showed the same result, so that the great difference in the zeitgeber strengths is statistically significant.

Similar experiments were performed with the same light intensities but with constantly lengthening zeitgeber period. The results corresponded to those with the shortening protocol: no synchronization with relative light-dark of 300:30 lux but full synchronization up to periods of about 29 h with that of 3000:300 lux, and subsequent free-run with internally synchronized rhythms. This result is illustrated in Fig. 29 by showing the courses of the urinary melatonin (with the same indications as in Fig. 23). In the left panel (with the lower light level) sleep-wake and the rhythm of urinary melatonin (and likewise the rhythm of body temperature) ran freely during the entire experiment, i.e., the range of entrainment of this zeitgeber did not even include the initial period of 25.0 h. In the right panel

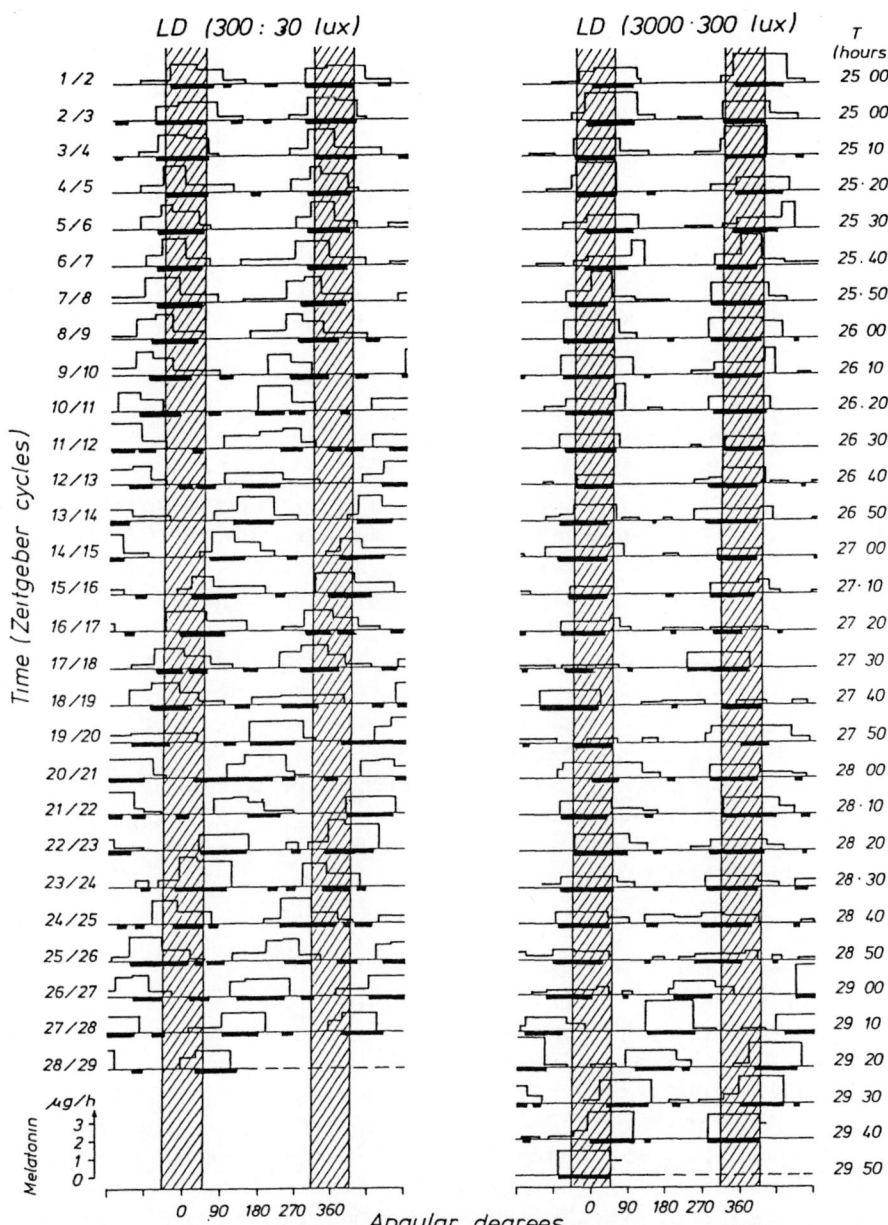

Fig. 29. Results of two experiments in which a 38-year-old man (*left*) and a 28-year-old woman (*right*), lived without environmental time cues but under the influence of artificial zeitgebers (relative light-dark with a ratio of light intensities of only 10:1) with constantly lengthening periods (beginning with a cycle duration of 25.0 h, every subsequent cycle was 10 min longer than the previous one). Presented are the courses of the sleep episodes and urinary melatonin in the same way as in Fig. 23. *Left*, light-dark 300:30 lux; no synchronization to the zeitgeber at all, i.e., free-running (including the sleep-wake rhythm) during the entire experiment. *Right*, light-dark 3000:300 lux; full synchronization to the zeitgeber up to a period of 29:00 h and free-running (including the sleep-wake rhythm) thereafter

(with the higher light level) sleep-wake and urinary melatonin (and likewise body temperature) ran synchronously with the zeitgeber up to a period of 29:00 h, and only thereafter did they run freely internally synchronized. These experiments, therefore, also indicate a (nearly) lacking zeitgeber effectiveness with the lower light level (i.e., staying in light as well as in "dark" below the threshold of effectiveness) but a powerful light-dark zeitgeber with the higher light level (i.e., alternating between values above and below the threshold). Furthermore, the (at least temporary) free-run also of the sleep-wake rhythm indicates the absence of a behavioral component; these experiments (together with the six others showing the same results) therefore confirm a powerful effect of light with intensities above 3000 lux on human circadian rhythms (Wever 1989 a).

The right panel of Fig. 29, in addition, shows suppression of melatonin excretion during the first 26 cycles of the experiment, i.e., during that time when the melatonin rhythm remained synchronized to the zeitgeber (approximating the entrainment limit). From the day on which the free-running starts (cycle number 27, i.e., with a zeitgeber period of 29:10 h), melatonin excretion returned to its original value. This result confirms the previous finding (see Fig. 23) of melatonin suppression under the influence of a zeitgeber which operates close to the entrainment limit. Here (under the influence of the strong bright-light zeitgeber), this entrainment limit is at about 29 h; in Fig. 23 (under the influence of the much weaker normal-light zeitgeber which is effective due to its behavioral component), the entrainment limit (at about 27 h) is much closer to the free-running period. This means, again, that normal melatonin excretion is suppressed to about 30% when the system is under the pressure of any zeitgeber which forces synchronization in a borderline case. Normal melatonin excretion can be observed only when the circadian system is free of tension, i.e., either synchronized to a period close to its free-running period (i.e., about in the middle of the range of entrainment) or free-running (Wever 1989 a).

How Long Must Humans Be Exposed to Bright Light?

These experiments show unmistakably that bright light is a powerful stimulus in controlling the human circadian system. However, all these zeitgeber experiments used bright-light fractions of three quarters of the full cycle, i.e., bright light for 18 h in the 24-h day (supplementing 6 h of dark); the question of the necessary duration of the bright-light phase to constitute an effective zeitgeber therefore remains open (a zeitgeber is effective when it is strong enough to overcome the difference between the common free-running period of about 25 h and the period of the natural day of 24 h; the bright-light zeitgeber used so far is stronger than necessary for practical purposes). Since preliminary studies had shown that a bright-light fraction of only 3 h is too short to be effective, different types of experiments were performed using 6 h of bright light per cycle. The middle panel of Fig. 28 shows a typical example of an experiment using relative light-dark alternation (to exclude the participation of a behavioral component) with only 6 h of bright light. The light intensities are identical to those in the right panel (3000:300 lux), and the temporal protocol was the same as in the other panels of Fig. 28 except for the temporal ratio between the light and the "dark" phases, which was reversed (not 75%:25% as in the other panels, but 25%:75%). The result is clear. The limit of entrainment of all rhythms (i.e., with maintaining internal synchronization) with a bright-light fraction of 25% is not at a period of 20.5 h as it is with a bright-light fraction of 75% (right panel) but only at a period of about 23 h. This means that a bright-light zeitgeber with a light fraction of 25% of the full cycle, or 6 h in the 24-h day, is sufficient to overcome the common difference between the free-running period and the day-night cycle. The same result was obtained in several lengthening studies: an entrainment limit of the temperature rhythm with a period about 1.5 h longer than the free-running period also needs a bright-light zeitgeber with a light fraction of 25%, or 6 h in the 24-h day.

A similar result follows from experiments with an absolute light-dark alternation. These experiments were all performed using the same temporal protocol (constant lengthening of the zeitgeber period by 10 min/cycle), and they are based on the behavioral zeitgeber (absolute light-dark 300:0.03 lux plus seven request cues per cycle, which constituted the same behavioral component in all experiments). Consequently, in all these experiments the sleep-wake rhythm maintained synchronously with the zeitgeber during the entire experiment. In detail, the experiments were varied in four steps. First, experiments were identical to the one shown in Fig. 22, lower panel; they resulted in an upper entrainment limit of the physiological variables of about 27 h (due only to the behavioral component). In the last step the normal light during the full light phase was substituted by bright light (3000 lux) as it was in Fig. 27, lower panel; this means that the behavioral zeitgeber component was complemented by a strong direct effect of light. The result was synchronization of the rhythms of the physiological variables during the entire experiment (i.e., the upper entrainment limit was at a period longer than 29 h). In the most crucial intermediated steps, only during one-third of the light phases was the normal light substituted by bright light (i.e., 6 h each in a 24-h day while the remaining 12 h maintained with normal light). The results were limits of entrainment that were about 1 h longer than with the initial light intensity and hence considerably shorter than with the bright-light zeitgeber. This means that 6 h of bright light are sufficient to enlarge the range of entrainment to an extent that is adequate for zeitgeber effectiveness in the natural 24-h day.

A closer inspection showed clear differences in the entrainment limits between different positions of the bright-light section within the light phase. If the 6-h section of bright light (normalized to a 24-h day) is at the beginning of the light phase (and hence is followed by 12 h of normal light) the upper entrainment limit is between about 27.5 and 28 h. If the 6-h section of bright light is at the end of the light phase (and hence is preceded by 12 h of normal light) the upper entrainment limit is between about 28 and 28.5 h; this means that, with regard to zeitgeber periods longer than the free-running period, bright light at the end of the light phase is more effective in synchronizing physiological rhythms than light at the beginning of the light phase (Wever 1989a).

The results of these experiments are confirmed by those of experiments with the same zeitgeber modalities but shortening protocols. Here also 6 h of bright light of 3000 lux per cycle (supplemented by 12 h of light of normal intensity of 300 lux) is necessary (and sufficient) to shift the lower entrainment limit for about 1 h to shorter periods. However, in this case a position of the bright-light section at the beginning of the light phase is more effective than a position at the end of the light phase. This difference in the phase-shifting ability of bright light depending on the phase of the rhythm hit by the bright-light fraction is in accordance with predictions deduced from phase (and amplitude) response curves of human circadian rhythms to bright light (Wever 1989 a). In summary, the results of the experiments with absolute light-dark alternations are in agreement with the results of the experiments with relative light-dark alternations (Fig. 28): 6 h of bright light per cycle is necessary and sufficient to extend the range of entrainment to either side for about 1 h.

Conclusions

Bright-Light Zeitgeber Versus Information Zeitgeber

These investigations have shown that the bright-light zeitgeber is the strongest known zeitgeber in controlling human circadian rhythms. However, it is not the most relevant zeitgeber because its effectiveness is bound to conditions which are hard to fulfill in our modern industrial society. Subjects must be exposed to bright light exceeding a threshold of about 2500 lux (which is commonly not available indoors or under artificial light but only outdoors on not overly cloudy days) and for not less than about 6 h per day. It is not yet known whether the exposure to light of considerably higher intensity (e.g., to 30000 lux, as is reached in natural sunshine without shadow) would shorten the span of exposure time necessary for a shift of the rhythm. This question, however, is not very relevant to most applications because it would be impossible for technical reasons artificially to generate light of such intensity in a whole room, mainly because of heat problems. Therefore, the most relevant zeitgeber in humans is behavioral in nature, that of social contacts. This is true – in spite of the fact that this zeitgeber is not the strongest – because it is ubiquitous. This is the case at least in healthy subjects without special problems such as the necessity of shift work or transmeridian flights.

Applications to Elderly and Ill Patients

A well-known problem in the elderly is their lack of social contacts. On the basis of the new knowledge concerning zeitgeber effects, this lack may not only lead to psychological defects (which exclusively have been considered up to the present) but may also take on a physiological dimension. This is the case when social contacts are too weak to guarantee full synchronization of all rhythms to the 24-h day (Wever 1975). The problem is aggravated by the fact that the only rhythm that is recognizable without special facilities, i.e., the sleep-wake rhythm, is also the rhythm which needs the least strongest zeitgeber for synchronization (and hence is synchronized to the 24-h day in nearly all these cases). The physiological rhythms, on the other hand, which need considerably stronger zeitgebers to become synchronized cannot be measured without expensive long-term investigations (see Fig. 16), which are particularly complicated in the elderly and the ill – where they are needed. Thus, the danger lies not in complete external desynchronization (which would be easy to recognize) but in only partial external synchronization which is, moreover, always combined with internal desynchronization. Similar problems arise in patients suffering from certain, particularly mental, diseases. The danger may also arise in these patients that the circadian rhythms are not fully but only partially synchronized to the 24-h day and are hence internally desynchronized.

The present investigations have shown that the tendency to rhythm disorders such as internal desynchronization increases with advanced age and certain mental disorders (see "The Multioscillator Concept"). On the other hand, it has been shown, though only in flies (Aschoff et al. 1971; Wever 1975), that rhythm disorders lead to accelerated aging processes resulting eventually in a shortening of the life span. This means that the special danger of a vicious circle arises which amplifies the initial diseases (Wever 1975). Every therapy must therefore begin by breaking this circle; this means that the rhythm disorder must be corrected. With the new knowledge concerning the characteristics of human circadian rhythms and their disorders such correction should be possible in many cases.

In the described groups of elderly or ill patients, the – insufficient – behavioral zeitgeber must be supplemented, or even substituted, by a more effective zeitgeber to overcome these problems. Apart from an intensification of social contacts, this can only be the bright-light zeitgeber (Wever 1985 d). Precisely these groups find it difficult to stay, or even walk, outdoors for as many hours as would be necessary to make use of natural bright light as a zeitgeber. Consequently, one should consider installing a lounge with artificial bright-light facilities in hospitals, where the patient can spend many hours. In most of these cases the social contacts are not completely ineffective but only too weak for full entrainment. If they have, for instance, only half the strength necessary for entrainment, only the missing half must be substituted by the bright light, since it has been shown that the effects of the different zeitgeber modes are virtually additive (Wever 1989 a). Subjects therefore must not necessarily be exposed to the bright light for 6 h per day, but shorter periods may suffice. It is to be expected that such a type of bright light therapy will assist in improve the quality of life in these patients; for instance, it is the distinct hope that rhythmically repeated sleep disorders, as are typical in these patients, would be cured (bright-light therapy in patients suffering from Seasonal Affective Disorders using similar conditions has shown promising results; it is not yet fully clear whether these results are based only on a strengthening of the overall zeitgeber).

Applications to Shift Work

A problem which particularly concerns healthy persons is shift work, which obviously is often unavoidable in modern societies. During their night shifts workers must stay active at times when their circadian rhythms would normally indicate rest. Since their social contacts do not reverse, their rhythms stay largely unshifted. In most cases in which an adaptation of rhythms to the shifted working schedule has been described, a masking effect of considerable extent was seen to be present; Wever 1985 c. A shift worker must thus be alert at times when his alertness is necessarily reduced, and when, for instance, his reaction time is lengthened and the probability for errors is increased; moreover, working in opposition to his internal clock may in the long run lead to special health disorders. Up to the present, the only way of trying to minimize adverse effects is using rapidly rotating shift systems and selecting prospective shift workers (the tolerance to rhythm disorders of the type under consideration is individually different). In most cases a true adaptation of circadian rhythms to shifted working schedules has not hitherto been possible (Wever 1985 c).

With the new knowledge concerning the effects of bright light it becomes possible to help shift workers reduce their problems. By applying bright-light zeitgebers, it is possible to shift circadian rhythms and adapt them to any working schedule, even against the influence of social contacts, so that the workers must no longer remain in conflict with their circadian system (Wever 1985 d). Workers can be exposed to bright light during their work shifts (depending on the position of the working shift, the bright light can be used before and/or after the shift, i.e., during leisure). To supplement this, during the time opposite to the shifts the workers should avoid bright light. Of course, such a lighting program is meaningful only when the (presently preferred) rapidly rotating shift system is replaced by a slowly rotating system. Even under bright light it may take a few days before the rhythms have fully adapted and have thus reached a new steady state; it is only during such a steady state that the advantages of this adaptation can be realized.

Applications to Jet Lag

A problem similar to that of shift work is jet lag following transmeridian flights. While it has been possible hitherto to measure the interindividually varying tolerance to the jet lag syndrome (Wever 1980), it was not been possible to overcome the problem. Exposure to bright light can alleviate the problem (Wever 1985 d). It is an old experience that the duration of reentrainment after phase shifts of a zeitgeber depends on the strength of the controlling zeitgeber; a stronger bright-light zeitgeber should therefore lead to a shorter duration of reentrainment than the weaker normal-light zeitgeber (see above). Experimental simulations of zeitgeber shifts have confirmed this predicted shortening. Figure 30 presents in the left panels the results of such experiments. The upper panel shows the course of an experiment. Two successive 6-h "westward" shifts were simulated at intervals of 2 weeks (this direction of the zeitgeber shift had been selected because reentrainment in this direction is slower than in the other direction and hence, the discrimination power is greater after shifts in this direction; see "Phase Shifts of the Zeitgeber: Jet Lag Simulation"). In the first shift the subject lived under a normal-light zeitgeber (relative light-dark plus regular request cues; i.e., under a zeitgeber that has been shown to be of similar strength to that of the natural zeitgeber; see "Relative Light-Dark Supplemented by Regular Request Cues") and in the second shift under a bright-light zeitgeber (which had been shown to be much stronger than the natural zeitgeber; see "Relative Light-Dark alternations of Bright Light"). The

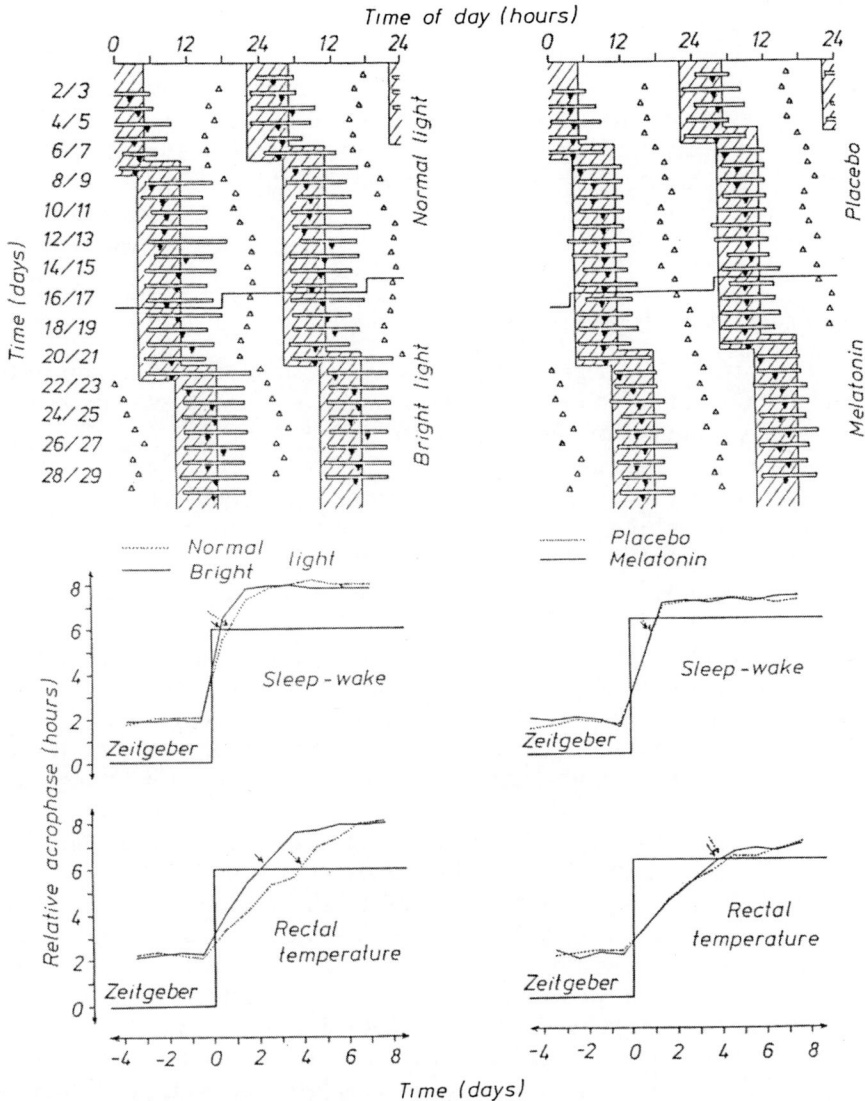

Fig. 30. Results of experiments in which subjects lived without environmental time cues but under the influence of artificial zeitgebers (relative light-dark, supplemented by seven regular request cues per cycle), with a period of 24.0 h and two successive delaying time shifts of the zeitgebers for 6 h each (simulating westward flights over 6 time zones each). *Left*, the first time shift was under a normal-light zeitgeber (300:0.03 lux) and the second under a bright-light zeitgeber (3000:0.03 lux). *Right*, both time shifts were, coincidingly, under a normal-light zeitgeber (300:0.03 lux), but the first was under placebo and the second under the administration of melatonin (5 mg orally, taken every day 1 h before going to bed). *Above*, courses of experiments with a 19-year-old man (*left*) and a 25-year-old woman (*right*) with the same designations as in Fig. 16, left. *Below*, averaged courses (from several identical experiments each) of the acrophases of the rhythms of sleep-wake (*upper*) and body temperature (*lower*) drawn separately for the two shifts each; the duration of reentrainment was half as long under bright light as under normal light (*left*), but the durations were identical with placebo and melatonin (*right*). Thus, the exposure to bright light speeds up the reentrainment process considerably, but the administration of melatonin is without effect on this process

rate of reentrainment is different for both rhythms as usual (see Fig. 18). Primarily, however, the subject adapted to both shifts with different rates (as shown in the lower panel, which presents courses of acrophases of the two rhythms, averaged from several experiments of the same type); this rate is, on average, twice as great under bright light as it is under normal light for both rhythms. The advice to a traveler after a long-distance flight is therefore to go outdoors after his arrival for several hours (though not necessarily in bright sunshine) to shorten the time needed to overcome jet lag (Wever 1985 d).

Possible Effects of Melatonin

By comparison, the right panels of Fig. 30 show the effect of melatonin administration on the duration of reentrainment (melatonin has often been seen as the ideal substance for overcoming jet lag). In experiments using the same temporal protocol as in the left panels, subjects were exposed to the normal-light zeitgeber during the entire experiment. For the first 2 weeks they received placebo and during the second 2 weeks 5 mg melatonin. The time of oral administration was 1 h before going to sleep; control was by analysis of urinary melatonin. Again, the subjects adapted to both shifts (as the lower panel shows); however, in contrast to the left panel the rates of reentrainment were indistinguishable from one another (Wever 1986). In addition, these coincided with the rate as common under the normal-light zeitgeber (left panel). Consequently, in contrast to the exposure to bright light, the administration of melatonin has no effect on reentrainment after a long-distance flight. This result is supported by inspection of the educed cycles of the rhythm of body temperature. The mean cycles are indistinguishable in both sections, i.e., under placebo and under melatonin, while the two sections in the left panel, under the normal-light and under the bright-light zeitgeber, show clear differences: under bright light the amplitude is clearly smaller and the reliability clearly lower than under normal light. Moreover, the mean value is slightly higher under bright than under normal light, and the wave shapes are different in the two conditions. This result, which is in agreement with results in all other experiments (in particular with results in experiments without phase shifts), indicates again the clear influence of bright light and the lack of influence of melatonin on human circadian rhyhtms. The subjective feeling of the subjects was also not influenced. After the experiment no subject could say in which section he received placebo and in which melatonin (during the experiment the subjects were convinced of receiving melatonin all the time). Of course, these statements are valid only with the dose of melatonin used and with its time of administration (possibly also with the shift direction used).

The results of these melatonin experiments are in full agreement with other types of experiments in which subjects also received melatonin. The latter experiments were performed with the technique of fractional desynchronization (see Fig. 22); these used the normal-light zeitgeber in the usual absolute light-dark fashion; in addition, however, the subjects received melatonin (again 5 mg orally every day 1 h before going to sleep). If the administration of melatonin had an independent zeitgeber effect, it should extend the range of entrainment of the physiological rhythms in comparison to those without melatonin administration (which is determined by the behavioral nature of the effective zeitgeber; see "Absolute Light-Dark with Constantly Changing Zeitgeber Period: Fractional Desynchronization"). However, it does not extend the range of entrainment; the results of the melatonin experiments did not differ in any respect from those of corresponding experiments without administration of melatonin (Wever 1986). One can therefore conclude that the administration of melatonin does not show any zeitgeber effectiveness (or any other influence on the circadian system; Wever 1989c). This result thus also means that bright light, which exerts a great effect on the circadian system, cannot operate physiologically via an effect of light on the metabolism of melatonin.

References

Aschoff J, v. Saint Paul U, Wever R (1971) Die Lebensdauer von Fliegen unter dem Einfluß von Zeit-Verschiebungen. Naturwissenschaften 58:574

Aschoff J, Hoffmann K, Pohl H, Wever R (1975) Re-entrainment of circadian rhythms after phase shifts of the zeitgeber. Chronobiologia 2:23–78

Aschoff J, Wever R, Wildgruber C, Wirz-Justice A (1984) Circadian control of meal timing during temporal isolation. Naturwissenschaften 71:534

Folkard S, Wever RA, Wildgruber CM (1983) Multi-oscillatory control of circadian rhythms in human performance. Nature 305:223–226

Lewy AJ, Wehr TA, Goodwin FK, Newsome DA, Markey SP (1980) Light suppresses melatonin secretion in humans. Science 210:1287–1289

Wever R (1975) Die Bedeutung der circadianen Periodik für den alternden Menschen. Verh Dtsch Ges Pathol 59:160–180

Wever RA (1979) The circadian system of man. Springer, Berlin Heidelberg New York

Wever RA (1980) Phase shifts of human circadian rhythms due to shifts of artificial zeitgebers. Chronobiologia 7:303–327

Wever RA (1981) On varying work-sleep schedules: the biological rhythm perspective. In: Johnson LC, Tepas DI, Colquhoun WP, Colligan MC (eds) Biological rhythms, sleep and shift work. Spectrum, New York, pp 35–60

Wever RA (1982) Behavioral aspects of circadian rhythmicity. In: Brown FM, Graeber RC (eds) Rhythmic Aspects of Behavior. Erlbaum, Hillsdale, pp 105–171

Wever RA (1983a) Fractional desynchronization of human circadian rhythms: a method for evaluating entrainment limits and functional interdependences. Pflügers Arch 396:128–137

Wever RA (1983b) Organization of the human circadian system: internal interactions. In: Wehr TA, Goodwin FK (eds) Circadian rhythms in psychiatry. Boxwood, Pacific Grove, pp 17–32

Wever RA (1984a) Toward a mathematical model of circadian rhythmicity. In: Moore-Ede MC, Czeisler CA (eds) Mathematical Models of the circadian sleep-wake cycle. Raven, New York, pp 17–97

Wever RA (1984b) Properties of human sleep-wake cycles: parameters of internally synchronized freerunning rhythms. Sleep 7:27–51

Wever RA (1984c) Sex differences in human circadian rhythms: intrinsic periods and sleep fractions. Experientia 40:1226–1234

Wever RA (1985a) Internal interactions within the human circadian system: the masking effect. Experientia 41:332–342

Wever RA (1985b) Circadian aspects of sleep. In: Kubicki S, Herrmann WM (eds) Methods of sleep research. Fischer, Stuttgart, pp 119–151

Wever RA (1985c) Man in temporal isolation: basic principles of the circadian system. In: Folkard S, Monk TH (eds) Hours of work. Wiley, New York, pp 15–28

Wever RA (1985d) Use of light to treat jet lag: differential effects of normal and bright artificial light on human circadian rhythms. In: The medical and biological effects of light. Ann N Y Acad Sci 453:282–304

Wever RA (1985e) Modes of interaction between ultradian and circadian rhythms: toward a mathematical model of sleep. Exp Brain Res [Suppl] 12:309–317

Wever RA (1986) Characteristics of circadian rhythms in human functions. J Neural Transm [Suppl] 21:323–373

Wever RA (1987) Mathematical models of circadian one- and multi-oscillator systems. In: Carpenter GA (ed) Some mathematical questions in biology: circadian rhythms. American Mathematical Society, Providence, pp 205–265

Wever RA (1988) Order and disorder in human circadian rhythmicity: possible relations to mental disorders. In: Kupfer DJ, Monk TH, Barchas JD (eds) Biological rhythms and mental disorders. Guilford, New York, pp 254–346

Wever RA (1989a) Light effects on human circadian rhythms: a review of recent Andechs experiments. J Biol Rhythms 4:161–185

Wever RA (1989b) Geschlechtsunterschiede von Schlafparametern. In: Saletu B (ed) Biologische Psychiatrie. Thieme, Stuttgart, pp 375–379

Wever RA (1989c) Schlaf und Melatonin. In: Saletu B (ed) Biologische Psychiatrie. Thieme, Stuttgart, pp 397–401

Wever RA, Polasec J, Wildgruber CM (1983) Bright light affects human circadian rhythms. Pflügers Arch 396:85–87

Wirz-Justice A, Wever RA, Aschoff J (1984) Seasonality in freerunning circadian rhythms in man. Naturwissenschaften 71:316–319

Diurnal Variations
in Cardiac Rhythms

Diurnal Heart Rate Rhythms in Small Mammals: Species-Specific Patterns and Their Environmental Modulation

K. Eisermann and W. Stöhr

Introduction

Temporal variations in the cardiovascular system are not only a problem of chronobiological research but are of considerable practical interest to any study of cardiovascular parameters, especially in laboratory animals. The choice of suitable animal models and of well-controlled housing conditions is an inevitable prerequisite for obtaining valid results. In our studies of social influences upon heart rate we concentrated mainly on four animal species: tree shrews (*Tupaia belangeri*), wild European rabbits (*Oryctolagus cuniculus*), Mongolian gerbils (*Meriones unguiculatus*), and guinea pigs (*Cavia aperea f. porcellus*). Some further heart rate data are available on laboratory mice (*Mus musculus*) and yellow-toothed cavies (*Galea musteloides*).

From all these species continuous heart rate measurements over several months were obtained, giving a total of more than 100000 h of heart rate recordings. Based on these data the basal diurnal heart rate patterns of these species and some widespread environmental disturbances of these patterns are presented in this paper.

Methods

Heart rates of all animals were measured radiotelemetrically using a system described by Stöhr (1988). Heart rate transmitters weighed between 1.0 and 4 g (depending on the battery used) and had lifetimes of 3–9 months. The duration of R-R interbeat intervals was measured continuously from the transmitted ECGs and recorded on chart strip recorders or stored on computers throughout the transmitter's lifetime.

Tree shrews, gerbils, and guinea pigs were housed in climatized rooms under artificial 12 L/12 D light cycles with food and fresh water ad libitum. Further details of the housing conditions are given by von Holst (1986), Probst et al. (1987), and Sachser and Lick (1989) for tree shrews, gerbils, and guinea pigs, respectively. Rabbits were kept in groups of two to four adults in a 100 m² open-air enclosure with free access to food and fresh water as described by Eisermann

Schmidt/Engel/Blumchen (Eds.)
Temporal Variations of the Cardiovascular System
© Springer-Verlag Berlin Heidelberg 1992

(1988). Yellow-toothed cavies lived in pairs in two interconnected tree shrew cages (described in v. Holst 1986) placed in an open-air enclosure. Food and fresh water were available ad libitum.

Results

While in all rodent species that we studied there is no clear diurnal heart rate pattern, rabbits and tree shrews show very distinct diurnal patterns of heart rate (Fig. 1). The diurnal fluctuations superimposed upon the heart rate pattern in *Galea* were caused by the cycle of ambient temperature and were not present in indoor environment with stable temperature. The heart rate of laboratory mice is not displayed in Fig. 1, but it shows a pattern similar to that of mongolian gerbils with even higher oscillations. It should be emphasized that the lack of diurnal variations in heart rate has no implication for the diurnal variability of behavioral or hormonal parameters. Despite their erratic heart rate fluctuations, mongolian gerbils, for instance, show very clear diurnal rhythms of serum testosterone concentration, scent marking, and open-field locomotor activity (Probst et al. 1987).

The distinct diurnal patterns of heart rate are closely related to the patterns of locomotor activity, hormonal parameters (von Holst, personal communication) and body temperature (Stöhr 1982) in tree shrews and to locomotor activity in

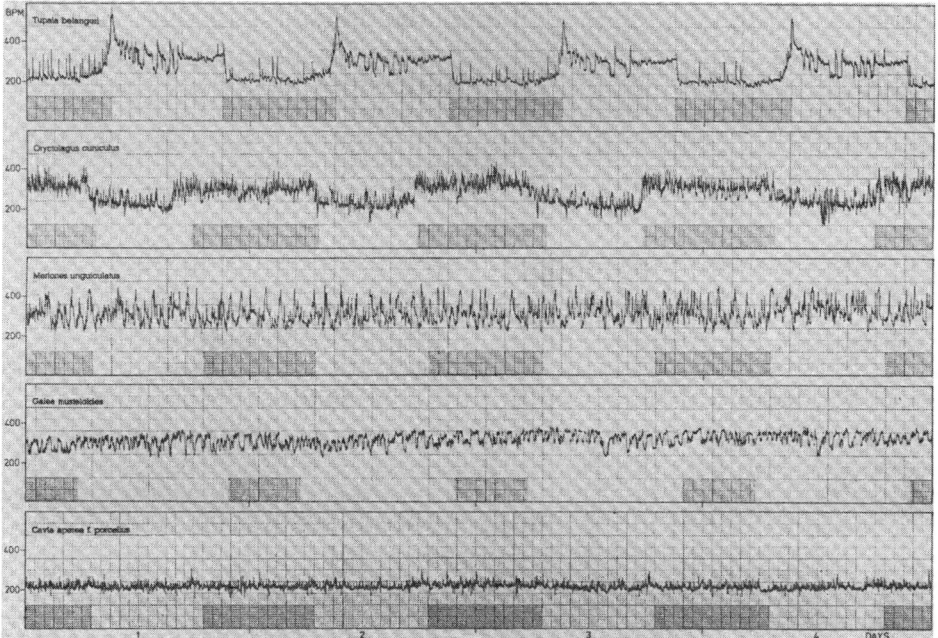

Fig. 1. Four days (0000–2400) of heart rate measurement in a tree shrew, a rabbit, a Mongolian gerbil, a yellow-toothed cavie, and a guinea pig (*from above*). *Shadowed areas:* the dark phase

rabbits (Eisermann 1988). Therefore, onset and cessation of the activity phase in these species may be determined from a sharp rise or drop in the animals heart rate cycle. In tree shrews the laboratory activity was almost exclusively confined to the light phase of an artificial 12 L/12 D light cycle. In rabbits, however, onset and cessation of activity were found to be independent of the annual variations of daylight and seemed rather to be coupled to a constant zeitgeber. Probably the animals synchronized their activity cycle with some anthropogen disturbances in the vicinity of their enclosure (Eisermann 1988). In animal studies one should always be well aware of the fact that light regimen is only one possible zeitgeber, and that, for instance, the animals may also be synchronized with feeding times, working hours in the laboratory, or cyclic fluctuations in ambient temperature.

As long as a stable environment is provided, the diurnal heart rate pattern is also very stable for all individuals of a species, and it may even be characteristic for each individual (Stöhr 1988). However, maintaining an absolutely stable environment is almost impracticable under normal laboratory conditions and is completely impossible if the animals must be studied in their natural environment. Therefore in daily practice it is interesting to note that there are considerable species-specific differences in susceptability to environmental disturbances. The heart rate of guinea pigs, for example, is usually not affected by environmental noise, although the animals show a behavioral response. Even the breaking down of walls in a laboratory adjacent to the housing room did not substantially alter the guinea pigs heart rate, and our experiments could continue. Tree shrews, on the other hand, are extremely sensitive to noise, and even a short knocking may cause a massive an prolonged cardioacceleration that is prominent in the animal's diurnal heart rate pattern. Similar relationships hold true for the reactions of these two species to other standard laboratory disturbances such as handling, supply of food and water, and cleaning the cages.

Blood sampling is another routine procedure carried out during numerous different experiments. Again, tree shrews show the most pronounced reaction, and their heart rate may remain elevated for up to 2 weeks upon one multiple blood sampling (Fig. 2). Blood sampling in tree shrews may even be used as a test stimulus for the reactivity of the sympathico-adrenomedullary system (von Holst 1986). In rabbits blood sampling causes a disturbance of the diurnal heart rate pattern that is very similar to the reaction upon merely capturing and handling the animal, and blood sampling does not influence the rabbits heart rate for more than 1 day. In guinea pigs there may sometimes be a minimal heart rate reaction to blood sampling, but it hardly changes the diurnal pattern, even on the day when the sample is taken.

All disturbances of the diurnal heart rate pattern discussed up to now are results of interference by the experimenter and may be controlled during crucial phases of an experiment. Unfortunately, there are other factors disturbing the animals heart rate patterns that are not so easily detected, especially if the animals are housed in open-air enclosures. The influence of ambient temperature, for instance, feigned a diurnal heart rate pattern in *Galea* that is absent at constant environmental conditions. The heart rate of wild rabbits, on the other hand, does not seem to be temperature dependent under open-air housing conditions. Even more difficult to detect are heart rate changes by rare weather situations such as smog, as was

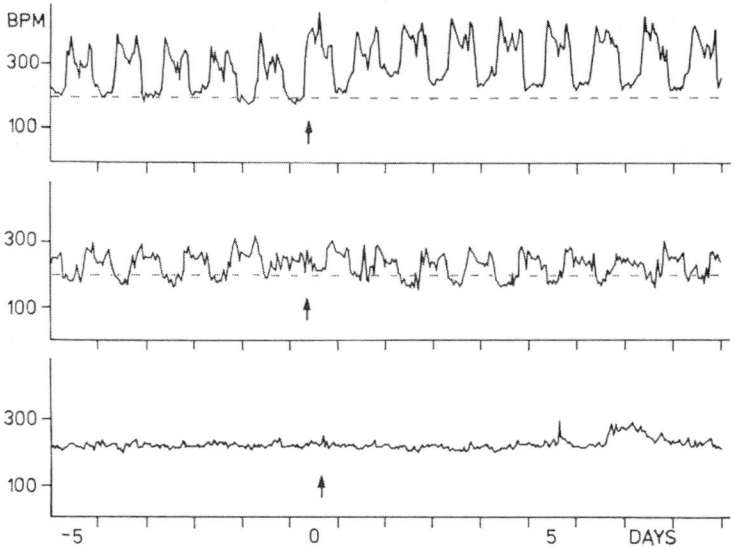

Fig. 2. Heart rate reaction of a tree shrew, a rabbit, and a guinea pig (*from above*) to multiple blood sampling at day 0 (*arrows*). Displayed are the hourly means of heart rate. In the tree shrew and the rabbit recordings, *dashed lines* indicate 200 BPM for ease of orientation

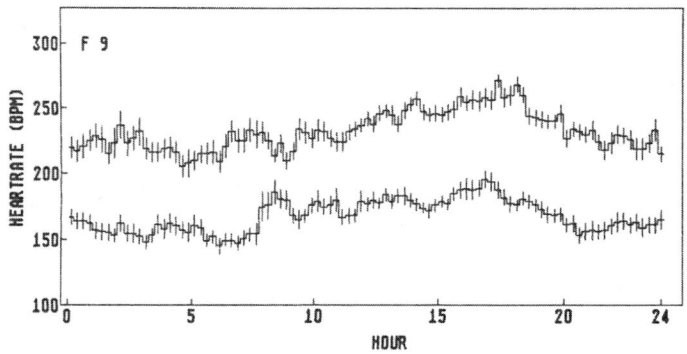

Fig. 3. Hourly means ± SEM of heart rate in a rabbit based on 30 days when the animal was fed on turnips (*above*) or exclusively on hay (*below*)

observed in a rabbit (Stöhr 1988). The lack of a diurnal cycle in ambient temperature is characteristic of another weather situation that repeatedly caused a complete breakdown in the heart rate pattern of rabbits, and that might also be related to cardiovascular malfunction in humans (Eisermann 1988). Up to now this kind of disturbance has been observed only in female rabbits, indicating that things may be further complicated by sex-specific or individual components.

A shift not in the pattern but in the level of heart rate is observed in rabbits if the availability of high-quality food is reduced. With hay as the only food the animals show about 30 % lower heart rates than rabbits fed with grass, turnips, or pellets (Fig. 3). In guinea pigs the spout size of the drinking bottles determines to a certain extent the amount of water consumed, and though the animals show no sign of thirsting, they consume less water and have slightly elevated heart rates if spout size is reduced.

Of course, an animal's internal physiological state also determines its heart rate rhythm. This fact is widely accepted for changes by social and nonsocial stress, but little is known about the consequences of pregnancies, for example. In rabbits during the last phase of pregnancy heart rate steadily rises, and the variation in heart rate between acitivity and rest is markedly dampened. A normal diurnal heart rate pattern is resumed after parturition.

Conclusions

Of course, the list of factors influencing diurnal heart rate cycles, given in this paper, is by no means complete. Even if the species-specific heart rate patterns are very stable over long periods, valid experimental results can be obtained only in an extremely stable environment or – even better – if heart rate is continuously controlled throughout the entire experimental phase. Continuous long-term measurement of the heart rate also gives rise to an entirely new experimental approach to the study of diurnal rhythms. Understanding climatic influences upon the heart rate pattern or the obvious discrepancy between the erratic heart rate fluctuations and the clearly diurnal behavioral and hormonal rhythms in rodents would surely contribute to our knowledge about the regulation of diurnal patterns.

References

Eisermann K (1988) Seasonal and environmental influences upon the diurnal heart rate pattern in wild rabbits living under seminatural conditions. Physiol Behav 43:559–565

Probst B, Eisermann K, Stöhr W (1987) Diurnal patterns of scent-marking, serum testosterone concentration and heart rate in male Mongolian gerbils. Physiol Behav 41:543–547

Sachser N, Lick C (1989) Social stress in guinea pigs. Physiol Behav 46:137–144

Stöhr W (1982) Telemetrische Langzeituntersuchungen der Herzfrequenz von *Tupaia belangeri*: Basalwerte sowie phasische und tonische Reaktionen auf nichtsoziale und soziale Belastungen. Thesis, University of Bayreuth

Stöhr W (1988) Longterm heart rate telemetry in small mammals: a comprehensive approach as a prerequisite for valid results. Physiol Behav 43:567–576

von Holst D (1986) Vegetative and somatic components of tree shrews behavior. J Auton Nerv Syst [Suppl] 657–670

Long-Term Changes of Heart Rate in Tree Shrews: Indicators of Social Stress?

W. Stöhr

Introduction

Tree shrews (Tupaia belangeri) are small, diurnal mammals about the size of small squirrels and are found throughout Southeast Asia. Originally considered primates, it now seems likely that they are a model of the common ancestor of all living placental animals (Martin 1968). In nature they live in pairs in territories which they defend vigorously against intruders of the same sex (Kawamichi and Kawamichi 1979). This dominance behavior can also be induced in the laboratory by simply putting two animals of the same sex into one enclosure (von Holst 1972, 1977; von Holst et al. 1983). Furthermore, tree shrews are – in contrast to most other laboratory animals – closely related to primates and strictly diurnal like humans. Thus tree shrews are an interesting animal model for studies of social stress in humans.

This chapter deals with the differentiated heart rate responses of tree shrews in different social situations.

Materials and Methods

The tree shrews used in this study were either captured in Thailand or bred in our animal house. If not otherwise specified the animals were housed singly in cages (floor area 70 × 70 cm, height 50 cm); adjacent animals were deprived of physical and visual contact by removable wooden partitions. All animals were kept at an artificial day–night cycle of 12:12 h; room temperature was $25 \pm 0.5\,°C$ relative humidity was about 55%. Food (*Tupaia*-Standard Diät 8010, Altromin, Lage FRG) and water were provided ad libitum. The tree shrews could be watched from an adjacent room through one-way windows, and frequently their behavior was recorded on video.

As tree shrews are quite small (about 200 g) and extremely active animals (about 15 km per day of horizontal locomotion alone), we had to develop a very small transmitter system to be able to record heart rate reliably over long periods of time. The transmitters weighed about 1 g and had a range of more than 5 m and a lifetime of about 4 months. They were implanted subcutaneously on the back of

Schmidt/Engel/Blümchen (Eds.)
Temporal Variations of the Cardiovascular System
© Springer-Verlag Berlin Heidelberg 1992

the animals with the electrodes extending to the thorax (for details see Stöhr 1988). Heart rate was determined as the inverse of the intervals between two consecutive R waves, either electronically or by computer. Heart rate was recorded continuously, day and night, from the implantation to the end of transmitter function.

After the implantation of the transmitter, the animals were left undisturbed until their heart rate had stabilized to the individual level of the specific animal. This usually took about 2 weeks. The animals were then left undisturbed for another week, and mean heart rates during the day and night of these 7 days were taken as the baseline heart rate of this specific animal.

Results and Discussion

Although the cardiovascular system of the *Tupaias* is very reactive and heart rate extremes range from 100 to 650 beats/min (bpm), the heart rate changes over consecutive days are only minimal as long as the animals live absolutely undisturbed in a stable environment (Fig. 1). Each animal has an individual, distinctive pattern of heart rate fluctuations which is extremely stable over long periods of time. Even if an animal is subjected to various tests and social confrontations, its heart rate eventually returns to the individual pattern if the animal is left undisturbed for a sufficient amount of time (Fig. 2).

Heart rate is very low in tree shrews during the night, so mean heart rate during the day exceeds the night values by about 50 %. About 2 h before lights-on, the heart rate begins to rise and reaches its maximum at lights-on when the animals leave their nest box and start to explore and mark their cage. Throughout the day there are alternating phases of rest and rapid arousals, with consecutive exploration and marking phases which are interspersed with periods of high

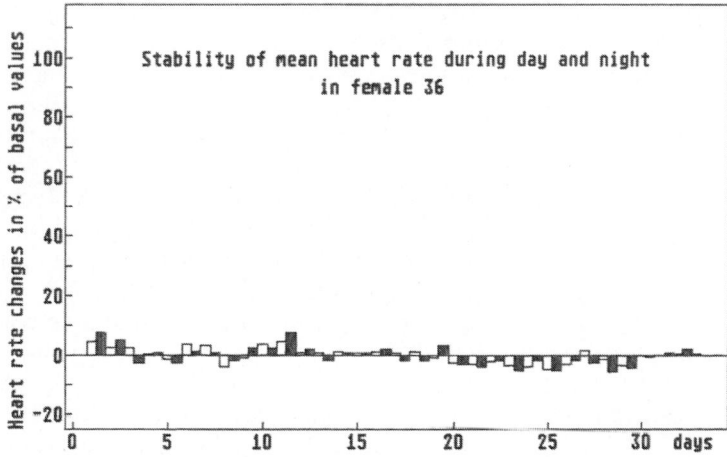

Fig. 1. Heart rate changes in a tree shrew living under stable, undisturbed conditions (*open blocks* mean day heart rate; *shaded blocks* mean night heart rate)

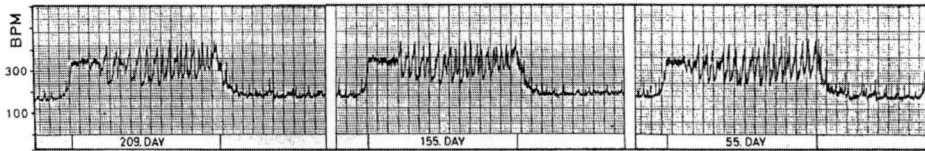

Fig. 2. Long-term stability of heart rate pattern in a tree shrew under stable, undisturbed conditions. Original registration on days 55, 155, and 209 after implantation of the transmitter. To be read from right to left (*shaded areas*; dark cycle)

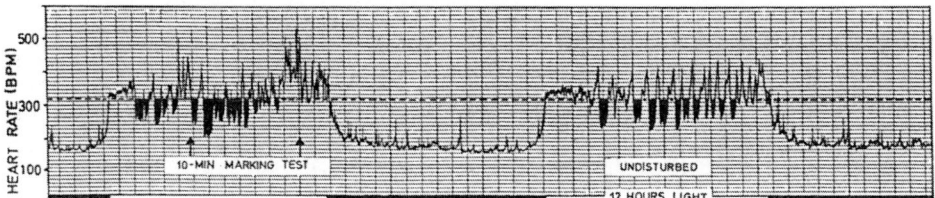

Fig. 3. Heart rate pattern of a tree shrew on a day with marking tests (mean, 318 bpm) in comparison with that during an undisturbed day (mean, 323 bpm). Original registration, to be read from right to left. Heart rates below mean day heart rate level are emphasized in *black*

locomotor activity. All these activities are clearly detectable by their characteristic heart rate profiles. Before heart rate drops rapidly to night values after lights-out, there is usually a prolonged phase of high locomotor activity (see also Fig. 2).

Tree shrews react to any kind of handling with drastic heart rate increases. If, however, an animal is familiar with the experimental procedure, it will show a transient response, but its heart rate will return to normal quickly and compensate the elevation by prolonged phases of low heart rate for the rest of the day. Mean heart rates of 7 consecutive days with marking tests (mean, 330.3 bpm) and 7 days without marking tests (mean, 331.6 bpm) did not differ significantly, although each test caused a prominent tachycardia (Fig. 3). Interestingly, the animals also compensate for other parameters such as marking, resting, and locomotor activity as long as they are not exposed to any kind of stress. It seems that tree shrews possess an innate knowledge of the amount of activity which is optimal for them.

In contrast to nonsocial stimuli, social contact invariably elicits a drastic, long-lasting heart rate response. In the case of male/female confrontations, the male immediately initiates sexual following which can go on for hours until the female either submits to copulation or rejects the male aggressively. The female's response to a specific male is highly individual, and we could not predict it. Only about 20 % of arbitrary couplings result in a harmonious couple; the rest are characterized by persistent following of the female by the male and more or less intense defense behavior of the female. Naturally during such a vigorous activity, the heart rate patterns in both animals are changed. While the male's heart rate is raised only temporarily during acute pursuit, however, his mean heart rate during the day is hardly elevated. Though less pronounced, the female's heart rate shows similar tachycardias during pursuit, but, in contrast to the male, its mean heart

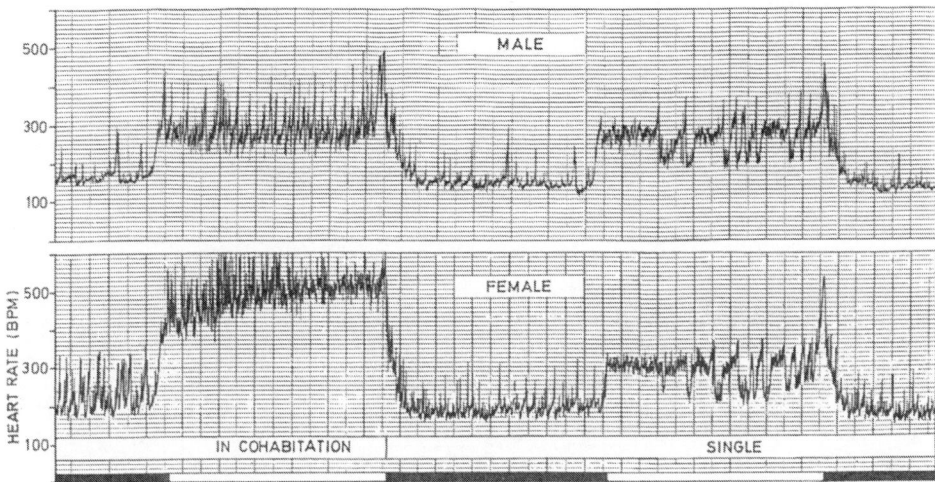

Fig. 4. Heart rate pattern of a male and a female tree shrew on the first day of an incompatible cohabitation. Original registration, to be read from right to left

rate is drastically elevated by up to 70 % throughout the whole day (Fig. 4). This shows clearly that it is not physical activity which causes heart rate elevations, but rather the emotional stress exerted upon the female by the male. As one would expect for diurnal animals, any interaction ceases with the end of the light cycle, when both animals retreat to separate nest boxes to sleep. Heart rate during the night is not significantly elevated in either animal. In an incompatible cohabitation, the situation described above can prevail for long periods of time. In the example shown in Fig. 4, the female's heart rate remained elevated for 23 days until the animals were separated. After termination of such an incompatible cohabitation the female's heart rate will frequently show an overshoot reaction. Basal values are sometimes only regained only after 1 to 2 weeks.

When two male tree shrews are put together, there is usually an immediate fight for dominance. Naturally the heart rates of both animals are drastically elevated for the duration of the fighting. If one animal is clearly dominant, the opponent is quickly subdued and fighting ceases. From this point on the dominant's heart rate quickly returns to prefight levels, whereas the subdominant retains a permanently elevated heart rate, up to nearly 100 % above baseline values. In contrast to male/female confrontations, the heart rate of subdominants is elevated drastically during the night. In some cases, nocturnal heart rate exceeded previous daytime levels, even though the animals were sleeping in separate nest boxes and there was no direct threat from the antagonist. The previously distinct diurnal rhythm broke down completely (von Holst 1983). If in a fight there is no clear winner and loser, the animals gradually come to some arrangement, and a relative dominance results: both animals have an elevated heart rate which is inversely correlated to their degree of dominance. The subdominant animal controls a smaller portion of the cage, yields upon the approach of the dominant animal, and rarely enters the dominant animal's portion of the cage.

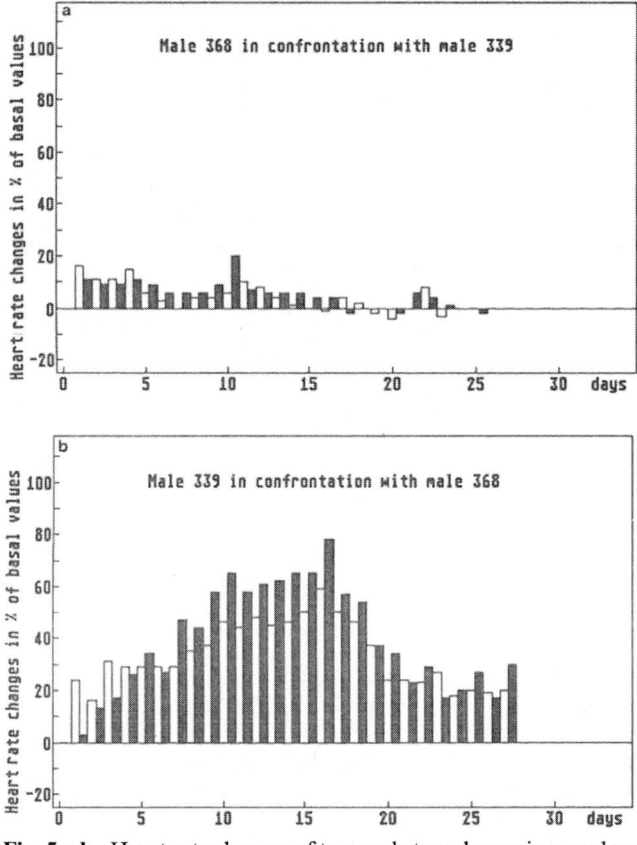

Fig. 5a, b. Heart rate changes of two male tree shrews in a prolonged confrontation (*open blocks*, mean day heart rate; *shaded blocks*; mean night heart rate)

Figure 5 shows an unusual confrontation in which both animals were reluctant to fight right away. Accordingly, during the first few days neither animal showed drastic increases in heart rate until on day 5 male 339 gained a relative superiority. From then on, its heart rate was reduced, while the subdominant's heart rate rose steadily to day 10. After this, fighting was reduced, and the subdominant's heart rate stabilized at about 50 % above baseline values. On day 16, the subdominant male 368 in a last encounter tried to expand its territory without success and was from then on completely ignored by the dominant. Its heart rate slowly fell to a moderately elevated level until on day 28 the two animals were separated. In this confrontation, there were neither severe fights nor drastic heart rate elevations, but its slow progress enables us to see clearly the subtle heart rate responses to changes in the dominance relation. Furthermore, it demonstrates that only a more severe stress (from day 8 to day 16) causes heart rates to be elevated during the night more than during the day. In really antagonistic confrontations, mean nocturnal heart rate will exceed former daytime heart rate, and thus the diurnal pattern of heart rate completely breaks down. After termination of such a

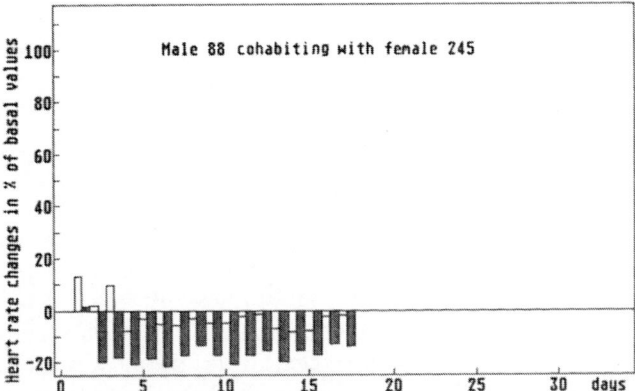

Fig. 6. Heart rate changes of a male tree shrew in a harmonious cohabitation with a female (*open blocks*; mean day heart rate; *shaded blocks*; mean night heart rate)

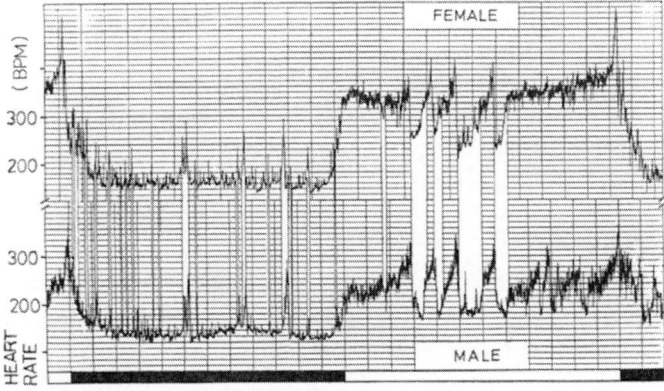

Fig. 7. Heart rate pattern of two harmoniously cohabiting tree shrews. Original registration, to be read from right to left. Corresponding heart rate changes are emphasized in *white*

confrontation, heart rate takes many days to return to baseline values. Elevated nocturnal heart rate is thus a precise indicator of persistent stress, especially as it is not affected by physical activity as is diurnal heart rate.

The great significance of nocturnal heart rate levels has its counterpart in harmonious cohabitations of males and females. Here we found heart rate levels significantly lower in both animals than when the same animals lived singly and undisturbed. Again, this effect of social support was more prominent during the night than during the daytime (Fig. 6). While stress was seen to break down diurnal rhythms, in harmonious couples both animals synchronized their rhythms of rest and activity and even their nocturnal tachycardias. This can be seen clearly in the heart rate readings (Fig. 7).

Conclusions

Tree shrews have a very reactive cardiovascular system, and their heart rate ranges from 100 bpm to 650 bpm. They can perform their complete activity program at heart rates between 250 and 350 bpm, while maximums of 650 bpm are only reached in emotionally excited situations, regardless of activity. Mean heart rate is very stable from day to day as long as the animals live in a stable environment. Tree shrews have a distinct, individual pattern of heart rate fluctuations, which is also very stable in undisturbed animals. Tree shrews are strictly diurnal animals with mean day heart rates 50 % higher than night heart rates.

Heart rate responses to familiar, nonsocial stimuli are compensated by prolonged phases of low heart rate, so means are not changed. In contrast, social threat causes drastic, persistent heart rate responses which hardly habituate. If the social situation stabilizes, heart rate stabilizes as well, at a level correlated with the level of social stress. The heart rate responses hardly decrease, however, if two animals are confronted repeatedly on consecutive days. In a dominance relation, heart rate is inversely correlated to relative dominance. Severe stress is more prominent in nocturnal heart rate than in diurnal heart rate, although the animals sleep in separate nest boxes and there is no threat from the antagonist. After termination of social stress, heart rate returns only very slowly to basal values, and frequently there is an overshoot reaction. In harmonious couples of the opposite sex, the heart rate of both animals is persistently lower than when the same animals live singly and undisturbed.

References

Kawamichi T, Kawamichi M (1979) Spatial organisation and territory of the tree shrews (*Tupaia glis*) Anim Behav 27:381–393

Martin RD (1968) Reproduction and ontogeny in tree shrews (*Tupaia belangeri*) with reference to their general behavior and taxonomic relationship. Z Tierpsychol 25:409–495, 505–532

Stöhr W (1988) Long-term heart rate telemetry in small mammals: A comprehensive approach as a prerequisite for valid results. Physiol Behav 43:567–576

von Holst D (1972) Renal failure as the cause of death in *Tupaia belangeri* exposed to persistent social stress. J Comp Physiol 78:236–273

von Holst D (1978) Social stress in tree-shrews: problems, results and goals. J Comp Physiol 120:71–86

von Holst D, Fuchs E, Stöhr W (1983) Physiological changes in male *Tupaia belangeri* under different types of social stress In: Dembroski TM, Schmidt TH, Blümchen G (eds.) Biobehavioral bases of coronary heart disease. Karger, Basel, pp. 382–390

Spectral Analysis of Heart Rate During Different States of Activity *

H.-H. Abel, D. Klüßendorf, E. Koralewski, R. Krause, and R. Droh

Introduction

The momentary mean heart rate results from an interaction of several different mechanisms. The reticular activating system which generates the basic drive for somatomotor, respiratory, and cardiovascular control systems (Magoun 1950; Moruzzi 1972) exerts excitatory influences on cardiomotor neurons and, therefore, "unspecifically" drives the chronotropic cardiac innervation. Conversely, limbic structures specifically control heart rate when organizing the autonomic components of ongoing behavior (Hess 1949). With increasing activity, afferent information processing from various receptor sites contribute to the adequate adjustment of the heart rate to changing metabolic demands. Especially during low physical activation, heart rate, as an effector of the blood pressure control system, is affected by baroreceptor activity via a negative feedback loop (Bristow et al. 1971).

A characteristic phenomenon of heart beat time courses during physical rest is the more or less pronounced beat-to-beat variability. This physiological "arrhythmia" of the heart depends on age and physical capacity (Schlomka and Reindell 1936; Schlomka 1937) and is diminished with several diseases which are accompanied by autonomic disturbances (Gunderson and Neubauer 1977; Burgess 1982). The deterministic nature of heart rate variability becomes evident when the specific time structure of the heart rate is analyzed (Peňáz et al. 1968; Hyndman et al. 1971; Sayers 1973). Several preferential frequency ranges of heart rate fluctuations are described. Heart rate rhythmicity in the frequency range of respiration, the so-called respiratory sinus arrythmia, is based on intracentral coupling between inspiratory, sympathetic, and parasympathetic neurons (Koepchen and Thurau 1959; Gilbey et al. 1984), on respiratory modulated afferents from cardiovascular and pulmonary receptors (Anrep et al. 1936; Melcher 1976), and on respiratory phase-dependent baroreceptor processing (Koepchen et al. 1961; Eckberg and Orshan 1977). The 0.25 Hz rhythmicity is primarily mediated by the parasympathetic innervation of the heart (Katona et al. 1970; Akselrod et al. 1981). Heart rate oscillations in the 0.1 Hz frequency range depend on both the

* This research was supported by a grant from Sporthilfe e.V., Federal Republic of Germany.

Schmidt/Engel/Blümchen (Eds.)
Temporal Variations of the Cardiovascular System
© Springer-Verlag Berlin Heidelberg 1992

parasympathetic and the sympathetic components of the chronotropic control of the heart (Pomeranz et al. 1985). An expression of an endogeneous reticular rhythm generator (Langhorst et al. 1984), oscillations in the baroreceptor feedback loop (Guyton and Harris 1951), or reflection of autonomous vascular smooth muscle rhythmicity (Seller et al. 1967) are explanations for the 0.1 Hz rhythmicity. Contradictory results exist concerning the direction of change in heart rate rhythmicity during behavior accompanied by sympathetic activation. An increase in 0.1 Hz and a decrease in 0.25 Hz heart rate rhythmicity has been described during mental load as well as physical work (Pagani et al. 1986). However, a diminution of rhythmicity in both frequency ranges has also been seen (Mulder and Mulder 1981; Abel et al. 1988).

The aim of this study was an indirect, noninvasive analysis of the relationship between mean value and rhythmicity in the human chronotropic cardiac control during different states of central nervous activation and a brief review of interpretatory approaches which hypothesize the relationship between heart rate rhythmicity and autonomic "tone".

Methods

The study consisted of three series of experiments (Table 1). In series A, the volunteers were examined during 44 min of physical rest. In series B they were tested during 44 min of physical rest and 1 week later during a 14-min pretest period, a 14-min Raven test period, and a subsequent 14-min recovery period. The solution of the Raven test tasks requires mental performance to complete geometrical patterns quickly and accurately. In series C, endurance trained athletes were examined during 44 min of physical rest and 1 week later during a physical performance test in which a crank handle ergometer was used. After a 10-min prework period, the work load was increased stepwise every 3 min to 30, 70, 110, and 150 W; 20 min after the work ended, the athletes were examined during 44 min of recovery. The volunteers' anthropometric data demonstrated that all groups were of comparable age (Table 2). This fact is important for the interpretation of the results of the heart rate variability and rhythmicity analysis because these parameters are age-dependent (Schlomka 1937; Weise et al. 1987). All experiments were carried out with subjects in a sitting position. During rest

Table 1. Experimental protocol

	Series A (physical rest)	Series B (mental stress)	Series C (physical work)
Step 1	44 min physical rest	44 min physical rest	44 min physical rest
Step 2 (1 week later)	–	14 min pretest 14 min Raven test 14 min posttest	10 min prework 3 min 30 W 3 min 70 W 3 min 110 W 3 min 150 W
Step 3 (20 min later)	–	–	44 min postwork

Table 2. Anthropometric data

	Sex		Age (years)		Height (cm)		Weight (kg)	
	Sex	n	Mean	SEM	Mean	SEM	Mean	SEM
Series A	m	9	23.6	0.7	180.3	2.6	74.3	3.3
(n = 17)	f	8	23.0	0.5	171.0	1.3	58.5	1.6
Series B	m	13	22.4	0.7	185.3	1.9	75.5	3.3
(n = 16)	f	3	21.3	0.3	169.3	0.7	64.7	2.3
Series C	m	19	21.0	0.8	182.5	1.6	78.6	1.6
(n = 19)								

m, male; f, female.

and recovery periods, the volunteers listened to background music. The electro-cardiogram recordings, together with registrations of respiratory movements, were continuously made throughout every session. The following calculations were performed from consecutive 2-min recording periods. The intervals between successive R waves were computed beat to beat and 2-min mean values were calculated. Differences between neighboring R-R intervals were computed, and their 2-min mean values were also calculated. This heart rate parameter, Δ R-R interval, represents a trend-corrected measurement of heart rate variability (Eckoldt 1984). The electrocardiogram was transformed into an R-R interval signal. After fast Fourier transformation, the power spectra were computed from 122.9-s recording periods. The typical power spectrum calculated from the resting heart rate shows two prominent peaks which occur at about 0.1 Hz and about 0.25 Hz (Fig. 1). Like other authors (Akselrod et al. 1981; Sayers 1973), we defined two frequency ranges: the 0.1 Hz band from 0.05 Hz to 0.15 Hz and the 0.25 Hz band from 0.15 Hz to 0.37 Hz. The areas under the respective spectrum segments were computed in absolute units and were taken as measurements of 0.1 Hz

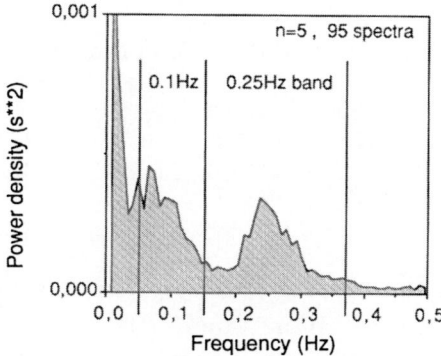

Fig. 1. Analysis of heart rate rhythmicity. The mean power spectrum of 95 spectra from five resting athletes is computed from the R-R interval signal. It exhibits two prominent peaks at about 0.1 Hz and 0.25 Hz ($T_0 = 122.9$ s). Therefore, in two frequency bands, areas under the spectrum were calculated in absolute units as measurements of heart rate rhythmicity: area in the 0.1 Hz band from 0.05 to 0.15 Hz and area in the 0.25 Hz band from 0.16 to 0.37 Hz

rhythmicity and 0.25 Hz rhythmicity. For some analysis procedures, the individual 2-min mean values of R-R intervals and of ΔR-R intervals and the values of the areas in the 0.1 Hz band and 0.25 Hz band were transformed into relative values by dividing them by the total mean value of the individual experiment. Because heart rate variability as well as rhythmicity depend on respiratory frequency (Hirsch and Bishop 1981; Ahmed et al. 1982), the respiratory cycle time was computed breath-to-breath by a respiratory pattern analysis (Abel et al. 1989a), averaged over 2-min recording periods and related to the heart rate parameters.

Results

Relationship Between Heart Rate and Its Time Structure During Physical Rest

Mean time courses of the relatively transformed parameters R-R interval, ΔR-R interval, area in the 0.1 Hz band, and area in the 0.25 Hz band were computed from 22 successive 2-min recording periods of the series A (Fig. 2). The time courses were fitted polynomially or linearly. All heart rate parameters changed spontaneously and demonstrated a significant positive linear trend during 44-min physical rest (F test, $p < 0.01$). The correlations between the variable R-R interval and the variables ΔR-R interval, area in the 0.1 Hz band, and area in the 0.25 Hz band were significantly positive (Fig. 3). This means that during resting behavior, a "spontaneous" increase in heart rate was normally accompanied by a decrease in heart rate variability and rhythmicity and vice versa.

Relationship Between Heart Rate and Its Time Structure During Mental Stress

In comparison to physical rest, all heart rate parameters had already decreased during the prestart phase of the Raven test (Fig. 4). The diminution of the area in the 0.25 Hz band (-20.2%) was more pronounced than the diminution of the area in the 0.1 Hz band (-8.0%). Mental performance was accompanied by a further decrease in the heart rate and its variability and rhythmicity. The change in the 0.25 Hz rhythmicity (-58.8%) again exceeded the change in the 0.1 Hz rhythmicity (-28.1%).

Relationship Between Heart Rate and Its Time Structure During Physical Work

In order to provoke more extended changes in the chronotropic control of the heart, six athletes were examined under physical work conditions. During the prestart phase, all heart rate parameters decreased by up to 35.3% in comparison to the resting session (Fig. 5). This tendency continued with the onset of work.

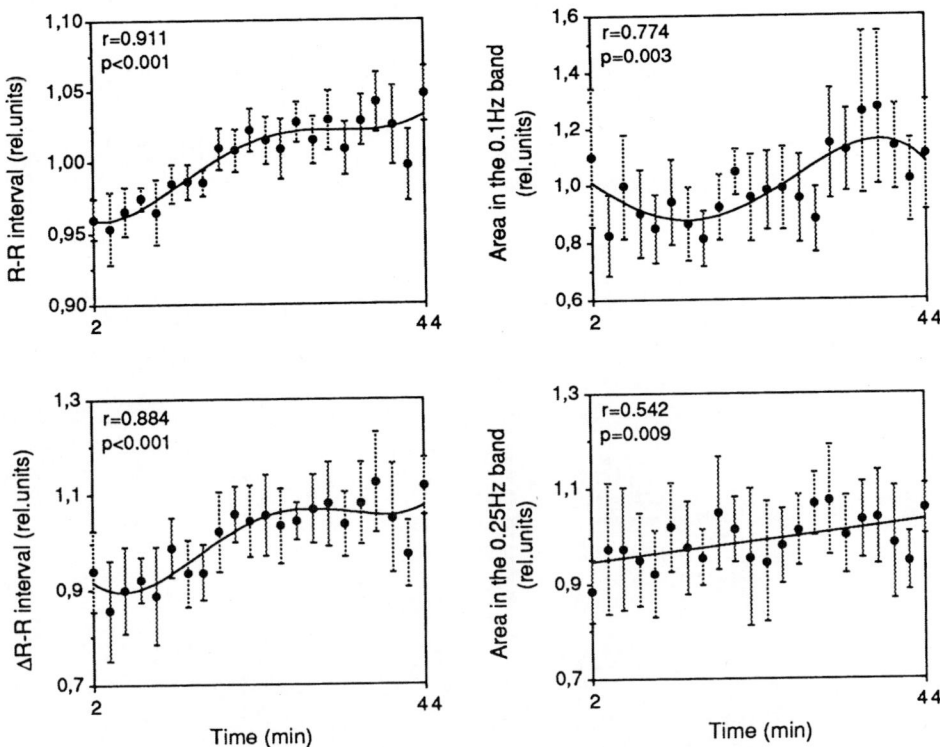

Fig. 2. Relative time courses of heart rate parameters during physical rest. The 44-min experimental session was partitioned into 22 segments. In each 2-min segment, volunteers' mean value and standard deviation of the parameters R-R interval, Δ R-R interval, area in the 0.1 Hz band, and area in the 0.25 Hz band were calculated from the relatively transformed heart rate parameters (division by the individual mean value of the session). The time courses were fitted polynomially $(y = a + bx + cx^2 + dx^3)$ or linearly $(y = a + bx)$. Over time, "spontaneous" changes occurred in all heart rate parameters

Even at a very light work load of 30 W, the area in the 0.25 Hz band was already diminished by 90.7%. As with mental stress, the decrease in the 0.25 Hz rhythmicity was more pronounced than that in the 0.1 Hz rhythmicity. Above 110 W performance, heart rate rhythmicity was practically absent in both frequency ranges. Summarizing the relationship between the mean R-R interval and its variability and rhythmicity during mental and physical activity, the variables Δ R-R interval, area in the 0.1 Hz band, and area in the 0.25 Hz band, computed in absolute units, declined exponentially when the mean R-R interval was shortened (Fig. 6). Another interesting aspect is a distinct intersubject variance of both R-R interval variability and rhythmicity at low heart rate which decreased with increasing heart rate.

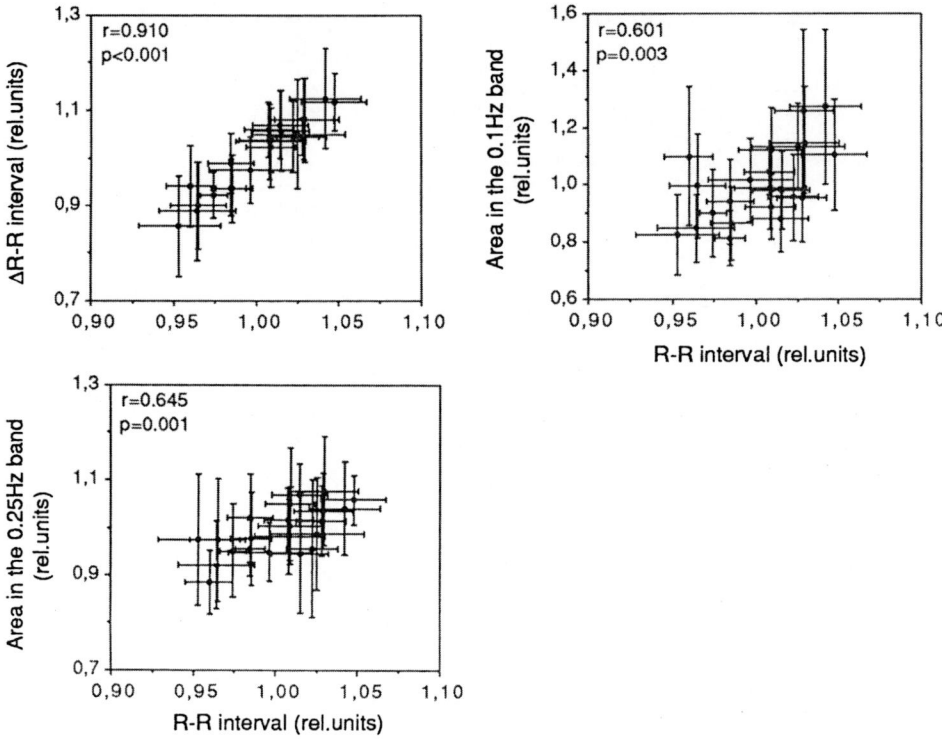

Fig. 3. Relationship between heart rate parameters during physical rest. Correlation analysis of the relative heart rate parameter time courses shows that all correlations between the variable mean R-R interval and the variables Δ R-R interval, area in the 0.1 Hz band, and area in the 0.25 Hz band were significant ($\alpha = 0.05$). This means that with decreasing mean R-R interval, its beat-to-beat variability and its rhythmicity in both frequency ranges also decreased

Changes in the Relationship Between Heart Rate and Its Time Structure

The basic relationship between the mean R-R interval and its variability and rhythmicity is altered under certain circumstances. The resting session of series A was compared with the resting session of series B, the latter preceding the Raven test session. The only difference between the two was the subjects' anticipation of performing the Raven test 1 week later in series B. There were no significant differences between either series for the variables R-R interval and Δ R-R interval (Mann-Whitney test, $\alpha = 0.05$) (Fig. 7). However, in comparison to series A, the areas in the 0.1 Hz band and the 0.25 Hz band were significantly diminished in series B. Thus, the expectancy of mental stress was accompanied only by a changed time structure of the chronotropic cardiac control; the mean heart rate remained unchanged. A further example of a changed relationship between the mean R-R interval and the variables Δ R-R interval and area in the 0.25 Hz band is the recovery period following maximum physical work. The analyzed recovery

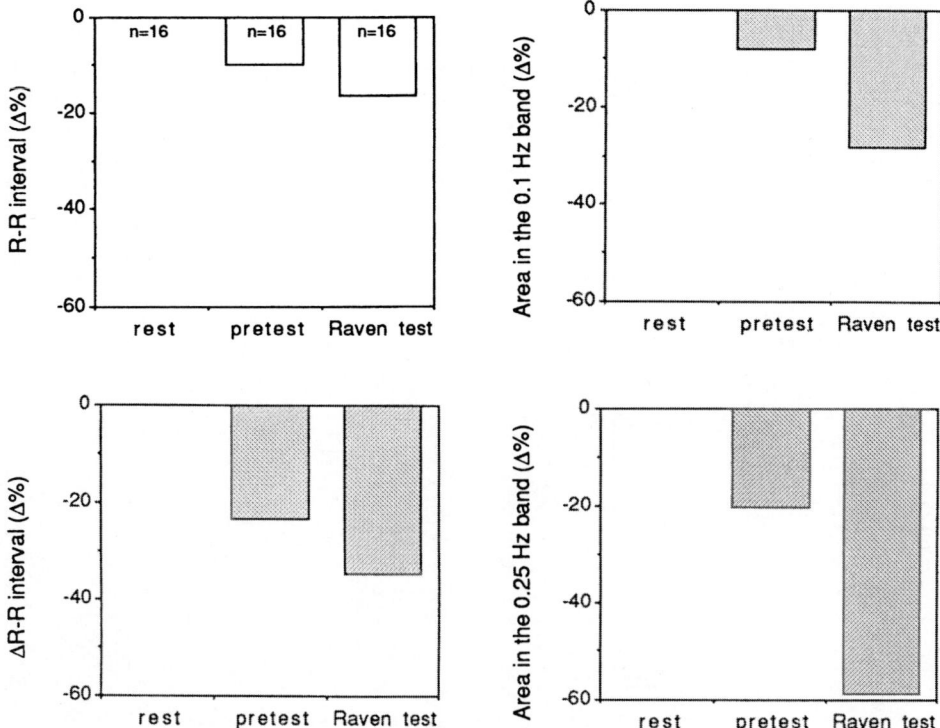

Fig. 4. Percentage changes of heart rate parameters during mental stress. Mean values of the parameters R-R interval, Δ R-R interval, area in the 0.1 Hz band, and area in the 0.25 Hz band were calculated in absolute units during the situations pretest and Raven test in series B. Divided by the respective mean value of the resting session, they were expressed as percentage changes. For further explanation see text

period began 20 min after the work ended and lasted 44 min. Compared with physical rest, the variables Δ R-R interval and area in the 0.25 Hz band were significantly diminished during the recovery period at the same mean R-R interval (Mann-Whitney test, $\alpha = 0.05$) (Fig. 8). This means that after physical work, mean heart rate and its time structure, primarily of parasympathetic origin, returned to resting values, but with a different delay. Nevertheless, in both the situations rest and postwork, the variables Δ R-R interval, area in the 0.1 Hz band, and area in the 0.25 Hz band differed significantly between R-R interval ranges (Kruskal-Wallis test, $\alpha = 0.05$). Bot heart rate variability and heart rate rhythmicity increased as the mean R-R interval lengthened. The delayed return of heart rate variability as well as heart rate rhythmicity was not observed in the recovery period following mental stress (Fig. 9). The variables Δ R-R interval, area in the 0.1 Hz band, and area in the 0.25 Hz band did not differ significantly between the situations physical rest and recovery from mental stress within the same R-R interval ranges (Mann-Whitney test, $\alpha = 0.05$). However, in both situations, the characteristic relationship between heart rate and its variability and rhythmicity

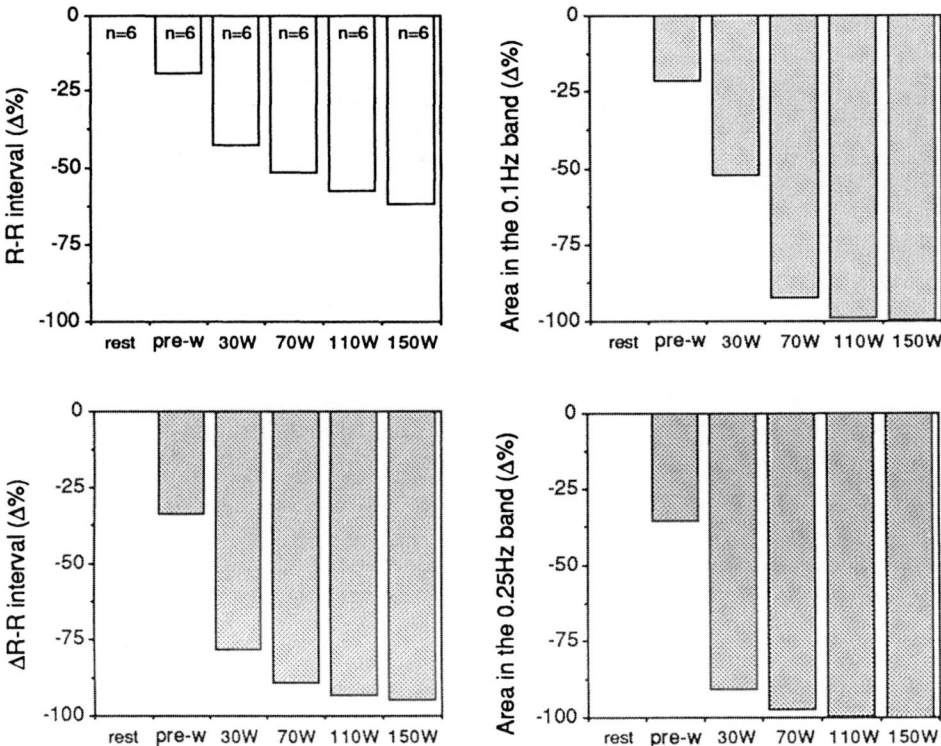

Fig. 5. Percentage changes of heart rate parameters during physical work. Mean values of the parameters R-R interval, Δ R-R interval, area in the 0.1 Hz band, and area in the 0.25 Hz band were calculated in absolute units during the situations prework and physical work (30, 70, 110, 150 W) in series C. Divided by the respective mean value of the resting session, they were expressed as percentage changes. For further explanation see text

was present. The variables Δ R-R interval, area in the 0.1 Hz band, and area in the 0.25 Hz band increased significantly with lengthening of the mean R-R interval, as shown above for the situations rest and recovery from physical work (Kruskal-Wallis test, $\alpha = 0.05$).

Discussion

Spontaneous Fluctuations in Chronotropic Cardiac Control at Rest and Subthreshold Adaptations to Increased Central Nervous Activation

It is well known that the ongoing heart rate is the result of a precise autonomic balance between the parasympathetic and the sympathetic chronotropic control of the heart (Levy and Zieske 1969). During behavioral activation, the heart rate pattern as one part of a generalized change in the vegetative innervation

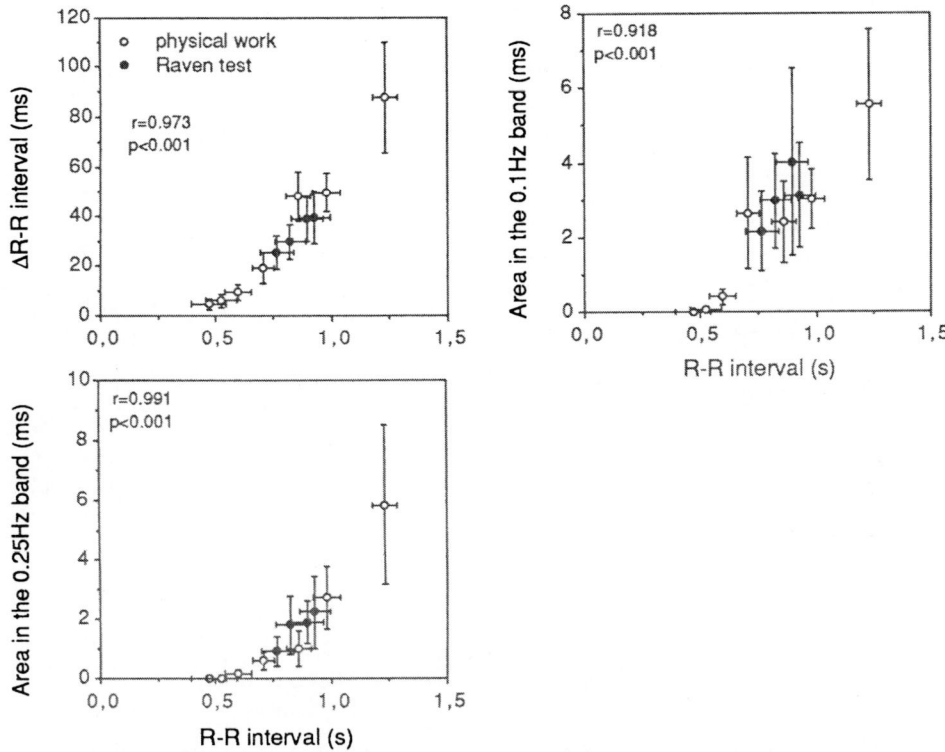

Fig. 6. Relationship between mean R-R interval and its variability and rhythmicity, respectively, during activation. Mean values with standard deviation of the parameters R-R interval, ΔR-R interval, area in the 0.1 Hz band, and area in the 0.25 Hz band were computed in absolute units from the situations rest, pretest, Raven test, and post-test in series B as well as from the situations rest, prework, 30 W, 70 W, 110 W, 150 W and postwork in series C. As R-R intervals shortened, their beat-to-beat variability (ΔR-R interval) as well as their rhythmicity in both frequency bands (0.1 Hz band, 0.25 Hz band) decreased exponentially independent of the kind of activation

is generated primarily by central autonomic control systems (Ranson and Magoun 1939). Additional excitatory influences come from various peripheral receptor sites via the reticular activating system (Magoun 1950; Moruzzi 1972) which also have an important role for the vegetative adaptation to physical work (e.g., Mitchell and Schmidt 1983). We suggest that the significant continuous slowing of the mean heart rate, observed during the 44-min resting period, is an expression of a centrally organized resting behavior accompanied by an alteration in the relation between parasympathetic and sympathetic cardiac control. The conspicuous scattering in the individual R-R interval time courses is hypothesized to be caused by "spontaneously" generated central vegetative events as adaptations to physical performance. However, during this momentary rudimentary behavior, the somatomotor behavioral component remains subthreshold. Thus, the description of the entity physical rest by mean values seems to be incomplete without an analysis of its inherent dynamics.

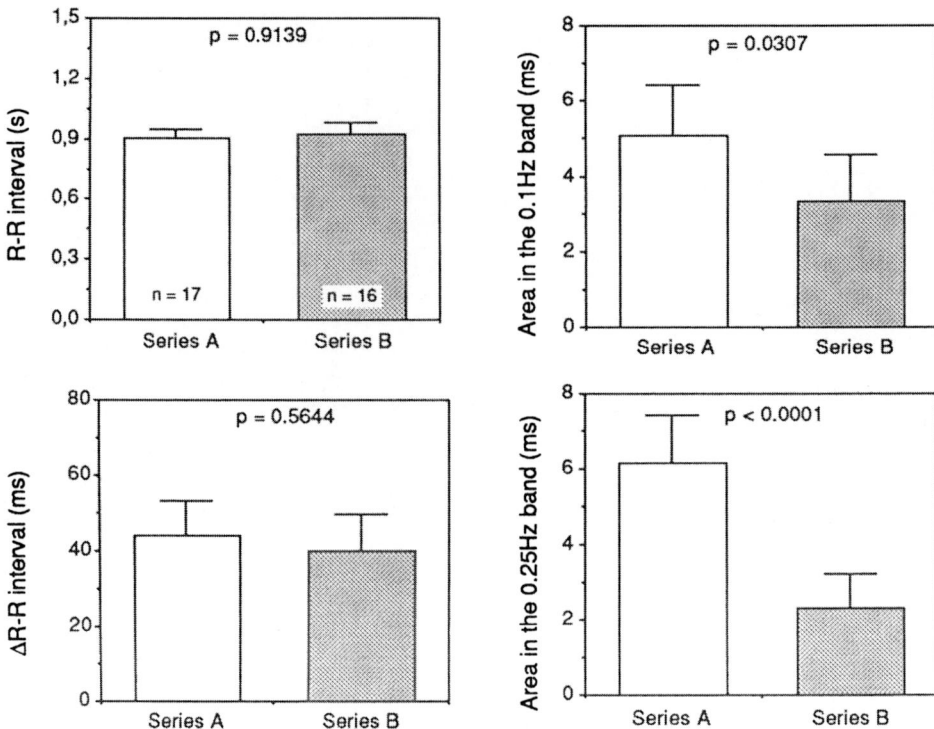

Fig. 7. Comparison of heart rate parameters during expectancy of mental stress. Mean values with standard deviation of the parameters R-R interval, ΔR-R interval, area in the 0.1 Hz band, and area in the 0.25 Hz band were computed in absolute units from the 44-min resting sessions of series A and B. The volunteers in series B who took part in the Raven test 1 week later showed a significantly diminished heart rate rhythmicity in both frequency ranges during physical rest (Mann-Whitney test, $\alpha = 0.05$)

Characteristic Relationship Between Mean Value and Time Structure of the Chronotropic Cardiac Control

At rest, short-term heart rate variability depends on mean heart rate (Schlomka 1937). Our differentiated analysis of heart rate variability, regarding its intrinsic time structure, shows that with lengthening of the mean R-R interval, heart rate fluctuations rose at about 0.25 Hz as well as at about 0.1 Hz. Thus, because of the primarily parasympathetic nature of the respiration-related heart rate variability (Katona and Jih 1975; Fouad et al. 1984), the increase in 0.25 Hz rhythmicity during elevated parasympathetic tone is suggested to be an expression of enhanced rhythmic modulations in the parasympathetic cardiac control (Abel et al. 1989b). This conclusion concurs with findings that parasympathetic blockade removes heart rate rhythmicity in the 0.25 Hz range (Akselrod et al. 1981; Pomeranz et al. 1985). The increased heart rate fluctuations in the respiratory frequency range can be explained by an enhancement of the efficiency of the baroreceptor input when parasympathetic tone is elevated (Koepchen et al. 1961). The volunteers' mean respiratory rate of 0.30 Hz occurred in the 0.25 Hz band, and its changes remained

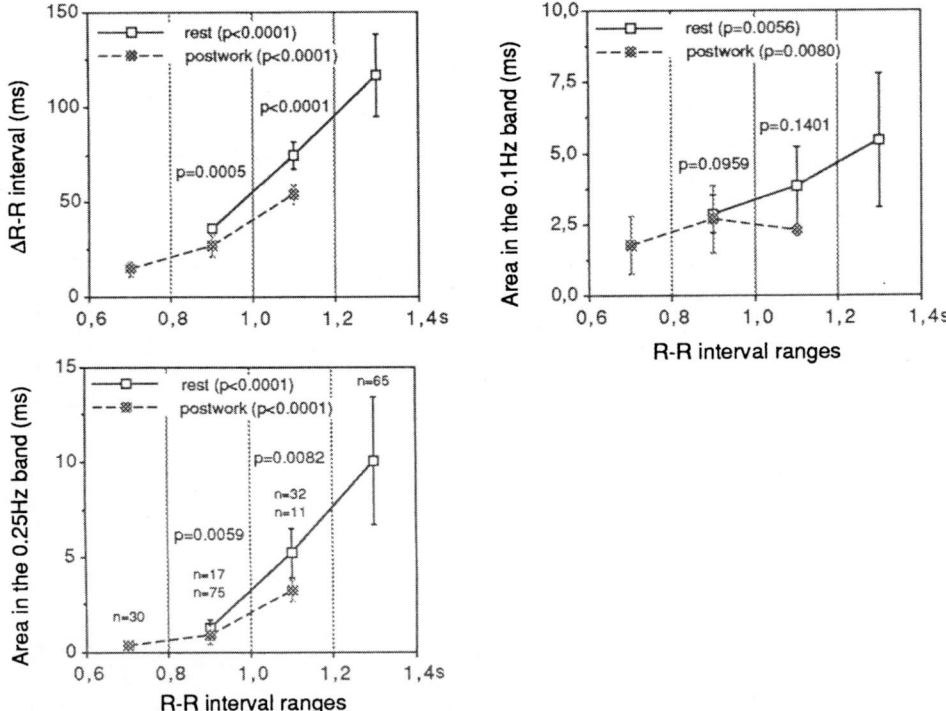

Fig. 8. Comparison of the relationship between heart rate parameters during physical rest and recovery from physical work. In series C, the 2-min mean values of the parameter ΔR-R interval and the corresponding 2-min values of the parameters area in the 0.1 Hz band, and area in the 0.25 Hz band (computed in absolute units) were divided into four classes according to the 2-min mean values of the R-R interval: $0.6 \leq$ R-R < 0.8 s, $0.8 \leq$ R-R < 1.0 s, $1.0 \leq$ R-R < 1.2 s, and $1.2 \leq$ R-R ≤ 1.4 s. Statistical comparisons of the variables ΔR-R interval, area in the 0.1 Hz band, and area in the 0.25 Hz band between the four R-R interval classes were made by use of the Kruskal-Wallis test ($\alpha = 0.05$), comparisons between physical rest and the recovery period after physical work (postwork) by use of the Mann-Whitney test ($\alpha = 0.05$). For further explanation see text

in this frequency range. According to previous results, it has been suggested that these alterations in the spontaneous resting respiratory pattern have a negligible influence on the heart rate rhythmicity (Abel et al. 1991 a). However, as shown in other studies, when the voluntarily decelerated respiratory frequency leaves the 0.25 Hz band and reaches the 0.1 Hz band, the amplitude of respiratory heart rate fluctuations increases resonance-like (Angelone and Coulter 1964; Ahmed et al. 1982).

Diminution of Rhythmicity in the Chronotropic Cardiac Control During Behavioral Activation

In our experiments, as expected, the mean R-R interval shortened with increasing central nervous activation during mental stress or physical work. This indicates a

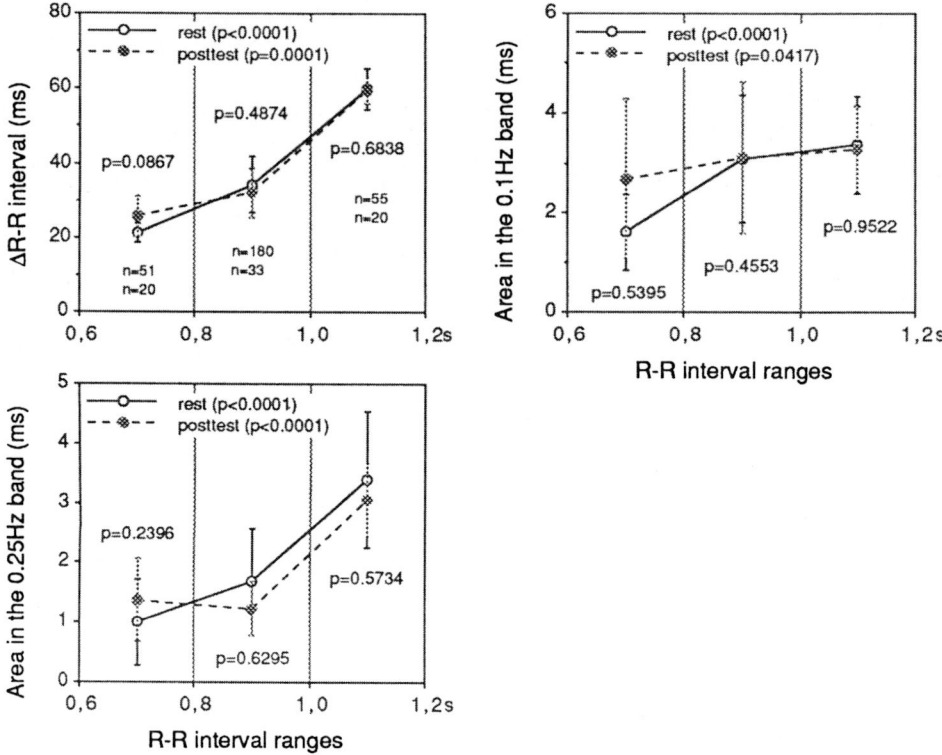

Fig. 9. Comparison of the relationship between heart rate parameters during physical rest and recovery from mental stress. In series B, the 2-min mean values of the parameter ΔR-R interval and the corresponding 2-min values of the parameters area in the 0.1 Hz band and area in the 0.25 Hz band (computed in absolute units) were divided into four classes according to the 2-min mean values of the R-R interval: $0.6 \leqq$ R-R < 0.8 s, $0.8 <$ R-R < 1.0 s, $1.0 \leqq$ R-R < 1.2 s, and $1.2 \leqq$ R-R $\leqq 1.4$ s. Statistical comparisons of the variables ΔR-R interval, area in the 0.1 Hz band, and area in the 0.25 Hz band between the four R-R interval classes were made using the Kruskal-Wallis test ($\alpha = 0.05$), and comparisons between physical rest and the recovery period after the Raven test (post-test) using the Mann-Whitney test ($\alpha = 0.05$). For further explanation see text

decreased parasympathetic tone and an increased sympathetic tone. Under these conditions, heart rate variability as well as rhythmicity in both frequency ranges, measured in absolute units, declined as schematically summarized in Fig. 10. These results are in agreement with other studies (Mulder and Mulder 1981; Arai et al. 1989). During low level activation, the more pronounced decrease in 0.25 Hz rhythmicity results from a withdrawal of predominantly parasympathetic chronotropic control of the heart, compared with the 0.1 Hz rhythmicity. The absence of heart rate rhythmicity in this frequency range at higher work loads is then caused by a complete withdrawal of parasympathetic chronotropic activity. Beside the parasympathetic involvement (Akselrod et al. 1981; Pomeranz et al. 1985), we assume that the progressive decrease of 0.1 Hz heart rate rhythmicity is related to increased nonrhythmic excitatory inputs from central autonomic

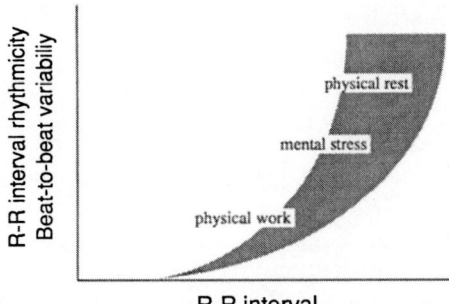

Fig. 10. Scheme of the relationship between heart rate, heart rate variability, and heart rate rhythmicity. During increasing activity from quiet physical rest to heavy physical performance, the shortening of R-R intervals is related to a diminution of beat-to-beat R-R interval variability (Δ R-R interval) as well as short-term R-R interval rhythmicity (area in the 0.1 Hz band and area in the 0.25 Hz band). Both are accompanied by a pronounced decrease in their scattering

control systems and peripheral receptor sites which override rhythmic inputs from other sources, including central rhythm generators. The diminution of baroreceptor sensitivity during increasing physical work (Pickering et al. 1972), which indicates a changed relation between blood pressure waves and their reflection in the heart rate as respective rhythmic fluctuations, also explains the decreased 0.1 Hz heart rate rhythmicity.

Alterations in the Relationship Between Mean Value and Time Structure of the Chronotropic Cardiac Control

After physical performance, the return of beat-to-beat variability and heart rate rhythmicity in the 0.1 Hz and 0.25 Hz bands towards resting values is delayed compared with the return of the mean R-R interval (Pfeifer et al. 1977; Abel et al. 1988). In the same narrow R-R interval range, heart rate rhythmicity in both frequency ranges is diminished during recovery from exercise. We assume that different mechanisms are involved. Overlasting effects of the stimulated energy metabolism such as decreased intramuscular pH generate continuous increased activity from peripheral afferents which interact with the chronotropic control. This is supported by our findings that, after mental stress, no changes occur in the relationship between mean R-R interval and its rhyhtmicity in both frequency bands compared with physical rest. During mental strain the increase in energy metabolism with accompanying effects in the recovery period is significantly less than changes during heavy physical work. In addition, central autonomic mechanisms may also play a significant part. One week before the Raven test, heart rate rhyhtmicity in the 0.1 Hz band as well as in the 0.25 Hz band was diminished during physical rest without any changes in the mean R-R interval. Emotional activation as behavioral anticipation could be responsible for the altered chronotropic cardiac control.

Heart Rate Rhythmicity as a Predictor of Autonomic "Tone"?

In human experiments, two basic approaches were chosen for testing the hypothesis that certain components of heart rate rhythmicity could be employed in order to assess sympathetic tone and parasympathetic tone (Zwiener 1979; Akselrod et al. 1981; Abdul-Satter and Young 1983; Pomeranz et al. 1985; Pagani et al. 1986; Weise et al. 1987). Differentiated autonomic blockade was used to pharmacologically separate the effects of sympathetic and parasympathetic chronotropic activity on short-term heart rate variability. Passive orthostatic load acted as a stimulus for inducing a reciprocal alteration of the autonomic cardiac innervation with sympathetic activation and parasympathetic withdrawal. This vegetative pattern is an expression of the homeostatic feedback blood pressure control. A third approach used stimuli which elicit vegetative components of physiological behavior (Mulder and Mulder 1981; Eckoldt 1985; Abel et al. 1989 a). Mental, emotional, and physical performance lead to changes in the autonomic balance in the chronotropic cardiac control. In order to quantify heart rate rhythmicity in different frequency ranges by power spectral analysis, areas under the respective spectrum segments were computed either in absolute units or in normalized form. The transformation was carried out by dividing the single spectral component by the total power of the spectrum or by the sum of the computed areas.

It is well established that the 0.25 Hz rhythmicity may be deemed a suitable indicator of the parasympathetic chronotropic control of the heart. This suggestion based on the strong correlation between the neural firing frequency in fibers of the cardiac vagus nerve and the duration of heart beats (Iriuchijima and Kumada 1964; Jewett 1964; Katona et al. 1970) and the findings that the so-called respiratory sinus arrhythmia is predominantly mediated by the vagus nerves (Katona and Jih 1975). Parasympathetic blockade not only decreases mean R-R interval, but also has a striking effect on the pattern of fluctuations at respiratory frequencies. The heart rate rhythmicity in the 0.25 Hz range practically disappears (Akselrod et al. 1981; Pomeranz et al. 1985). Similar results were obtained by orthostasis (Zwiener 1979; Abdul-Satter and Young 1983; Pomeranz et al. 1985; Pagani et al. 1986; Weise et al. 1987) and behavioral interventions (Mulder and Mulder 1981; Koepchen et al. 1985; Abel et al. 1991 b) which were accompanied by a withdrawal of parasympathetic chronotropic activity of the heart.

The hypothesis that spectral analysis of heart rate variability could provide an assessment of sympathetic tone (Malliani et al. 1986) originated from increased heart rate fluctuations in the 0.1 Hz range during standing when the mean R-R interval is shortened. The autospectra of systolic arterial pressure variability with subjects standing also demonstrated to predominant 0.1 Hz rhythmicity compared with when subjects were supine (Pagani et al. 1986). Various hypotheses, including central rhythm generators, peripheral feedback mechanisms, resonance-like disturbances, and vascular smooth muscle oscillations, were advanced for the interpretation of cardiovascular 0.1 Hz rhythmicity (Peňáz 1978; Koepchen 1984). Thus, increased 0.1 Hz blood pressure waves in the upright position could elicit the marked increase in heart rate fluctuations in the 0.1 Hz range via the feedback baroreflex loop. This suggestion is supported by atrial pacing experiments (Akselrod et al. 1985). In contrast to blood pressure variability in the 0.25 Hz range, which largely depends on 0.25 Hz heart rate fluctuations, 0.1 Hz blood pressure waves do not seem to be primarily caused by respective heart rate oscillations because of their persistance during the atrial pacing period. Autonomic blockade experiments demonstrated a sympathetic as well as a parasympathetic contribution to the genesis of 0.1 Hz heart rate rhythmicity (Akselrod et al. 1981; Pomeranz et al. 1985; Weise et al. 1987). The pronounced decrease in power density in the 0.1 Hz band after parasympathetic blockade indicates that these oscillations cannot be caused exclusively by the sympathetic chronotropic control of the heart. The pattern of the 0.1 Hz and 0.25 Hz heart rate fluctuations during orthostasis were independent of their computation in absolute or normalized units. But conspicuous differences were observed during behavioral activation. As shown in our results, heart rate increases during mental load and physical work were accompanied by decreases in 0.1 Hz and 0.25 Hz heart rate rhythmicity which was computed in absolute units (see also Mulder and Mulder 1981; Arai et al. 1989). Conversely, an increase in 0.1 Hz heart rate fluctuations was observed during mental stress (Pagani et al. 1989). In that study, heart rate rhythmicity was calculated in normalized form by dividing each spectral component by the total power of the spectrum. These findings represent only apparently conflicting results. With regard to our study, when normalizing the 0.1 Hz rhythmicity by dividing it by the sum of the areas in the 0.1 Hz and 0.25 Hz band, the relative 0.1 Hz rhythmicity increases during the Raven test as well as 30-W ergometer performance (Fig. 11). Therefore, in these situations, short-term heart rate fluctuations decrease, but the diminution of 0.25 Hz rhythmicity is more pronounced than that of the 0.1 Hz rhythmicity. When computing normalized heart rate rhythmicity, it has to be considered that changes in a single spectral

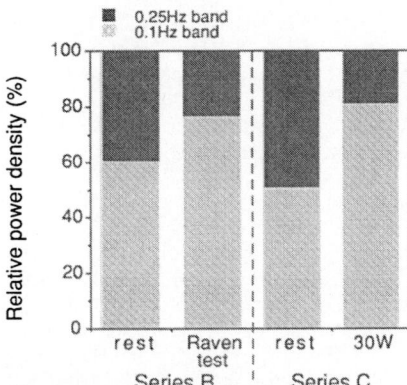

Fig. 11. Relation between 0.1 Hz rhythmicity and 0.25 Hz rhythmicity during physical rest and low-level activation. The heart rate rhythmicity parameters area in the 0.1 Hz band and area in the 0.25 Hz band were computed for the situations rest and Raven test in series B as well as for the situations rest and 30 W performance in series C. The relative portion of the absolute 0.1 Hz and 0.25 Hz rhythmicity of the total power density in the spectrum between 0.05 Hz and 0.37 Hz was calculated by dividing each frequency band area by the sum of both frequency band areas. During the Raven test as well as 30 W work load, the relative portion of the 0.1 Hz rhythmicity increased in comparison to physical rest, whereas that of the 0.25 Hz rhythmicity consequently decreased

component can also be caused by changes in other spectral components. For example, a more pronounced diminution of rhythmicity in the 0.25 Hz band than in the 0.1 Hz band would lead to an increase in the normalized 0.1 Hz band power, as shown during the prework phase and the lowest work intensity (see Fig. 5).

Because of the different pattern of 0.1 Hz heart rate rhythmicity during orthostasis and behavioral activation, both of which are accompanied by increased sympathetic activity, because of the uncertainty in the interpretation of changes in the normalized 0.1 Hz spectral component, and the largely parasympathetic mediation of heart rate fluctuations in the 0.1 Hz range, the problem of approaching the sympathetic tone has to be reinvestigated. It has also to be considered that power spectral analysis represents a tool for analyzing the time structure of the chronotropic cardiac control and that the mean value and its overlying rhythmic modulations can behave independently (see Figs. 7, 8).

References

Abdul-Satter N, Young S (1983) Effects of posture on the heart rate pattern in man. J Physiol 343:54P–55P

Abel H-H, Krause R, Klüßendorf D, Miltenberger M, Koepchen HP (1988) Differentiation of heart rate parameters during recovery from maximum physical work. Pflügers Arch 411:R18

Abel H-H, Klüßendorf D, Koepchen HP (1989a) New approach of analysing the neurovegetative state in man. In: Droh R, Spintge R (eds) Innovations in physiological anaesthesia and monitoring. Springer, Berlin Heidelberg New York, pp 21–34

Abel H-H, Klüßendorf D, Koepchen HP (1989b) Relation between tone and rhythmicity of cardiac chronotropic innervation. Pflügers Arch 413:R11

Abel H-H, Klüßendorf D, Droh R, Koepchen HP (1991a) Cardiorespiratory relations in human heart rate pattern. In: Koepchen HP, Huopaniemi T (eds) Cardiorespiratory and motor coordination. Springer, Berlin Heidelberg New York, pp 307–318

Abel H-H, Krause R, Klüßendorf D, Berger R, Droh R, Koepchen HP (1991b) Inference about cardiac chronotropic innervation during varying levels of physical activity by power spectral analysis of heart rate. In: Bachl N, Graham TE, Löllgen H (eds) Advances in ergometry. Springer, Berlin Heidelberg New York, pp 325–331

Ahmed AK, Harness JB, Mearns AJ (1982) Respiratory control of heart rate. Eur J Appl Physiol 50:95–104

Akselrod S, Gordon D, Ubel FA, Shannon DC, Barger AC, Cohen RJ (1981) Power spectrum analysis of heart rate fluctuation: a quantitative probe of beat-to-beat cardiovascular control. Science 213:220–222

Akselrod S, Gordon D, Madwed JB, Snidman NC, Shannon DC, Cohen RJ (1985) Hemodynamic regulation: investigation by spectral analysis. Am J Physiol 249:H867–H875

Angelone A, Coulter NA (1964) Respiratory sinus arrhythmia: a frequency dependent phenomenon. J Appl Physiol 19:479–482

Anrep GV, Pascual W, Rössler R (1936) Respiratory variations of the heart rate. I – The reflex mechanism of the respiratory arrhythmia. Proc R Soc Lond (B) 119:191–217

Arai Y, Saul JP, Albrecht P, Hartley LH, Lilly LS, Cohen RJ, Colucci WS (1989) Modulation of cardiac autonomic activity during and immediately after exercise. Am J Physiol 256:H132–H141

Bristow JD, Brown EB Jr, Cunningham DJC, Howson MG, Peterson ES, Pickering TG, Sleight P (1971) Effect of bicycling on the baroreflex regulation of pulse interval. Circ. Res 28:582–592

Burgess ED (1982) Cardiac vagal denervation in hemodialysis patients. Nephron 30:228–230

Eckberg DL, Orshan CR (1977) Respiratory and baroreceptor reflex interactions in man. J Clin Invest 59:780–785

Eckholdt K (1984) Verfahren und Ergebnisse der quantitativen automatischen Analyse der Herzfrequenz und deren Spontanvariabilität. Dtsch Gesundh Wesen 39:856–863

Eckholdt K (1985) Herzfrequenzvariabilität und deren spektrale Komponenten bei unterschiedlichen autonomen Funktionszuständen. Ergebn exp Med 46:106–116

Fouad FM, Tarazi RC, Ferrario CM, Fighaly S, Alicandri C (1984) Assessment of parasympathetic control of heart rate by a noninvasive method. Am J Physiol 246:H838–H842

Gilbey MP, Jordan D, Richter DW, Spyer KM (1984) Synaptic mechanisms involved in the inspiratory modulation of vagal cardio-inhibitory neurones in the cat. J Physiol 356:65–78

Gunderson HJG, Neubauer B (1977) A long-term diabetic autonomic nervous abnormality. Reduced variations in resting heart rate measured by a simple and sensitive method. Diabetologia 13:137–140

Guyton AC, Harris JW (1951) Pressoreceptor-autonomic oscillation: a probable cause of vasomotor waves. Am J Physiol 165:158–166

Hess WR (1949) Das Zwischenhirn. Syndrome, Lokalisationen, Funktionen. Schwabe, Basel

Hirsch JA, Bishop B (1981) Respiratory sinus arrhythmia in humans: how breathing pattern modulates heart rate. Am J Physiol 241:H620–H629

Hyndman BW, Kitney RI, Sayers BMcA (1971) Spontaneous rhythms in physiological control systems. Nature 233:339–341

Iriuchijima J, Kumada M (1964) Activity of single vagal fibers efferent to the heart. Jpn J Physiol 14:479–487

Jewett DL (1964) Activitiy of single efferent fibers in the cervical vagus nerve of the dog with special reference to possible cardio-inhibitory fibers. J Physiol 175:321–357

Katona G, Poitras J, Barnett O, Terry B (1970) Cardiac vagal efferent activity and heart period in the carotid sinus reflex. Am J Physiol 218:1030–1037

Katona PG, Jih F (1975) Respiratory sinus arrhythmia: noninvasive measure of parasympathetic cardiac control. J Appl Physiol 39:801–805

Koepchen HP (1984) History of studies and concepts of blood pressure waves. In: Miyakawa K, Koepchen HP, Polosa C (eds) Mechanisms of blood pressure waves. Japan Scientific Society and Springer, Berlin Heidelberg New York, pp 3–23

Koepchen HP, Thurau K (1959) Über die Entstehungsbedingungen der atemsynchronen Schwankungen des Vagustonus (Respiratorische Arrhythmie). Pflügers Arch 269:10–30

Koepchen HP, Wagner P-H, Lux HD (1961) Über die Zusammenhänge zwischen zentraler Erregbarkeit, reflektorischem Tonus und Atemrhythmus bei der nervösen Steuerung der Herzfrequenz. Pflügers Arch 273:443–465

Koepchen HP, Abel H-H, Klüßendorf D (1985) Heart-rate dynamics in healthy humans before, during and after a mental test. Pflügers Arch 405:R50

Langhorst P, Schulz G, Lambertz M (1984) Oscillating neuronal network of the "common brainstem system". In: Miyakawa K, Koepchen HP, Polosa C (eds) Mechanisms of blood pressure waves. Japan Scientific Society and Springer, Berlin Heidelberg New York, pp 257–275

Levy MN, Zieske H (1969) Autonomic control of cardiac pacemaker activity and atrioventricular transmission. J Appl Physiol 27:465–470

Magoun HW (1950) Caudal and cephalic influences of the brain stem reticular formation. Physiol Rev 30:459–474

Malliani A, Lombardi F, Pagani M, Cerutti S (1986) The problem of approaching the sympathetic and vagal "tone". J Autonom Nerv Syst [Suppl] 191–196

Melcher A (1976) Respiratory sinus arrhythmia in man. A study in heart rate regulating mechanisms. Acta Physiol Scand [Suppl] 435:1–31

Mitchell JH, Schmidt RF (1983) Cardiovascular reflex control by afferent fibers from skeletal muscle receptors. In: Shepherd JT, Abboud FM, Geiger SR (eds) Handbook of physiology, Sect. 2: The Cardiovascular System, vol III, part 2. American Physiological Society, Bethesda, Maryland, pp 623–658

Moruzzi G (1972) The sleep-waking cycle. Ergebn Physiol 64:1–165

Mulder G, Mulder LJM (1981) Information processing and cardiovascular control. Psychophysiology 18:392–402

Pagani M, Lombardi F, Guzzetti S, Rimoldi O, Furlan R, Pizzinelli P, Sandrone G, Malfatto G, Dell'Orto S, Piccaluga E, Turiel M, Baselli G, Cerutti S, Malliani A (1986) Power spectral analysis of heart rate and arterial pressure variabilities as a marker of sympathovagal interaction in man and conscious dog. Circ Res 59:178–193

Pagani M, Furlan R, Pizzinelli P, Crivellaro W, Cerutti S, Malliani A (1989) Spectral analysis of R-R and arterial pressure variabilities to assess sympatho-vagal interaction during mental stress in humans. J Hypert 7 [Suppl] 6:S14–S15

Peňáz J (1978) Mayer waves: history and methodology. Automedica 2:135–141

Peňáz J, Roukens J, Waal HJ van der (1968) Spectral analysis of some spontaneous rhythms in the circulation. Biokybernetic I:233–236

Pfeifer B, Cammann H, Dinter W, Eckoldt K, Schädlich M, Schubert E (1977) Herzrhythmik und metabolische Größen bei und nach Ergometerbelastung. Med Sport 17:143–145

Pickering TG, Gribbin B, Petersen ES, Cunningham DJC, Sleight P (1972) Effects of autonomic blockade on the baroreflex in man at rest and during exercise. Circ Res 30:177–185

Pomeranz B, Macaulay RJ, Caudill MA, Kutz I, Adam D, Gordon D, Kilborn KM, Barger AC, Shannon DC, Cohen RJ, Benson H (1985) Assessment of autonomic function in humans by heart rate spectral analysis. Am J Physiol 17:H151–H153

Ranson SW, Magoun HW (1939) The hypothalamus. Ergebn Physiol 41:56–163

Sayers BMcA (1973) Analysis of heart rate variability. Ergonomics 16:17–32

Schlomka G (1937) Untersuchungen über die physiologische Unregelmäßigkeit des Herzschlages. III. Mitteilung. Über die Abhängigkeit der respiratorischen (Ruhe-)Arrhythmie von der Schlagfrequenz und vom Lebensalter. Z Kreislaufforsch 29:510–524

Schlomka G, Reindell H (1936) Untersuchungen über die physiologische Unregelmäßigkeit des Herzschlages. Z Kreislaufforsch 28:473–492

Seller H, Langhorst P, Polster J, Koepchen HP (1967) Zeitliche Eigenschaften der Vasomotorik. II. Erscheinungsformen und Entstehung spontaner und nervös induzierter Gefäßrhythmen. Pflügers Arch 296:110–132

Weise F, Heydenreich F, Runge U (1987) Contributions of sympathetic and vagal mechanisms to the genesis of heart rate fluctuations during orthostatic load: a spectral analysis. J Autonom Nerv Syst 21:127–134

Zwiener U (1979) The influence of orthostatic load upon coherence and phase spectra of autonomic rhythms in healthy volunteers and patients suffering from neurocirculatory asthenia. Automedica 3:57–61

The Neurovegetative System as a Link Between Internal and External Environments

M. Pagani and A. Malliani

Opening Remark: Extrapolations and the Environment

The pious Naruddin used to take his five blind brothers to the caravanserrai once a year, on the occasion of the town restivities.

At the end of the day, all the brothers gathered again at the gates. The five blind men were all excited, every one of them claiming to have encountered the most extraordinary creature living on earth.

One had met a bird which, upon touching, felt like the leaves of the banana tree.

A second had found a bird, capable of spitting at a distance large amounts of water.

The third had met a huge bird, shaped like a barrel.

The fourth had stumbled on a snake that could fly.

The fifth brother had got hold of four sturdy animals, that seemed attached to the ground as if they had strong roots.

After sunset, on the return journey the blind men were still quarelling, while Naruddin was silently wondering how to help his brothers realize that they had all encountered the same animal: an elephant (From G. I. Gurdjeff: Meetings with Remarkable Men, 1963).

The Subject and His Environment

In classical physiology the interpretation of basic life properties has been profoundly influenced by Claude Bernard's concept of the *fixité du milieu intérieur* and Walter Cannon's concept of homeostasis, whereby the organism's biochemical and physiological parameters tend to remain stable in spite of a continuously changing environment. In this context, the emphasis has usually been laid on the study of the multifarious adaptive mechanisms and on the individual responses to external stimuli. The circular (Fig. 1) and dynamic nature of the relationship between the subject and his environment, as well as the possibility that physiological changes may supervene in the absence of overt environmental stimuli, are usually less well appreciated. In this article we concentrate in particular on the problem of assessing the physiological changes attending psychological stimuli.

Schmidt/Engel/Blümchen (Eds.)
Temporal Variations of the Cardiovascular System
© Springer-Verlag Berlin Heidelberg 1992

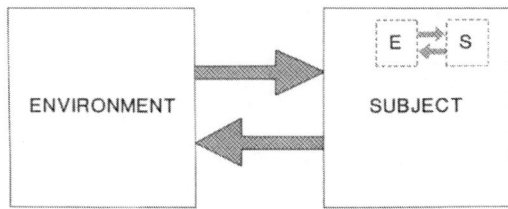

Fig. 1. Schematic representation of the circular relationship between the subject and his environment. *Boxes in broken lines*, the simultaneous subjective perception, which is not directly accessible to the observer

From a psychological point of view it is important to consider beforehand the possible confounding role of autoreferenciality [1], an aspect that we must deal with whenever subjective feelings come into play. Indeed the perception of any given situation depends on a complex amalgam of often ill-defined concepts and constructions usually reflecting the unique personal history [2]. Other important sources of uncertainty should also be considered, such as the origin of emotions,

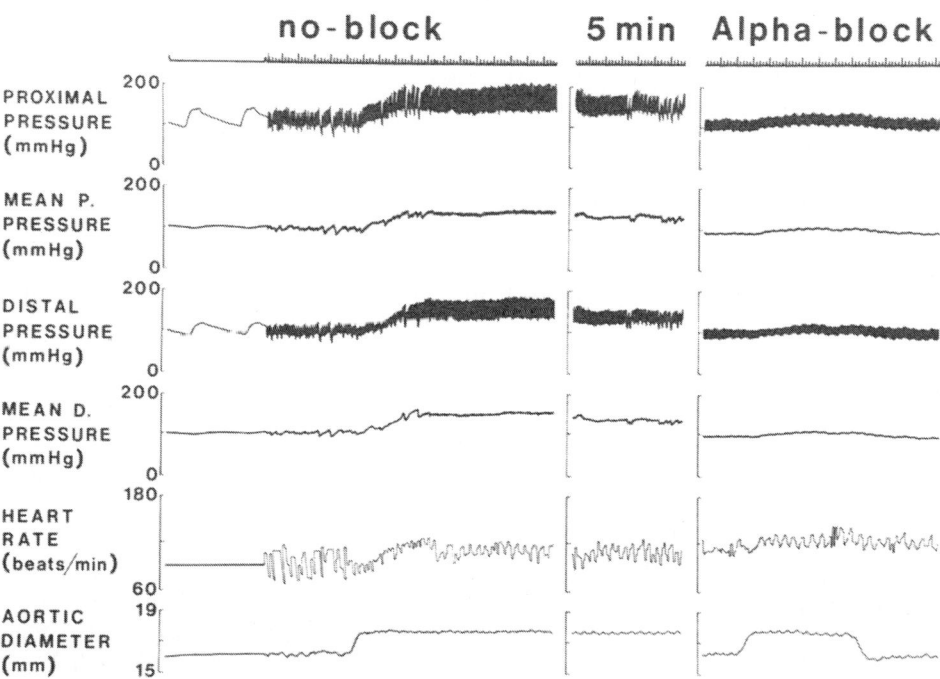

Fig. 2. Pressor and heart rate responses to stretch of the descending thoracic aorta in a conscious dog. The initiation of aortic stretch (*left*) is indicated by the increase in aortic diameter. Note the similar increase in both proximal and distal pressures, indicating the lack of direct mechanical obstruction to blood flow by aortic distension. After 5 min (*middle*), the pressor and heart rate responses are still maintained. α-Adrenergic blockade (phentolamine 1 mg/kg; *right*) virtually abolishes the pressor response to aortic stretch, while an increase in heart rate is still present. (From [10])

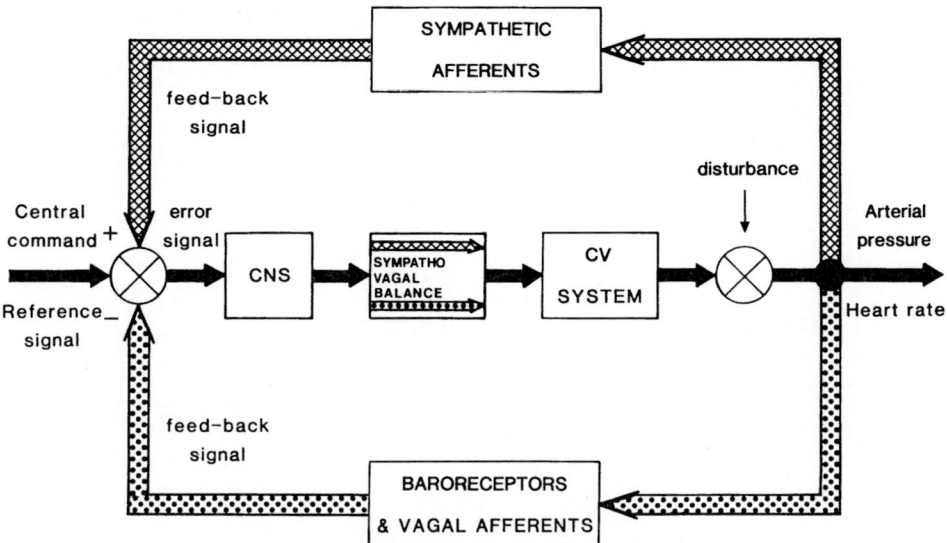

Fig. 3. Schematic representation of the neural control of the circulation, modeled as a continuous interaction between two opposing sympathetic and vagal feedback loops, operating with a positive and a negative sign

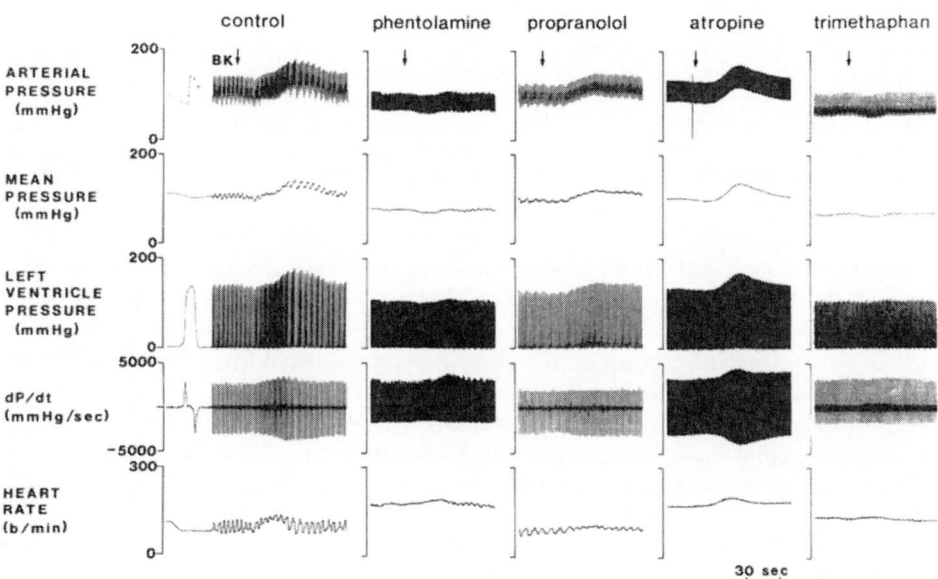

Fig. 4. Hemodynamic effects of intracoronary bradykinin in a conscious dog in control conditions and during various autonomic blockades. Injections (100 ng/kg; *arrow*) performed on separate days. (From [12])

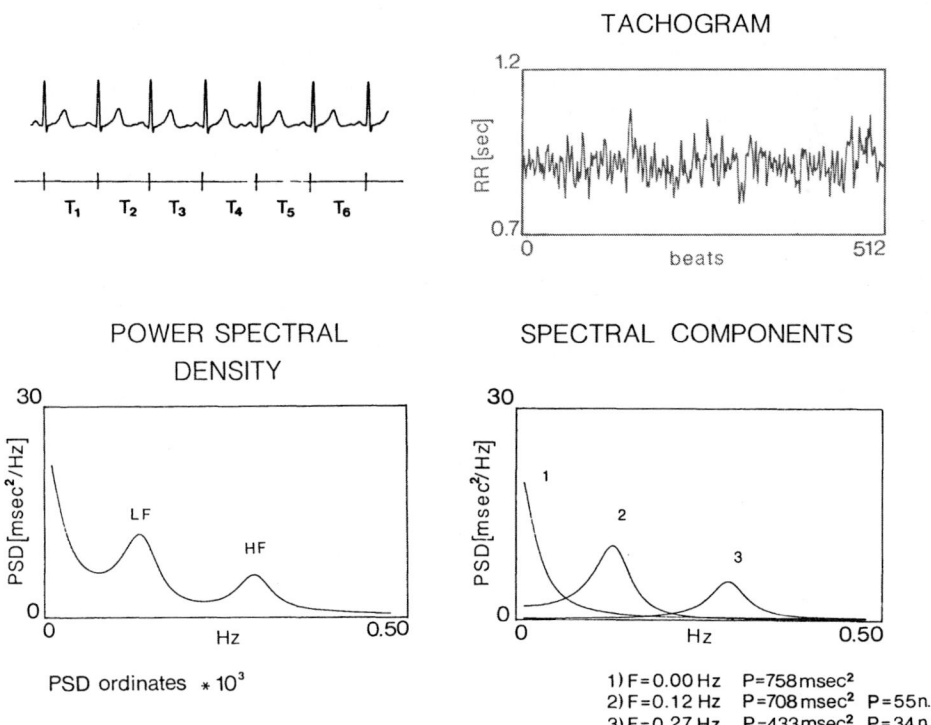

Fig. 5. Schematic representation of the method used for the spectral analysis of R-R interval variability. From the surface electrocardiogram (*top left panel*), the program computes the individual R-R intervals T_1-T_6 and stores them in memory as the tachogram. From the tachogram, the power spectral density estimate is computed. Two major components, low frequency (*LF*) and high-frequency (*HF*), are usually recognized as well as a large and variable fraction of very slow oscillations (below 0.03 Hz), which are not considered in the analysis. Note that the computer program automatically recognizes and prints out for each component the center frequency and associated power in absolute and normalized units (*n.u.*). Power spectral ordinates should be multiplied by 10^3. *PSD*, Power spectral density. (From [14])

some theories seeing them originating in the peripheral and some in the central nervous system. On the other hand, the observation that feelings and emotions may also produce visible changes in the body is as old as Aristotle [3], who pointed out that the relationship with their bodily expression is complex and depends on the individual's disposition to react, as emotions may at times be expressed vividly in the absence of overt environmental clues, or vice versa. In brief, every "affection of the soul" must be defined according to the pattern of corresponding bodily changes, which usually comprise alterations in cardiac activity [4].

The Physiological Approach

Regarding the physiological approach to this problem it should be recalled that the study of visceral behavior has been influenced to a great extent by early

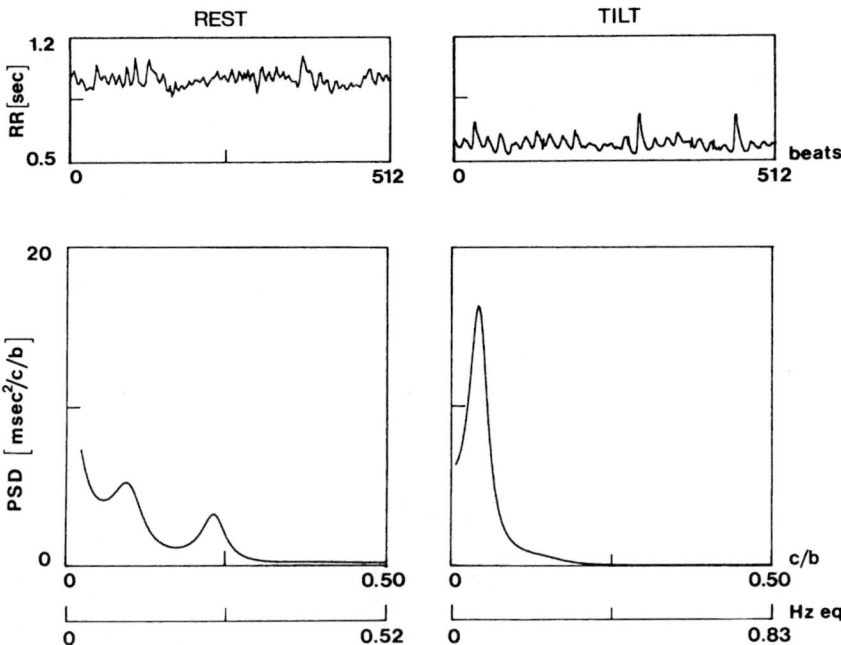

Fig. 6. R-R interval series, i.e., tachogram at rest and during passive upright 90° tilt. On the autospectra (*bottom panels*), two clearly separated low- and high-frequency components are present at rest. During tilt, the low-frequency component becomes preponderant. (From [12])

experiments on anesthetized preparations, particularly in the case of the circulation. Koch in the 1930s [5] described a profound calming effect on animal behavior by the stimulation of the carotid bifurcation in conscious dogs. At about the same time, Heyman's [6] work on anesthetized animals provided the initial evidence for the still dominant concept of circulatory homeostasis. His observations indicated that increases in arterial pressure, limited to the carotid bifurcations, were accompanied by reflex systemic hypotension and bradycardia. From this and subsequent experiments [7], the theory developed that neural control of the circulation is based on potent negative feedback reflexes which are mediated primarily by afferent nerve fibers impinging upon supraspinal structures, and which tend to oppose any external disturbances [8].

On this basis, however, it was difficult to account for the observation that in free-moving animals, arterial pressure and heart rate very often increase simultaneously, such as during exercise or emotion. To account for such etherostasis other mechanisms were necessary. In our group we have demonstrated that an additional circuit, based on sympathetic afferent and efferent nerve fibers, may subserve such a role; this is operatively based on a positive feedback mechanism [9]. For example, the stimulation of vascular areas innervated by sensory afferents belonging to the negative feedback system (i.e., the carotid bifurcation) causes a reflex reduction in systemic arterial pressure and in heart rate [6]; the contrary, i.e., an increase in arterial pressure and heart rate, follows the stimulation of afferents belonging to the positive feedback system, such as

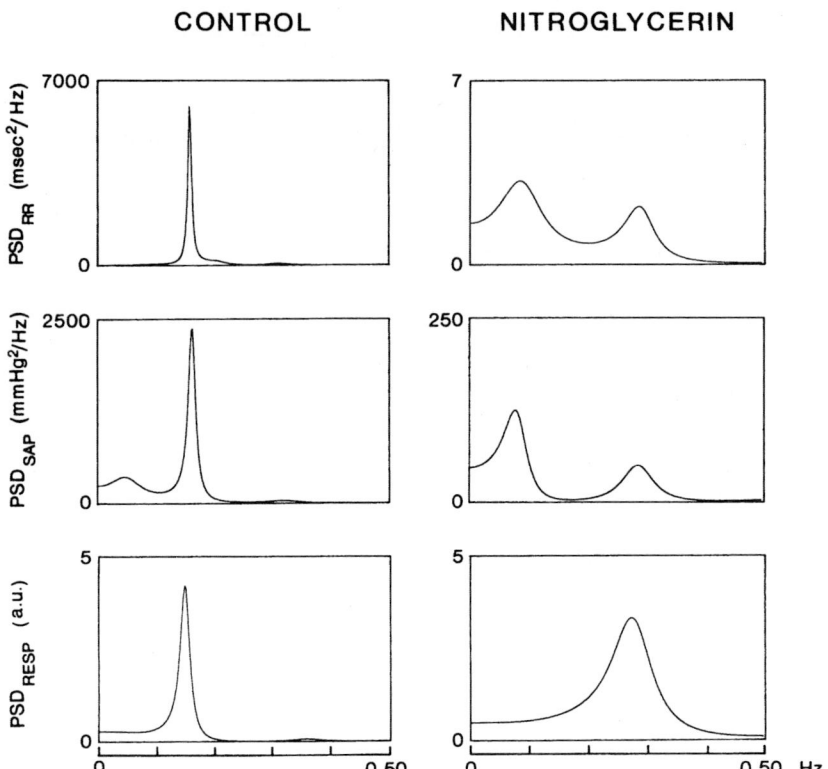

Fig. 7. Effects of $32 \,\mu g \,kg^{-1} \,min^{-1}$ intravenous nitroglycerin on R-R and systolic arterial pressure *(SAP)* variabilities and on respiration *(RESP)*. Note marked predominance of respiratory component in both R-R and SAP autospectra *(PSD$_{RR}$* and *PSD$_{SAP}$)* at control, and note appearance of a large low-frequency component during nitroglycerin infusion. (From [17])

the descending thoracic aorta, i.e., a vascular area innervated by sympathetic afferents (Fig. 2).

It would therefore appear that neural control of the circulation depends on the continuous interaction of mechanisms of opposite feedback signs, positive and negative, in a system which can be modeled as a simplified closed loop (Fig. 3). The performance of such a double-loop feedback control system, in terms of sign, amplitude, and speed of response to a given disturbance, is thus under the potential control of the central nerve structures. Indeed, we observed that the same stimulus, i.e., the intracoronary injections of bradykinin, which stimulates both vagal and sympathetic cardiac sensory endings, produces an excitatory reflex in animals that had fully recovered from the prior surgery, necessary for their instrumentation, while before full recovery inhibitory responses could also be observed [11] (Fig. 4).

More recently the clinical role of the visceral nervous system has come to the forefront as the one component that is responsible for generating and maintaining the functional integration among the various constituents of the organism. Therefore, the assessment of its function might provide an important practical

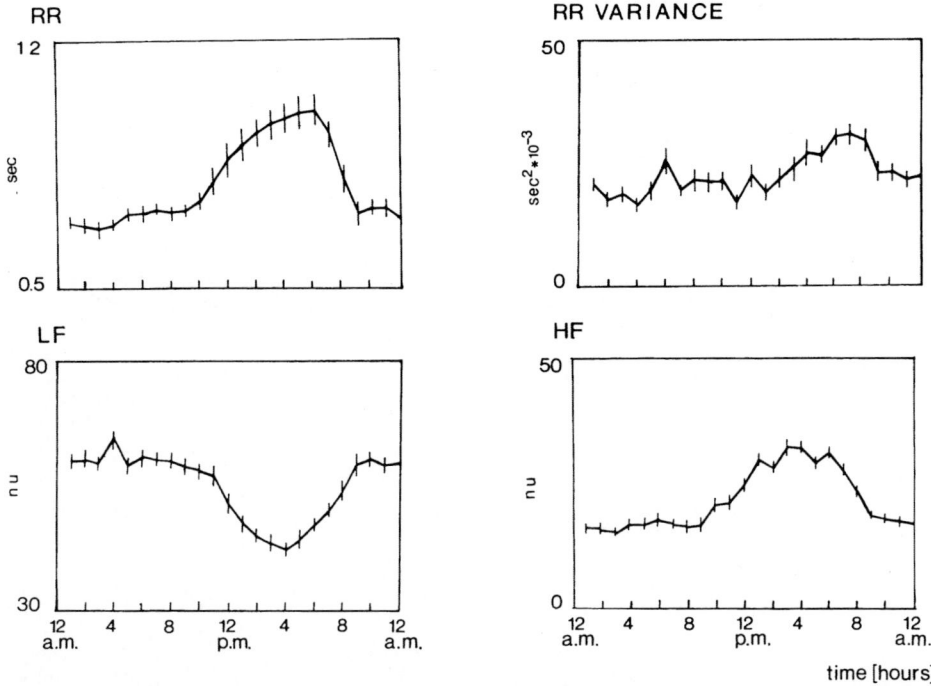

Fig. 8. Plots of average hourly values of R-R interval, of its variance (in absolute units), and of low- (*LF*) and high-frequency (*HF*) components (in normalized units) during 24 h in a group of nonhospitalized subjects free to move. (From [14])

tool for interpreting the dynamics of the interaction between the opposing mechanisms governing bodily functions in various pathophysiological conditions.

We have approached the study of the tonic activity of the visceral nervous system in intact conscious animals and man since 1983 by using spectral analysis of cardiovascular variabilities, as a tool capable of providing markers, from both noninvasive and invasive measurements, of sympathetic and vagal control activities, and of their interaction. We focused initially on R-R interval variability, as a variable reflecting neural control of the SA node [12], and on systolic arterial pressure variability, as reflecting sympathetic vasomotor activity [13].

In general, two major oscillatory components were present in both variability signals, and in the case of R-R variability (Fig. 5) [14] the high-frequency (HF) respiratory-related component provided a marker mostly of vagal activity [12–16] while the low-frequency (LF; 0.1 Hz) component reflected mostly sympathetic activity and its changes. In our laboratory, HF and LF powers are usually assessed in normalized units, which are obtained by dividing the power of individual HF or LF components by total variance, cleared by the power of the component with a center frequency at about 0 Hz (and below 0.03 Hz) [12]. Increases in sympathetic activity were associated with increases in LF (Figs. 6, 7), while, conversely, increases in vagal activity were associated with increases in HF and vice versa [12, 13]. Therefore, the dynamics of the changing balance between sympathetic and

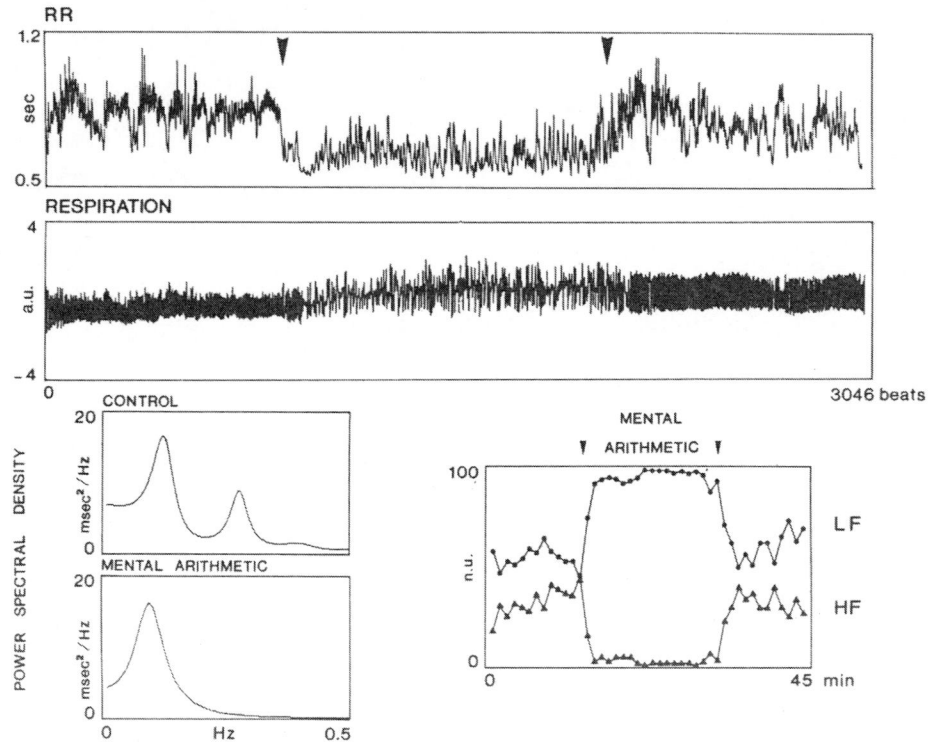

Fig. 9. Effects of mental arithmetic on spectral analysis of R-R variability. *Above*, continuous representation of the successive R-R intervals (*upper trace*) and of the respiration signal (*lower trace*). Note the reduction of the R-R interval during mental arithmetic (*arrows*). *Lower left*, autospectra of R-R interval variability at control (*upper*) and during mental arithmetic (*lower*). *Lower right*, continuous representation of the power of the low-frequency (*LF*) and high-frequency (*HF*) components of R-R variability during control, mental arithmetic (*arrows*) and recovery. (From [25])

vagal activities could be appreciated by a continuous analysis, up to 24 h, of R-R interval variability [14] (Fig. 8).

A similar analysis was performed on the arterial pressure variability signal, recorded invasively with high-fidelity methods [17] in the case of dynamic and ambulatory conditions and also with a noninvasive approach with the appropriate precautions in the laboratory. Cross-spectral analysis of simultaneous R-R interval and arterial pressure variabilities provided a quantitative assessment of the neural link between them [18], without the need of resorting to disturbances from the outside, as in the case of phenylephrine or collar techniques. When applied to physiological conditions, this approach not only permitted assessment of the increases in sympathetic activity attending single bouts of exercise, both in conscious dogs [19] and in human subjects [20], but also changes in the complex baroreceptor control of the circulation produced by physical training in mild hypertensives [18].

As to the analysis of disease processes, it was possible to describe a continuum of increases in markers of sympathetic activity in parallel with the rising values of resting arterial pressure [21] in a group of subjects with pressure values ranging from normotension to hypertension. The alteration in neural control of heart rate present in myocardial infarction [22], diabetes [23], or Chagas' disease [24] were also well described by this approach.

Spectral analysis of cardiovascular variabilities also appears a promising technique for studying the possibility that the central nervous system per se promotes changes in neural control of the circulation, even in the absence of variations in environmental variables or stimuli acting on reflexogenic areas. Indeed, the preliminary studies on conscious dogs and human subjects subjected to experimental psychological stress, a condition most likely characterized by an enhanced sympathetic drive, we have observed a marked increase in the LF component, i.e., a marker of sympathetic excitation (Fig. 9) [24–26]. Since this methodology can also be applied to data obtained with portable Holter tape recorders or with telemetric equipment, it appears particularly well suited in the field, under various behavioral conditions where the restrictions imposed by the instrumentation should be kept to a minimum.

Concluding Remarks

In the continuous domain of the health/disease process, the subject/environment relationship, cleared of subjective elements, can be simplistically described as a series of quantitative relationships among defined classes of components.

Considering subjects' behavior as comprised of motor, visceral, and verbal components all described in quantitative terms, it follows that any verbal self-report must be analyzed separately as an independent indicator of the level of self-awareness (whatever this means) and employed as an additional component to the whole description. Motor behavior, at least grossly, can be considered self-evident while changes in visceral behavior as a first approximation could be assessed using the dynamic changes in the balance between sympathetic and vagal control mechanisms that attend any change in visceral functions.

Thus, spectral analysis of cardiovascular variabilities seems to provide a convenient tool to describe the visceral changes that may occur spontaneously or accompany overt behavior independently of any self-report by the subject under study.

References

1. Lazarus RS, Delongis A, Folkman S, Gruen R (1985) Stress and adaptational outcomes. Am Psychol: 770–779
2. Lown B (1986) Clinical studies of the relation behavioral factors and sudden cardiac death. In: Lown B, Malliani A, Prosdocimi M (eds) Neural mechanisms and cardiovascular disease. Liviana, Padova, pp 495–512 (Fidia research series, vol 5)
3. Aristotle (1964) On the soul. Harvard University Press, Cambridge
4. Harvey W (1628) De motu cordis
5. Koch E (1932) Die Irradiation der pressoreceptorischen Kreislaufreflexe. Klin Wochenschr 6
6. Heymans C (1929) Le sinus carotiedien. Lewis, London
7. Heymans C, Neil E (1958) Reflexogenic areas of the cardiovascular system. Churchill, London

8. Abboud FM, Thames MC (1983) Interaction of cardiovascular reflexes in circulatory control. In: Shepherd JT, Abboud FM (eds) The cardiovascular system. Am Physiol Soc, Bethesda, pp 675–754 (Handbook of Physiology)
9. Malliani A, Pagani M, Lombardi F (1986) Positive feedback reflexes. In: Zanchetti A, Tarazi RC (eds) Pathophysiology of hypertension – regulatory mechanisms. Elsevier, Amsterdam (Handbook of hypertension, vol 8)
10. Pagani M, Pizzinelli P, Bergamaschi M, Malliani A (1982) A positive feedback sympathetic pressor reflex during stretch of the thoracic aorta in conscious dogs. Circ Res 50:125–132
11. Pagani M, Pizzinelli P, Furlan R, Guzzetti S, Rimoldi O, Sandrone G, Malliani A (1985) Analysis of the pressor sympathetic reflex produced by intracoronary injections of bradykinin in conscious dogs. Circ Res 56:175–183
12. Pagani M, Lombardi F, Guzzetti S, Rimoldi O, Furlan R, Pizzinelli P, Sandrone G, Malfatto G, Dell'Orto S, Piccaluga E, Turiel M, Baselli G, Cerutti S, Malliani A (1986) Power spectral analysis of heart rate and arterial pressure variabilities as a marker of sympatho-vagal interaction in man and conscious dog. Circ Res 59:178–193
13. Rimoldi O, Pierini S, Ferrari A, Cerutti S, Pagani M, Malliani A (1990) Analysis of short-term oscillations of R-R and arterial pressure in conscious dogs. Am J Physiol 258:H967–H976
14. Furlan R, Guzzetti S, Crivellaro W, Dassi S, Tinelli M, Baselli G, Cerutti S, Lombardi F, Pagani M, Malliani A (1990) Continuous 24-hour assessment of the neural regulation of systemic arterial pressure and R-R variabilities in ambulant subjects. Circulation 81:537–547
15. Akselrod S, Gordon D, Ubel FA, Shannon DC, Barger AC, Cohen RJ (1981) Power spectrum analysis of heart rate fluctuation: a quantitative probe of beat-to-beat cardiovascular control. Science 213:220–222
16. Pomeranz B, Macaulay RJB, Caudill MA, Kutz I, Adam D, Gordon D, Kilborn KM, Barger AC, Shannon DC, Cohen RJ, Benson H (1985) Assessment of autonomic function in humans by heart rate spectral analysis. Am J Physiol 248:H151–H153
17. Pagani M, Furlan R, Dell'Orto S, Pizzinelli P, Lanzi G, Baselli G, Santoli C, Cerutti S, Lombardi F, Malliani A (1986) Continuous recording of direct high fidelity arterial pressure and electrocardiogram in ambulant patients. Cardiovasc Res 20:384–388
18. Pagani M, Somers V, Furlan R, Dell'Orto S, Conway J, Baselli G, Cerutti S, Sleight P, Malliani A (1988) Changes in autonomic regulation induced by physical training. Hypertension 12:600–610
19. Rimoldi O, Pagani M, Pagani MR, Baselli G, Malliani A (1990) Sympathetic activation during treadmill exercise in the conscious dog: assessment with spectral analysis of heart period and systolic pressure variabilities. J Auton Nerv Syst 30:129–132
20. Furlan R et al. (to be published)
21. Guzzetti S, Piccaluga E, Casati R, Cerutti S, Lombardi F, Pagani M, Malliani A (1988) Sympathetic predominance in essential hypertension: a study employing spectral analysis of heart rate variability. J Hypertens 6:711–717
22. Lombardi F, Sandrone G, Pernpruner S, Sala R, Garimoldi M, Cerutti S, Baselli G, Pagani M, Malliani A (1987) Heart rate variability as an index of sympathovagal interaction after acute myocardial infarction. Am J Cardiol 60:1239–1245
23. Pagani M, Malfatto G, Pierini S, Casati R, Masu AM, Poli M, Guzzetti S, Lombardi F, Cerutti S, Malliani A (1988) Spectral analysis of heart rate variability in the assessment of autonomic diabetic neuropathy. J Auton Nerv Syst 23:143–153
24. Guzzetti S, Josa D, Pecis M, Bonura L, Prosdocimi M, Malliani A (1990) Effects of sympathetic activation on heart rate variability in Chagas' patients. J Auton Nerv Syst 30:79–82
25. Pagani M, Furlan R, Pizzinelli P, Crivellaro W, Cerutti S, Malliani A (1989) Spectral analysis of R-R and arterial pressure variabilities to assess sympatho-vagal interaction during mental stress in humans. J Hypertens 7 [Suppl 6]:S14–S15
26. Pagani M, Mazzuero G, Ferrari A, Liberati D, Cerutti S, Vaitl D, Tavazzi L, Malliani A (1991) Sympatho-vagal interaction during mental stress: a study employing spectral analysis of heart rate variability in healthy controls and in patients with a prior myocardial infarction. Circulation 83 [Suppl II]:II-43–II-51

The Relationship Between Cardiovascular Responses in the Laboratory and in the Field: The Importance of "Active Coping" *

D. W. Johnston, P. Anastasiades, C. Vögele, D. M. Clark, C. Kitson, and A. Steptoe

Introduction

The cardiovascular response to psychological stimuli is central to current research and theorising on the psychophysiological and neurogenic aspects of cardiovascular disease. It is implicated in the development of hypertension (Folkow 1982; Obrist 1981; Fredrikson and Matthews 1990), coronary atherosclerosis (Manuck et al. 1983), and as the physiological mechanism linking type A behaviour and coronary heart disease or even as a risk factor in its own right (Krantz and Manuck 1984). Outside the area of cardiovascular disease, cardiovascular reactivity is related to the development and maintenance of anxiety and panic disorders (Clark 1986; Ehlers et al. 1988).

At present most research on the cardiovascular effects of stress is laboratory based. The assumption is that the laboratory measures relate to the cardiovascular responses to real life stressors and are thus analogues of significant aspects of cardiovascular functioning, i.e. a similar process occurs at other times, in the same people, to a similar extent and with significant frequency. If this is not so, then the relevance of laboratory studies to the understanding and assessment of disease is drastically reduced.

In this paper we present the results of an ongoing research programme which is directed at the following five issues:

(a) the measurement of cardiovascular reactivity,
(b) the nature of the laboratory stressors that predict reactivity in the field,
(c) the relationship between cardiovascular activation and stress in real life,
(d) models of cardiovascular hyperreactivity in real life, and
(e) the psychological and physiological processes mediating the relationship between reactivity in the laboratory and in the field.

* Much of the research reported in this paper was supported by the Medical Research Council of Great Britain.

Schmidt/Engel/Blümchen (Eds.)
Temporal Variations of the Cardiovascular System
© Springer-Verlag Berlin Heidelberg 1992

The Measurement of Cardiovascular Reactivity

Cardiovascular reactivity in the field is most often measured using ambulatory non-invasive blood pressure and heart rate recorders. Attempts to relate such measures to laboratory-defined hyperreactivity have not been strikingly successful (Matthews et al. 1986; Harshfield et al. 1988), almost certainly because the measurement is too infrequent (four times per hour at most) and so constrains the subject that ongoing behaviour is disrupted. Studies using continuous invasive measurement of blood pressure in hypertensives have obtained rather stronger relationships, with Floras et al. (1987) reporting correlations of 0.53 between the response to a reaction time task and blood pressure variability. Parati et al. (1988) report correlations of a similar order between the response to mental arithmetic and blood pressure variability in the field. It is, of course, also possible that the relationship between laboratory and field responses is greater in hypertensive patients, perhaps because of structural changes in the blood vessels, compared to the normotensives usually studied. No attempt was made in any of these studies to allow for the effects of ongoing or recently completed physical activity, which has a profound effect on heart rate and to a slightly lesser extent on blood pressure.

Four characteristics distinguish the research described here from most of the published literature:

(a) the use of continuous cardiovascular measure in the field,
(b) the measurement of physical activity in the field,
(c) the use of times series methods to allow for serial dependency in the field measures and for the effects of activity on heart rate, and
(d) the use of the peak rather than the average response to laboratory stressors.

The primary ambulant measure in our studies is heart rate measured from a continuous ECG. Heart rate was chosen because of its ease of measurement, relevance to cardiovascular disease and responsiveness to laboratory stressors. Until very recently there has been no viable continuous non-invasive measure of blood pressure (but see Langewouters et al., this volume).

If subjects respond to everyday challenges in the same manner as they respond to laboratory challenge, with substantial cardiac acceleration, then more responsive subjects should show more variable heart rate during the waking day. However heart rate varies as a result of many intrinsic and extrinsic factors, such as ambient temperature, baroreceptor sensitivity and, above all else, the varying metabolic demands placed on the heart as a result of physical activity. If this is not taken into account, measures of heart rate variability may be seriously inaccurate or insensitive as measures of psychological effects on the heart. We have shown (Anastasiades and Johnston 1990) that the electromyogram (EMG) measured from the thigh is a sensitive and robust measure of activity which reliably differentiates, on an individual basis, sitting and standing from walking, which is distinguishable from running. Sitting and standing are not distinguishable. We have incorporated this measure in all our studies, and it has proved a valuable method for estimating the effect of extraneous factors on heart rate. An example of a typical heart rate and activity record is shown in Fig. 1. The data shown are of heart rate and activity averaged over successive 6-min periods, the interval that we have used in all the studies to be reported. The close covariation between heart rate and activity is apparent.

Continuous records of cardiovascular activity, while obviously much more informative than discontinuous records, present particular problems of analysis and interpretation. The data almost invariably display strong serial dependency, with heart rate and blood pressure related to preceding values. Measures of reactivity derived from such series, including common measures of variability such as the standard deviation, can be seriously distorted by such dependencies and also by any temporal trends in the records. For example, if a subject, rather improbably, produced a heart rate record that increased steadily by 1 bpm every minute for 30 min, i.e. 61, 62, 63 etc. to 90 bpm, the standard deviation would be equal to that in a subject who produced the same 30 readings in a random order, e.g. 70, 84, 61, 67, 77 bpm etc. Few would want to regard the two series as displaying identical variability. In a less dramatic form such issues arise in all continuous cardiovascular records and must be resolved if appropriate measures of variability are to be derived and justifiable measures of statistical significance determined.

Our solution to this problem has been heavily influenced by our desire to establish and allow for the relationship between heart rate and activity and consists of non-stochastic, autoregressive modelling incorporating the current and delayed effects of variables. The basic assumption of this approach is that there is a proportional relationship between activity (ACT) and heart rate (HR), and that a general autoregressive distributed lag relationship exists between the two variables (Hendry and Richard 1983; Hendry et al. 1983). The simplest case, which in fact held in most of our data, takes the form:

$$HR_t = \alpha_0 + \alpha_1 HR_{t-1} + \beta_0 ACT_t + \beta_1 ACT_{t-1} + \varepsilon_t$$

with ε representing error, which should in an adequate model be white noise, i.e. random. For those not familiar with regression analysis, the model essentially asserts that current heart rate is a linear function of a constant, the immediately preceding heart rate, the current level of activity, the immediately preceding level of activity, and error. The variability in the measure of error, the residual difference between the observed and expected observation, is the data that we are attempting to predict from the response to laboratory challenge. The same methods can also be used to allow for serial dependency in the absence of activity. In this case the simplest and by far the most common model becomes:

$$HR_t = \alpha_0 + \alpha_1 HR_{t-1} + \varepsilon_t$$

Again, the variability in the residual error is taken as the measure of reactivity in the field. Doubtless other approaches to these problems are also viable, including simpler methods based on successive differencing (Schachinger et al. 1989) and more complex techniques of non-linear modelling (Box and Jenkins 1976). We offer our approach as a realisable method that has been tested and found valuable.

The measurement of reactivity in the laboratory has been the subject of extensive debate over many years (Fahrenberg et al. 1985), but it has become common to rely on comparatively simple change scores in which the average level, for example, of blood pressure, during a baseline period is subtracted from the average level during a task. While this is appropriate for characterising the overall response to a challenge, we doubt whether it is the most sensitive measure of responsiveness, and we have focused on the peak response to either individual tasks or to classes of tasks. This may be a better measure of the subject's capacity or potential to respond to psychological challenge with a large physiological change and hence a more relevant measure to relate to reactivity in the field. Our own findings, as well as those of others (e.g. Floras et al. 1987; Parati et al. 1988) appear to support this view.

In our first study on this topic (Johnston et al. 1990) we expressed the response to the psychological challenge as a proportion of the response to a standard physical challenge in the belief that this might take into account some of the purely peripheral factors that might affect reactivity. We hoped that this might produce a measure with some of the positive features of "additional heart rate", (Carroll et al. 1987; Turner 1988). Later research has not confirmed the advantages of allowing for the effects of physical activity in this simple way, although measuring additional heart rate in the conventional manner by taking oxygen consumption into account might well generate a particularly appropriate measure of reactivity.

The Nature of the Laboratory Stressors that Predict Reactivity in the Field

Laboratory stressors can be classified in a number of ways, for example, by procedure or by psychological or physiological processes. In this area of research it has been most fruitful to classify them either by psychological or physiological process. The main psychological process used to differentiate laboratory stressors is that of effortful "active coping" versus "passive coping" (Obrist 1981). Active coping is invoked when the task requires that the subject make a continuous behavioural response to cope with a demanding and rapidly changing situation; tasks such as video games or paced versions of choice reaction time are typical examples. Passive coping involves situations in which no continuous behavioural adjustment is required, and the stress must simply be endured; the cold pressor test is an example of such a task.

Classification by physiological process has focused on whether the cardiovascular changes are primarily cardiac or non-cardiac (i.e. vascular), sympathetic or parasympathetic, and if sympathetic, whether the β- or α-adrenergic receptors are primarily involved. Active coping tasks have been shown to be primarily cardiac (involving increases in heart rate and cardiac output) and β-adrenergic (Obrist et al. 1978; Langer et al. 1985). Passive coping may be more vascular and α-adrenergic (Obrist et al. 1978). Some tasks that cannot be readily classified psychologically can be grouped physiologically. Very recent research has shown that mirror drawing has a substantial non-cardiac α-adrenergic component (M. Gellman 1990, personal communication) while difficult auditory mental

Table 1. Correlations between peak responses, indices and field measures (experiment 1)

Field measure	Task			
	ACR	PCR	ACI	PCI
	Heart rate			
1	0.20	−0.09	0.26	0.17
2	0.01	−0.18	0.01	0.14
3	0.26	0.02	0.35	−0.02
4	0.30	0.25	0.44	0.31
5	0.29	0.06	0.50	0.17
6	0.23	0.15	0.36	0.20
	Pulse transit time			
1	−0.03	−0.20	−0.05	−0.07
2	0.21	−0.11	0.18	0.14
3	−0.13	0.17	−0.22	−0.02
4	−0.35	−0.06	−0.47	−0.28
5	−0.58	−0.04	−0.51	−0.15
6	−0.41	−0.04	−0.35	−0.13

$r \geq 0.35$; $p < 0.05$

1, Waking HR; 2, sleeping HR; 3, waking-sleeping HR; 4, SD of raw HR; 5, SD of residuals of: $HR_t = f(HR_{t-1}$ etc.$)$; 6, SD of residuals of: $HR_t = f(HR_{t-1}$ etc., ACT, ACT_{t-1} etc.$)$;
ACR, peak response during active coping; PCR, peak response during passive coping; ACI, active coping Index (peak during active coping: peak during exercise); PCI, passive coping Index (peak during passive coping: peak during exercise).

arithmetic, which is regarded as involving active coping, appears primarily cardiac and β-adrenergic (Brod et al. 1959).

These classifications should be born in mind when considering three studies that have recently been completed in our laboratories in London and Oxford.

In experiment 1 (Johnston et al. 1990) 32 unselected young men underwent a battery of laboratory stressors while heart rate, pulsed transit time and various non-cardiovascular measures were taken. Heart rate and activity were also monitored over a continuous 24 h period using standard Medilog cassette recorders. The laboratory tasks consisted of soccer-style video games, mental arithmetic (spoken aloud), the cold pressor test and dynamic and isometric exercise. The video games and mental arithmetic were regarded as active coping tasks, the cold pressor as involving passive coping. The peak heart rate and the peak pulse transit time to any of the active coping tasks expressed as a proportion of the peak response to exercise correlated reliably with heart rate variability in the field, during the waking day. The correlations (Table 1) were significant even when serial dependency and activity were taken into account. The peak responses to either the cold pressor or physical exercise did not relate to heart rate variability in the field. The heart rate and activity records for a hyperreactive and a non-reactive subject are shown in Figs. 1 and 2. The heart rate response to the laboratory tasks is shown in the insets. As can be seen, the two subjects differ markedly in their response to active coping but not to the cold pressor or exercise. During the day the hyperreactive subject has a much more variable heart rate, despite apparently

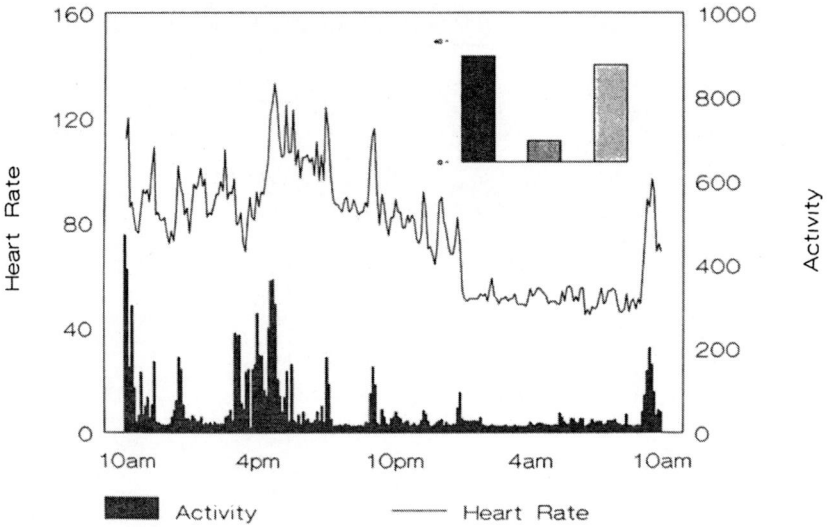

Fig. 1. This typical hyperreactive subject has a very variable heart rate throughout the day. His increase in heart rate during active coping (*left most column of insert*) is much larger than his response to passive coping (*middle column*) and comparable to the response to exercise

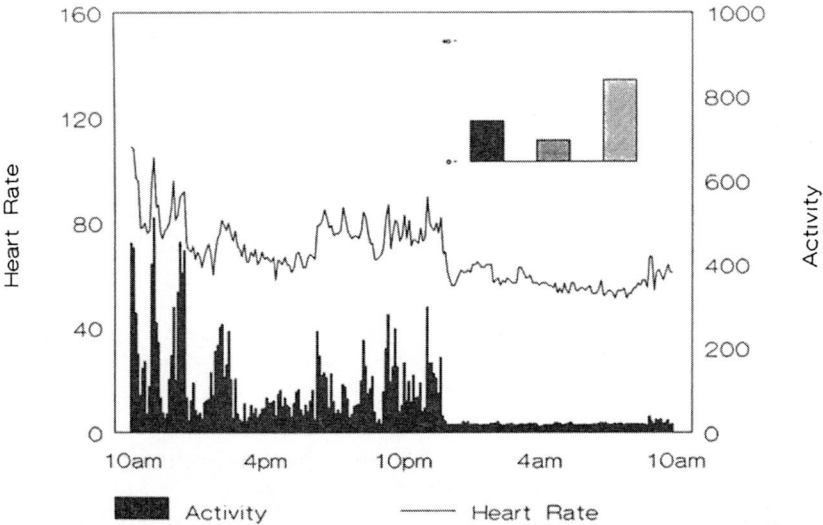

Fig. 2. This hyporeactive subject has a much less variable heart rate during the day than the subject in Fig. 1, despite having an apparently more active day. His response to active coping is also much less, although his responses to passive coping and exercise are comparable

Table 2. Correlations between peak responses and field measures (experiment 2)

Field measure	Task		
	MAR	MDR	CPR
	Heart rate		
1	0.17	0.34	0.13
2	0.01	0.15	0.16
3	0.25	0.36	0.02
4	−0.05	0.06	−0.07
5	−0.01	−0.01	−0.18
6	0.02	0.00	−0.12
	Systolic blood pressure		
1	0.02	0.08	0.12
2	0.07	0.09	0.13
3	−0.06	0.02	0.03
4	−0.05	−0.13	−0.13
5	−0.01	−0.05	−0.27
6	0.05	0.01	−0.17
	Diastolic blood pressure		
1	−0.07	−0.04	0.04
2	0.04	−0.03	0.02
3	−0.15	−0.03	0.05
4	0.00	0.12	0.13
5	−0.05	0.22	−0.10
6	−0.09	0.15	−0.03

$r \geq 0.35$; $p < 0.05$

1, Waking HR; 2, sleeping HR; 3, waking-sleeping HR; 4, SD of raw HR; 5, SD of residuals of: $HR_t = f(HR_{t-1}$ etc.$)$; 6, SD of residuals of: $HR_t = f(HR_{t-1}$ etc., ACT, ACT_{t-1} etc.$)$;
MAR, peak response during mental arithmetic; MDR, peak response during mirror drawing; CPR, peak response during cold pressor.

having a less active day. Overall, the subjects' activity explained approximately 50% of the heart rate variability that was not explained by serial dependency.

In experiment 2 the subjects were 34 male medical students selected from a larger group so that they had resting blood pressure at the top and bottom of the normal blood pressure distribution. Heart rate and activity were measured as already described. The laboratory tasks were a silent form of mental arithmetic, a mirror-drawing task in which the subjects traced a star shape seen in a mirror, the cold pressor and exercise. The measures were heart rate and systolic and diastolic blood pressure measured continuously at the finger using the FINAPRES system (Wesseling et al. 1982). Autoregressive analysis of the heart rate and activity were conducted in the same way as in experiment 1. The results on the laboratory/field relationships are shown in Table 2. It is clear that the peak heart rate and blood pressure responses did not relate to heart rate variability in the field. It should be noted that in neither of these studies did the response to the cold pressor or physical exercise relate to the heart rate variability in the field.

Table 3. Correlations between peak heart rate responses and field measures (experiment 3)

Field measure	Task		
	AC/ANX.	NEUT.	EX
1	0.25	0.10	0.13
2	0.51	0.09	0.20
3	0.12	0.03	0.05
4	0.30	0.14	−0.09
5	0.59	0.05	−0.15
6	0.49	0.01	−0.10

$r \geq 0.44$; $p < 0.05$

1, Waking HR; 2, sleeping HR; 3, waking-sleeping HR; 4, SD of raw HR; 5, SD of residuals of: $HR_t = f(HR_{t-1}$ etc.); 6, SD of residuals of: $HR_t = f(HR_{t-1}$ etc., ACT, ACT_{t-1} etc.); AC/ANX, peak HR response to active coping/anxiogenic tasks; NEUT, peak HR response to neutral tasks; EX, peak HR response to exercise.

The subjects in experiment 3 were 20 panic disorder patients fulfilling DSM-III-R criteria for this disorder with no or mild to moderate agoraphobia. Although the primary abnormality in panic is likely to be cognitive (e.g. the catastrophic misinterpretation of bodily sensations; Clark 1986), cardiovascular reactivity may be implicated (as a vulnerability factor) in the development and maintenance of panic attacks (Anastasiades et al. 1990; Ehlers et al. 1988). The field measures in this study were heart rate and activity as described above. The laboratory tasks included an example of active coping in the form of mental arithmetic spoken aloud and physical exercise. As this was a clinical sample, tasks that were specifically anxiogenic for panic patients were also used. These were derived from the cognitive model of panic and consisted of false feedback of rapid heart rate increase (50 bpm over 30 s) and a paired associates task, in which subjects were asked to read and dwell on pairs of symptom and catastrophe words, such as "breathlessness – suffocate", "palpitations – dying" (Clark et al. 1988). Panic patients find these tasks particularly stressful and anxiety provoking, exhibiting significantly greater cardiovascular activation than controls. For each of these tasks a neutral, non-threatening version of the task was also employed. The results on the relationships between the peak heart rate responses and field measures are shown in Table 3. The results were broadly consistent with those of experiment 1. The peak heart rate response to the active coping or anxiogenic tasks correlated significantly with field heart rate variability, particularly when serial dependency and activity were allowed for. The responses to the physical exercise and the neutral tasks again failed to show any association with the field measures of heart rate responsiveness. It may be postulated that the common mechanisms mediating the effects of instances of active coping and intense anxiety are mobilization for action and enhanced sympathetic activation in response to psychological challenge. Similar processes may also underlie the laboratory-field relationship.

In addition to these three experiments the same methods of autoregressive analysis have been applied to daytime heart rate and activity records in 32 subjects characterised as either extreme hyper- or hypocardiovascular reactors to a complex multiple-choice reaction time task. This study was conducted in collaboration with Dr. Thomas Schmidt of Hanover Medical School. Essentially it replicated the findings of experiments 1 and 3. Hyperreactive subjects had more variable heart rates, particularly when serial dependency and activity were allowed for.

It can be seen that our results generate the hypotheses that laboratory tasks which primarily invoke active coping and/or substantial β-adrenergic input to the heart (video games, mental arithmetic, intense anxiogenic tasks) predict heart rate reactivity in real life. Tasks that involve passive coping (cold pressor) or α-adrenergic input to the vasculature (mirror drawing) do not, nor do neutral tasks or physical exercise. The failure of the response to the silent form of mental arithmetic in experiment 2 to predict reactivity in the field is anomalous.

The Relationship Between Heart Rate and Stress in Real Life

In assessing the relationship between cardiovascular responses in the laboratory and in real life we have assumed that a significant proportion of heart rate variability in the field, after activity is controlled for, is stress related. While the correlations between laboratory and field measures of heart rate responsiveness support this, more direct evidence is required. As an initial test of this we have examined the relationship between heart rate and moods that may reflect the subjective effects of stress, measured every 30 min.

The most satisfactory methods of relating stress and heart rate is on a within-subject basis by covarying mood and heart rate measure at the same time. Obviously the problems of serial dependency discussed above arise in an acute form in such analyses, and it is very likely that the simple correlation of mood and heart rate does not represent the true relationship accurately, and that the usual tests of significance are not appropriate. We attempted to deal with this by correlating subjective mood state with, in addition to raw heart rate, the residual left after allowing for serial dependency and such dependencies and activity Johnston and Anastasiades (1990). This may well be a rather conservative procedure since such residuals are most insensitive to enduring periods of high or low heart rate, although these might genuinely be associated with persistent periods of high or low subjective stress. This is because the autoregressive model ensures that the residuals are minimal during periods of stable heart rate. Residuals are large when heart rate has just changed, and the autoregressive adjustments have not yet come into play. It can be seen from Table 4 that there were comparatively few significant relationships between the various stress-related moods and heart rate, and that these became even less frequent when allowance was made for serial dependency and activity. In experiment 2 comparable methods were applied. In this case the mood measures were analogue scales of anxiety, anger and frustration (chosen to match ratings the subjects gave after the laboratory stressors). Even fewer of the correlations were significant in this case (Table 5). The subjects also rated how physically active they were. This did relate to heart rate, as one might expect, indicating that such analogue scales can be used to detect significant relationships.

Table 4. Significant correlations between heart rate, heart rate residuals and mood recorded every 30 min (experiment 1)

Mood	n	Heart rate		Heart rate residuals		Heart rate residuals (allowing for activity)	
		Positive	Negative	Positive	Negative	Positive	Negative
Arousal	31	5	2	0	2	2	2
Stress	31	8	2	4	0	2	1
Time pressure	30	5	1	2	1	4	0

Table 5. Significant correlations between heart rate, heart rate residuals and mood recorded every 30 min (experiment 2)

Mood	n	Heart rate		Heart rate residuals		Heart rate residuals (allowing for activity)	
		Positive	Negative	Positive	Negative	Positive	Negative
Anxiety	33	3	1	2	0	0	0
Anger	25	2	2	0	1	1	1
Frustration	32	2	1	1	0	1	1
Activity	33	0	4	1	3	3	1

The results suggest that the relationship between stress and heart rate in real life is weak. This is consistent with the results of others using similar procedures for assessing stress (Sokolow et al. 1970). However, the weakness of methods for measuring real life stress must be acknowledged. Stress was measured infrequently and was assessed purely in terms of its subjective effects. More frequent objective measures are clearly required to supplement the subjective.

Models of Cardiovascular Hyperreactivity in Real Life

The issue of what mechanisms mediate the relationship between cardiovascular reactivity in the laboratory and in the field can be approached in various ways. One approach is to examine the nature of the psychological and physiological processes mediating the relationship. This is discussed in the next section. Another approach is at the more descriptive level, in which simple models are formulated to depict the possible relationship between responses in the laboratory and in real life.

In this study we examined three such basic models that have been proposed in the literature. The first two are opposing theoretical models proposed by Manuck and Krantz (1984), and the third is a synthesis of the two proposed by Light (1987). They all revolve around the issue of whether heightened activation is evident throughout the day or in particular periods only.

The first model, labelled the recurrent activation model, proposes that specific episodes of enhanced physiological activity, such as increased heart rate, are observed in response to everyday demands and challenges while at other, rest, periods heart rate returns to a consistently low baseline level. Laboratory hyperreactors are distinguished from low reactors by higher episodic peaks but are not different in apparent baseline level. Thus the model predicts no difference in resting (or minimum) heart rate level but does predict that laboratory haperreactors should exhibit greater heart rate fluctuations and hence greater heart rate variability during the waking day. The model is also consistent with elevated average heart rate values, resulting indirectly from the larger episodic responses.

The second model described by Manuck and Krantz, the prevailing state model, suggests that there are no episodic peaks during the day but instead a rise in heart rate soon after awakening, reaching a level that is steadily maintained throughout the day as long as the subject is alert and functioning. Hyperreactors would thus have elevated heart rate throughout the day. An implication of this proposition is that any point during the day is representative and should discriminate between low and high reactors. There is, however, abundant evidence of substantial fluctuations in level throughout the day (e.g. Pickering et al. 1982). Thus the assumption of a constant prevailing state is untenable. Nevertheless, the essential feature of this model is that basal level or tone would be elevated in high reactors. All subjects may show fluctuations in level but the magnitude of these fluctuations would be comparable in high and low reactors. The fluctuations, however, are superimposed on different basal levels; minimum heart rate levels should be higher in hyperreactors.

The third model, that proposed by Light (1987), combines features from both the simple models and is influenced by some laboratory observations from her work with Obrist (e.g. Light and Obrist 1980). They had observed that laboratory hyperreactors exhibited elevated "pre-stress" baselines but similar "relaxation" baselines. According to Light's combined model, laboratory hyperreactors would be expected to show both elevated heart rate baselines in the field and enhanced heart rate peaks and responses and thus greater overall heart rate variability. Resting heart rate levels would be particularly elevated during the working day as hyperreactors anticipate the upcoming events of the day and experience the cumulative effects of these events but may be similarly low later in the evening as subjects are resting at home.

The comparison of high and low laboratory reactors on basal heart rate level and overall heart rate variability affords a sufficient basis for discriminating between the three models.

The models were tested in the study of 32 young volunteers undergoing laboratory and field measurements as described above in experiment 1. The subjects were categorised as high or low reactors according to their peak heart rate response to active coping tasks (video games and mental arithmetic). Despite the marked differences in their response to the active coping task high and low reactors showed very similar heart rate and pulse transit time responses to the passive coping and exercise tasks.

High reactors were compared with low reactors in terms of their overall heart rate values and overall heart rate variability during the day (Table 6). High reactors had similar average heart rate levels during sleep and only marginally elevated levels while awake but a significantly greater heart rate increase from

Table 6. Comparison of high and low laboratory reactors on overall mean ($\pm$SD) heart rate values in the field

Field measure	High reactors	Low reactors	p
1	86.3 $\pm$ 10.6	81.0 $\pm$ 8.8	n.s.
2	55.7 $\pm$ 6.2	55.4 $\pm$ 6.1	n.s.
3	30.6 $\pm$ 7.6	25.6 $\pm$ 6.2	< 0.05
4	11.8 $\pm$ 2.7	9.9 $\pm$ 1.9	< 0.05
5	7.6 $\pm$ 1.4	6.6 $\pm$ 1.2	< 0.05
6	5.9 $\pm$ 1.7	4.8 $\pm$ 1.2	< 0.05

1, Waking HR; 2, sleeping HR; 3, waking-sleeping HR; 4, SD of raw HR; 5, SD of residuals of: $HR_t = f(HR_{t-1}$ etc.); 6, SD of residuals of: $HR_t = f(HR_{t-1}$ etc., ACT, ACT_{t-1} etc.).

Table 7. Comparison of high and low laboratory reactors on lowest mean ($\pm$SD) heart rate values during the day

Field measure	High reactors	Low reactors	p
1	68.0 $\pm$ 9.6	65.4 $\pm$ 7.6	n.s.
2	12.3 $\pm$ 6.5	10.0 $\pm$ 5.6	n.s.
3	$-$ 7.9 $\pm$ 3.6	$-$ 9.3 $\pm$ 5.1	n.s.
4	$-$ 6.3 $\pm$ 3.4	$-$ 6.7 $\pm$ 4.0	n.s.
Physical activity	$-$ 0.5 $\pm$ 0.1	$-$ 0.6 $\pm$ 0.2	n.s.
Stress	2.3 $\pm$ 3.3	2.3 $\pm$ 2.3	n.s.
Arousal	3.9 $\pm$ 1.3	4.3 $\pm$ 1.6	n.s.

1, Raw HR level; 2, HR level $-$ sleeping HR; 3, HR residuals of: $HR_t = f(HR_{t-1}$ etc.); 4, HR residuals of: $HR_t = f(HR_{t-1}$ etc., ACT, ACT_{t-1} etc.).

sleep. More importantly, high reactors exhibited significantly higher variability of both raw heart rate level and of heart rate residuals after allowing for serial dependency and activity effects. High and low reactors reported very similar levels of stress and arousal during the day (assessed by mood rating scales every 30 min).

While the greater average heart rate increase from sleep shown by laboratory hyperreactors is consistent with the prevailing state model; the greater heart rate variability reflecting larger fluctuations and enhanced episodic activity is not. This pattern of results is, however, consistent with the predictions stemming from both the recurrent activation and combined models. The differentiation of these two models requires the comparison of baseline heart rate levels.

Baseline or resting heart rate values were defined as occurring in the 6-min period with the lowest mean heart rate level, as long as the subject reported being alert. Table 7 illustrates the comparison between high and low laboratory reactors on the various parameters associated with this period. It is clear that no comparison was significant or even approached significance. High and low reactors had similar resting heart rate, whether this was expressed as heart rate tonic level, heart rate change from sleep or heart rate residuals. Furthermore, none of the potentially confounding variables during this period were different. Both physical activity and mood (stress and arousal) were very similar in the two groups.

As a single 6-min heart rate value might be considered unrepresentative of the distribution of low heart rate levels shown by a subject, the bottom 5 % of heart rate values were also extracted. The results were consistent with the above findings; the lowest 5 % of all heart rate values were similar in the two groups. For example, the mean of the lowest 5 % of heart rate levels was 69.9 bpm for the high reactors and 67.0 bpm for the low reactors. The corresponding comparisons for the heart rate residuals after serial dependency was allowed for was -7.0 versus -6.9 bpm, and when activity was also taken into account -5.4 versus -5.0 bpm. None of these comparisons was significant. It can thus be safely concluded that high and low reactors did not differ in their resting heart rate. These results are again contrary to the predictions of the prevailing state model. They are also inconsistent with the combined model but are quite in accordance with the specifications of the recurrent activation model.

A further test of the combined versus the recurrent activation model was conducted, examining the effect of time of day. As the combined model proposes that high reactors are more likely to show their lowest heart rate in the evening, there is the obvious danger that the similarity in resting heart rate levels between the two groups was attributable to the high reactors experiencing their minimum heart rate in the evening. An examination of the temporal distribution of the periods with the lowest heart rate demonstrated that this was definitely not the case. Approximately the same number of subjects experienced their minimum heart rate in the morning/noon (six high versus six low reactors), afternoon (six versus five) and evening (four versus five).

In summary, the results produced a clear and consistent pattern. Laboratory hyperreactors exhibited significantly greater heart rate fluctuations and variability during everyday life than low reactors, but the two groups did not differ in their resting or basal heart rate level. This pattern of results is entirely contrary to the prevailing state model and offers only non-critical support for the combined model. The results are most consistent with the recurrent activation model. They suggest that laboratory hyperreactors are primarily distinguished from low reactors in terms of their enhanced episodic activity in response to everyday demands and challenges.

This suggestion was further specifically tested by comparing the heart rate response of high and low reactors to episodes of heightened stress in the field. The subject's mood ratings of stress were used as the basis for identifying such instances. For each subject, the period in which peak stress was reported was used. The results of this analysis are presented in Table 8 and, as can be seen, produced the clearest differentiation between high and low laboratory reactors. High reactors showed higher heart rate levels, greater increases from sleep, a larger increase from their minimum heart rate, a markedly larger "phasic" heart rate response (defined as the change from the lowest 6-min mean heart rate in the preceding 30 min) and higher values of heart rate residual both after serial dependency and after activity were taken into account. No difference in physical activity or levels of stress and arousal were found. Both groups reported similarly high levels of maximal stress. It is worth noting that the two groups were not as clearly differentiated in overall peak heart rate (regardless of whether the peak was stress related or not).

Table 8. Comparison of high and low laboratory reactors on mean ($\pm$SD) heart rate response to peak stress

Field measure	High reactors	Low reactors	p
1	113.6 ± 20.0	96.2 ± 13.7	< 0.01
2	57.9 ± 21.0	40.8 ± 12.9	< 0.01
3	45.6 ± 18.1	30.8 ± 14.0	< 0.01
4	28.0 ± 10.9	15.6 ± 7.9	< 0.001
5	18.8 ± 9.4	11.1 ± 7.1	< 0.05
6	14.3 ± 8.9	8.0 ± 7.0	< 0.05
Physical activity	1.3 ± 1.8	0.6 ± 1.3	n.s.
Stress	7.5 ± 2.1	6.6 ± 2.2	n.s.
Arousal	4.5 ± 1.3	4.0 ± 1.6	n.s.

1, Raw HR level; 2, HR level – sleeping HR; 3, HR level – minimum HR; 4, phasic HR response (see text); 5, HR residuals of: $HR_t = f(HR_{t-1}$ etc.); 6, HR residuals of: $HR_t = f(HR_{t-1}$ etc., ACT, ACT_{t-1} etc.).

Thus laboratory hyperreactors did show an enhanced cardiac response to specific stress episodes in real life. This provides further support for the recurrent activation model and confirms the generalisation of the cardiac hyperreactivity to stress from the laboratory to the field. It raises the possibility that the same psychophysiological mechanisms operating in response to laboratory stressors, i.e. active coping, also mediate the response to naturalistic stressors and the overall cardiac variability during the day.

The Psychological and Physiological Processes Mediating the Relationship Between Reactivity in the Laboratory and in the Field

While we have demonstrated significant relationships between laboratory and field reactivity, the effects are not large and are specific to a few laboratory tasks, and we have encountered failures in finding strongly predicted relationships. The situation is unlikely to improve until the mechanisms underlying the relationships are established. It is, in fact, surprising that significant relationships are ever observed since we have no way of controlling the subject's behaviour in the field or characterising the relevant parameters. It is not unlikely that results will fail to replicate across studies in which subjects have widely differing patterns of activities and stressors. An understanding of the processes involved will provide the basis for more reliable, valid and appropriate measures of responsiveness in the field.

We are only now starting on our studies of mechanism, but it may be helpful to incidate the areas of investigation that may prove fruitful. The relationships that we have observed between cardiovascular responses in the laboratory and field could come about in the following ways:

1. Many of the stressors that one deals with in real life may involve active coping, and hence the responses provoked in the laboratory by active coping tasks are provoked to a similar extent by naturalistic stressors involving active coping.

2. Active coping stressors in the laboratory may involve a mechanism that is triggered by many stressors in real life, even if these do not involve the same behavioural processes as active coping. This could be a specific psychological process or may be a physiological one such as a form of β-adrenergic hyperresponsivity to stress. It has, for example, recently been shown that the cardiovascular response to laboratory challenge is enhanced in subjects with increased β-adrenergic receptor density on the lymphocytes (Mills et al. 1990).
3. Active coping may tap a more general β-adrenergic sensitivity that is the basis of much heart rate variability in real life, even of a non-stress-related origin.

We have not yet been able to explore these possibilities in any detail. Obviously our finding that hyperreactive subjects had particularly high heart rates at times of heightened stress suggests that active coping tasks are predicting stress-related activity in the field rather than elevated heart rates of any origin. However, the reliable relationships with so general a measure of responsiveness as heart rate variability, when much of the variability could be non-stress-related, suggests that more general mechanisms may also be involved. If this is so it is perhaps surprising that the response to other challenges, such as physical exercise, did not also tap the same mechanism.

It clearly follows from our contention that active coping tasks specifically predict heart rate responsiveness in the field and the considerable evidence that active coping produces cardiovascular changes of a primarily β-adrenergic origin that we would expect both reactions to share a common β-adrenergic origin. This was tested in the study with Schmidt by examining the laboratory/field relationships in subjects with the β-adrenergic system blocked pharmacologically. In brief, it was found that the relationship between the heart rate response to active coping and heart rate reactivity in the field was not significant during β-blockade whereas it was when the same subjects were not blockaded. This is clearly consistent with the view that there is a common β-adrenergic basis to both laboratory and field responses. However, there appeared to be some residual relationship between-laboratory and field responsiveness even during blockade. This could be due to incomplete blockade but may suggest that there is also a common non-β-adrenergic basis to laboratory/field reactivity. This is presumably parasympathetically mediated. This would hardly be surprising since it is likely that many laboratory challenges produce vagally mediated changes in heart rate (Grossman et al. 1990). Vagal effects are also implicated in the hyperreactivity seen in hypertension (Julius et al. 1971; Julius and Esler 1975; Drummond 1990). A synergistic combination of β-adrenergic activation and vagal withdrawal may therefore underlie cardiac hyperreactivity in the laboratory and in the field.

Concluding Remarks

We have argued that studies of the cardiovascular response to laboratory challenges would be put on a much firmer footing if such responses could be shown to relate to cardiovascular responses in real life, particularly if the field responses were also stress related. In a series of studies we have obtained results that generally support the view that the response to particular laboratory tasks which involve active coping, closely related behaviours and/or β-adrenergic input to the heart relate to heart rate reactivity in the field. Tasks which involve passive coping and/or α-adrenergic input to the vasculature do not. These relationships are seen most clearly when allowance is made for the serial dependency seen in the heart rate series and for concurrent activity. The heart rate responses in the field of laboratory hyperreactors show a pattern of periods of elevated heart rate, particularly at times of stress, but their lowest heart rates do not differ from those of hyporeactors. This is consistent with the recurrent activation model proposed by Manuck and Krantz (1984).

Future studies should formally test our contention that tasks involving active coping and β-adrenergic input to the heart best predict cardiovascular responsiveness in the field and extend the field measurement beyond heart rate to other cardiovascular parameters, most obviously blood pressure. Since we are in a period of rapid technical advance in ambulatory measurement, we can expect exciting developments in our knowledge of the physiological processes involved in cardiovascular arousal in the laboratory, in the field and in their relationship. A deeper understanding of the psychological and behavioural processes involved will require a rapid advance in behavioural assessment in the field. Developments in technology (such as computerised diaries and ambulatory monitors with onboard intelligence) will aid this, but ingenuity and persistence will be even more necessary.

References

Anastasiades P, Johnston DW (1990) A simple activity measure for use with ambulatory subjects. Psychophysiology 27:87–93

Anastasiades P, Clark DM, Salkovskis PM, Middleton H, Hackman A, Gelder MG, Johnston DW (1990) Psychophysiological responses in panic and stress. J Psychophysiol 4: 329–336

Box GEP, Jenkins GM (1976) Time series analysis: forecasting and control. Holden-Day, San Francisco

Brod J, Fencl W, Hejl Z, Jirka J (1959) Circulatory changes underlying blood pressure elevation during acute emotional stress (mental arithmetic) in normotensive and hypertensive subjects. Clinical Science 18:269–279

Carroll D, Turner JR, Rogers S (1987) Heart rate and oxygen consumption during mental arithmetic, a video game, and graded exercise. Psychophysiology 24:112–118

Clark DM (1986) A cognitive approach to panic. Behav Res Ther 24:461–470

Clark DM, Salkovskis PM, Gelder M, Koehler C, Martin M, Anastasiades P, Hackman A, Middleton M, Jeavons A (1988) Tests of a cognitive theory of panic. In: Hand I, Wittchen H (eds) Panic and phobias. Springer, Berlin Heidelberg New York, pp 149–158

Drummond PD (1990) Parasympathetic cardiac control in mild hypertension. J Hypertens 8: 383–387

Ehlers A, Margraf F, Roth WT (1988) Interaction of expectancy and physiological stressors in a laboratory model of panic. In: Hellhammer D, Florin I, Weiner H (eds) Neurobiology of human disease. Huber, Toronto, pp 379–384

Fahrenberg J, Schneider H-J, Foester F, Myrtek M, Muller W (1985) The quantification of cardiovascular reactivity in longitudinal studies. In: Steptoe A, Ruddel H, Neuss H (eds) Clinical and methodological issues in cardiovascular psychophysiology. Springer, Berlin Heidelberg New York, pp 106–119

Floras JS, Hassan MO, Jones JV, Sleight P (1987) Pressor responses to laboratory stresses and daytime blood pressure variability. J Hypertens 5:715–719

Folkow B (1982) Physiological aspects of primary hypertension. Physiol Rev 62:347–504

Fredrikson M, Matthews KA (1990) Cardiovascular responses to behavioral stress and hypertension: a meta-analytic review. Annals of Behavioral Medicine 12:30–39

Grossman P, Stemmler G, Meinhardt E (1990) Paced respiratory sinus arrhythmia as an index of cardiac parasympathetic tone during varying behavioral tasks. Psychophysiology 27:404–416

Harshfield GA, James GD, Schlussel Y, Yee LS, Blank SG, Pickering TG (1988) Do laboratory tests of blood pressure reactivity predict blood pressure change during everyday life? Am J Hypertens 1:168–174

Hendry DF, Richard J-R (1983) The econometric analysis of economic time series. Int Stat Rev 51:111–163

Hendry DF, Pagan AR, Sargan JD (1983) Dynamic specification. In: Griliches Z, Intriligator MD (eds) Handbook of econometrics. North-Holland, Amsterdam, pp 1022–1100

Johnston DW, Anastasiades P (1990) The relationship between heart rate and mood in real life. Psychosom Res 34:21–27

Johnston DW, Anastasiades P, Wood C (1990) The relationship between cardiovascular responses in the laboratory and in the field. Psychophysiology 27:34–44

Julius S, Esler M (1975) Autonomic nervous cardiovascular regulation in borderline hypertension. Am J Cardiol 36:685–696

Julius S, Pascual AV, London R (1971) Role of parasympathetic inhibition in the hyperkinetic type of borderline hypertension. Circulation 44:413–418

Krantz DS, Manuck SB (1984) Acute psychophysiologic reactivity and the risk of cardiovascular disease: a review and methodologic critique. Psychol Bull 96:435–464

Langer AW, McCubbin JA, Stoney CM, Hutcheson JS, Charlton JD, Obrist PA (1985) Cardiopulmonary adjustments during exercise and an aversive reaction time task: effects of beta-adrenoceptor blockade. Psychophysiology 22:59–68

Light KC (1987) Psychosocial precursors of hypertension: experimental evidence. Circulation 76:67–76

Light KC, Obrist PA (1980) Cardiovascular response to stress: effects of opportunity to avoid, shock experience, and performance feedback. Psychophysiology 17:243–252

Manuck SB, Krantz DS (1984) Psychophysiologic reactivity in coronary heart disease. Behav Med Update 6:11–15

Manuck SB, Kaplan JR, Clarkson TB (1983) Behaviourally induced heart rate reactivity and atherosclerosis in cynomolgus monkeys. Psychosom Med 45:95–108

Matthews KA, Manuck SB, Saab PG (1986) Cardiovascular responses of adolescents during a naturally occurring stressor and their behavioural and psychophysiological predictors. Psychophysiology 23:198–209

Mills P, Dimsdale J, Ziegler M, Berry C (1990) Beta-adrenergic receptors and cardiovascular reactivity to a psychosocial stress. Psychophysiology 27 (4a):S 52

Obrist PA (1981) Cardiovascular psychophysiology: a perspective. Plenum, New York

Obrist PA, Gaebelin CJ, Teller ES, Langer AW, Grignolo A, Light KC, McCubbin JA (1978) The relationship among heart rate, carotid dP/dT and blood pressure in humans as a function of the type of stress. Psychophysiology 15:102–115

Parati G, Pomidossi G, Casadei R, Ravogli A, Gropelli A, Cesana B, Mancia G (1988) Comparison of the cardiovascular effects of different laboratory stressors and their relationship with blood pressure variability. J Hypertens 6:481–488

Pickering TG, Harshfield GA, Kleinert HD, Laragh JH (1982) Ambulatory monitoring in the evaluation of blood pressure in patients with borderline hypertension and the role of the defense reflex. Clin Exp Hypertens [A] 4:675

Schachinger H, Langewitz W, Schmieder RE, Ruddel H (1989) Comparison of parameters for assessing blood pressure and heart rate variability from non-invasive twenty-four-hour blood pressure monitoring. J Hypertens 7 [Suppl 3]:S81–S84

Sokolow M, Werdegar D, Perloff DB, Cowan RM, Brenenstuhl H (1970) Preliminary studies relating portably recorded blood pressure to daily life events in patients with essential hypertension. In: Koster M, Musaph H, Visser P (eds) Psychosomatics in essential Hypertension. Karger, Basel, pp 164–189

Turner JR (1988) Inter-task consistency: an integrative re-evaluation. Psychophysiology 25: 235–238

Wesseling KH, De Wit B, Settels JJ, Klawer WH (1982) On the indirect registration of finger blood pressure after Penaz. Funk Biol Med 1:245–250.

Diurnal Variation and Triggers of Onset of Cardiovascular Disease

G. H. Tofler and J. E. Muller

Introduction

Recent information suggests that the onset of myocardial infarction and sudden cardiac death is frequently triggered by daily activities. The importance of physical or mental stress in triggering onset of coronary thrombosis is supported by the following findings:

(a) The frequencies of onset of myocardial infarction, sudden cardiac death, and stroke show marked diurnal variations with parallel increases in the period from 6 A.M. to noon.
(b) Transient myocardial ischemia shows a similar morning increase, and episodes are often preceded by mental or physical triggers.
(c) A ruptured atherosclerotic plaque, often nonobstructive by itself, lies at the base of most coronary thrombi.
(d) A number of physiologic processes that could lead to plaque rupture, a hypercoagulable state, or coronary vasoconstriction are accentuated in the morning; and
(e) aspirin and beta-adrenergic blocking agents that block certain of these processes have been shown to prevent disease onset.

It is proposed that occlusive coronary thrombosis occurs when:

(a) an atherosclerotic plaque becomes vulnerable to rupture;
(b) mental or physical stress causes the plaque to rupture; and
(c) increases in coagulability or vasoconstriction, triggered by daily activities, contribute to complete occlusion of the coronary artery lumen.

Recognition of the diurnal variation – and the possibility of frequent triggering – of onset of acute disease, suggests the need for pharmacologic protection of patients during vulnerable periods and provides clues to mechanism, the investigation of which may lead to improved methods of prevention.

Schmidt/Engel/Blümchen (Eds)
Temporal Variations of the Cardiovascular System
© Springer-Verlag Berlin Heidelberg 1992

History of the Triggering Concept

In 1910 Obraztsov and Strazhesko stated that activities frequently triggered infarction onset and presented graphic cases of triggering, such as infarct onset after a heated card game [1]. Their view was challenged in the 1930s as studies revealed that in many instances infarction occurred without an obvious precipitating event. A controversy developed with authors for [2, 3] and against [4, 5] the view that triggers were frequent. For many years the debate was suspended with widespread acceptance of the conclusion of Master, based on retrospective questionnaires, that activities are of little importance in triggering onset [6].

Concurrent with, and in some instances stimulated by, the recognition of the morning increase in infarction onset [7], there has been renewed study of the possibility of triggering. Sumiyoshi et al. reported on the activities prior to onset in 416 patients with infarction [8]. In patients without prior angina, 53% reported that their infarct began during a period of moderate-to-heavy exercise, emotional stress, or excitation. Our group has reviewed the incidence of reporting of possible triggers of infarction by patients enrolled in the Multicenter Investigation of the Limitation of Infarct Size (MILIS). It was found that 48.5% reported a possible trigger [9], a number similar to that reported by Sumiyoshi et al. [8]. An additional report has described anecdotal cases in which it was readily apparent that the infarct had been triggered (snow shoveling, extreme exertion, and emotional stress immediately prior to onset) [10]. The problem of biased recall complicates interpretation of these findings. Collection of appropriate control data presents the major difficulty in clarifying the role of potentially triggering activities in the onset of infarction. The methodologic problems involved in collection of such data have led to a proposal by Maclure that a case-crossover design be utilized in which each patient serves as his or her own control for relatively recent activities [11]. This method is now being utilized in an NHLBI-funded study entitled Determinants of the Onset of Myocardial Infarction in which over 3000 patients with infarction will be interviewed.

Epidemiologic Evidence that Morning Activities Trigger Onset

The proposal that daily activities are of importance in triggering myocardial infarction is supported by epidemiologic findings that infarction does not occur randomly throughout the day but shows a prominent circadian variation with a morning increase in frequency. Objective evidence obtained from MILIS [7] (Fig. 1) and from the Intravenous Streptokinase in Acute Myocardial Infarction (ISAM) study [12] clearly demonstrates that myocardial infarction is at least three times more likely to begin in the morning than in the late evening. Both studies determined the onset of myocardial infarction objectively on the basis of the time of first appearance of creatine kinase in the plasma. Their finding is supported by a larger number of studies [13] that used onset of pain as a marker of time of myocardial infarction onset. The earlier studies received limited attention because it was thought that the reported morning increase in incidence was simply the

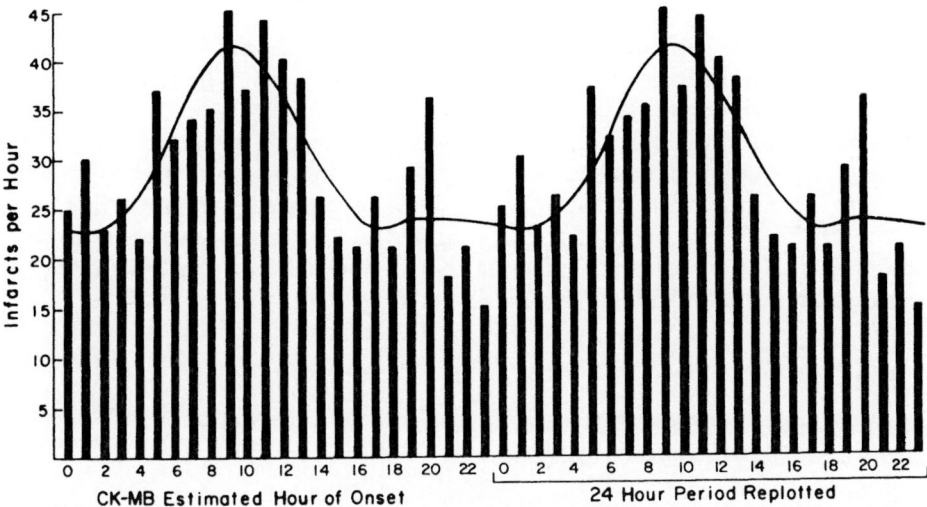

Fig. 1. *Left*, the number of infarctions beginning during each of the 24 h of the day; *right*, the identical data are plotted again to permit appreciation of the relationship between the end and the beginning of the day. A two-harmonic regression equation for the frequency of onset of myocardial infarction has been fitted to the data (*curved line*). A prominent circadian rhythm is present, with a primary peak incidence of infarction at 9 A.M. and a secondary peak at 8 P.M. (From [7] with permission)

result of delayed reporting of onset of myocardial infarction which actually began during the night while the patient was sleeping.

Several features of this morning increase have recently been explored. Hjalmarson et al. have found that the morning increase is blunted or abolished in subgroups of patients with characteristics such as advanced age, diabetes, smoking history, and prior infarction [14], while Goldberg et al. have reported that the increase in incidence occurs in the first 4 h after awakening [15].

The finding that nonfatal myocardial infarction has a prominent morning increase in onset is supported by, and in turn is supportive of, the finding that sudden cardiac death, a condition often caused by coronary thrombosis, has a similar diurnal pattern [16–19]. Stroke, a third condition often resulting from occlusive arterial thrombosis, has a similar morning increase [20, 21].

Timing of Transient Myocardial Ischemia

Data indicating the increased morning incidence of onset of the relatively infrequent cardiovascular disasters – myocardial infarction, sudden cardiac death, and stroke – have been supported by information about the much more frequent and more easily studied disorder of transient myocardial ischemia. With episodes of transient ischemia occurring so frequently, and with continuous Holter monitoring eliminating the possibility of bias resulting from unobserved periods, it has been possible to determine the timing of episodes of transient ischemia with great certainty. These studies have consistently demonstrated a peak incidence of episodes occurring between the hours of 6 A.M. and 12 noon [22–24]. Furthermore, Rocco et al. were able to adjust the timing of episodes for wake time and demonstrate that the increase in frequency occurs in the first 4 h after awakening and beginning the day's activities [23], a finding similar to that reported for myocardial infarction onset [15]. Detailed study indicates that episodes are often triggered by activities causing a transient coronary vascoconstriction and transient increases in heart rate and/or systemic arterial pressure [25]. Clarification of the phenomenon of triggering may lead to improved means of prevention, not only of transient ischemia, but of the related conditions of myocardial infarction and sudden death.

Autopsy and Angiographic Data Pertinent to Triggering of Onset of Myocardial Infarction

In 1980 DeWood et al. convincingly demonstrated that occlusive coronary artery thrombosis is the cause of most Q-wave myocardial infarctions [26]. Furthermore, patients with rest pain and unstable angina, who frequently progress to myocardial infarction, have been found to have a high frequency of nonocclusive coronary thrombosis [27, 28]. The linkage of this knowledge of the presence of thrombus to the concept of triggering results from information on the cause of the thrombus. With the use of serial histologic sections Constantinides discovered that in the majority of cases the thrombus had formed over a ruptured atherosclerotic plaque [29]. This pathologic finding has recently been supported by angiographic studies in patients demonstrating the presence of an outpouching of contrast media indicative of plaque rupture [30].

Two mechanisms of plaque rupture have been proposed: Constantinides has advanced the concept that the rupture occurs from the lumen *into the plaque* [29], while Barger et al. have proposed that rupture may occur from the plaque *into the lumen* [31]. Richardson et al. [32] have recently reported that in 63% of cases rupture of the plaque occurred at the junction of a lipid pool with normal tissue. Further study is needed of the plaque characteristics and processes external to the plaque that might cause rupture. Although autopsy studies generally reveal severe atherosclerotic stenosis at the base of a fatal coronary thrombosis [33], there is angiographic evidence that in many patients surviving a myocardial infarction, the degree of stenosis is relatively mild, and obstructive thrombus accounts for the majority of the obstruction to blood flow. Brown et al. reported that the degree of "original" stenosis in patients with myocardial infarction observed following treatment with streptokinase was under 60% in two-thirds of cases [34]. Other investigators support this view that the site of occlusion frequently does not have severe underlying stenosis [35, 36]. Rapold et al. have reported signs of increased activity of the clotting system and platelets in patients with infarction later found to have no angiographically visible coronary atherosclerosis [37]. These findings may explain the absence of prior symptoms in many patients presenting with acute myocardial infarction and indicate that attempts to identify and modify triggers of thrombus formation may have great clinical benefit [38].

Morning Increase of Physiological Processes
that Might Trigger Myocardial Infarction

A coronary atherosclerotic plaque is exposed to a number of systemic physiologic processes which could, if the plaque were vulnerable, cause disease onset. Many of these processes are accentuated in the morning. Accentuation of these processes could, alone or in combination, account for the morning increase in myocardial infarction onset (Fig. 1) through a variety of mechanisms (Fig. 2).

The morning arterial pressure surge [39] could cause plaque rupture. The coronary arterial tone increase [40] could worsen the flow reduction produced by a fixed stenosis. The arterial pressure increase and the tone increase could result in increased shear stress (force directed against the endothelium resulting from increased coronary blood flow velocity) [41] predisposing to plaque rupture and increased platelet deposition [42]. The increase in blood viscosity [43], increased platelet aggregability [44] (resulting from assumption of the upright posture [45]) and an insufficient countervailing increase in circulating t-PA activity [46–48] could produce a state of relative hypercoagulability. Such a thrombotic tendency could increase the likelihood that an otherwise harmless mural thrombus overlying a small plaque fissure would propagate and occlude the coronary lumen. Although serum cortisol levels are falling during the period of increased disease onset, they are increased above basal levels [49]. This increase could enhance the sensitivity of the coronary arteries to the vasoconstrictor effects of catecholamines [50], which have a prominent surge after assumption of the upright posture [45].

Although a 24-h periodicity of disease onset (Fig. 1) and physiologic processes (Fig. 2) is well established, the degree to which this periodicity results from a true, endogenous circadian rhythm versus the daily rest-activity cycle is only partially characterized. Cortisol secretion, for example, is well known to be an endogenous circadian process not dependent on daily activity [49], while the morning platelet aggregability increase is abolished if the subjects remain at bedrest [44]. The rest-activity cycle appears to be a major determinant of disease onset since adjustment for time of awakening shows that infarction onset [15] and transient ischemia increases [23] follow awakening, but such adjustment could also align the population for their endogenous circadian rhythms. There may also be an interaction between circadian and rest-activity cycles; for example, assumption of the upright posture leading to sympathetic activation may be more likely to cause intense vasoconstriction when endogenously controlled cortisol levels are high [50].

Although attention has been focused on the morning as the time of peak incidence of disease onset, it is likely that similar physiological processes trigger disease onset at other times of the day. A secondary evening peak in infarct onset observed in the MILIS data may result from synchronization of the population for a trigger such as the evening meal. For other periods of the day, exposure of the population to potential triggers is random, and no other prominent peaks of incidence are observed.

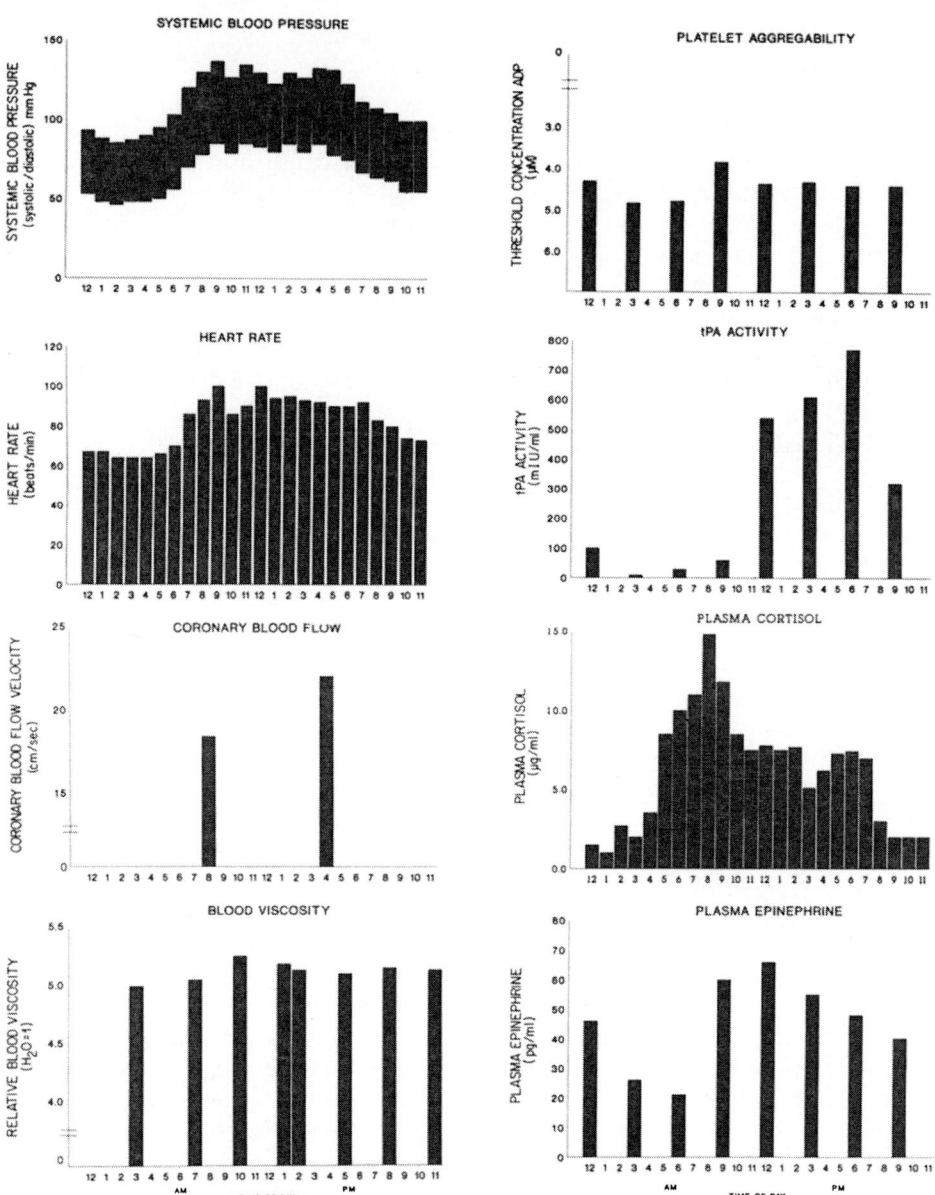

Fig. 2. The variation during a 24-h period of eight physiologic processes possibly contributing to the increased morning frequently of acute cardiovascular disease. (Reprinted from [57], with permission)

Ability of Agents that Block Potential Triggering Processes to Prevent Myocardial Infarction

The theories advanced above are indirectly supported by the demonstrated efficacy of aspirin therapy and beta-adrenergic blockade in preventing myocardial infarction [51, 52]. Aspirin, which presumably acts primarily as an antiplatelet agent, is thought to reduce the occurrence of myocardial infarction by preventing coronary thrombosis [51]. In a recent detailed analysis of this beneficial effect by Ridker et al. it was found that aspirin exerted a selective effect – a 59 % reduction – during the morning interval when platelet activity is increased [53]. This prevention of infarction by elimination of a potential triggering mechanism – a platelet activity surge – supports the assertion that platelet activity surges are harmful, suggests that increased basal platelet activity in individuals is an unrecognized risk factor for infarction, and demonstrates the potential value of identifying other triggering processes.

Beta-adrenergic blocking agents have been shown to prevent myocardial infarction and sudden cardiac death even though these agents do not have potent antithrombotic or antiarrhythmic properties. A clue to the mechanism is provided by the observations in the MILIS and the ISAM databases that beta-blockade eliminated the morning peak in incidence of myocardial infarction [7, 12]. In addition, in the Beta Blocker Heart Attack Trial there was a morning increase in sudden cardiac death in the placebo group but not in the group randomly assigned to beta-blockade therapy, suggesting that the beneficial effect was achieved by blockade of the morning surge in sympathetic activity [54]. Beta-blockade, but not a short-acting calcium blocker, has been shown to attenuate the morning increase in silent myocardial ischemia [55], and a recent review has summarized the inability of previously available calcium blocker preparations to provide a cardioprotective effect [56]. It has been suggested that the beta-blockers may prevent rupture of atherosclerotic plaques, just as they are considered to exert a beneficial effect in dissecting aneurysm by prevention of rupture of the aortic wall. With increased knowledge of triggering mechanisms, it is likely that the impressive gains already achieved by aspirin and beta-blockade therapy can be increased.

General Theory of Triggering of Coronary Thrombosis

Our group has proposed a general hypothesis of the manner in which daily activities might trigger coronary thrombosis [57]. The hypothesis presented in Fig. 3 adds the concept of triggering activities to the general scheme of the role of thrombosis in the acute coronary syndromes advanced by Falk [33], Davies and Thomas [58], Fuster et al. [59] and Willerson et al. [60]. It is proposed that the initial step in the process leading directly to coronary thrombosis is the development, with advancing age, of what can be termed a *vulnerable* atherosclerotic plaque. Plaque vulnerability is defined functionally as the susceptibility of a plaque to rupture. Development of such vulnerability is a poorly understood process, but it is presumably a dynamic, potentially reversible disorder caused by changes in the constituents of the plaque, its blood supply via vasa vasorum, and/or the functional integrity of the overlying endothelium. The

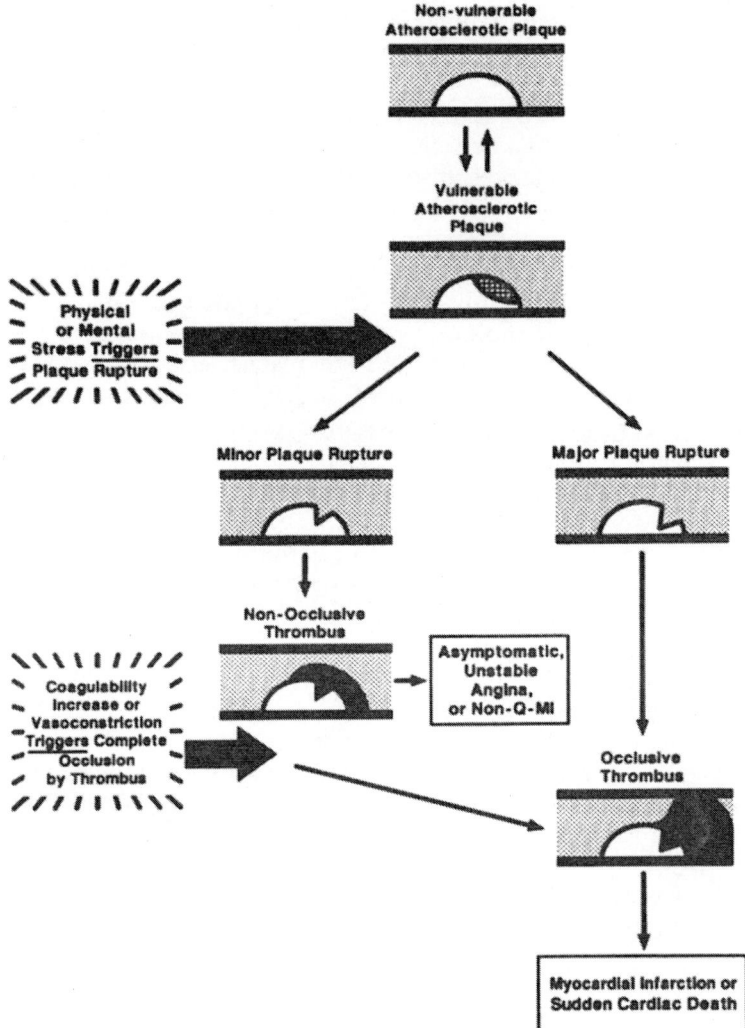

Fig. 3. A hypothetical presentation of the manner in which daily activities may trigger coronary thrombosis. Three triggering mechanisms – (a) physical or mental stress producing hemodynamic changes leading to plaque rupture, (b) a coagulability increase, and (c) vasoconstriction – have been added to the well-known scheme depicting the role of coronary thrombosis in unstable angina, myocardial infarction, and sudden cardiac death. See text for detailed discussion. (Reprinted from [51] with permission)

theory that onset of thrombosis is unrelated to daily activities would presumably attribute disease onset solely to evolution of the plaque, and the diagram would therefore lead directly from the plaque to occlusive coronary thrombosis. In the present formulation, however, it is proposed that onset might frequently begin when a physical or mental stress triggers a hemodynamic change sufficient to rupture a vulnerable plaque. (If such a trigger does not occur during vulnerability, the plaque may change and become nonvulnerable).

The rupture in the plaque may be major or minor, depending on factors such as the amount and type of collagen exposed [61]. A major plaque rupture produces a thrombogenic focus sufficiently intense to cause occlusive coronary thrombosis leading directly to myocardial infarction or sudden cardiac death. A minor rupture leads only to a mural thrombus which fails to produce or leads to unstable angina or non-Q-wave myocardial infarction. At this point, mental stress or physical activity may trigger increases in coagulability or vasoconstriction [62, 63]. Such a coagulability increase may trigger growth of the thrombus, or vasoconstriction may lead to complete occlusion of an already compromised lumen leading to infarction or sudden death. Since normal individuals and even patients with coronary artery disease are constantly exposed to potentially triggering activities which do not produce coronary thrombosis, it seems likely that development of plaque vulnerability is the rarest event in the chain of causation described above.

It is likely that there is an inverse relationship between the degree of plaque vulnerability and the intensity of the triggering stimulus required to produce rupture. For instance, an elderly individual with a severe fixed stenosis in a coronary artery and an extremely vulnerable plaque may develop thrombosis with only a minor stress, while a young individual with only a luminal irregularity might require a major stress (such as heavy lifting producing markedly increased arterial pressure) to trigger plaque rupture and coronary thrombosis. Sumiyoshi et al. reported that younger patients were more likely than older patients to report unusual stress prior to onset, but control data on the relative frequency of unusual stress in older versus younger individuals are not available [8]. A synergistic combination of triggering activities may account for thrombosis. For example, the combination of physical exertion (producing a minor plaque rupture) followed by cigarette smoking (producing an increase in coronary artery vasoconstriction and a relatively hypercoagulable state) [64] may be needed to cause disease onset. Thus, the onset of infarction in some cases may be the result of the unfortunate simultaneous occurrence of several events each by itself of little consequence, but catastrophic when occurring together.

Significance

The primary immediate value of recognition of the diurnal variation of acute onset of myocardial infarction is the emphasis that can be placed on pharmacologic protection during the morning hours for patients already receiving anti-ischemic therapy. Although no scientific studies have been performed to test the hypothesis, it seems reasonable that long-acting anti-ischemic agents would have an advantage over short-acting agents in providing protection against myocardial infarction in the morning when the effects of short-acting agents taken the night before may begin to attenuate.

The finding that infarcts appear to be triggered in the morning raises questions about the desirability of exercise in the morning. At present the evidence that exercise is beneficial in reducing the risk of infarction [65] is substantial, and although theoretical concerns can be raised, there is no evidence that exercise in the morning is more hazardous than exercise at other times of the day. A controlled trial of thousands of individuals randomized to exercise in the morning or the evening would be needed to resolve the issue conclusively.

Even complete elimination of the morning increase in onset of myocardial infarction by optimal timing of exercise and effective therapy would prevent only a small fraction of the total morbidity and mortality caused by this disease. Although the incidence of disease onset is greatest in the 6 A.M. to noon period, the majority of infarcts occur at other times of the day, and their prevention requires a broader approach. For this reason, it is likely that the primary significance of the recognition of diurnal variation of disease onset is the support that it provides for the broader concept that the onset of infarction *at any time of the day* is frequently triggered by activities of the patient. This concept provides a number of clues to the mechanisms of disease onset – clues which suggest a value of studies ranging from the epidemiologic to the molecular level.

On the epidemiologic level, studies must be conducted in which patients who experience a nonfatal myocardial infarction are interviewed to determine whether the event had an identifiable trigger. Since potentially triggering activities occur frequently without producing an event, the studies must be controlled for the frequency of potential triggers at times when an event did not occur.

The certainty with which an activity can be identified as a trigger will also vary in individual cases. In a patient whose plaque is only slightly vulnerable, the activity required to produce disease onset may be extreme, and the activity can be recognized as a trigger by its intensity. Other features which may aid in the recognition of an activity as a trigger are its occurrence immediately before the event, its ability to produce physiologic changes likely to trigger thrombosis, and its absence as part of the patient's routine activity. However, in a patient with an extremely vulnerable plaque, even nonstrenuous, routine, daily activities such as eating a heavy meal may be sufficient to trigger the cascade leading to infarction [66]. In such instances, it may be impossible to identify the triggering activity even though it was present. Thus, the group of patients with *identifiable* triggers will be a subset of those in whom external triggering actually occurred.

On the clinical level, increased study of the relationship between daily activities and potentially triggering physiologic responses could clarify the manner in which these processes cause disease onset.

On the basic science level, there is a need for characterization of the control mechanisms of potentially adverse and potentially beneficial physiologic changes. When these mechanisms are understood more fully, it may be possible to eliminate potentially detrimental surges in arterial pressure, vasoconstriction, and coagulability that contribute to disease onset and increase the activity of potentially beneficial processes such as the fibrinolytic system. Further study is also needed of the factors determining plaque vulnerability, and the possibility that reduction in clinical events recently achieved by marked lowering of plasma cholesterol [67] might result not only from reduction of the tendency of coronary artery stenosis but partially from a reduction in the formation of lipid pools within plaques that might increase the susceptibility of the plaque to rupture [32]. A more complete understanding of triggering mechanisms should permit progress in prevention of myocardial infarction. The means of prevention would not be to eliminate potential triggering activities – an undesirable and unattainable goal – but to design regimens that can be evaluated in randomized studies for their ability to sever the link between a potential triggering activity and an acute cardiac event.

Acknowledgement. We are grateful for the assistance of Ms. Kathleen Carney in the preparation of the manuscript.

References

1. Obraztsov VP, Strazhesko ND (1910) The symptomatology and diagnosis of coronary thrombosis. In: Vorobeva VA, Konchalovski MP (eds) Works of the 1st congress of Russian therapists. Comradeship typography of Mamontov AE, pp 26–43
2. Fitzhugh G, Hamilton BE (1933) Coronary occlusion and fatal angina pectoris. Study of the immediate causes and their prevention. JAMA 100:475–80
3. Sproul J (1936) A general practitioner's views on the treatment of angina pectoris. N Engl J Med 215:443–452
4. Parkinson J, Bedford DE (1928) Cardiac infarction and coronary thrombosis. Lancet 1:4–11
5. Phipps C (1936) Contributory causes of coronary thrombosis. JAMA 106:761–762
6. Master AM (1960) The role of effort and occupation (including physicians) in coronary occlusion. JAMA 174:942–948
7. Muller JE, Stone PH, Turi ZG, Rutherford JD, Czeisler CA, Parker C, Poole WK, Passamani E, Roberts R, Robertson T, Sobel BE, Willerson JT, Braunwald E, and the MILIS Study Group (1985) Circadian variation in the frequency of onset of acute myocardial infarction. N Engl J Med 313:1315–1322
8. Sumiyoshi T, Haze K, Saito M, Fukami K, Goto Y, Hiramori K (1986) Evaluation of clinical factors involved in onset of myocardial infarction. Jpn Circ J 50:164–173
9. Tofler GH, Stone PH, Maclure M, Edelman E, Davis VG, Robertson T, Antman EM, Muller JE, and the MILIS Study Group (1989) Analysis of possible triggers of acute myocardial infarction (MILIS Study). Am J Cardiol 66:22–27
10. Muller JE, Tofler GH, Edelman E (1989) Probable triggers of onset of acute myocardial infarction. Clin Cardiol 12:473–476
11. Maclure M (1991) The case-crossover design: a method for studying transient effects on the risk of acute events. Am J Epidemiol 133:144–153
12. Willich SN, Linderer T, Wegscheider K, Leizorovicz MD, Alamercery I, Schroder R, and the ISAM Study Group (1989) Increased morning incidence of myocardial infarction in the ISAM Study: absence with prior beta-adrenergic blockade. Circulation 80:853–858
13. Thompson DR, Blandford RL, Sutton TW, Marchant PR (1985) Time of onset of chest pain in acute myocardial infarction. Int J Cardiol 7:139–46
14. Hjalmarson A, Gilpin E, Nicod P, Dittrich H, Henning H, Engler R, Blacky AR, Smith SC Jr, Ricou F, Ross J Jr (1989) Differing circadian patterns of symptom onset in subgroups of patients with acute myocardial infarction. Circulation 80:267–275
15. Goldberg R, Brady P, Chen Z, Gore J, Flessas A, Greenberg J, Thedosiou G, Dalen J, Muller JE (1990) Time of onset of acute myocardial infarction after awakening (abstract). Am J Cardiol 66:140–144
16. Muller JE, Ludmer PL, Willich SN, Tofler GH, Aylmer G, Klangos I, Stone PH (1987) Circadian variation in the frequency of sudden cardiac death. Circulation 75:131–138
17. Willich SN, Levy D, Rocco MB, Tofler GH, Stone PH, Muller JE (1987) Circadian variation in the incidence of sudden cardiac death in the Framingham Heart Study Population. Am J Cardiol 60:801–806
18. French AJ, Dock W (1944) Fatal coronary arteriosclerosis in young soldiers. JAMA 124:1233–1237
19. Moritz AR, Zamcheck N (1946) Sudden and unexpected deaths of young soldiers. Diseases responsible for such deaths during World War II. Arch Pathol 42:459–494
20. Tsementzis SA, Gill JS, Hitchcock ER, Gill SK, Beevers DG (1985) Diurnal variation of and activity during the onset of stroke. Neurosurgery 17:901–904

21. Marler JR, Price TR, Clark GL, Muller JE, Robertson T, Mohr JP, Hier DB, Wolf PA, Caplan LR, Foulkes MA (1989) Morning increase in onset of ischemic stroke. Stroke 20:473–476
22. Selwyn AP, Shea M, Deanfield JE, Wilson R, Horlock P (1986) Character of transient ischemia in angina pectoris. Am J Cardiol 58:21B–25B
23. Rocco MB, Barry J, Campbell S, Nabel E, Cook EF, Goldman L, Selwyn AP (1987) Circadian variation of transient myocardial ischemia in patients with coronary artery disease. Circulation 75:395–400
24. Nademanee K, Intarachot V, Josephson MA, Singh BN (1987) Circadian variation in occurrence of transient overt and silent myocardial ischemia in chronic stable angina and comparison with Prinzmetal's angina in men. Am J Cardiol 60:494–498
25. Barry J, Selwyn AP, Nabel EG, Rocco MB, Mead K, Campbell S, Rebecca G (1988) Frequency of ST-segment depression produced by mental stress in stable angina pectoris from coronary artery disease. Am J Cardiol 61:989–993
26. DeWood MA, Spores J, Notske R, Mouser LT, Burroughs R, Golden MS, Lang HT (1980) Prevalence of total coronary occlusion during the early hours of transmural myocardial infarction. N Engl J Med 303:897–902
27. Ambrose JA, Winters SL, Stern A, Eng A, Teichholz LE, Gorlin R, Fuster V (1985) Angiographic morphology and the pathogenesis of unstable angina pectoris. J Am Coll Cardiol 5:609–616
28. Sherman CT, Litvack F, Grundfest W, Lee M, Hickey A, Chaux A, Kass R, Blanche C, Matloff J, Morgenstern L, Ganz W, Swan HJC, Forrester J (1986) Coronary angioscopy in patients with unstable angina pectoris. N Engl J Med 315:913–919
29. Constantinides P (1966) Plaque fissure in human coronary thrombosis. J Atheroscler Res 1:1–17
30. Nakagawa S, Hanada Y, Koiwaya Y, Tanaka K (1988) Angiographic features in the infarct-related artery after intracoronary urokinase followed by prolonged anticoagulation: role of ruptured atheromatous plaque and adherent thrombus in acute myocardial infarction in vivo. Circulation 78:1335–1344
31. Barger AC, Beeuwkes R, Lainey LL, Silverman KJ (1984) Hypothesis: vasa vasorum and neovascularization of human coronary arteries. N Engl J Med 310:175–177
32. Richardson PD, Davies MJ, Born GVR (1989) Influence of plaque configuration and stress distribution on fissuring of coronary atherosclerotic plaques. Lancet 2:941–944
33. Falk E (1983) Plaque rupture with severe pre-existing stenosis precipitating coronary thrombosis. Br Heart J 50:127–134
34. Brown BG, Gallery CA, Badger RS, Kennedy JW, Mathey D, Bolson EL, Dodge HT (1986) Incomplete lysis of thrombus in the moderate underlying atherosclerotic lesion during intracoronary infusion of streptokinase for acute myocardial infarction: quantitative angiographic observations. Circulation 73:653–661
35. Little WL, Constantinescu M, Applegate RJ, Kutcher MA, Burrows MT, Kahl FR, Santamore WP (1988) Can coronary angiography predict the site of a subsequent myocardial infarction in patients with mild-to-moderate coronary artery disease. Circulation 78:1157–1166
36. Haft JI, Haik BJ, Goldstein JE (1987) Catastrophic progression of coronary artery lesions, the common mechanism for coronary disease progression (abstract). Circulation 76 [Suppl IV]:IV-168
37. Rapold HJ, Haeberli A, Kuemmerli H, Weiss M, Baur HR, Straub WP (1989) Fibrin formation and platelet activation in patients with myocardial infarction and normal coronary arteries. Eur Heart J 10:323–333
38. Oliver MF (1986) Prevention of coronary heart disease – propaganda, promises, problems, and prospects. Circulation 73:1–9
39. Millar-Craig MW, Bishop CN, Raftery EB (1978) Circadian variation of blood pressure. Lancet 1:795–797
40. Fujita M, Franklin D (1987) Diurnal changes in coronary blood flow in conscious dogs. Circulation 76:488–491

41. Vita JA, Treasure CB, Ganz P, Cox DA, Fish RD, Selwyn AP (1989) Control of shear stress in the epicardial coronary arteries of humans: impairment by atherosclerosis. J Am Coll Cardiol 14:1193–1199
42. Badimon L, Badimon JJ (1989) Mechanisms of arterial thrombosis in nonparallel stream-lines: platelet thrombi grow on the apex of stenotic severely injured vessel wall: experimental study in pig model. J Clin Invest 4:1134–1144
43. Ehrly AM, Jung G (1973) Circadian rhythm of human blood viscosity. Biorheology 10:577–583
44. Tofler GH, Brezinski DA, Schafer AI, Czeisler CA, Rutherford JD, Willich SN, Gleason RE, Williams GH, Muller JE (1987) Concurrent morning increase in platelet aggregability and the risk of myocardial infarction and sudden cardiac death. N Engl J Med 316:1514–1518
45. Brezinski DA, Tofler GH, Muller JE, Pohjola-Sintonen S, Willich SN, Schafer AI, Czeisler CA, Williams GH (1988) Morning increase in platelet aggregability: association with assumption of the upright posture. Circulation 78:35–40
46. Rosing DR, Brakman P, Redwood DR, Goldstein RE, Beiser GD, Astrup T, Epstein SE (1970) Blood fibrinolytic activity in man: diurnal variation and the response to varying intensities of exercise. Circ Res 27:171–184
47. Andreotti F, Davies GJ, Hackett DR, Khan MI, De Bart ACW, Aber VR, Maseri A, Kluft C (1988) Major circadian fluctuations in fibrinolytic factors and possible relevance to time of onset of myocardial infarction, sudden cardiac death, and stroke. Am J Cardiol 62:635–637
48. Speiser W, Langer W, Pschaick A, Selmayr E, Ibe B, Nowacki PE, Muller-Berghaus G (1988) Increased blood fibrinolytic activity after physical exercise: comparative study in individuals with different sporting activities and in patients after myocardial infarction taking part in a rehabilitation sports program. Thromb Res 51:543–555
49. Weitzman ED, Fukushima D, Nogeire C, Roffwang H, Gallagher TF, Hellman L (1971) Twenty-four hour pattern of the episodic secretion of cortisol in normal subjects. J Clin Endocrinol 33:14–22
50. Sudhir K, Jennings GL, Esler MD, Korner PI, Blombery PA, Lambert GW, Scoggins B, Whitworth JA (1989) Hydrocortisone-induced hypertension in humans: pressor responsiveness and sympathetic function. Hypertension 13:416–421
51. Steering Committee of the Physicians' Health Study Research Group (1989) Final report on the aspirin component of the ongoing Physicians' Health Study. N Engl J Med 321:129–135
52. Beta-blocker Heart Attack Trial Research Group (1982) A randomized trial of propranolol in patients with acute myocardial infarction. Mortality results. JAMA 247:1707–1714
53. Ridker PM, Manson JE, Buring JE, Muller JE, Hennekens CH (1991) Circadian variation of acute myocardial infarction and the effect of low-dose aspirin in a randomized trial of physicians. Circulation (to be published)
54. Peters RW, Muller JE, Goldstein S, Byington R, Friedman LM (1988) Propranolol and the circadian variation in the frequency of sudden cardiac death: the BHAT experience (abstract). Circulation 76 [Suppl IV]:IV-364
55. Mulcahy D, Keegan J, Cunningham D, Quyyumi A, Crear P, Park A, Wright C, Fox K (1988) Circadian variation of total ischemic burden and its alteration with anti-anginal agents. Lancet 2:755–759
56. Held PH, Yusuf S, Furberg CD (1989) Calcium channel blockers in acute myocardial infarction and unstable angina: an overview. Br Med J 299:1187–1192
57. Muller JE, Tofler GH, Stone PH (1989) Circadian variation and triggers of onset of acute cardiovascular disease. Circulation 79:733–743
58. Davies MJ, Thomas AC (1985) Plaque fissuring – the cause of acute myocardial infarction, sudden ischemic death, and crescendo angina. Br Heart J 53:363–373
59. Fuster V, Steele PM, Chesebro JH (1985) Role of platelets and thrombosis in coronary atherosclerotic disease and sudden death. J Am Coll Cardiol 5 [Suppl]:175B–184B
60. Willerson JT, Campbell WB, Winniford MD, Schmitz J, Apprill P, Firth BG, Ashton J, Smitherman T, Bush L, Buja LM (1984) Conversion from chronic to acute coronary artery disease: speculation regarding mechanisms. Am J Cardiol 54:1349–1354 (editorial)
61. Badimon L, Badimon JJ, Turitto VT, Vallabhajosula S, Fuster V (1988) Platelet thrombus formation on collagen type I. A model of deep vessel injury. Influence of blood rheology, von Willebrand factor, and blood coagulation. Circulation 78:1431–1432

62. Rebecca G, Wagner R, Zebede T, D'Adamo A, Hanlon B, Sandor T, Ganz P, Selwyn A (1986) Pathogenetic mechanisms causing transient myocardial ischemia with mental arousal in patients with coronary artery disease (abstract). Clin Res 34:338A

63. Ogston D (1964) Fibrinolytic activity and anxiety and its relation to coronary artery disease. J Psychosom Med 8:219–222

64. Belch JJF, McArdle BM, Burns P, Lowe GDO, Forbes CD (1984) The effects of acute smoking on platelet behaviour, fibrinolysis, and haemorrheology in habitual smokers. Thromb Haemost 51:6–8

65. Ekelund LG, Haskell WL, Johnson JL, Whaley FS, Criqui MH, Sheps DS (1988) Physical fitness as a predictor of cardiovascular mortality in asymptomatic North American men. The Lipids Research Clinics Mortality Follow-up Study. N Engl J Med 319:1379–1384

66. Kelbaek H, Gjorup T, Christensen NJ, Munck O, Godtfredsen J (1989) Central hemodynamic changes after ingestion of a meal in patients with coronary artery disease. Arch Intern Med 149:363–365

67. Brown BG, Lind JT, Schaeder SM, Kaplan CA, Dodge HT, Albers JJ (1989) Niacin or lovostatin, combined with colestipol, regress coronary atherosclerosis and prevent clinical events in men with elevated apolipoprotein B (abstract). Circulation 80 [Suppl II]:II-267

Daily Variations in ST Segment Depression in Patients with Coronary Heart Disease

G. Blümchen and M. Jetté

Introduction

For some time, we have observed and reported on what appears to be a diurnal rhythm, or a temporal variation, with respect to episodes of angina pectoris and ST segment deviation during exercise stress tests when conducted at different times during the day (Henkels and Blümchen 1977; Henkels et al. 1977). Patients who were tested during the morning hours were more likely to develop angina, dyspnea, exhaustion, and ST segment depression, and at a lower threshold, than when tested during the late morning or afternoon.

Recently, a number of authors have reported on an apparent diurnal variation in the manifestations of acute myocardial infarctions and sudden death. These events would seem to begin more often during the morning hours in comparison to other time periods (Muller et al. 1987, 1989; Willich et al. 1987, 1989 a, b; Bogarty and Waters 1988; Muller 1989; Hohnloser et al. 1990) with a lower peak in the evening between 1800 and 0000 hours (Mulcahy et al. 1988; Hjalmarson et al. 1989). However, in their study, Gnecchi Ruscone et al. (1987) indicated that the lowest percentage of patients developing acute myocardial infarction was during the period of 0000–0600 hours while there were no significant differences in frequency distribution during the remainder of the day. Also, a report by Barash et al. (1989) indicated that although the percentage of patients admitted to their hospital from 1200 to 1600 hours accounted for only 17% of their caseload, these patients showed a significantly higher incidence of acute myocardial ischemia (76% versus 28%) and death (47% versus 9%) than patients admitted at other times of the day. Notwithstanding, utilizing ambulatory monitoring of the electrocardiogram, Deanfield et al. (1983) demonstrated quite convincingly that the frequency of symptomatic and asymptomatic episodes of ischemic ST segment depression in patients with coronary disease is maximal in the early morning hours.

Early Morning Susceptibility to Myocardial Ischemia

This observation of a diurnal cycle in ischemia became apparent when we started evaluating the prolonged effects of the new long-acting anti-ischemic

Schmidt/Engel/Blümchen (Eds.)
Temporal Variations of the Cardiovascular System
© Springer-Verlag Berlin Heidelberg 1992

drugs, where repeated exercise tests were administered during the course of a 12- to 16-h period. A clinical study was designed to assess the effect of nifedipine on work tolerance in patients with known coronary insufficiency (Henkels et al. 1977). Twenty patients were evaluated on a progressive cycle ergometer test in the supine position four times during the course of a single day: 0800, 1100, 1400, and 1700 hours. Significant differences were seen among the four tests. Basically, the lowest workloads achieved by the patients were those performed at 0800 hours while the best workloads were those performed at 1100 hours. In addition, mean work tolerance in these patients was superior when the test was repeated on a 2nd day, a phenomenon which we attributed to an adaptation effect. As a result of this study, we cautioned clinicians to take into account the diurnal effect on work tolerance and ischemia in coronary patients when prescribing medication, due to the apparent vulnerability of patients in the early morning hours.

Shortly after, Yasue et al. (1978) reported the results of their study involving 13 patients with Prinzmetal's variant angina. The patients performed a first treadmill exercise test between 0500 and 0800 hours and a second test between 1500 and 1600 hours. All of their 13 patients reported anginal pain during the morning session, which was shown to be associated with ST segment elevations. However, during the afternoon testing, not only did the patients achieve a higher work intensity, but only 2 of the 13 patients reported angina. The authors reported that angiographic evaluation in similar patients indicated that epicardial coronary vessel caliber was smaller in the early morning, and that nitroglycerin appeared to have a greater dilating effect in the morning than in the afternoon. On the basis of their studies, Yasue et al. (1989) suggested that temporal variations in vasomotor tone of the large coronary arteries, via alpha-adrenergic-mediated vasoconstriction, would partially explain the clinical variability in symptoms and exercise response in patients with variant angina. As indicated by Bassenge and Busse (1988), under normal physiological conditions, the tone of the epicardial coronary arteries plays a minimal role in the regulation and distribution of myocardial blood flow. However, under pathological conditions and especially in coronary heart disease even small changes in tone may play a significant role.

Mattioli et al. (1986) studied 187 subjects for the diurnal rhythm of chest pain attacks for 7 days without therapy (placebo) and 7 days with therapy (nifedipine, metropolol, or isosorbide dinitrate). During the placebo period most of the attacks occurred between 0500 and 0800. Although a reduction of painful episodes was observed during the period with therapy, the diurnal distribution remained unchanged.

Rocco et al. (1987a) have reported that although the number of episodes of ischemia that occurred during the morning hours was approximately twice the number that occurred during the evening hours, there were no significant differences in maximal ST depression, heart rate at onset of ST depression, or level of physical activity. Notwithstanding, when they established the threshold heart rate at ST depression, patients were more likely to develop ischemia when they reached this threshold during the morning hours than in the evening. It was suggested that this observation could possibly account for patients demonstrating more ischemia in the morning than in the evening hours.

Levy et al. (1987) investigated the diurnal variation in pulmonary artery diastolic pressure in 6 normal subjects, 18 patients with coronary heart disease, 5 with variant angina, and 6 with syndrome X. Episodes of ST segment change occurred predominantly in the early morning (0000–0600 hours) in variant angina whereas in syndrome X all episodes were recorded during the day. In coronary artery disease, both painful and painless episodes were distributed throughout the day. Their findings indicated that pulmonary artery diastolic pressure and therefore left ventricular enddiastolic pressure, is greatest in the early morning and would represent the background hemodynamic state in which other factors lead to myocardial ischemia during the hours of vulnerability.

Recently, Khurmi and Raftery (1988) examined diurnal variations in 41 patients aged 53–75 years with established chronic stable angina on two occasions 5 days apart, at 1000 and 1600 hours. On day 1, the mean $\pm$ standard error of the mean exercise time was 5.0 ± 0.4 min at 1000 hours and 5.1 ± 0.5 min at 1600 hours, while on the 2nd day it was 5.6 ± 0.4 min at 1000 hours and 5.5 ± 0.4 min at 1600 hours. There were no statistical differences among these values. Also, the time to the development of 1-mm ST segment depression and maximal ST depression did not show any statistical differences during any of the testing sessions. Heart rate at rest was 79 ± 3 bpm at 1000 hours and 81 ± 3 bpm at 1600 hours on day 1, while on day 2 it was 78 ± 2 bpm at 1000 hours and 80 ± 3 bpm at 1600 hours (non-significant). There were also no significant changes observed in maximal heart rate or rate-pressure product at peak exercise.

Fox et al. (1989), in an experiment designed to study evidence for the occurrence, pathophysiology, and diurnal distribution of ischemic episodes, demonstrated that episodes of ST segment depression show a diurnal rhythm similar to that seen for heart rate and cathecholamine release. The basic pattern showed a low incidence of ischemia at night followed by a primary peak on rising, a decrease at midday, and then a secondary peak in the evening, with a final decrease again at night.

In summary, a number of studies which have evaluated myocardial ischemia during the course of repeated testing on the same day report that the ST segment depression, particularly during exercise, appears to be greater during the early morning hours. Furthermore, the exercise intensity that can be tolerated during this period is lower and occurs at a lower threshold. These observations would indicate that patients are more vulnerable during this period of the day. This is of particular interest, since this period is similar to that reported for onset of myocardial infarction and cardiac sudden death. Whether a risk exists for coronary patients to participate in exercise programs during the early morning hours has yet to be investigated.

Pathophysiology of Early Morning Susceptibility Ischemia

A number of factors have been advanced to explain the higher incidence of early morning myocardial ischemia (Gottlieb 1988). At the root of this explanation is a disturbance in the balance between myocardial oxygen supply (primary ischemia) and demand (secondary ischemia) or both (mixed ischemia) during the early morning hours (Cohn 1986). Both internal and external factors are suspected (Rocco et al. 1987b).

With respect to external factors, early morning hours are associated at times with a rude awakening, changes in environmental stimuli such as light, ingestion of food (at times saturated with fat), caffeine, and in some cases nicotine. These stimuli may be accompanied with a reacquaintance of one's occupational and personal problems. Another major external factor relevant to this topic is the performance of physical activity including the exercise stressor utilized in the evaluation of myocardial ischemia.

A number of cardiovascular endogenous responses, due to enhanced sympathetic activity, have been reported to be greater in the early morning hours, such as plasma cortisol and cathecholamines, platelet aggregation, and CK-MB isoenzyme along with a decrease in fibrinolytic activity. These changes have also been shown to cause constriction of epicardial coronary vessels, hypercoagulation, coronary spasm, and increased left ventricular end-diastolic pressure resulting in a decrease in the regulation and distribution of myocardial blood flow.

Conclusions

Coronary patients appear to be more prone to myocardial ischemia during the early morning hours and particularly so during exercise testing. The pathophysiology of this phenomenon remains unclear. However, it appears to be related to enhanced sympathetic activity leading to an increase in the sensitivity of epicardial coronary vessel tone. This would result in either a disturbance in the oxygen supply and demand ratio and a consequent disturbance in the regulation and distribution of myocardial blood flow or to coronary spasm.

Acknowledgements. We would like to extend our appreciation to the Verein zur Bekämpfung von Gefäßerkrankungen e. V., Engelskirschen, and the LVA Rheinprovinz, Düsseldorf, FRG.

References

Barash D, Silverman RA, Gennis P, Budner N, Matos M, Gallagher EJ (1989) Circadian variation in the frequency of myocardial infarction and death associated with acute pulmonary edema. J Emerg Med 7:119–121

Bassenge E, Busse R (1988) Endothelial modulation of coronary tone. Prog Cardiovasc Dis 30:349–380

Bogarty P, Waters DD (1988) Circadian patterns in coronary disease: the mournfulness of morning. Can J Cardiol 4:5–11

Cohn PF (1986) Total ischemic burden: definition, mechanisms, and therapeutic implications. Am J Med 81:2–6

Deanfield JE, Selwyn AP, Chierchia S, Maseri A, Ribiero P, Kricler S, Morgan M (1983) Myocardial ischaemia during daily life in patients with stable angina: its relation to symptoms and heart rate changes. Lancet 2:753–758

Fox K, Mulcahy D, Keegan J, Wright C (1989) Circadian patterns of myocardial ischemia. Am Heart J 118:1084–1086

Gottlieb SO (1988) Circadian patterns of myocardial ischemia: pathophysiologic and therapeutic considerations. J Cardiovasc Pharmacol 12 [Suppl 7]:S18–21

Gnecchi Ruscone T, Guzzeti S, Piccaluga E, Di Mattia D (1987) Circadian variation in the frequency of myocardial infarction and death associated with acute pulmonary edema. Int J Cardiol 16:161–167

Henkels U, Blümchen G (1977) Tageszeitliche Schwankungen der Belastungs-Koronar-insuffizienz. Münch Med Wochenschr 119:59–63

Henkels U, Blümchen G, Ebner F (1977) Zur Problematik von Belastungsprüfungen in Abhängigkeit von der Tageszeit bei Patienten mit Koronarinsuffizienz. Herz Kreisl 9: 343–347

Hjalmarson A, Gilpin EA, Nicod P, Dittrich H, Henning H, Engler R, Blacky AR, Smith SC Jr, Ricou F, Ross J Jr (1989) Differing circadian patterns of symptom onset in subgroups of patients with acute myocardial infarction. Circulation 80:267–275

Hohnloser SH, Just H, Zehender M (1990) Zirkadiane Variationen verschiedener Manifesta-tionsformen der koronaren Herzkrankheit. Intensivmedizin 27:451–453

Khurmi NS, Raftery EB (1988) Lack of diurnal variation in maximal symptom-limited exercise test response in chronic stable angina. Am J Cardiol 61:38–42

Levy RD, Cunninghan D, Shapiro LM, Wright C, Mockus L, Fox KM (1987) Diurnal variation in left ventricular function: a study of patients with myocardial ischemia, syndrome X and of normal controls. Br Heart J 57:148–153

Mattioli G, Cioni G, Andreoli C (1986) Time sequence of anginal pain. Clin Cardiol 9:165–169

Mulcahy D, Keegan J, Cunningham D, Quyyumi A, Crean P, Park A (1988) Circadian variation of total ischaemic burden and its alteration with anti-anginal agents. Lancet 2:755–759

Muller JE (1989) Morning increase of onset of myocardial infarction. Implications concerning triggering events. Cardiology 76:96–104

Muller JE, Ludmer PL, Willich SN, Tofler GH, Aylmer G, Klangos I, Stone PH (1987) Circadian variation in the frequency of sudden cardiac death. Circulation 75:131–138

Muller JE, Tofler GH, Stone PH (1989) Circadian variation and triggers of onset of acute cardiovascular disease. Circulation 79:733–743

Rocco MB, Nabel EG, Selwyn AP (1987a) Circadian rhythms and coronary artery disease. Am J Cardiol 59:13C–17C

Rocco MB, Barry J, Campbell S, Nabel E, Cook EF, Goldman L, Selwyn AP (1987b) Circadian variation of transient myocardial ischemia in patients with coronary artery disease. Circulation 75:395–400

Willich SN, Levy D, Rocco MB, Tofler GH, Stone PH, Muller JC (1987) Circadian variation in the incidence of sudden cardiac death in the Framingham Heart Study population. Am J Cardiol 60:801–806

Willich SN, Linderer T, Wegscheider K, Schröder R (1989a) Circadian variation in the incidence of myocardial infarction. New perceptions about the mechanisms of acute coronary disease. Dtsch Med Wochenschr 114:613–617

Willich SN, Linderer T, Wegscheider K, Leizorovicz A, Alamercery I, Schröder R (1989b) Increased morning incidence of myocardial infarction in the ISAM Study: absence with prior beta-adrenergic blockade. Circulation 80:853–858

Yasue H, Omote S, Takizawa A, Nagao M, Miwa K, Kato H, Tanaka S, Akiyama F (1978) Circadian variation of exercise capacity in patients with Prinzmetal's variant angina: role of exercise-induced coronary arterial spasm. Circulation 59:938–948

Yasue H, Ogawa H, Okumura K (1989) Coronary artery spasm in the genesis of myocardial ischemia. Am J Cardiol 63:29E–32E

Nocturnal Hemodynamic Responses to Chronic, Mild Atrial Demand Pacing in Nonhuman Primates

B. T. Engel

We have described a stable diurnal pattern of hemodynamic function in monkeys characterized by a progressive nighttime fall in cardiac output [3, 4] and central venous pressure [4]. The nocturnal fall in output is mediated primarily by a fall in heart rate since stroke volume is relatively unchanged. Blood pressure also is lower at night than it is during the evening and morning hours; this effect is characterized by an initial fall early in the evening, a sustained lower level throughout the night, and an early morning rise. These changes in flow and pressure result in a rise in total peripheral resistance [3, 4]. All of these hemodynamic patterns are extremely reliable and highly reproducible since they are based on month-long studies of continuous, beat-to-beat measurements of intraarterial blood pressure from a catheter in the distal aorta, central venous pressure from a catheter placed in or near the right atrium, and stroke volume from a probe placed at the root of the aorta. Similar hemodynamic patterns have been reported in the rat [9] except that the trends are shifted by 12 h since the rat sleeps during the day and is active at night. In addition, Miller and Horvath [7] have reported a nocturnal fall in cardiac output in normal man which is independent of sleep stage.

While autoregulation associated with a fall in oxygen need could cause a fall in regional blood flow and a rise in peripheral resistance, this mechanism by itself would be associated with a redistribution of plasma volume to the venous circulation and a concomitant rise in central venous pressure. The fall in venous pressure that we observed could have been mediated by a redistribution of blood volume or by an actual fall in plasma volume. Studies with α- and β-sympathetic blocking agents revealed that blockade exacerbated the nocturnal rate of fall in cardiac output and rise in peripheral resistance [10]. The level of central venous pressure rises during total sympathetic blockade; however, the nocturnal fall is identical to that seen during control studies [4]. Therefore, we believe that the fall in cardiac output is mediated, in part, by a fall in plasma volume, and that the rise in total peripheral resistance is probably the result of a compensatory hemodynamic adjustment which acts to maintain blood pressure. The fall in plasma volume occurs, in part, because urine continues to be produced at night even though the animals do not drink [8]. It is noteworthy that plasma volume has been shown to fall about 5% overnight in normal man [1, 6] and about 12% in hypertensive patients [2].

Schmidt/Engel/Blümchen (Eds.)
Temporal Variations of the Cardiovascular System
© Springer-Verlag Berlin Heidelberg 1992

Since the fall in cardiac output in our animal model always was mediated by a fall in heart rate with little or no change in stroke volume, we hypothesized that if heart rate was not allowed to fall, stroke volume would fall in order to accommodate the reduction in plasma volume. To test this hypothesis, we implanted an atrial demand pacemaker into the right atrium at the time that we implanted the flow probe. After allowing adequate time for the animals to recover from surgery, we studied each of four animals for 2 months. During the 1st month we monitored beat-to-beat levels of heart rate, stroke volume, arterial pressure and central venous pressure 18 h/day for 20 consecutive days, from 1800 hours to 1200 hours the following day. After these baseline studies were completed, we repeated the studies while at the same time pacing the atrium at a rate sufficient to prevent the night-time fall in heart rate but not so great as to exceed normal daytime rates. The rate we chose was about 10 beats/min faster than the fastest average rate during any hour of the 20-day control period. When heart rate was prevented from falling overnight, stroke volume fell, whereas in the control condition stroke volume did not change (Fig. 1). These findings confirmed our hypothesis. However, a number of other changes occurred that were unexpected. The overall levels of cardiac output, blood pressure, and central venous pressure were elevated; stroke volume was elevated early in the evening but was below control level by morning, whereas peripheral resistance was at control level early in the evening but then rose so that by morning it was significantly elevated [5]. To

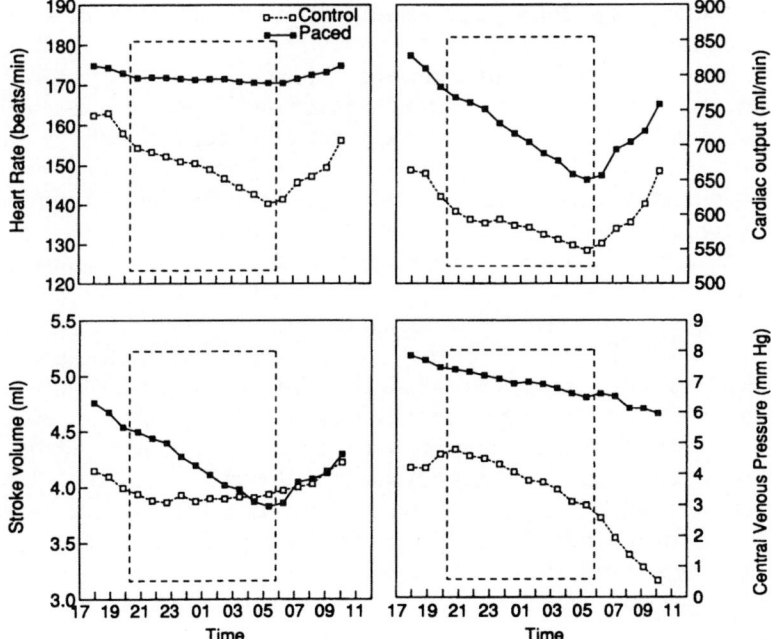

Fig. 1. Diurnal patterns of heart rate, stroke volume, cardiac output, and central venous pressure during control (*open circles*) and atrial demand pacing (*closed circles*)

understand these nocturnal changes more clearly, we analyzed the day-to-day and week-to-week changes in greater detail [11].

We blocked the 20 days of data into four, 5-day segments, which for convenience we shall call "weeks." In the subsequent paragraphs we shall report on the week-to-week patterns of cardiovascular change and also the day-to-day patterns within the 1st week. This analysis is limited to the 10-h interval from 2100 hours to 0700 hours the following morning. This interval comprises the major portion of the 12-h nighttime period when the room lights were off.

The overall levels of stroke volume, cardiac output, and blood pressure were significantly higher, and total peripheral resistance was significantly lower during pacing than during control throughout the first 5 days of pacing; however, by the 4th day, the level of cardiac output had begun to decline (Fig. 2). The level of central venous pressure was below control level during the first 2 days and then became significantly elevated, especially by the 5th day (Fig. 2). Thus, during the first 2 days cardiac output and arterial pressure rose without any change in plasma volume. However, by the 3rd day there was a rise in central venous pressure which probably reflected a rise in total plasma volume since cardiac output and arterial pressure remained elevated. The increase in total blood volume coupled with an increase in blood flow reflected in the elevated cardiac output and reduced peripheral resistance, compensated for the reduced vis a tergo gradient; however, this mechanism apparently was not sufficient since by the 4th day cardiac output had begun to decline. The decline in output coupled with a marked rise in central venous pressure indicates the presence of early signs of cardiac decompensation.

During the 2nd and 3rd weeks of pacing, cardiac output was maintained since the decrease in venous return resulting from the elevated central venous pressure was compensated by an increase in mean filling pressure (Fig. 3). This effect was probably mediated by an additional increase in total plasma volume since the elevated total peripheral resistance precluded a shift in plasma volume to the venous compartment. The elevated resistance was probably, in part, a result of autoregulation triggered by the reduced demand for oxygen during the night; however, it may also reflect an increase in vasomotor tone. During the 4th week of pacing, central venous pressure rose even higher and stroke volume fell from earlier levels, suggesting a progression of the cardiac decompensation seen at the end of the 1st week.

Of special interest is the nocturnal pattern of change in cardiac performance. If one plots Starling curves for the night-time hours (2100–0700 hours) for each of the 4 weeks, it can be seen that the week-to-week graph of stroke volume as a function of central venous pressure displaces to the right; however, the slopes of the curves are similar, suggesting a progressive decline in cardiac performance (Fig. 4). Inspection of Fig. 4 reveals that the level of stroke volume in the early evening, from 2100 to 2300 hours, does not change from the 1st week of pacing to the 4th week; thus, it would appear that the shift in cardiac performance is adequately compensated. However, if one examines the level of stroke volume during the early morning hours, from 0500 to 0700 hours, one can see that stroke volume is falling even though central venous pressure is rising over the weeks. This pattern is confirmed by statistical comparisons of the slopes of the lines of best fit through the early evening and early morning points. The trend of the evening

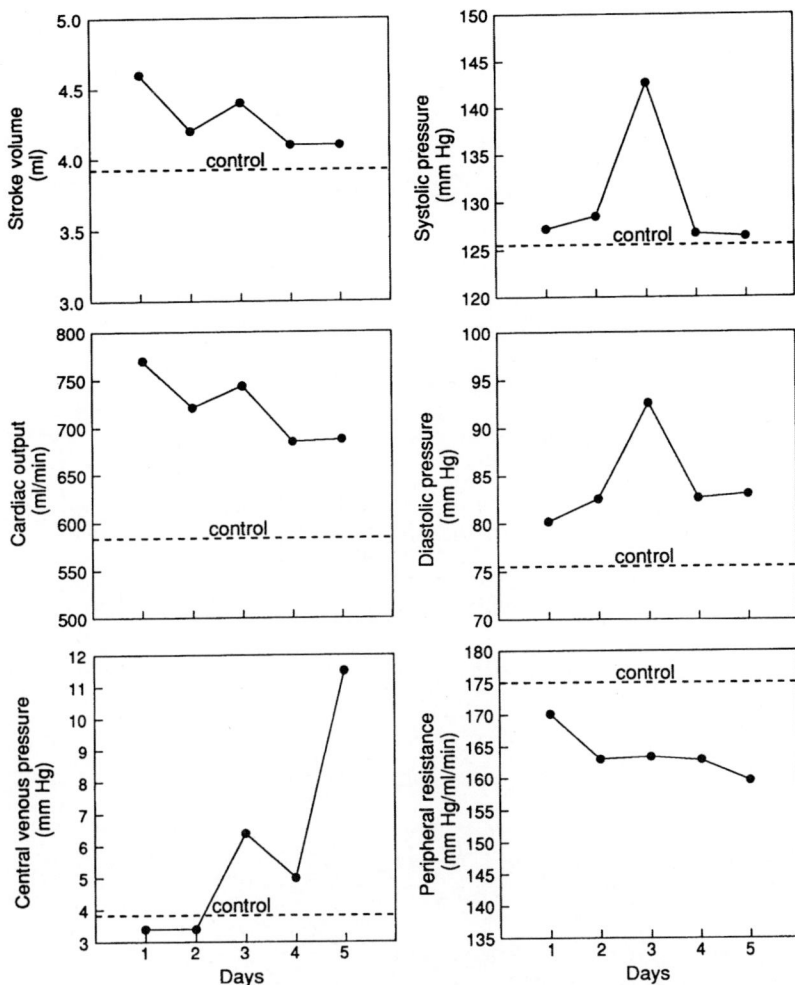

Fig. 2. Average nocturnal levels of stroke volume, cardiac output, central venous pressure, systolic and diastolic blood pressure, and total peripheral resistance during the first 5 days of atrial demand pacing. *Dashed lines*, prepacing control levels

values over the 4 weeks is not different from zero, whereas the trend of the morning values is significantly negative and significantly different from the evening trend. Thus, what appears to be a compensated, high output heart failure throughout the day and into the early evening, becomes a more serious-appearing, decompensated failure by early morning.

The results of this study were surprising to us. We had set the pacemaker at a relatively modest level – approximately 10 beats/min above the highest average daytime rate – because we wanted to test the hypothesis that if we prevented the fall in heart rate overnight, stroke volume would fall because there is a normal nocturnal fall in total plasma volume. We believe that the pacemaker did not even fire throughout most of the day; in fact, it was turned off from 1200 until 1700

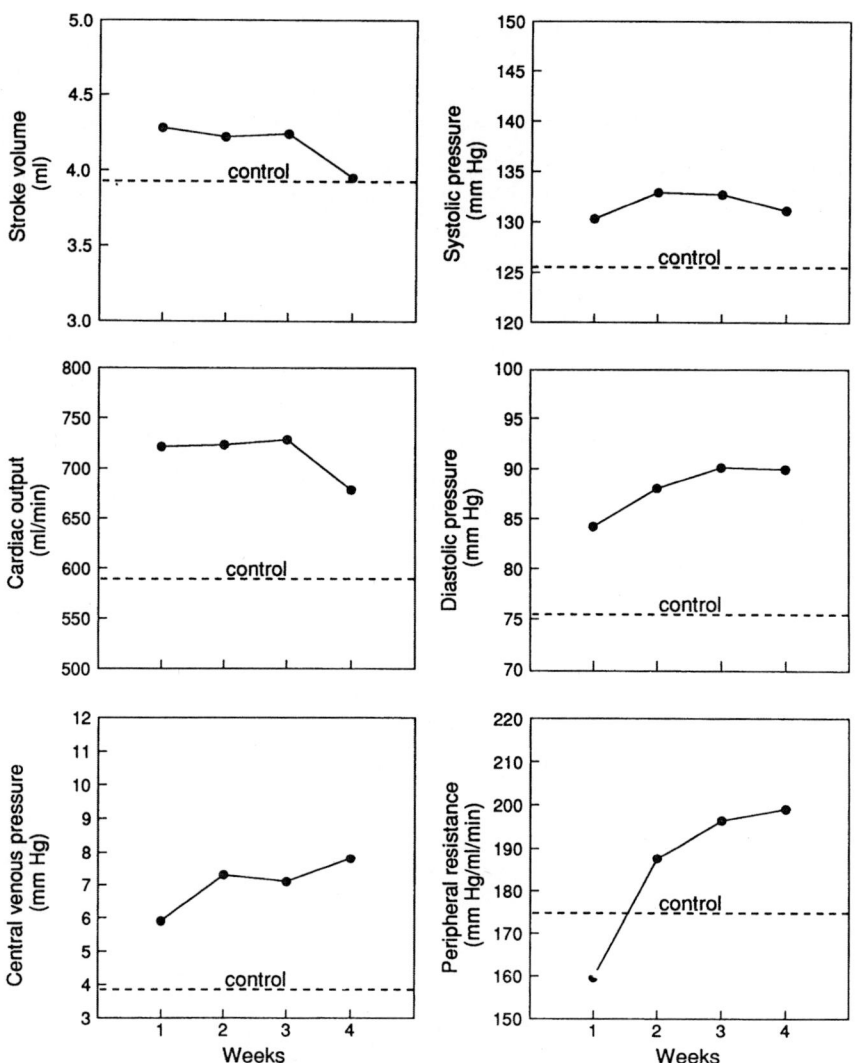

Fig. 3. Average nocturnal levels of stroke volume, cardiac output, central venous pressure, systolic and diastolic blood pressure, and total peripheral resistance during 4 weeks of atrial demand pacing. *Dashed lines*, prepacing control levels

hours each day. Our hypothesis was confirmed since the pacemaker-mediated constraint on heart rate did not allow the nocturnal fall, and stroke volume did fall instead. The average heart rate during pacing was less than 9% above the control level at 1800 hours. The normal nocturnal fall in heart rate which pacing prevented is about 10%–15%. By preventing this seemingly small fall in rate over the 4 weeks of study we observed an average increase of 8% in mean arterial pressure, 23% in cardiac output, and 27% in left ventricular work. It would appear that the heart needs to rest at night!

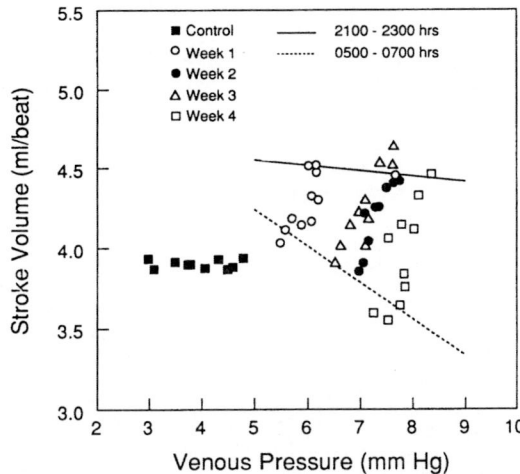

Fig. 4. Week-to-week Starling curves showing progressive shifts in the nighttime levels of central venous pressure. Note that during the early evening hours stroke volume is similar across weeks; however, during the early morning hours stroke volume falls across weeks even though central venous pressure is elevated. Prepacing, control values are included to provide reference levels

The emergence of what appears to be a high output, progressive heart failure that is worse in the early morning than it is in the early evening was totally unexpected. Thus, we do not have measurements of plasma volume, blood electrolytes, and heart size that would help to clarify the clinical aspects of our findings. Furthermore, we are aware that atrial demand pacing has been used clinically for many years, and we know of no known reports of heart failure in these patients. Nevertheless, we believe that the present findings warrant further study of cardiac function in patients who are fitted with atrial demand pacemakers. Especially needed are studies comparing cardiac performance at various times of day and at different rates of pacing.

References

1. Cranston WI (1964) Diurnal variation in plasma volume in normal and hypertensive subjects. Am Heart J 68:427–428
2. Cranston WI, Brown W (1963) Diurnal variation in plasma volume in normal and hypertensive subjects. Clin Sci 25:107–114
3. Engel BT, Talan MI (1987) Diurnal patterns of hemodynamic performance in nonhuman primates. Am J Physiol 253 (Regulatory Integrative Comp Physiol 22):R779–R785
4. Engel BT, Talan MI (1991) Diurnal variations in central venous pressure. Acta Physiol Scand 141:273–278
5. Engel BT, Talan MI, Chew P (1992) Effect of nocturnal atrial demand cardiac pacing on diurnal hemodynamic patterns. J Appl Physiol (in press)
6. Greenleaf JE (1984) Physiological responses to prolonged bed rest and fluid immersion in humans. J Appl Physiol 7 (Respiratory Environmental Exercise Physiol):619–633
7. Miller JC, Horvath SM (1976) Cardiac output during human sleep. Aviat Space Environ Med 47:1046–1051

8. Moore-Ede MC, Herd JA (1977) Renal electrolyte circadian rhythms: independence from feeding and activity patterns. Am J Physiol 232 (Renal Fluid Electrolyte Physiol): F 128–F 135
9. Smith TL, Coleman TG, Stanek KA, Murphy WR (1987) Hemodynamic monitoring for 24 hour in unanesthetized rats. Am J Physiol 253 (Regulatory Integrative Comp Physiol 22): R 779–785
10. Talan MI, Engel BT (1989) Effect of sympathetic blockade on diurnal variation of hemodynamic patterns. Am J Physiol 256 (Regulatory Integrative Comp Physiol 25): R 778–R 785
11. Talan MI, Engel BT, Chew P (1992) Systemic nocturnal demand pacing results in high output heart failure. J Appl Physiol (in press)

Diurnal Variations
in Blood Pressure Rhythms

Feasibility of Continuous Noninvasive 24-h Ambulatory Finger Blood Pressure Measurement with Portapres: Comparison with Intrabrachial Pressure *

G. J. Langewouters, B. de Wit, G. M. A. van der Hoeven, B. P. M. Imholz, G. Parati, G. A. van Montfrans, and K. H. Wesseling

Introduction

To date, the great majority of ambulatory blood pressure recordings are made with noninvasive intermittent devices (O'Brien et al. 1989). For several years, however, continuous noninvasive measurement of blood pressure has been possible in the finger with Finapres, based on the volume-clamp (vascular unloading) method of Peñáz (Peñáz 1973; Peñáz et al. 1976) and the physiocal criteria of Wesseling (Wesseling and de Wit 1983; Wesseling 1983, 1990). Several studies have shown that Finapres is an accurate alternative for intra-arterial blood pressure measurements (Smith et al. 1985; Molhoek et al. 1984; Imholz et al. 1988, 1990a, 1991; Parati et al. 1989). In 1984 TNO raised the following question: Is it possible to develop a portable version of Finapres? Recently, the project aiming to develop such a device, called Portapres, resulted in a clinically acceptable prototype Portapres model 1 (Langewouters et al. 1990). The objective of this paper is to present the major characteristics of the device and to show some intermediate results of the field study in which 24-h Portapres finger blood pressure is compared to simultaneously measured intrabrachial pressure (IBP; see also Imholz et al. 1990b). The results of the complete study in 24 subjects are described in the MD-thesis of Imholz (1991).

Methods

The stationary Finapres device was made suitable for ambulatory purposes by solving three major problems, namely:

– a significant reduction in size, weight, and power consumption;
– the development of a hydrostatic height compensation system to allow for free movement of the measured hand;

* This study was supported in part by a research grant from the Netherlands Heart Foundation (grant 87068). Travel grants were obtained from the Commission of the European Communities, Concerted Action I.3.1: Breakdown in Human Adaptation.

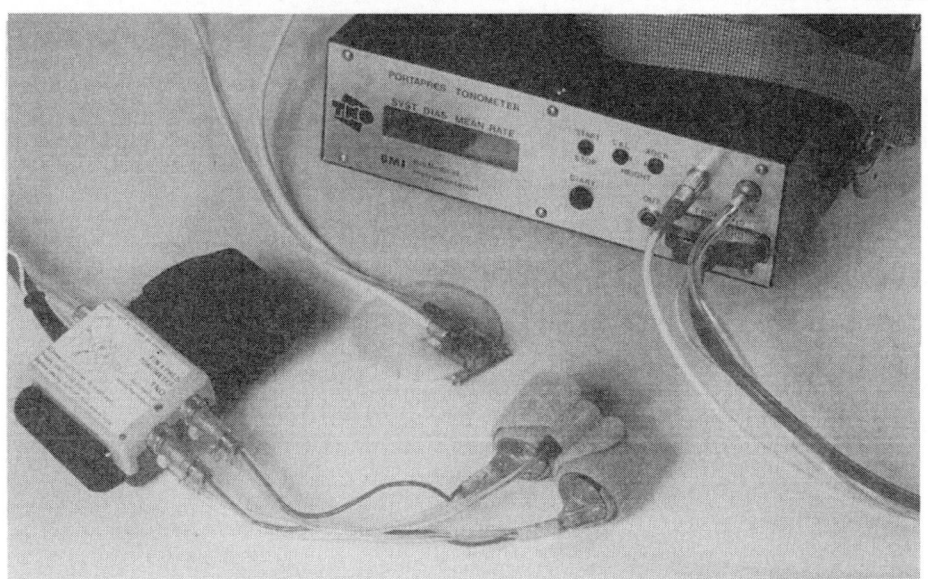

Fig. 1. Overview of prototype Portapres model 1, showing the front panel of the main unit, the patient front-end box with the two cuffs and the height correction system. A liquid cristal display is situated on the left side of the front panel showing the beat-to-beat values of systolic (*SYST*), diastolic (*DIAS*), mean pressure (*MEAN*), and heart rate (*RATE*) during the first 5 min of the measurement. Thereafter the display is blanked and shows the time after starting upon pressing the diary marker button (*DIARY*). The device is controlled through three hidden push-buttons. Once a measurement is started, it continues automatically until it is stopped manually

– the development of a two-finger switching system to monitor two adjacent fingers in alternation every 30 min.

Size, Weight, Power. A significant reduction in size could be realized due to the innovative redesign of major components such as the servovalve to control cuff pressure and the air pump to generate supply pressure. Figure 1 shows an overview of the front panel of the Portapres main unit, the patient front-end box, and the height correction system. The front panel contains a two-line by 16-character liquid cristal display, three hidden keys to control the device, a diary marker, and several connectors. The main unit of prototype model 1 contains the air pump, the BMI-88 computer board, and a proprietary analog electronics board, the battery pack, and a 4- (or 7-)channel, commercially available, TEAC cassette FM instrumentation tape recorder (see Fig. 2).

The recorded signals are the noninvasive continuous finger blood pressure (PORTAP) and the height signal (HEIGHT). One channel is used for noise compensation. The fourth channel is used in our field study to record IBP measured by the Oxford system. The main unit measures $240 \times 200 \times 60$ mm and weighs about 3000 g, including the tape recorder and the battery pack. The patient front-end box measures $60 \times 45 \times 30$ mm and weighs about 350 g. With special lithium battery packs measurement times of up to 36 h are possible. The main unit

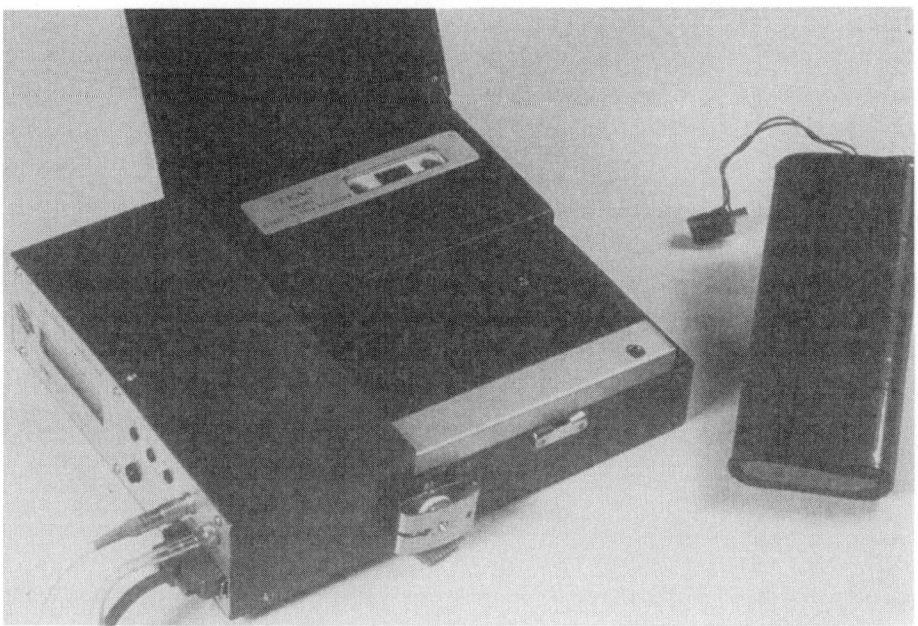

Fig. 2. A door in the main unit of Portapres model 1 can be opened to give access to the built-in four- or seven-channel commercially available cassette FM instrumentation tape recorder and the battery compartment to accommodate a 15 Ah at 14.5 V DC lithium battery pack for up to 36 h of uninterrupted blood pressure measurements

of Portapres can be worn on the stomach by means of two belts (one removable) or hung from the shoulder with only one belt. The patient front-end box is worn on the back of the hand or on the wrist and fixed by means of Velcro adhesive. The height correction transducer is taped to the subject at the chosen reference level, while the tube ending is fixed with Velcro adhesive to the two finger cuffs.

Height Correction. During ambulatory conditions the free movement of the hand on which pressure is measured in mandatory. However, movement of the hand causes a hydrostatic pressure in the finger with respect to the reference point at heart level. Consequently, a system is needed to correct for the effect of height changes on the recorded pressure. The prototype height correction system consists of a Gould pressure tranducer fixed at heart level and a flexible liquid-filled tube of 90 cm length. The end of the tube is closed by means of a small high-compliance bag contained in a rigid cover which is fixed to the cuffed fingers with Velcro adhesive. Some results obtained during ambulatory conditions are shown in Fig. 3.

Two-Finger Switching. During long-term finger blood pressure measurement in a cuffed finger, the blood supply to the finger tip distal from the cuff is reduced but not completely stopped. Consequently, venous congestion in the finger tip occurs

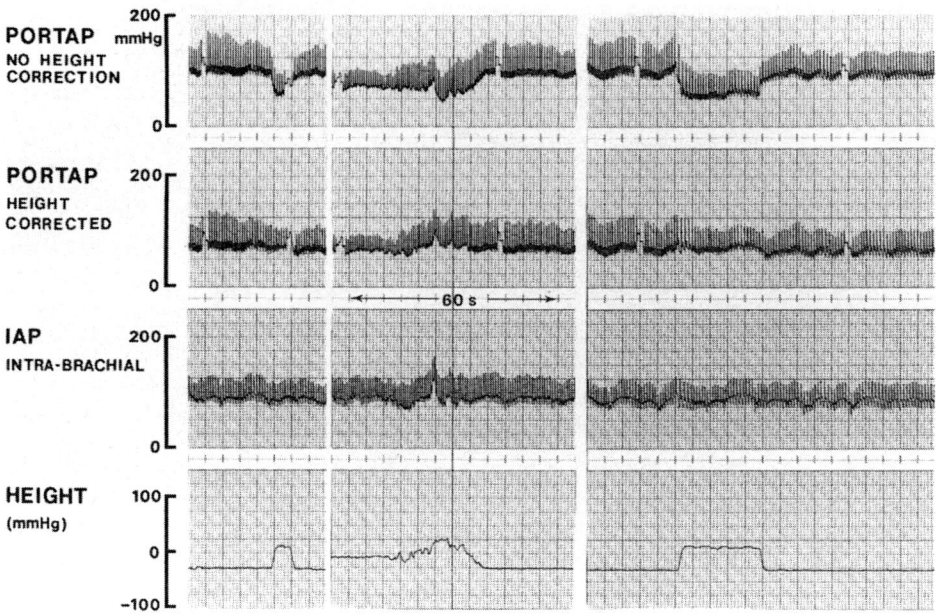

Fig. 3. Some practical examples of the effects of the height correction system on the recorded blood pressure signal. *Upper panel,* PORTAP signal when no height correction is used. The hydrostatic effects of height changes (*HEIGHT; lowest panel*) are clearly recognized. After height correction (*second panel*) the PORTAP signal closely resembles the simultaneoulsy measure intra-brachial pressure (*IAP; third panel*)

which might give a feeling of discomfort if associated with a low oxygen saturation of the blood (Gravenstein et al. 1985). For this reason Portapres is equipped with a two-finger switching device that automatically switches between two adjacent fingers every 30 min in alternation.

Field Study

To test Portapres a field study was designed in which Portapres finger pressure was measured simultaneously with IBP (Oxford method) in healthy volunteers and in hypertensive patients in two clinics: the Ospedale Maggiore in Milan and the Academic Medical Centre in Amsterdam. A standardized protocol was used, starting at 1300 hours, including a 2-h siesta period from 1400 to 1600 hours on day 1, followed by a 30-min period of 50-W cycloergometry. Also included was a 1-h walk outside the hospital. All subjects kept a diary. Diary messages were marked on tape by means of a diary marker, producing a brief staircase signal on the HEIGHT signal. Figure 4 shows an example of such a 24-h simultaneous measurement.

Recently a computer system for the analysis of 24-h blood pressure measurements has become available. Figure 5 shows some of the results of this analysis system. Note the high degree of correspondence between the invasive IBP and the

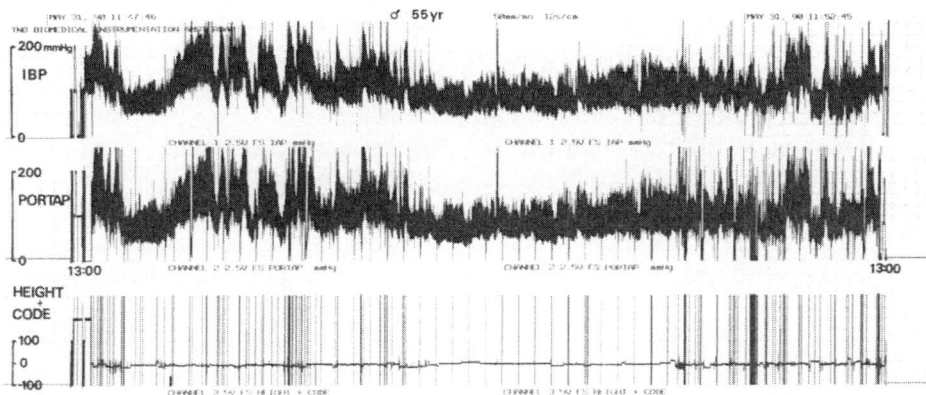

Fig. 4. Example of a 24-h continuous noninvasive finger blood pressure profile (*PORTAP*) in a 55-year-old man with labile blood pressure due to an afferent lesion in the baroreflex arc. Note the large excursions of the blood pressure, especially in the first part of the registration. Intrabrachial pressure (*IBP*) was measured simultaneously with an Oxford system. *Lowest panel*, shows the hydrostatic height signal (*HEIGHT*) on which coded messages are superimposed. Note the switching to another finger every 30 min marked by the regular downward spikes in the PORTAP signal

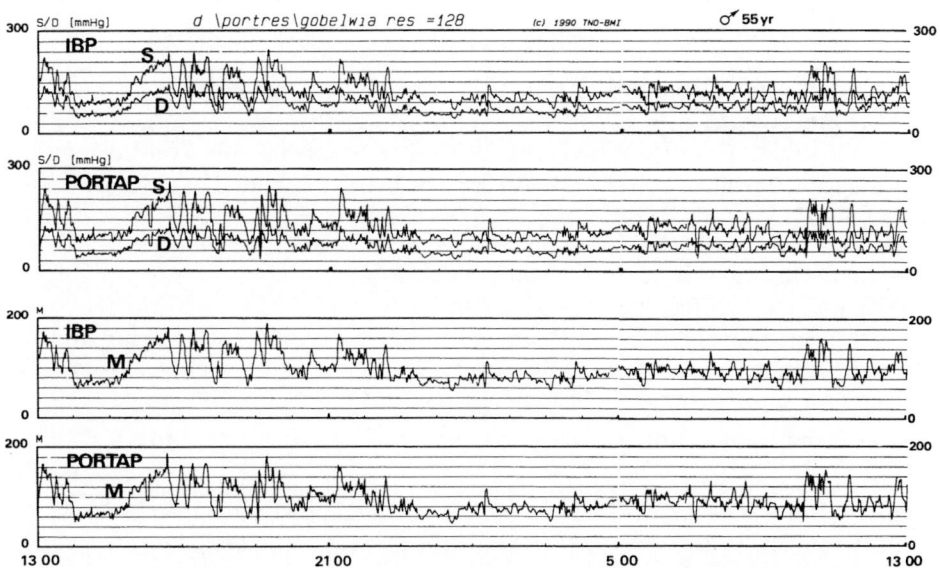

Fig. 5. The 128 beat averaged values of systolic (*S*), diastolic (*D*), and mean pressure (*M*) as obtained by computer analysis after replay of the taped 24-h noninvasive finger blood pressure (*PORTAP*) and the simultaneously measured intrabrachial pressure (*IBP*). Same patient as in Fig. 4. Note the high degree of correspondence between the PORTAP and IBP profiles

noninvasive PORTAP blood pressures. Since this analysis is time consuming, in this paper only the results of the first nine measurements (six volunteers and three hypertensive patients) are described. A less sophisticated analysis was used to obtain initial results of this subset of nine measurements. Upon playback of the 24-h tapes mean PORTAP and mean IBP measurements were obtained by electronic filtering on a Gould RS 3800 paper recorder. Their difference was obtained by subtraction. Then, 30-min averages were computed per subject and averaged over the nine subjects. A day-night comparison was also made. Finally, the results on the ring finger were compared with those on the middle finger.

Some Results

From spontaneous reactions, subject observations, and specific questioning we concluded that all subjects accepted the apparatus quite well despite the size and weight. All subjects except one reported having slept as usual.

PORTAP Compared to IBP. Figure 6 shows a plot of sequential 30-min values of mean IBP averaged over nine subjects. Note the dip in pressure during the siesta in the beginning to values as low as during the night period. Figure 6 also shows the difference between PORTAP and IBP for each 30-min period.

The results of the subset of nine measurements can be summarized as follows:

- Portapres underestimates mean IBP by about 9 mm Hg (range − 22 to + 0.7 mm Hg).
- Within subjects the PORTAP-IBP difference is remarkably constant with a standard deviation SD (PORTAP-IBP) of 6.2 mm Hg (range 3.8 – 11.5 mm Hg).
- Average daytime PORTAP-IBP difference is − 8.2 mm Hg (range − 22 to − 2 mm Hg), which is not significantly different from average nighttime PORTAP-IBP difference at − 12.5 mm Hg (range − 25 to − 2 mm Hg).
- On average PORTAP-IBP differences do not differ between the ring and the middle finger. In four subjects, however, significant differences were found, on average 8 mm Hg (range 4 – 11 mm Hg).

Similar values were found for the whole group of 24 subjects (see Imholz, 1991).

Artifacts. For PORTAP the fraction of monitoring time lost due to artifacts in the first nine subjects was 16%. PORTAP artifacts were associated mainly with the following circumstances:

- brisk walking while swinging one hand;
- rapid movements of the measured hand;
- cold fingers during outside walking with subsequent loss of signal.

Substantial improvement (about 50% reduction in time) was obtained by covering the hand with a glove or coat while being outside, and by instructing the subjects to limit movements of the hand by keeping it steady near heart level

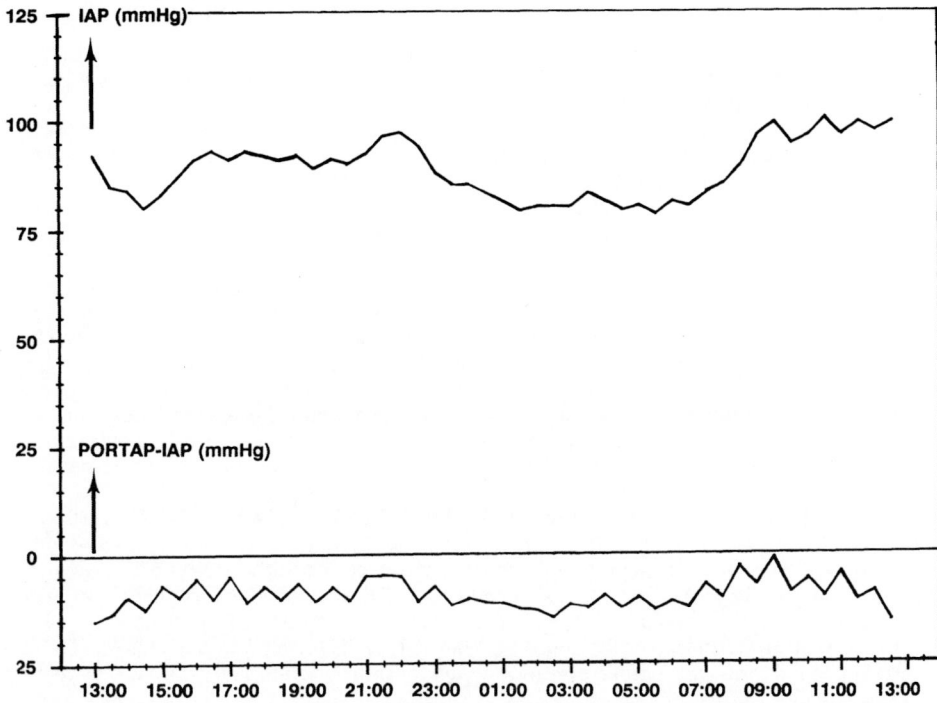

Fig. 6. Average 30-min mean values of intrabrachial pressure (*IAP*) averaged over nine subjects, showing the well-known circadian variation in blood pressure. The difference between the two pressures (PORTAP − IAP) is also shown, indicating that Portapres underestimates mean blood pressure (on average by about 9 mm Hg)

during walking. Thus the fraction reduced to 8.4% for the whole group of 24 measurements. For IBP the fraction of monitoring time lost was 10%, due mainly to pump artifacts during sleep.

Concluding Remarks

The results presented here indicate that prolonged 24-h noninvasive recording of finger blood pressure is possible. Taking simple precautions, the percentage monitoring time lost is of the same order of magnitude as that of IBP measurements with the Oxford system – around 10%. In general, the Portapres finger blood pressure profile closely resembles the IBP profile, but with an offset of about 9 mm Hg due to the fact that finger blood pressure is lower than IBP.

The great advantage of Portapres is, of course, the fact that it provides information on the blood pressure and its variability noninvasively. It provides a new means, among other things, to study 24-h blood pressure variability on a beat-to-beat basis.

References

Gravenstein JS, Paulus DA, Feldman J, McLaughlin G (1985) Tissue hypoxia distal to a Peñáz finger blood pressure cuff. J Clin Monit 1:120–125

Imholz BPM, van Montfrans GA, Settels JJ, van der Hoeven GMA, Karemaker JM, Wieling WW (1988) Continuous, non-invasive blood pressure monitoring: reliability of Finapres device during the Valsalva manoeuvre. Cardiovasc Res 22:390–397

Imholz BPM, Settels JJ, van den Meiracker AH, Wesseling KH, Wieling W (1990a) Noninvasive beat-to-beat finger blood pressure measurement during orthostatic stress compared to intra-arterial pressure. Cardiovasc Res 24:214–221

Imholz BPM, van Montfrans G, Parati G, Villani A, Gropelli A, Langewouters G, Wesseling K, Mancia G, Wieling W (1990b) First experience with Portapres: continuous noninvasive ambulatory finger blood pressure compared to intra-brachial blood pressure. J Hypertens 8 [Suppl 3]:S87

Imholz BPM (1991) Noninvasive Finger Arterial Pressure Waveform Registration: evaluation of Finapres and Portapres. MD-thesis, University of Amsterdam, The Netherlands

Langewouters GJ, de Wit B, van der Hoeven GMA, van Montfrans GA, Imholz BPM, Wieling W, Wesseling KH (1990) Feasibility of continuous noninvasive 24h ambulatory measurement of finger arterial blood pressure with Portapres. J Hypertens 8 [Suppl 3]:S88

Molhoek GP, Wesseling KH, Settels JJ, van Vollenhoven E, Weeda HWH, de Wit B, Arntzenius AC (1984) Evaluation of the Peñáz servo-plehysmo-manometer for the continuous non-invasive measurement of finger blood pressure. Basic Res Cardiol 79:598–609

O'Brien E, Cox JP, O'Malley K (1989) Editorial Review. Ambulatory blood pressure measurement in the evaluation of blood pressure lowering drugs. J Hypertens 7:243–247

Parati G, Casadei R, Groppelli A, DiRienzo M, Mancia G (1989) Comparison of finger and intra-arterial blood pressure monitoring at rest and during laboratory testing. Hypertension 13:647–655

Peñáz J (1973) Photoelectric measurement of blood pressure, volume and flow in the finger. Digest of the 10th international conference on medical and biological engineering, Dresden, p 104

Peñáz J, Voigt A, Teichmann W (1976) Beitrag zur fortlaufenden indirekten Blutdruckmessung. Z Inn Med 31:1030–1033

Smith NT, Wesseling KH, de Wit B (1985) Evaluation of two prototype devices producing non-invasive, pulsatile, calibrated blood pressure measurement from a finger. J Clin Monit 1:17–29

Wesseling KH (1983) A method and device for correcting the cuff pressure in measuring the blood pressure in a part of the body by means of a plethysmograph. European Patent: EP 0080778 A1, Bulletin 83/23

Wesseling KH (1990) Finapres, continuous noninvasive finger arterial pressure based on the method of Peñáz. In: Meyer-Sabellek W, Anlauf M, Gotzen R, Steinfeld L (eds) Blood pressure measurement. Steinkopff, Darmstadt, pp 161–172

Wesseling KH, de Wit B (1983) Method and device for controlling the cuff pressure in measuring the blood pressure in a finger by means of a photo-electric plethysmograph. European Patent EP 0078090 B1, Bulletin 83/18

A New Dimension of Blood Pressure Measurement in Man: 24-h Ambulatory Continuous Noninvasive Recording with Portapres

T. F. H. Schmidt, T. Steinmetz, J. Wittenhaus, P. Piccolo, and H. Lüpsen

Introduction

Portapres is a new portable device, recently developed by TNO, Amsterdam, which enables continuous 24 hour finger blood pressure recordings in ambulatory subjects. Like Finapres it is based on the volume-clamp method of Peñáz (vascular unloading) (Peñáz 1973; Peñáz et al. 1976) and the physiocal criteria of Wesseling (Wesseling et al. 1986, 1990). It is an attractive and accurate noninvasive alternative for intraarterial ambulatory 24 hour blood pressure measurement in man (Imholz 1990 a, b; Langewouters et al. 1990, 1992 in this volume). Here we shall report our first experience with Portapres and demonstrate some applications it can be used for in cardiovascular research.

Major Characteristics of Portapres

Portapres consists of a main unit including a tape recorder and battery-pack, a patient fronted box with two finger cuffs, and a height compensation system (see also previous chapter Langewouters et al. 1992). The prototype Portapres model 1 we used measures $255 \times 210 \times 60$ mm and weighs about 3000 g. The main unit contains the necessary electronics, a commercially available seven-channel TEAC cassette FM instrumentation recorder (HR 30J) and a Lithium battery pack with an energy content of 14 Ampere hours, specially designed for at least 24 hours of uninterrupted measurement. Portapres can also be run by an AC adapter, connected by a long cable (~ 12 m), allowing the subjects to move about somewhat inside a building without using the battery. It can be switched automatically from the battery to the AC adapter and vice versa while measuring without interruption and without any other adaptation. This helps to reduce the still expensive battery costs (~ 0.32 DM/minute).

The recorded signals are the noninvasive continuous finger blood pressure (PORTAP), the height compensation signal (HEIGHT) on which additionally error codes and a marker signal are superimposed, as well as beat-to-beat systolic, diastolic and mean arterial blood pressure as well as heart rate. Instead of mean arterial pressure other additional signals from an external input can be recorded such as integrated thigh-EMG as a measure of physical activity. One channel is used for noise compensation. The main unit of Portapres can be worn on the

Schmidt/Engel/Blümchen (Eds.)
Temporal Variations of the Cardiovascular System
© Springer-Verlag Berlin Heidelberg 1992

stomach by means of two belts (one removable), or hung from the shoulder with only one belt. Another well proven way is to put the unit into a rucksack which can be carried on the back during various activities such as bicycling etc. and which the patient can put down next to her-/himself when working in a sitting position for some time or during sleep at night.

The patient frontend box measures $60 \times 45 \times 30$ mm and weighs about 350 g. It is worn on the back of the non-dominant hand or on the wrist and is fixed by means of Velcro adhesive tape. Portapres is equipped with a two-finger switching device that automatically switches measurements every 30 minutes in alternation between two cuffs applied to two adjacent fingers. Usually the middle and ring-finger of the non-dominant hand are measured.

During ambulatory conditions the movement of the hand on which pressure is being measured causes a hydrostatic pressure in the finger with respect to the reference point at heart level. An elevation or lowering of the measured hand by 13 cm in the vertical direction causes a hydrostatic blood pressure change of 10 mm Hg. A prototype height correction system consisting of a Gould disposable pressure transducer and a liquid-filled flexible tube of 90 cm length corrects for such height changes in the recorded pressure. The height correction transducer is taped to the subject at the chosen reference level (left anterior axillar line at the height just below the processus xyphoideus of the sternum), while the tube ending is fixed with Velcro adhesive tape to the two finger cuffs. This height correction system is also available for the TNO Finapres model 5.

Portapres is operated from the main unit's front panel by three hidden keys to control the different functions of the device. The front panel further contains a two-line by 16-character liquid cristal display (LCD), a diary marker, and several connectors. For later analyses of taped data a 7-channel TEAC replay (MR-30AC) unit is necessary as well as computer equipment (analog-digital converter etc.) and adequate software.

By avoiding rapid movements of the measured hand and situations which provoke severe contraction of finger arteries, such as extended exposure to cold, the percentage monitoring time lost due to artefacts can be minimized. By keeping the measured hand steady and near heart level during walking and by covering the hand with a glove or coat when outside at low temperatures, it has been shown that the percentage monitoring time lost is with 10% of the same order of magnitude as that of intrabrachial measurements by the Oxford system (Langewouters et al. 1992, in this volume).

Methods

Procedure

In a first study we investigated 16 young healthy male subjects with Portapres during two 24 hour periods in everyday life as well as in two standardized laboratory test procedures, once in the morning (between 8.30–9.30 AM) and once in the afternoon (between about 5.30–6.30 PM) during each investigation day. It was designed as a randomized, placebo controlled, double blind, cross-over study in order to test the effect of one week of oral administration of 2.5 mg Cilazapril, an ACE-inhibitor newly developed by Hoffmann-La Roche (Investigational Drug Brochure 1989), on diurnal blood pressure and heart rate. According to the accepted basis for clinical trial ethics (current revision of the Helsinki declaration 1989) the subjects volunteered (Table 1) and gave informed consent to participate in the study, which was evaluated and approved by the Hannover Medical School ethical committee. After the subjects had taken Cilazapril or placebo respectively for seven days once in the morning with a wash-out-between-phase of one week between these two phases, Portapres measurements took place on the seventh day of both medication phases. The order of medication was randomized by Hoffmann-La Roche, Basel, Switzerland. 8 subjects started the medication with placebo in the first phase and Cilazapril in the second, whereas the other 8 subjects started the medication with Cilazapril followed by placebo. A double blind test procedure was guaranteed. A more detailed description of the effects of Cilazapril is published elsewhere (Schmidt et al. 1992, in press), but here we shall rather focus on some possible applications of Portapres.

Physiological Measurements

Continuous finger blood pressure was recorded using Portapres together with a continuous measure of physical activity (EMG of the left thigh) on the two experimental days for 24 hours during everyday life as well as during the two laboratory sessions. The thigh-EMG was assessed with the BIOPORT system (ZAK 1982) as the integral of EMG impulses. This measure allows major effects of physical activity to be controlled. The EMG electrodes were taped on the left thigh over the musculus quadriceps femoris, positioned between the upper and middle as well as between the middle and lower third of the thigh (Anastasiades and Johnston 1990). It was made certain that these electrodes were placed on the same positions on both testing days, enabling a somewhat more accurate comparison between different days of this relative measure of physical activity.

The continuous Portap finger blood pressure curve, the height signal, the beat-to-beat systolic and diastolic blood pressure and heart rate were recorded on tape on the 7-channel TEAC recorder (HR 30 J) together with the EMG signal. During the laboratory sessions these variables were also taped on a stationary TEAC 7-channel recorder and replay unit (MR-30 AC) and additionally recorded as 1 second mean values in a Macintosh plus computer by using a MacAdios Model 411 AD converter and special software developed for this purpose by P. Piccolo. For the analyses of 24 hour measurements tapes were replayed on the TEAC 7-channel replay unit. Systolic and diastolic blood pressure, heart rate and EMG were transformed to 64 second mean values by using the MacAdios AD converter, the Macintosh plus together with the above mentioned software. After correcting for artefacts there were about 3% missing data.

Subjects

Sixteen healthy young male subjects, aged 23–28 years, were selected in a pretest. In Table 1 means $\pm$ standard errors and ranges of the subjects' ages, heights, weights, and body mass indeces (BMI = weight/height^2) are shown.

Table 1. Means ($\pm$SE) and ranges of age, height, weight, and body mass index of the 16 subjets

	Mean $\pm$SE	Range
Age (years)	25.3 ± 1.6	$23-28$
Height (cm)	186.2 ± 5.6	$173-197$
Weight (kg)	81.2 ± 7.1	$67.8-93.3$
BMI (kg/cm^2)	23.4 ± 1.5	$21.8-27.0$

The subjects were told to spend the experimental day as normally as possible. Every 30 minutes while they were awake the subjects reported activities, events and emotions occurring during the previous half hour in a diary designed for that purpose. To reduce battery costs subjects were asked to use the AC adapter whenever possible inside a building.

Laboratory Test Procedures

The laboratory test procedure was composed in such a way that the effect of different body postures on blood pressure and heart rate could be investigated at rest, as well as the effect of active coping tasks (reaction time task, mild physical exercise) and a more passive coping task, the diving test (i.e. putting the face into ice water) in alternation with breath holding as a control procedure.

The laboratory tests consisted of the following 13 different parts which were performed in a fixed order:

- Rest (sitting), 5 min;
- Multiple choice reaction time task (sitting), 5 min;
- Rest (prone), 10 min;
- Standing, 5 min;
- Breath holding test 1 (sitting), 20 s;
- Diving test 1 (sitting), 20 s;
- Breath holding 2, 20 s;
- Diving 2, 20 s;
- Breath holding 3, 20 s;
- Diving 3; 20 s;
- Breath holding 4, 20 s;
- Mild physical exercise (25 W on a bicycle ergometer, sitting position), 5 min;
- Rest (sitting), 5 min.

With regard to the laboratory test we shall focus mainly on the results of the diving test. As we wanted to investigate the effect of Cilazapril on cardiovascular reactivity this test was chosen, for diving and cold stimulation is known to stimulate a blood pressure rise by vasoconstriction (Andren and Hanson 1980), the mechanism that is acted upon by ACE-inhibitors (Fischli et al. 1989; Waterfall 1989). Therefore this test and its control procedure are described here in detail: As it is necessary to hold one's breath during diving, which has itself an effect on blood pressure and heart rate, the "breath holding test" was additional introduced as a kind of "placebo diving" during which all behavioral components were identical to those during the actual diving when only cold water ($+ 4\,°C$) and ice cubes were added.

During the breath holding test subjects were asked to hold their breath for exactly 20 seconds while they put their head face down into a bowl. They were instructed to hold their breath after inhaling fully and to exhale again to about a middle breathing position, i.e. not extremely inhaled or exhaled, to avoid major intrathoracic pressure effects by pressing or sucking during the procedure. This test was repeated four times alternating with the diving test by using two identical bowls during the two procedures: one bowl was empty (during holding breath) and the other was filled with cold water and ice cubes (during the actual diving)."Diving" in the empty bowl was used as the "placebo diving". This allowed the cardiovascular reactions during the actual diving to be compared and separated from those during breath holding. The intervals between 20 s breath holding and 20 s diving were 90 seconds.

On the experimental day the subjects took their last Cilazapril medication in the morning on average at around 7.27 h (± 3 min). Portapres measurements were started at 8 AM. The laboratory test procedure started in the morning about 72 ± 2 min and in the afternoon 592 ± 7 min after the last drug administration, and lasted for about 53 ± 1 min on average.

Statistical Analyses

Statistical analyses were performed on IBM 3084 by using BMDP statistical software, Los Angeles. The cross-over design was taken into consideration by analyses of variance (Grizzle 1965), which tested dependent variables (i.e. systolic and diastolic blood pressure, heart rate as well as their reactions etc.) for carry over effects, differences between placebo vs Cilazapril, day 1 vs day 2 etc. For the analyses of 24 hour measurements as well as the analyses of 20 second intervals during the diving test, an additional time factor was introduced into the analyses of variance to test for differences between 48 half hour mean values or 20 second intervals. Moreover, interactions between the various factors were calculated.

Results

Multimodal Assessment in Everyday Life – The First Case

For the simultaneous recording of physiological parameters such as blood pressure, heart rate, physical activity together with self-reports of behavior, moods and environmental events at regular intervals the term "Multimodal Assessment" has been coined (Fahrenberg 1987; Stemmler and Fahrenberg 1989). Figure 1 shows an example of such multimodel 24 hour ambulatory assessment in our first subject, a 23-year-old healthy male medical student (IA1). Systolic and diastolic blood pressure, heart rate and physical activity recordings with Portapres are averaged at 64 second intervals. Little interruptions in the curves indicate Portapres switching measurement from the middle to the ring finger and vice versa. Major moods (upper staff lines), activities and events etc. (lower staff lines) are reported in a diary at half hour intervals while awake.

The lowest staff line in Fig. 1 (*Location*) indicates various locations where the subject spends his time (in the laboratory, medical school, at home, visiting his girl friend), with the shaded areas representing times when on the way from one place to another, usually by bicycle. On the lines above the lowest one (*Activities*) various activities are represented. On the lowest of these lines activities are indicated either by word symbols ("Lect" for listening to a lecture) or icons which show whether the subject uses his bicycle (bike), eats (fork) or drinks (bottle) within the respective half hour interval. When the subject is tested in the laboratory the bike icon indicates mild physical exercise with the ergometer.

In the third line from below the icons relate walking (legs) and climbing stairs (stair case) to the respective half hour intervals. The icons on the fourth line from below show when the subject is talking or phoning. On the fifth line it is shown when the subject is studying/reading (open book), going to the toilet, urinating, cleaning the house (broom). Moreover, numbers indicate special events marked by the subject: At ① the subject looses balance while cycling and nearly falls down. At ② he realises that the battery is empty and that Portapres stops the blood pressure measurement when he disconnects the AC-adapter. He phones the lab and he is told to come. He takes the bike and arrives there just after 5 PM when the battery is exchanged. This part is indicated by a long break in the blood pressure and heart rate but not in the EMG recordings. The latter shows a peak during this time when the subject cycles to the lab. At ③ the subject cycles to the laboratory in the morning when a dog runs into his bike and he nearly falls down. During this event systolic blood pressure and heart rate exceed 200 mm Hg and 130 bpm.

On the sixth line from below (*Position*) the various body position(s) during each half hour interval are symbolized. In the lab sitting, standing and lying vary in a fixed order at intervals too short to be related to the exact times in this figure. During the daytime the subjects is both sitting and standing during most half hour intervals (indicated by dotted lines after the icons for sitting/standing) and sometimes just sitting. When he visits his girl friend at night (around 9.30 PM), they have a meal together before having intercourse. Again during this time sitting and lying positions change too rapidly to enable an accurate time relation.

The top line of the lower staff lines (*Company*) shows the number of persons (0, 1, 2, more than 2) the subject is together with at each half hour interval. Again the dotted lines indicate that the last number remains unchanged. The clefs above the lower top line indicate that the subject is listening to music (during various other activities). The last icon on this line symbolizes a radio he is listening to just before leaving his home.

In the upper staff lines changes of five of the subject's major moods (happy, tired, busy, angry and sexually excited) can be followed at half hour intervals during the day. When no symbol for the respective mood is given at a half hour

Fig. 1. Multimodal assessment of cardiovascular parameters (continuous finger blood pressure measurement with Portapres), physical activity (integrated thigh-EMG), moods (*upper staff lines*), behavior and events (*lower staff lines*) in a 23 year old male medical student (subject IA1) during everyday life. For further details see text

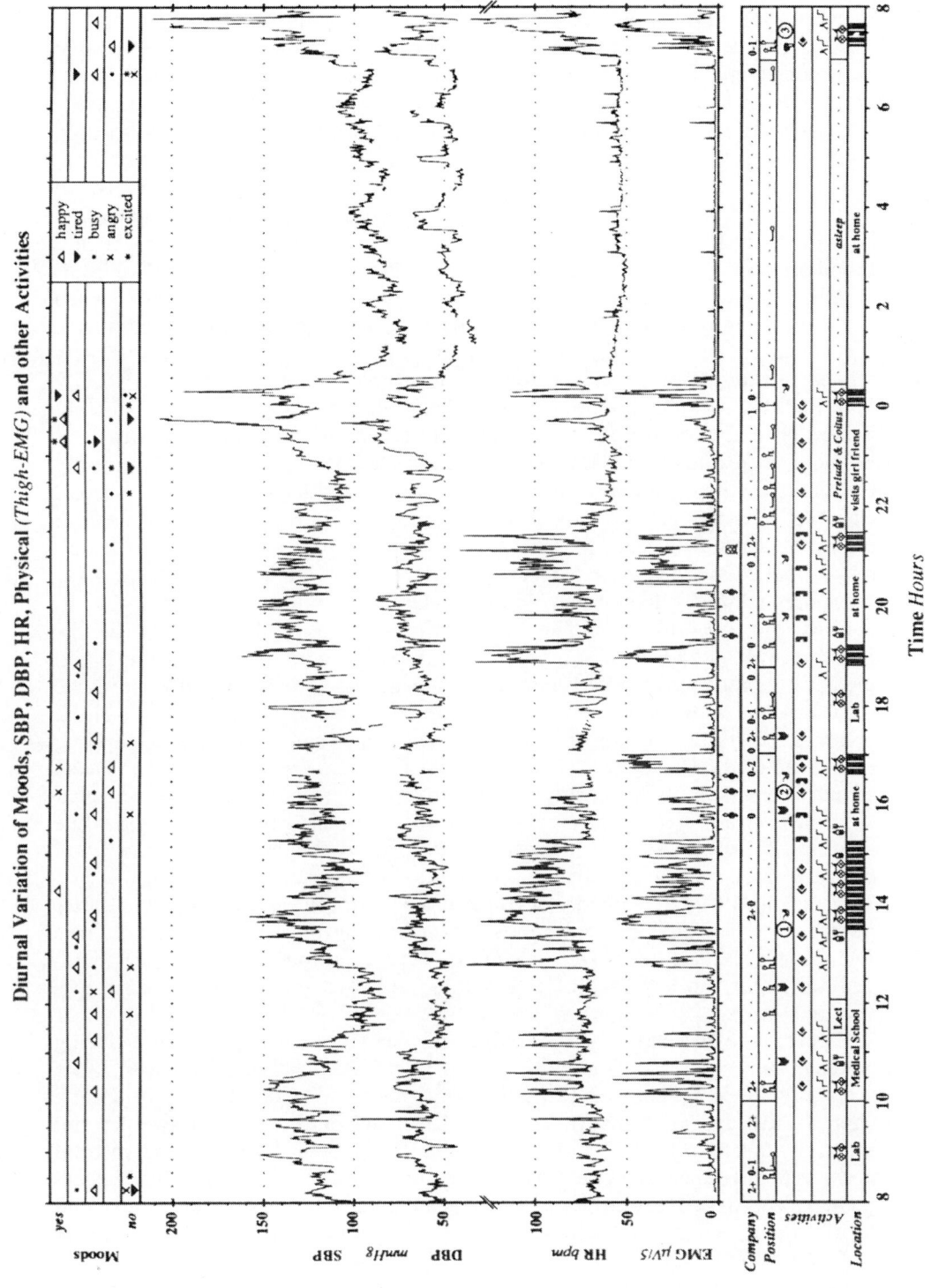

Diurnal Variation of Moods, SBP, DBP, HR, Physical *(Thigh-EMG)* and other Activities

interval it does not change. When the subject realizes in the afternoon that the Portapres batteries do not work anymore, it can be seen on his mood record that he becomes angry until the battery is exchanged in the laboratory. Moreover, visiting his girl friend at night he becomes exited and happy when he is sexually engaged with her, and tired afterwards when he cycles home where he falls asleep immediately.

The lowest blood pressure, heart rate and activity levels are seen, of course, at night during sleep. When awake low levels are found when he is studying and listening to the lecture, and during rest in the laboratory in the afternoon. Highest blood pressure peaks are to be seen during sexual intercourse, when the subject is cycling home afterwards and when he is cycling to the lab the next morning when the dog runs into his bike. Diastolic blood pressure is especially elevated during sexual activity and when the subject gets up in the morning. Heart rate is closely related to changes of physical activity as measured by integrated thigh-EMG.

In Figure 2 it can be seen that the major blood pressure peaks at night before going to bed are not just due to artefacts. Here 1-minute examples of continuous blood pressure and thigh-EMG recordings are shown at various activities: during the prelude (first example) just before as well as during the coitus (second example), during rest afterwards (third example), during cycling home (4th example), and during sleep at night (5th example). During the prelude when no major physical activity is displayed diastolic blood pressure exceeds 100 mm Hg most of the time, but systolic blood pressure does not reach 200 mm Hg. In contrast during coitus when the subject moves rhythmically (as shown in the EMG-recording) systolic blood pressure exceeds 200 mm Hg, but diastolic blood pressure remains well below 100 mm Hg. During the 35th second of the prelude recording and around the 40th second there are some artefacts (damped blood pressure recording). During coitus some arrhythmias can be seen. While cycling each tread of the left leg as well as free-wheeling can be recognized in the EMG signal. The shape of the Portap blood pressure curve is sometimes somewhat deformed during cycling, probably due to intrathoracic pressure changes while breathing forcefully. Also of interest are the differing shapes of the Portap blood pressure curve during the various activities.

Wesseling (1991) developed according to the pulse contour method a computer program for analysing the continuous intraarterial or finger blood pressure curve for beat-to-beat values of stroke volume, cardiac output and total peripheral resistance (for more details of this method see Wesseling et al. 1992, in this volume).

Figure 3 shows a beat-to-beat analysis of the hemodynamic responses during coitus in subject IA1. In this figure during the prelude total peripheral resistance is already somewhat elevated (around 2000 dyn $\times$ s/cm^5) from the very beginning (first 1200 heartbeats). During the very last part of this section systolic and especially diastolic blood pressure rises, due to a further large increase in total peripheral resistance. However, as soon as rhythmical physical movements start there is a rise in cardiac output produced by an increase of both stroke volume and heart rate, whereas total peripheral resistance decreases to below 1000 dyn $\times$ s/cm^5. This results in a further systolic blood pressure rise while diastolic blood pressure decreases. After orgasm blood pressure, heart rate, stroke

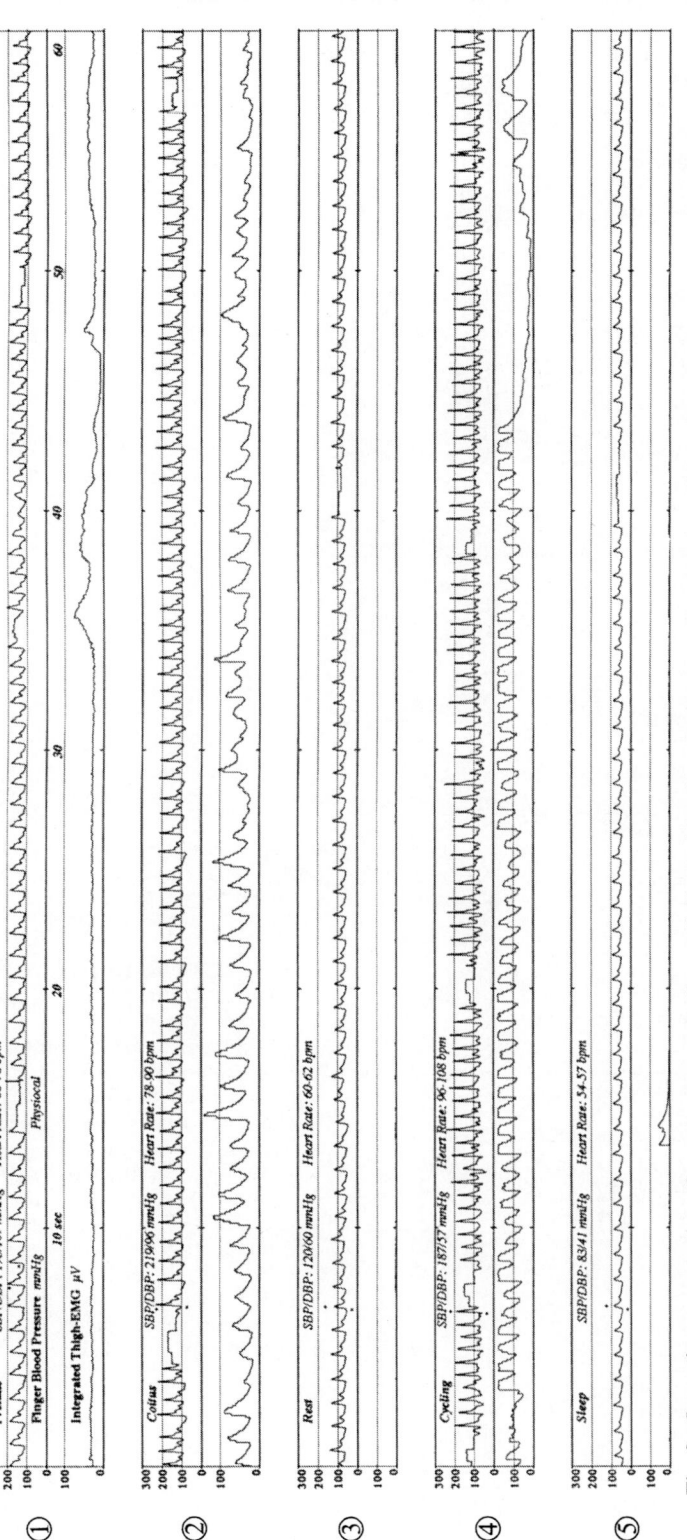

Fig. 2. One-minute examples of continuous recordings of finger blood pressure with Portapres and physical activity (integrated high-EMG) during subject IA1's various activities in everyday life: ① prelude (immediately before coitus), ② during coitus, ③ rest (afterwards), ④ cycling home, ⑤ sleep at night. These examples demonstrate that continuous finger blood pressure recordings with Portapres are possible in everyday life activities without major disturbances and artefacts

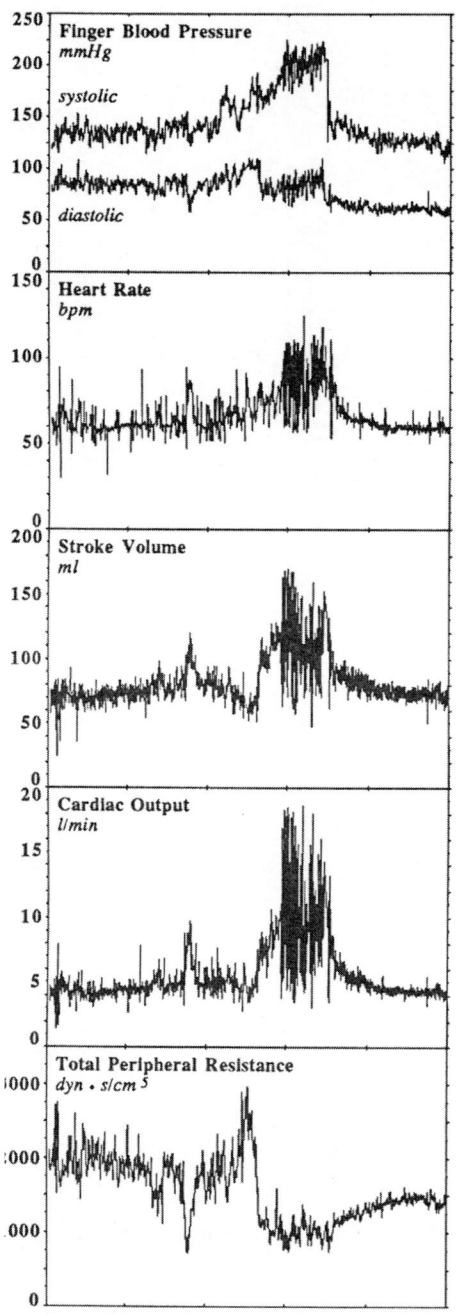

Fig. 3. Hemodynamic reactions during coitus (subject IA 1). Continuous finger blood pressure recordings with Porta-pres were analysed with the FAST system, a computer program developed by K. Wesseling (1991), which enables beat-to-beat analyses of systolic and diastolic blood pressure, heart rate, stroke volume, cardiac output, and total peripheral resistance according to the pulse contour method. The graph has been cleared of major artefacts (i.e. damped blood pressure recordings) such as mentioned in connection with fig. 2 during prelude. The various peaks/spikes in the beat-to-beat heart rate recording are due to arrhythmias

volume and cardiac output decrease rapidly to initial levels or below, while peripheral resistance rises slowly and remains below initial levels, pointing to a pronounced vasodilatation at rest afterwards.

This one example of 24 hour recording with Portapres clearly demonstrates in how much detail cardiovascular reaction patterns can now be analysed in everyday life. As behavior, emotions and environmental events strongly influence these patterns, it appears necessary to develop more sophisticated and reliable techniques to monitor these behaviors and events enabling a more accurate analysis of their relation to these cardiovascular parameters on a beat-to-beat basis.

24-Hour Recordings and the Effect of Physical Activity

Figure 4 shows the mean diurnal variation of systolic and diastolic blood pressure, heart rate and physical activity (as measured by integrated thigh-EMG) of 16 normotensive subjects during the placebo phase. Highest values of all four variables are found in the morning and afternoon. Lowest levels can be seen at night. While the activity measure reaches a bottom line at night, and both systolic and diastolic blood pressure decrease to their minimum quite rapidly, heart rate reaches its minimum only just before waking up again. The activity peaks in the first and second morning and in the afternoon correspond with the time when subjects either leave or come to the laboratory, for which purpose many subjects use their bicycle. Moreover, all subjects were asked not to use the elevator but rather to use the stairs when coming up to the laboratory on the fourth floor or when going down afterwards. So this effect can be seen as an activity synchronized somewhat between the different individuals during the 24 hour period, whereas other common activities spread over the day at different times, hiding their individual effects in the averaging process.

The night-time decrease in blood pressure, heart rate and activity is somewhat faster when the data are averaged after synchronisation for the individual times the subjects go to bed, which is shown in Fig. 5. During the last 4 1/2 hours before going to bed activity levels as well as blood pressure and heart rate are already somewhat reduced. Both systolic and diastolic blood pressure start to decrease about one hour before going to bed and reach their minimum about one hour afterwards, whereas the major changes of physical activity and heart rate are related somewhat more closely to the time of going to bed.

In the morning after synchronisation for the subjects' rising time activity, blood pressure and heart rate levels increase sharply and reach day-time levels within the first 30 minutes.

Another way to display 24 hour recordings are histograms which show the cumulative time the subjects spend on average at the various levels of blood pressure, heart rate and physical activity. In Fig. 6a each bar of each variable represents 1 unit (mm Hg, bpm or μV) and its height represents the cumulative minutes spent at this level during 24 hours. Values during day-time activity and night-time rest (indicated by white and black bars) are clearly separated in systolic and diastolic blood pressure as well as heart rate, whereas values of the physical activity measure overlap somewhat.

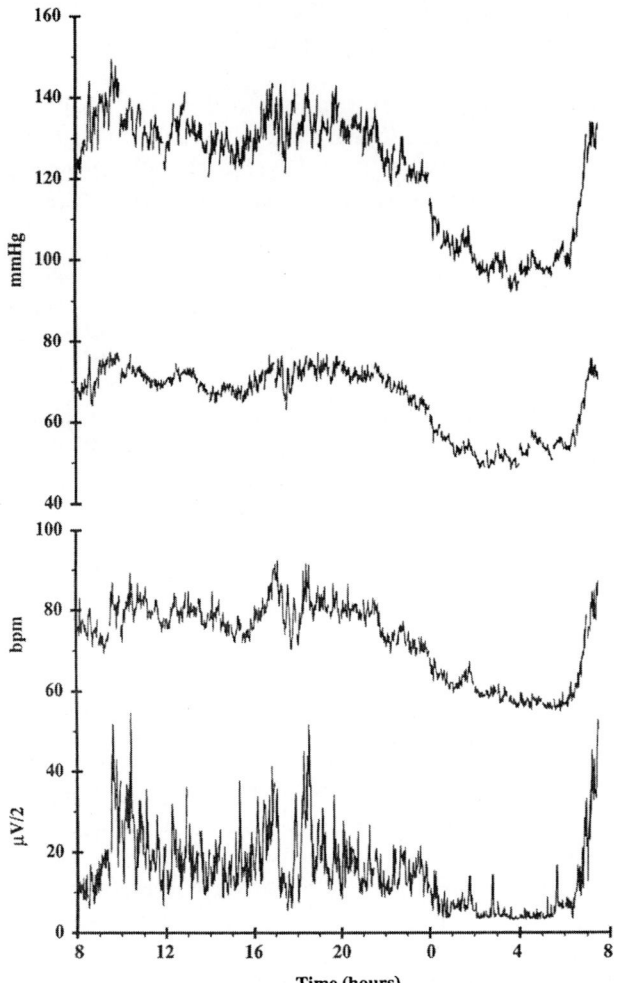

Fig. 4. Mean diurnal variation of systolic and diastolic blood pressure, heart rate, and physical activity as measured by integrated thigh-EMG of 16 young healty male subjects after placebo medication. Data are averaged as 64 second mean values in each subject

During activity systolic blood pressure levels range from 116–150 mm Hg on average during the day, with levels of 128–134 mm Hg most of the time, i.e. 60–80 minutes at each mm Hg in that range. For diastolic blood pressure the respective levels range from 62–78 mm Hg, with 70–73 mm Hg most of the time (i.e. 90–140 minutes). Average heart rate ranges between 67–93 bpm during activity, with levels of 76–81 bpm most of the time (i.e. 80–115 minutes).

During rest at night systolic blood pressure levels range from 92–115 mm Hg, with 97–100 mm Hg most of the time (i.e. 35–55 minutes). Average diastolic blood pressure levels range from 48–61 mm Hg, with 54–55 mm Hg most of the time (i.e. 45–65 minutes). Heart rate levels range at this time between 55–67 bpm,

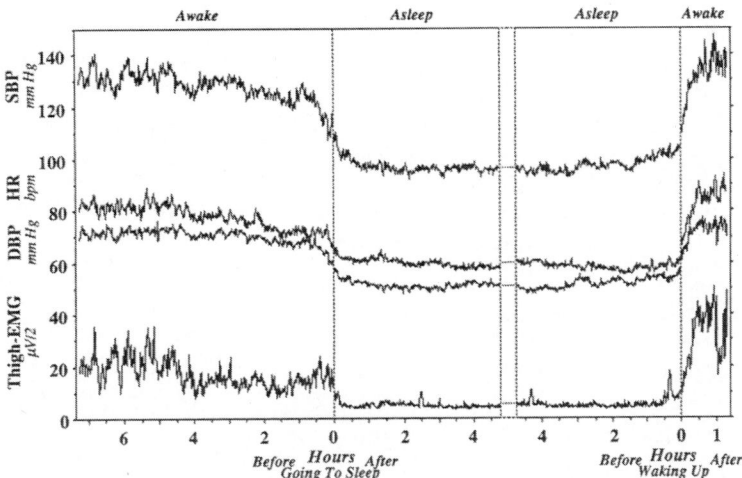

Fig. 5. Mean systolic and diastolic blood pressure, heart rate, and physical activity synchronized to the time of going to bed at night (*left*) and getting up in the morning (*right*). Averages of 64 second means of 16 young healty male subjects (after placebo medication)

most of the time being spent at 56–60 bpm (i.e. 40–60 minutes at each bpm in that range).

While active, systolic and diastolic blood pressure as well as heart rate and physical activity exhibit a broader range than during rest at night. Moreover, during the day blood pressure and heart rate columns are higher and/or comprise a larger area (the latter in the case of physical activity), indicating that within 24 hours a longer time is spent awake than asleep.

When four hours awake are compared to four hours asleep as in Fig. 6b all histograms during sleep are higher, i.e. a longer time is spent at a narrower range than while awake. This is because blood pressure, heart rate and physical activity vary more while awake. Such histograms can also be used to present drug or behavioral treatment effects on 24 hour blood pressure and heart rate (see Fig. 10).

Figure 1 gives a vivid impression of how highly blood pressure and heart rate are influenced by daily activities. Physical activity is one major source of their variation (van Egeren et al. 1992, in this volume). Using time series analysis it has been shown that thigh-EMG differentiates between different levels of physical activity such as running, walking and non-movement (Johnston et al. 1990a, b; Anastasiades and Johnston 1990). Moreover, it covaries closely with heart rate and appears to be a relatively more significant predictor of heart rate variance‧ than knowledge of the type of physical activity subjects are undertaking. It does not discriminate, however, between different postures (Anastasiades and Johnston 1990). The relationship between physical activity and blood pressure can now also be analysed in more detail with the continuous Portapres recordings.

If physical activity has a strong impact on blood pressure a methodological problem arises when the effect of an antihypertensive medication is to be evaluated. The drug might, for instance, cause tiredness without affecting blood

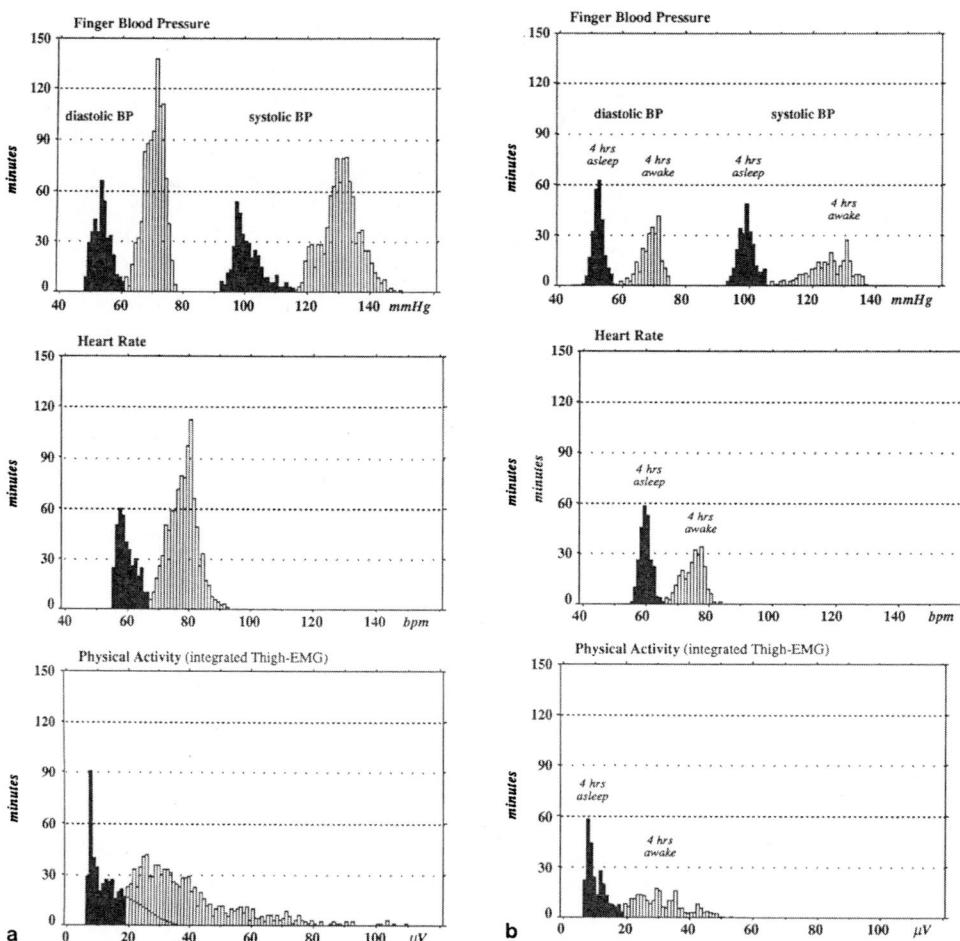

Fig. 6a. Cumulative time spent per unit (*minutes/mm Hg, bpm, µV*) within 24 hours at respective levels of systolic and diastolic blood pressure (*upper diagram*), heart rate (*middle diagram*) and physical activity (*lower diagram*). *White bars* indicate the time while awake and active, *black bars* the time while at rest and asleep at night. Based on 64 second averages of 16 young healthy male subjects (after placebo medication). **b.** Cumulative time spent per unit (*minutes/mm Hg, bpm, µV*) within 4 hours awake (*white bars*) and 4 hours asleep (*black bars*) at respective levels of systolic and diastolic blood pressure (*upper diagram*), heart rate (*middle diagram*) and physical activity (*lower diagram*). Based on 64 second averages of 16 young healthy male subjects (after placebo medication) synchronized for the time of going to bed

pressure directly. As subjects feel tired they are not as physically active as they are after placebo medication. The differing behavior might influence the blood pressure level significantly without the drug having any direct effect on blood pressure. Measuring physical activity as we have done with thigh-EMG in this investigation might help to control for such effects to some extent and to analyse this problem further.

Figure 7 shows the results of regression analyses predicting systolic and diastolic blood pressure (upper and middle diagram) as well as heart rate (lower

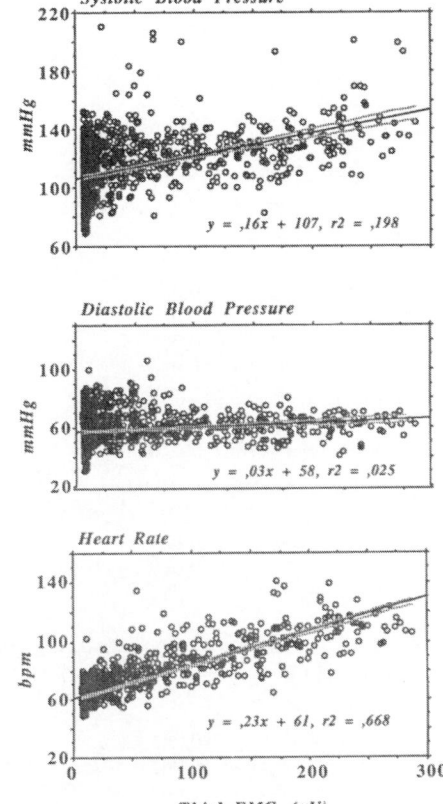

Fig. 7. Regression analyses of 24 hour systolic and diastolic blood pressure as well as heart rate in subject IA 1 on the basis of 64 second intervals. Physical activity (thigh-EMG) explains about 20% of systolic, 2.5% of diastolic blood pressure variance and 67% of heart rate variance. Dotted lines indicate 95% confidence bands for the true mean of y

diagram) by physical activity, as measured by thigh-EMG, in subject IA 1 using averaged 64-second-to-64-second intervals during 24 hours. In this subject physical activity explains 67% of heart rate variance within 24 hours, 20% of systolic and only 2.5% of diastolic blood pressure variance. The slope of each of the three regression lines is highly significant (p < 0.0001). This, however, does not take into account that physical activity has an effect upon these cardiovascular functions which may well last longer than just the 64 second interval during which these variables are averaged and related. By including the EMG-data additionally with time lags as possible predictors in stepwise multiple linear regression analyses this can be taken into consideration. Such analyses were performed by including 64 second EMG intervals with up to 10 and 20 time lags. This covers a total time of 10 minutes 40 seconds or 21 minutes 20 seconds in which a possible effect of physical activity can affect heart rate or blood pressure.

In Table 2 the results of multiple regression analyses for subject IA 1 are shown including up to 20 times lags as possible predictors. Prediction of heart rate variance by physical activity is improved through 6 different EMG predictors (at time lag 0, 13, 1, 4, 20, 10) by 11% up to a total explained variance of 77%. In systolic blood pressure prediction is improved when compared to the variance

Table 2. Stepwise multiple linear regression analyses of 24 hour systolic, diastolic blood pressure and heart rate at 64 second intervals in subject IA 1. Physical activity (thigh-EMG at 0 lag $\leq$ 20) explains about 30% of systolic and 9% of diastolic blood pressure variance within 24 hours as well as 77% of heart rate variance

Predictor	Regression Coefficient	Multiple R	R^2	F
Systolic Blood Pressure (24 h)				
EMG at lag				
2	0.049	0.476	0.227	336
5	0.052	0.512	0.262	55
0	0.063	0.531	0.282	31
14	0.036	0.540	0.292	17
3	0.038	0.543	0.295	6
Intercept 102.9				
Diastolic Blood Pressure (24 h)				
EMG at lag				
5	0.022	0.242	0.059	71
15	0.020	0.284	0.081	28
3	0.019	0.295	0.087	8
20	0.015	0.302	0.091	6
Intercept 55.7				
Heart Rate (24 h)				
EMG at lag				
0	0.141	0.818	0.668	2317
13	0.062	0.847	0.718	200
1	0.062	0.864	0.746	130
4	0.034	0.872	0.760	67
20	0.028	0.877	0.770	46
10	0.024	0.880	0.774	22
Intercept 57.7				

explained at lag 0 by 10% up to 30%, and in diastolic blood pressure by 7% up to 9%.

In Figure 8a for each of the 32 experimental days of the 16 subjects the heart rate, systolic and diastolic blood pressure variance within 24 hours explained by physical activity as measured by thigh-EMG including different time lags are shown. Including up to 20 time lags as possible predictors, covering a total time of 21 minutes and 20 seconds, physical activity explains 34–77% of heart rate variance (median 53%), 10–52% (median 31%) of systolic blood pressure variance and 4–38% (median 25%) of diastolic blood pressure variance. Prediction is improved above that at time lag 0 in all three variables between nearly 0 to 25%. On average prediction is improved in heart rate by 11%, in systolic blood pressure by 10% and in diastolic blood pressure by 14% (Fig. 8b). Including only up to ten time lags covering a time of 10 minutes and 40 seconds improves prediction up to 15–17% in heart rate and blood pressure for single cases.

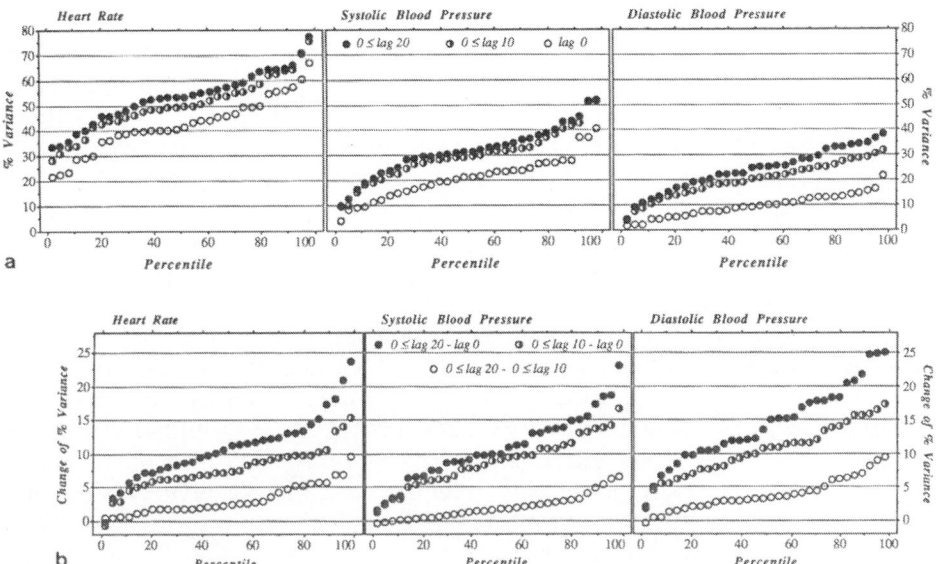

Fig. 8 a. Percentile plot of percentages of heart rate, systolic and diastolic blood pressure variances explained by physical activity (thigh-EMG) within 24 hours in a total of 32 experimental days in 16 subjects on the basis of 64 second intervals. Thigh-EMG at 0 lag $\leq$ 20 (*black circles*), at 0 lag $\leq$ 10 (half white, half black circles), and at lag 0 (*white circles*) were used as predictors in stepwise multiple linear regression analyses. **b** Percentile plot of percentage changes in heart rate, systolic and diastolic blood pressure variances explained by physical activity (thigh-EMG) within 24 hours at 0 lag $\leq$ 20 − lag 0 (black circles), 0 $\leq$ lag 10 − lag 0 (half white, half black circles), and 0 $\leq$ lag 20 − 0 $\leq$ lag 10 (black circles)

Physical activity appears to influence systolic and diastolic blood pressure in a more similar way than it does heart rate. This is indicated by the correlation coefficients between the systolic and diastolic blood pressure and heart rate variances explained by thigh-EMG. They are highest between systolic and diastolic blood pressure (r = 0.79), followed by systolic blood pressure and heart rate (r = 0.41), and diastolic blood pressure and heart rate (r = 0.27).

Thus, thigh-EMG appears to be an important measure which can be used to control for a powerful confounding variable, i.e. physical activity. On average more than half the heart rate variance within 24 hours is explained by this measure of physical activity, as also about 1/3 of systolic and 1/4 of diastolic blood pressure variance. However, it must be pointed out that physical activity alone might not be responsible for the variance explained by it. Other confounding variables which are related positively or negatively to this measure of physical activity might also contribute. For instance, it is known that body posture such as standing, sitting or a prone position has cardiovascular effects, for instance the heart rate being elevated when standing. Major physical activity will also only be recorded from thigh-EMG when the subject is erect; almost no activity will be recorded when the subject is sleeping in a prone position. This example also points to a number of other known and unknown confounders possibly contributing to the variance of these cardiovascular parameters explained within 24 hours by thigh-EMG.

Moreover, there are large differences in physical activity between individuals and days, explaining heart rate and blood pressure variance within 24 hours. The explained variance varies between different subjects and days by more than 40% in heart rate and systolic and avove 30% in diastolic blood pressure. Without regarding the time delayed effects, the explained variance is somewhat stable between the first and second experimental day in the 16 subjects in heart rate ($r = 0.75$) and systolic ($r = 0.74$) but not so much in diastolic blood pressure ($r = 0.23$). This points to the relatively greater importance, in this respect, of interindividual differences in the first two variables when compared to repeated days of the same subjects.

These results demonstrate that physical activity is a possible powerful confounding variable which may well effect results when evaluating antihypertensive therapies by 24 hour measurements. It remains for further analyses to determine why this activity measure explains such a large range of blood pressure and heart rate variance in different subjects and days. Other behavioral and environmental factors such as different patterns and kinds of activity, actions and movements with hands, body position, emotions and psychosocial stimuli etc. might play here an important role.

The thigh-EMG measure, however, appears to be valuable for controlling for the effects of physical activity to some extent not only in heart rate, but also in systolic blood pressure. In diastolic blood pressure prediction is improved especially when time delayed effects of physical activity are introduced. A somewhat higher percentage of variance might possibly be explained when time delayed effects for more than 21 minutes are allowed as predictors in the regression analyses. This is indicated by the fact that the 20th EMG time lag is quite often selected as significant predictor by regression analyses: in heart rate 23 times, in systolic blood pressure 16 times, and in diastolic blood pressure 21 times out of the 32 experimental days. However, the improvements between up to 10 and 20 time lags of the 64 second intervals are on average already small: 2% in systolic, 5% in diastolic blood pressure, and 3% in heart rate. Therefore only very small improvements could be expected by adding more time lags.

The Effect of Cilazapril on the Diurnal Variation of Blood Pressure and Heart Rate

Figure 9 shows the mean diurnal variation of systolic and diastolic blood pressure as well as heart rate and physical activity as measured by thigh-EMG during placebo and Cilazapril medication as 30 minute mean values.

In contrast to the pronounced diurnal variation the effect of Cilazapril appears to be rather small. Accordingly, analyses of variance reveal highly significant time effects for all four variables ($p < 0.0001$), but not Cilazapril or carry over effects when all 48 half hour mean values of each variable are analysed together at once. The cardiovascular variables show no significant interaction either between the effects of Cilazapril and time, i.e. the 48 half hour mean values. This indicates that no reliable effect of 2.5 mg Cilazapril on 24 hour blood pressure and heart rate can be demonstrated in this group of healthy young men after one week of medication.

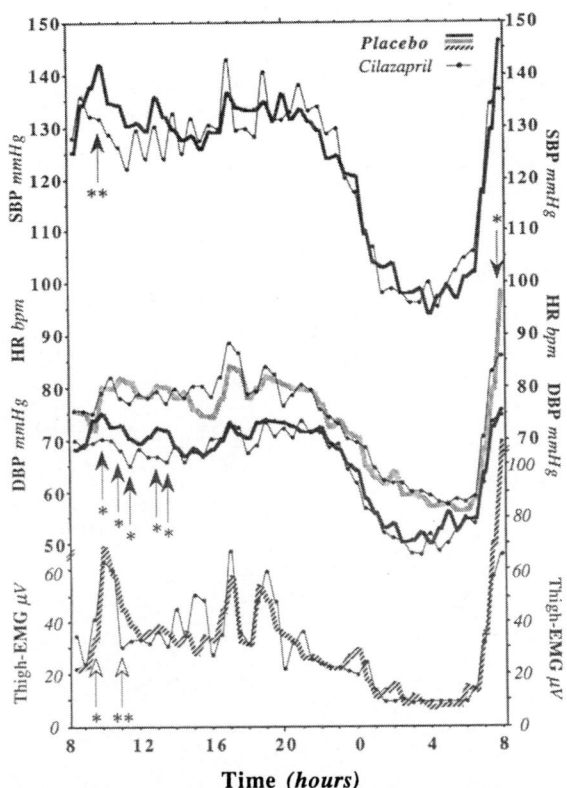

Fig. 9. Mean diurnal variation of systolic and diastolic blood pressure, heart rate, and physical activity as measured by thigh-EMG after placebo (*thick lines*) and after Cilazapril medication (thin lines) of 16 young healthy male subjects. Data are averaged as 30 minute means. *Arrows* indicate significant Cilazapril effects (*p < 0.05; **p < 0.01)

Although there has been no Cilazapril effect (neither as an overall main effect nor as an interaction effect with time) for exploratory reasons each half hour interval is analysed separately. These analyses of variance reveal few Cilazapril effects which are indicated in Fig. 9 by arrows. In Table 3 the exact differences and significance levels are shown for systolic and diastolic blood pressure for the first $3\frac{1}{2}-6$ hours. The results point to Cilazapril having an acute mainly diastolic blood pressure-lowering effect lasting only shortly, as most of the significant blood pressure differences are found in the morning up to six hours after the last Cilazapril medication.

Another way of presenting such treatment effects are histograms, in which the cumulative time spent at different blood pressure and heart rate levels within 24 hours is shown before and after treatment. Figure 10 shows the effect of Cilazapril (black/dotted area) vs placebo (white/dotted area) after one week's oral application in the 16 healthy male volunteers. The main drug effect appears to be on diastolic blood pressure: Cilazapril pushes both the day and night distributions to lower levels, i.e. more time is spent at lower diastolic blood pressure.

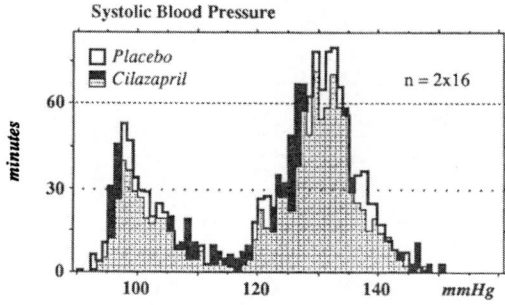

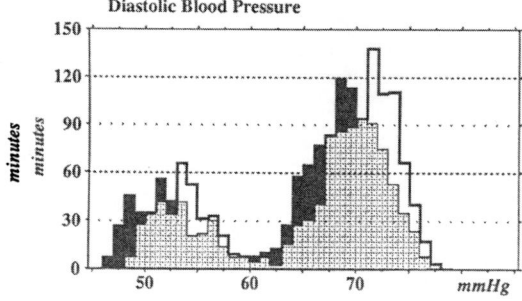

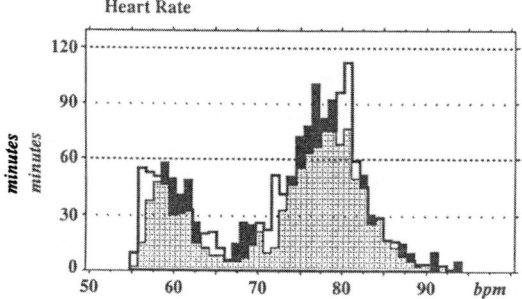

Fig. 10. Cumulative time spent per unit (*minutes/mm Hg, bpm*) within 24 hours at respective levels of systolic (*upper diagram*) and diastolic blood pressure (*middle diagram*) and heart rate (*lower diagram*) after placebo (*white/dotted*) and after Cilazapril medication (*black/dotted*). Based on 64 second averages of 2×16 subjects

It must be pointed out that performing so many significance tests (48 per variable) will also produce some significant results by chance. Moreover, confounding variables such as physical activity could have influenced the results. This may be the reason why only five out of eight possible half hour mean diastolic blood pressure differences between 9.30 AM and 1.30 PM are significant.

The possibility that the measure of physical activity, integrated thigh-EMG, could be a confounder is strongly supported by a significant interaction between the drug and time (i.e. 48 half hour intervals) effects in analysis of variance ($p < 0.001$) which can be seen in this variable in contrast to the cardiovascular parameters. This indicates that the pattern of physical activity during 24 hours is different after placebo and after Cilazapril medication. This, of course, can influence the results of how Cilazapril is affecting blood pressure and heart rate during different times of the day. Moreover, when half hour intervals are analysed separately in analyses of variance some significant differences can be seen during the first morning, indicated in Fig. 9 by unshaded arrows. However, it must be pointed out that EMG is not an absolute measure, which makes it difficult for different days to be compared even in the same subject. Therefore such comparisons must be handled with caution as it is not known to what extent such differences are caused by varying levels of physical activity or just be differing placements of the electrodes, although we tried to avoid such placement errors during the experiments. With an increasing number of subjects the influence of such errors becomes smaller. Furthermore, some EMG data are missing because of a loose contact in one subject. For this reason EMG analyses are based only on 15 instead of 16 subjects during the first morning, which is the time when Cilazapril mainly affects blood pressure. Differences in physical activity may especially confound drug effects if the investigated cardiovascular variables are very much dependent on this measure.

Control of Physical Activity

The thigh-EMG measure can be used to adjust the cardiovascular parameters to the varying impacts of physical activity in stepwise multiple linear regression analyses. Data of 64 second means of heart rate, systolic and diastolic blood pressure were taken as dependent (y), and 64 second means of thigh-EMG (e) as well as this thigh-EMG measure at time lag 1 to 20 as independent variables ($e_1, \ldots, e_{20}$), for the purpose of eliminating the influence of physical activity, including its time delayed effect, on these cardiovascular measures. Firstly the y-values, i.e. the parameters primarily under consideration, were adjusted for the influence of e, $e_1, \ldots, e_{20}$:

$$_{adjusted}y = y - b(e - \bar{e}) - b_1(e_1 - \bar{e_1}) - \ldots$$

with regression coefficients b for e, b_1 for e_1, and so forth, which is equivalent to adding the individual specific means of each dependent variable to the residuals of the above mentioned regression (Ostle 1969). The y adjusted in this way corresponds to a constant EMG for each individual over the 24 hour phase. But still the adjusted y corresponds to different levels of EMG from individual to individual. According to these calculations heart rate and blood pressure at 64 second intervals adjusted for the effect of physical activity were averaged as half hour means and used for further statistical analyses. It must be pointed out again that this procedure does not only adjust the cardiovascular parameters for the effect of physical activity, but also for all other confounding variables which are related positively or negatively to this thigh-EMG measure, such as for instance body posture.

In Figure 11, 24 hour systolic and diastolic blood pressure as well as heart rate thus adjusted for the effect of physical activity are shown after placebo and after Cilazapril medication. Compared to Fig. 9, blood pressure and heart rate peaks are lower during the day-time and especially early in the morning, when subjects quite often return to the laboratory by bicycle. Again, the diurnal variations override Cilazapril effects, which is indicated by analyses of variance. There are highly significant time effects (48 thirty minute means) for systolic and diastolic blood pressure and heart rate ($p < 0.0001$). However, the effect of Cilazapril is not

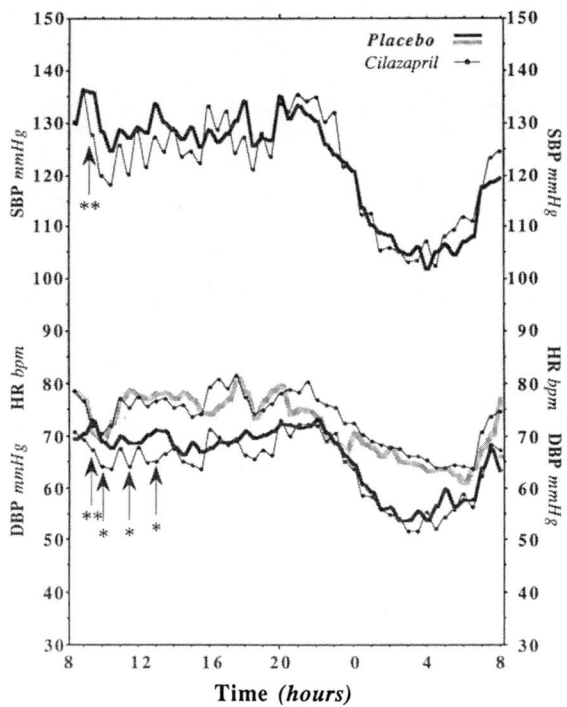

Fig. 11. Diurnal variation of systolic and diastolic blood pressure as well as heart rate adjusted for the effect of physical activity (thigh-EMG) after placebo (thick curves) and after Cilazapril medication (thin curves) as 30 minute means. *Arrows* indicate significant Cilazapril effects ($*p < 0.05$; $**p < 0.01$)

significant in systolic and diastolic blood pressure as well as heart rate. There are no significant interactions between the drug effect and time, and no carry over effects.

When, again for exploratory reasons, each half hour interval is analysed separately in analyses of variance, there are few significant Cilazapril effects, which are indicated by arrows in Fig. 11. In Table 3 also the exact differences and significance levels are shown for adjusted systolic and diastolic blood pressure for the first 3 1/2–6 hours. As before it must be pointed out that not each half hour interval could be calculated with all 16 subjects because of some missing EMG data caused by an occasionally loose contact.

Compared to the unadjusted data, the number of significant differences is reduced from 7 to 5 and there are changes in significance levels. However, in general, after additional control for physical activity the results confirm that in this group of healty young men one week of oral administration of 2.5 mg Cilazapril may have an acute effect, reducing mainly diastolic blood pressure by 4–6 mm Hg from about 1.5 h after oral application and lasting another 4 h during unrestricted daily life.

Cilazapril has been shown to lower systolic as well as diastolic 24 hour blood pressure in hypertensive patients reliably after 8 weeks of medication (mean dose

3.6 mg once daily), being most pronounced during the period being awake (19/12 mm Hg) (White et al. 1988). Moreover, according to Sanchez et al. (1988) a significant predose effect on sitting systolic and diastolic blood pressure was not seen before 4 weeks of 0.5–10 mg Cilazapril being applied once daily, whereas diastolic blood pressure was immediately significantly reduced two hours after the initial dose, with this reduction being further enhanced 2, 4, and 6 weeks later.

One week of oral Cilazapril application therefore appears too short for effects lasting 24 hours to be seen. In our study, however, we did not feel justified to treat healthy subjects for longer than one week at this stage of investigations. Therefore we had to accept the possibility of failing to demonstrate an effect lasting 24 hours.

As has been previously pointed out before, ambulatory blood pressure measurement during daily life is confounded by a great number of uncontrolled variables. Physical activity is just one of those and the variance it explains cannot only be attributed to this EMG measure which is definitely related to other confounding variables, such as for instance posture. Such variables might also contribute to the explained variance, but it is not known to what extent. Furthermore, physical activity of other body parts such as hands, arms, shoulder, head etc. are not measured by thigh-EMG, but might also influence blood pressure and heart rate to some extent (van Egeren et al. 1992, in this volume). Such and other uncontrolled behavioral confounders could be a reason why the effect of Cilazapril on diastolic blood pressure cannot be demonstrated in each half hour interval between 9 AM and 1 PM, even after adjustment for this thigh-EMG activity measure. An additional explanation could be that no adjustments were made for different days. As EMG is not on absolute measure such adjustments for different days were renounced. Furthermore, serial dependency of the cardiovascular variables has not yet been taken into account. Analyses aiming at dealing with this problem are in progress, and will be reported on later.

The fact that differing behaviors might play an important role in confounding the blood pressure lowering effect of Cilazapril is indicated by the subjects' diary reports. In Figure 11 systolic and diastolic blood pressure rises can be seen between 10.30–11.00 and 11.30–12.00 AM after Cilazapril medication which then reduces the assumed drug effects to nearly zero. By this time all subjects had left the laboratory. The subject showing the effect most contrary to the expected diastolic blood pressure lowering one between 10.30–11.00 AM (ΔSBP/ DBP$_{Cil-Pla}$ = +7.5/+8.4 mm Hg), a medical student (A 5), reports in his diary that he was quietly listening to a lecture during his first experimental day after having received placebo. After Cilazapril medication on his second experimental day he reported that during the same time interval he smoked 3 cigarettes, drank 3 cups of coffee, talked, read and climbed stairs – all behaviors known to raise blood pressure. Moreover, subject B 6, an engineering student, who exhibited the most opposing diastolic blood pressure drug effect between 11.30–12.00 AM (ΔSBP/ ΔDBP$_{Cil-Pla}$ = +21.4/+12.9 mm Hg) did not report behaving much differently at this time during both days: he was at home reading and preparing himself for his final examination and sometimes talking to his girl friend. On the first experimental day after having received the ACE-inhibitor he smoked a cigarette, and on the second experimental day after placebo medication he drank a cup of coffee during the same time interval. However, for some reason on the first day

Table 3a, b. Mean ($\pm$SE) 30 minute intervals of systolic (a) (between 8.00–11.30 AM) and of diastolic blood pressure (b) (between 8.00 AM–2.00 PM) after placebo and after Cilazapril medication not adjusted as well as adjustesd for the effect of physical activity (thigh-EMG)

a

Time		SBP$\pm$SE not adjusted (n = 16)	SBP$\pm$SE adjusted (n = 15)
8.00– 8.30	Placebo	125.3$\pm$2.3	130.2$\pm$2.6
	Cilazapril	128.0$\pm$4.2	130.3$\pm$4.4
	Diff. Cil-Pla	+2.7$\pm$3.3	+0.1$\pm$3.7
8.30– 9.00	Placebo	134.2$\pm$2.6	136.4$\pm$2.8
	Cilazapril	135.7$\pm$3.9	135.6$\pm$3.7
	Diff. Cil-Pla	+1.5$\pm$3.3	−0.8$\pm$3.5
9.00– 9.30	Placebo	137.7$\pm$2.4	136.2$\pm$2.7
	Cilazapril	132.2$\pm$3.1	127.6$\pm$3.0
	Diff. Cil-Pla	−5.6$\pm$2.7; $P = 0.054$	−8.6$\pm$2.3**; $P = 0.0067$
9.30–10.00	Placebo	141.9$\pm$2.4	127.3$\pm$3.7
	Cilazapril	131.7$\pm$3.4	119.9$\pm$3.5
	Diff. Cil-Pla	− 10.2$\pm$3.6**; $P = 0.0068$	−7.4$\pm$3.9; $P = 0.11$
10.00–10.30	Placebo	134.7$\pm$3.8	124.9$\pm$4.1
	Cilazapril	128.8$\pm$4.0	118.2$\pm$4.1
	Diff. Cil-Pla	−6.0$\pm$3.5; $P = 0.11$	−6.8$\pm$3.8; $P = 0.091$
10.30–11.00	Placebo	134.3$\pm$4.5	127.4$\pm$4.1
	Cilazapril	126.2$\pm$3.8	125.8$\pm$3.7
	Diff. Cil-Pla	−8.1$\pm$3.8; $P = 0.061$	−1.7$\pm$3.9
11.00–11.30	Placebo	130.5$\pm$4.5	127.2$\pm$4.1
	Cilazapril	122.1$\pm$3.7	120.0$\pm$3.7
	Diff. Cil-Pla	−8.4$\pm$3.9; $P = 0.066$	−5.6$\pm$3.7

(after Cilazapril) he reported in his diary that he felt somewhat busy, irritated, angry, and hurried at that time, – all moods which raise blood pressure to a greater extent than Cilazapril may lower it. When asked for the reason for his irritation and anger he reported that on the first day the AC adapter cable made him feel quite restricted in moving around his flat during the time in question. Therefore he preferred using the battery instead of the AC adapter on the second experimental day even when at home.

This, of course, is only accidental evidence, but points to the problem of behavioral confounders during everyday life when studying drug or other treatment effects in small groups. Such behavioral or emotional and environmental influences can easily override mild drug effects.

Using thigh-EMG in regression analyses cannot, of course, control for all potent behavioral influences. Nevertheless, by including this measure of physical activity at least one major confounding variable could be controlled for. Although somewhat restricted by some missing EMG data in this investigation, the way cardiovascular variables were adjusted for physical activity appears to be a

Table 3 b

Time		DBP ± SE *not adjusted* (*n* = 16)	DBP ± SE *adjusted* (*n* = 15)
8.00– 8.30	*Placebo*	68.2 ± 1.4	69.9 ± 1.3
	Cilazapril	69.9 ± 2.4	70.6 ± 3.0
	Diff. Cil-Pla	*+1.7 ± 2.1*	*+0.7 ± 2.3*
8.30– 9.00	*Placebo*	69.3 ± 1.5	70.2 ± 1.6
	Cilazapril	68.8 ± 2.1	69.2 ± 2.3
	Diff. Cil-Pla	*+0.5 ± 1.7*	*−1.0 ± 2.2*
9.00– 9.30	*Placebo*	73.8 ± 1.3	73.3 ± 1.3
	Cilazapril	69.5 ± 2.2	67.4 ± 2.1
	Diff. Cil-Pla	*−4.3 ± 2.1; P = 0.057*	*−6.0 ± 1.8**; P = 0.0094*
9.30–10.00	*Placebo*	75.1 ± 2.0	68.2 ± 1.8
	Cilazapril	70.1 ± 2.0	64.1 ± 2.0
	Diff. Cil-Pla	*−5.0 ± 1.8*; P = 0.012*	*−4.1 ± 1.7*; P = 0.033*
10.00–10.30	*Placebo*	72.6 ± 1.6	67.7 ± 2.0
	Cilazapril	70.0 ± 2.1	63.5 ± 2.2
	Diff. Cil-Pla	*−2.6 ± 1.9*	*−4.2 ± 1.9; P = 0.065*
10.30–11.00	*Placebo*	72.8 ± 2.1	69.0 ± 2.0
	Cilazapril	68.0 ± 1.9	67.4 ± 1.7
	Diff. Cil-Pla	*−4.8 ± 2.1*; P = 0.031*	*−1.6 ± 1.9*
11.00–11.30	*Placebo*	70.5 ± 2.4	68.4 ± 2.5
	Cilazapril	65.0 ± 2.1	64.0 ± 2.0
	Diff. Cil-Pla	*−5.5 ± 2.2*; P = 0.0182*	*−4.4 ± 2.3*; P = 0.026*
11.30–12.00	*Placebo*	69.5 ± 2.7	68.3 ± 2.9
	Cilazapril	68.2 ± 2.1	67.7 ± 2.2
	Diff. Cil-Pla	*−1.3 ± 2.3*	*−0.7 ± 2.1*
12.00–12.30	*Placebo*	70.6 ± 2.4	70.0 ± 2.5
	Cilazapril	66.8 ± 2.8	64.9 ± 2.6
	Diff. Cil-Pla	*−3.8 ± 3.3*	*−5.1 ± 3.2*
12.30–13.00	*Placebo*	72.4 ± 2.0	70.2 ± 2.0
	Cilazapril	66.7 ± 2.5	65.0 ± 2.6
	Diff. Cil-Pla	*−5.7 ± 2.2*; P = 0.028*	*−5.2 ± 2.1*; P = 0.05*
13.00–13.30	*Placebo*	72.0 ± 2.4	70.4 ± 2.3
	Cilazapril	65.7 ± 2.9	66.4 ± 2.8
	Diff. Cil-Pla	*−6.3 ± 2.7*; P = 0.047*	*−4.0 ± 2.8*
13.30–14.00	*Placebo*	68.6 ± 3.0	66.7 ± 2.8
	Cilazapril	68.7 ± 2.2	67.5 ± 2.2
	Diff. Cil-Pla	*+0.1 ± 3.0*	*+0.7 ± 3.0*

promising strategy, when the effect of an antihypertensive medication is to be evaluated with ambulatory continuous noninvasive blood pressure monitoring during 24 hours in nearly unrestricted everyday life. These adjustments may help to elaborate the true drug effect.

The Effect of Cilazapril on Blood Pressure and Heart Rate During Laboratory Tasks

Another and additional approach to assessing drug effects without the problem of major uncontrollable confounding variables which are unvoidable and during ambulatory monitoring are, of course, measurements during highly standardized laboratory tasks. Such tasks can be tailored to the desired study effects, and they can be repeated at different time intervals after drug administration. Repetition might bring up other confounding problems such as habituation which can be more severe in some tasks than in others. A further question is how relevant such tasks are, and to what extent they represent everyday life. A combination of the two, however, multimodal assessment in everyday life, i.e. ambulatory monitoring together with measurements during standardized laboratory tasks allows the strength of both methods to be combined and the results to be compared. This might be the best way of finding more comprehensive answers to the questions asked.

Figures 12a and b give a summary of the results of the morning and afternoon laboratory test sessions. The course of mean systolic and diastolic blood pressure and heart rate is shown after placebo as well as after Cilazapril medication during the various laboratory tasks. In systolic and diastolic blood pressure the highest levels are seen during the reaction time task (2) and the lowest levels during rest in a prone position (3). In heart rate comparably high levels are also found during the reaction time task (2), when standing (4), and during physical exercise (12), whereas low levels are seen during rest in a prone position (3) and during the breath holding procedures (5, 7, 9, 11).

In the morning session Cilazapril lowers systolic blood pressure significantly only during the last breath holding procedure (11) (p = 0.038) and during physical exercise (12) (p = 0.048); during the third breath holding procedure it misses the 5% significance level (p = 0.097). The most frequent significant effects can be seen in diastolic blood pressure. During all breath holding procedures (5, 7, 9, 11) (p < 0.005), the second and third diving tests (8, 10) (p < 0.03), mild physical exercise (12) (p = 0.0056) and rest afterwards (13) (p = 0.037), diastolic blood pressure is significantly lower after Cilazapril, that is 104–112 minutes after the last medication. During standing (4) this difference just misses the 5% significance level (p = 0.079). Heart rate is slightly but significantly elevated after Cilazapril only during the third breath holding procedure (9) (p = 0.046). During the first, second and fourth breath holding procedure (5, 7, 11) this difference just misses the 5% significance criterion (p < 0.1). These results show that Cilazapril lowers mainly diastolic blood pressure, but not before 100 minutes after its application. Furthermore, the results confirm that after seven days of medication in this group of young healthy men Cilazapril has no blood pressure effect lasting for 24 hours or longer. Otherwise significant differences should also be seen from the very beginning of the laboratory test session. Moreover, in the afternoon session there

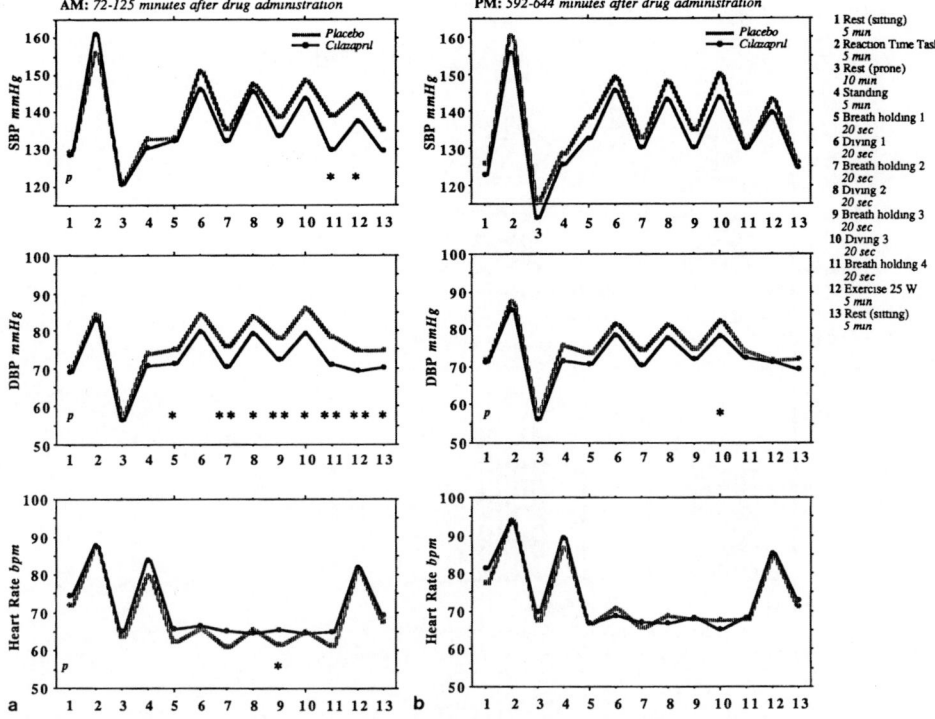

Fig. 12a, b. Mean systolic, diastolic blood pressure and heart rate during 13 different laboratory situations after placebo and Cilazapril medication in the morning (**a**) and afternoon test sessions (**b**); (n = 16; *p < 0.05; **p < 0.01)

are no significant differences at all in systolic blood pressure and heart rate, and in diastolic blood pressure a small but significant difference can only be seen during the last diving test (10) (p = 0.027); during the second breath holding procedure (7) (p = 0.086) and during standing (4) it just misses the 5% significance criterion (p = 0.059).

Figure 13 shows the effect of Cilazapril on systolic and diastolic blood pressure and heart rate during mild physical exercise (25 Watt). In the morning it lowers systolic and diastolic blood pressure by 7/5 mm Hg (= 0.048/p = 0.0056) but has no significant effect on heart rate or in the afternoon. A systolic and diastolic blood pressure lowering effect of Cilazapril during physical exercise without changing heart rate has also been shown in hypertensive patients (White et al. 1988) and is supported in this study.

The results of the laboratory test procedures confirm those already described for ambulatory monitoring. As in everyday life Cilazapril shows a mainly diastolic blood pressure lowering effect. It does not reach significance levels before about 104 minutes after Cilazapril administration but can be seen up to the end of the morning laboratory tests 125 minutes after drug application. Moreover, the morning and afternoon laboratory test sessions confirm that there is no general long lasting blood pressure lowering effect. This effect would otherwise have been

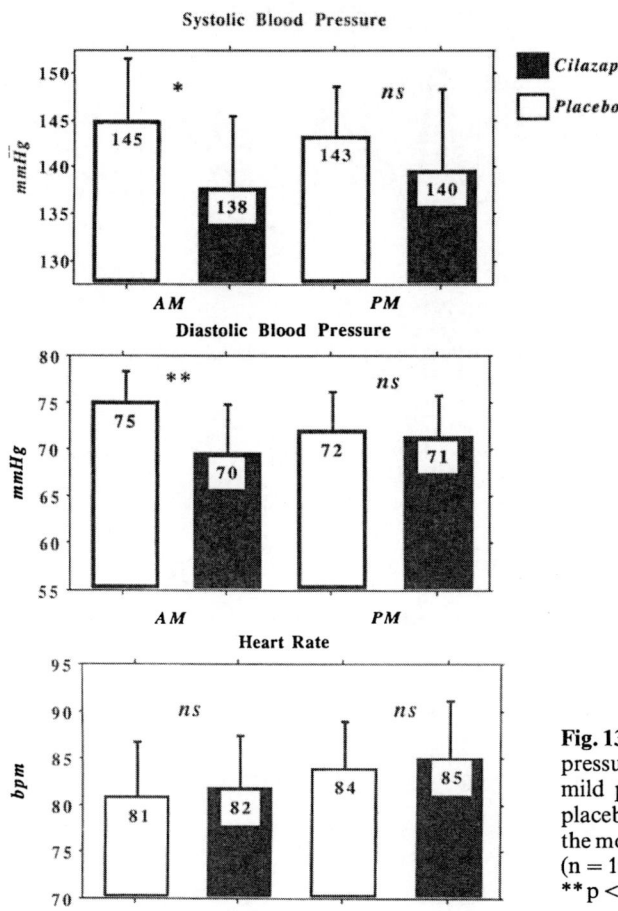

Fig. 13. Mean systolic, diastolic blood pressure and heart rate during 5 minute mild physical exercise (25 Watt) after placebo and Cilazapril medication in the morning and afternoon test sessions (n = 16) (*ns*, non significant; *p < 0.05; **p < 0.01)

demonstrable in the afternoon laboratory test session at approximately 10 hours after drug application, and during the first 4 sections of the morning laboratory test session 72–103 minutes afterwards.

The systolic blood pressure lowering Cilazapril effect which can be shown 1 1/2–4 hours after drug administration in the 24 hour recordings is also supported by the laboratory tests during the last breath holding procedure and during mild physical exercise. This systolic blood pressure lowering effect is about 6–10 mm Hg and seems to last for a somewhat shorter time than the effect on diastolic blood pressure. The more reliable and longer lasting effect of cilazapril on diastolic blood pressure might be due to the mechanisms by which this drug affects the cardiovascular system: it reduces the plasma angiotensin II level, thus preventing the vasoconstriction it would induce, i.e. it lowers total peripheral resistance. It might also be partly due to diastolic blood pressure being a more reliable Portapres/Finapres measure than systolic blood pressure (Imholz et al. 1988, 1991; Parati et al. 1989).

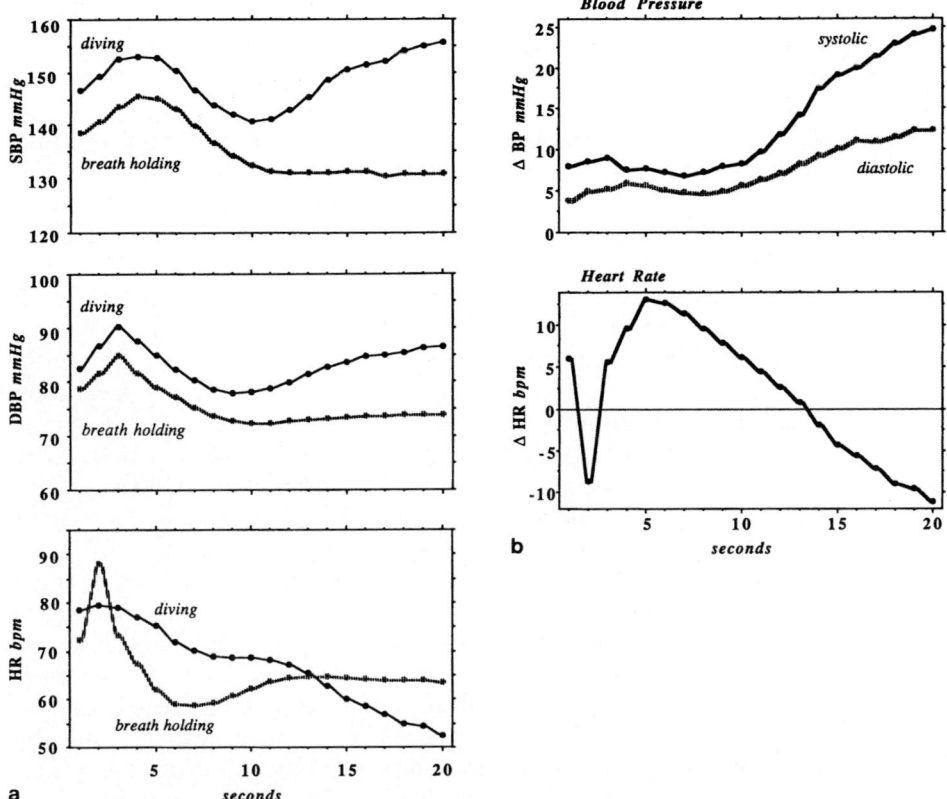

Fig. 14a, b. Mean 20 second intervals of systolic, diastolic blood pressure and heart rate during the breath holding and diving tests after placebo medication averaged for morning and afternoon test sessions (**a**), as well as corresponding blood pressure and heart rate differences *diving-breath holding test* (**b**)

Cardiovascular Responses During the Breath Holding and Diving Test

An excellent test in our experiment for investigating the effect of Cilazapril on blood pressure reactivity is the diving test and its control procedure, breath holding. Here, 104–112 minutes after drug administration, we could demonstrate reliable effects on diastolic blood pressure levels. For further detailed analyses all four breath holding and all three diving tests in the morning test session as well as separately those in the afternoon session were averaged for each of the 20 seconds of these procedures in each subject. These averaged data were used for further analyses.

Figure 14a shows the course of systolic, diastolic blood pressure and heart rate during both procedures after placebo medication. Here the data of each second of the 20 second intervals of all performed tests from the morning together with those from the afternoon session were averaged. Therefore each of the diving test curves is averaged across 96 trials (16 × 2 × 3) altogether and the breath holding curves across 128 trials ($16 \times 2 \times 4$) of the 16 subjects. In Figure 11 b the blood pressure and heart rate values recorded during the diving test are subtracted from those recorded during the breath holding procedure, averaged for all subjects in each of the 20 seconds.

As can be seen in Fig. 14 a, systolic and diastolic blood pressure rises by about 5 mm Hg during the first few seconds of both the diving and breath holding test, followed by a drop. Compared to the breath holding test, both pressures are about 8/4 mm Hg higher during the diving test right from the beginning (Fig. 14 b, upper diagram). This elevation might be an activation effect of knowing that the face has now to be put into cold water and not into an empty bowl. Only after the tenth second does the blood pressure change differently in both tests: it rises slowly by another 16/8 mm Hg when diving, but remains constant while holding the breath. This later blood pressure rise when diving is probably due to an increasing vascular resistance. The two tests show quite different heart rate changes from the very beginning. During breath holding it rises from an average of 72 bpm by more than 15 bpm for the first two seconds, followed by a drop of about 30 bpm until the sixth second and a slow rise up to the 12th second, when it remains constant at about 64 bpm. During the diving test the heart rate continues to drop from the first to the 20th second by altogether 28 bpm on average, due to an increasing vagal and perhaps also decreasing sympathetic activation. In the lower diagram of figure 14 b heart rate differences (diving minus breath holding test) above and below zero indicate a heart rate in the diving test above or below the heart rate recorded during the breath holding control procedure. Although continuously dropping during the diving test, the heart rate is not reduced below that measured during the breath holding procedure until the 14th second (with an exception during the 2nd second which is due to the heart rate peak during breath holding). This points both to a sympathetic stimulation and a vagal withdrawal in the initial part of the diving test, as can usually be seen during the defense reaction which is coordinated in the hypothalamic defense area. A sympathetic withdrawal below and/or a vagal stimulation above the sympathetic and/or vagal activation during the corresponding seconds of the breath holding test only takes place in the last 6 seconds of the diving test.

In Figures 15a, b, c the effects of Cilazapril on systolic and diastolic blood pressure as well as on heart rate are shown during the breath holding and diving test in the morning and afternoon. Analyses of variance reveal highly significant time effects ($p < 0.001$), i.e. differences between 20 second intervals, in all these cardiovascular variables during both tests in the morning as well as in the afternoon test session. During both test sessions, in the morning and afternoon, after Cilazapril application systolic blood pressure is somewhat but not significantly reduced in the breath holding as well as diving test (Fig. 15a). In the morning breath holding test the significance criterion is just missed ($p = 0.059$) for systolic blood pressure.

Fig. 15a–c. Mean 20 second intervals of systolic (a), diastolic blood pressure (b), and heart rate (c) during the breath holding and diving tests after placebo and Cilazapril medication in the morning and afternoon laboratory test sessions (*ns*, non significant; *$p < 0.05$; ***$p < 0.001$)

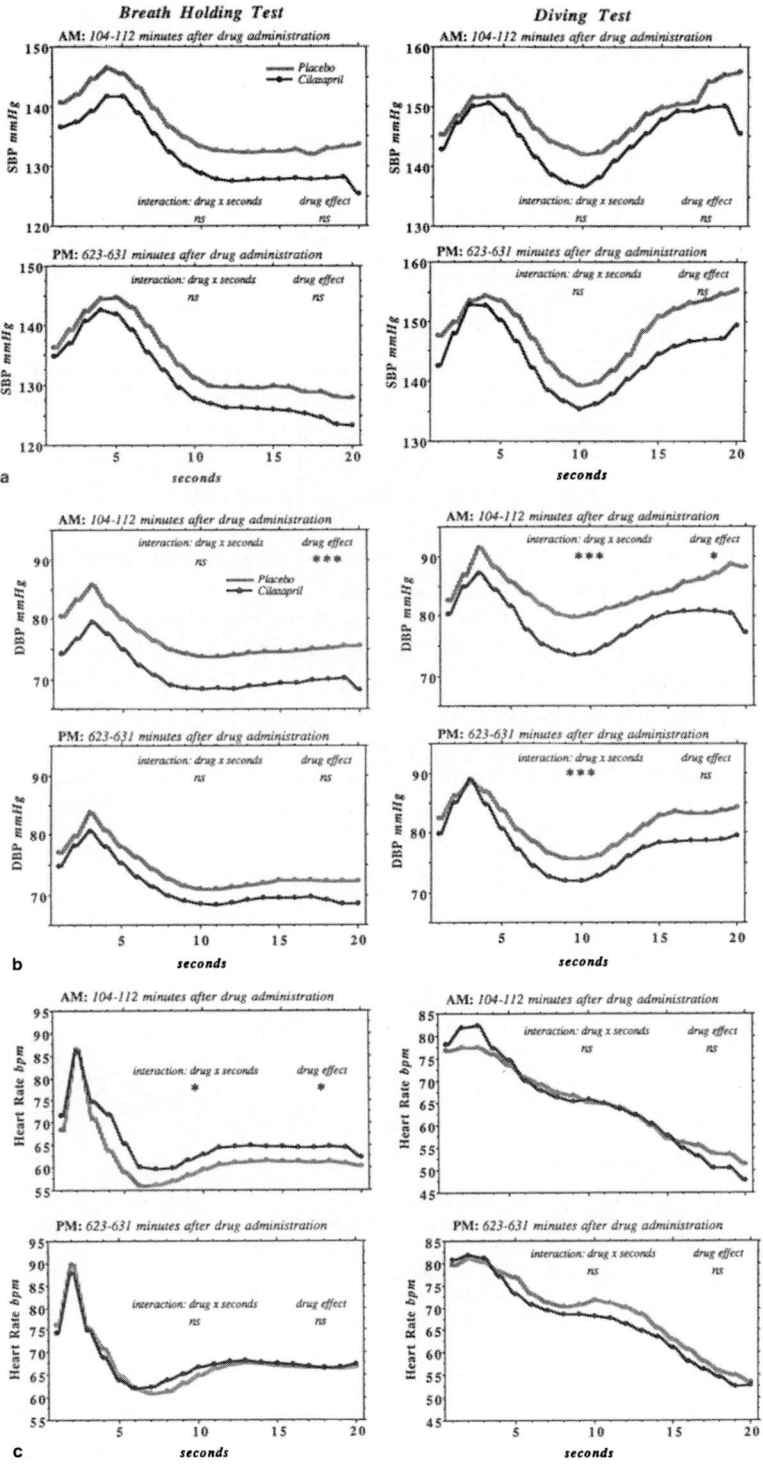

Cilazapril lowers diastolic blood pressure significantly during both tests in the morning: during the breath holding test by 5.7 ± 1.8 (p = 0.001) and during the diving test by 5.4 ± 2.4 mm Hg (p = 0.01). In the afternoon diastolic blood pressure is also somewhat lowered by Cilazapril, but the significance criterion is just missed during the diving test ($- 3.5 \pm 1.6$ mm Hg; p = 0.06) and the effect is not significant during breath holding test ($- 2.8 \pm 1.7$ mm Hg) (Fig. 15 b). Moreover, during the diving test in the morning and afternoon a significant interaction (p < 0.004) can be seen between the drug and time (i.e. 20 second intervals) effect. This indicates that in contrast to the breath holding test the time course of diastolic blood pressure is not the same before and after Cilazapril administration during this test.

This is illustrated in Figure 16 by showing the diastolic blood pressure lowering effect of the ACE-inhibitor (Cilazapril minus placebo) during each of the 20 second intervals for the breath holding (upper diagram) and diving test (lower diagram). Values below zero indicate a blood pressure lowering effect of Cilazapril. The upper diagram shows that the diastolic blood pressure differences during the breath holding test run parallel to the zero line in both the morning and afternoon. In the morning the averaged diastolic blood pressure difference is, as indicated before, significant, but not in the afternoon. In the diving test, however, the mean diastolic blood pressure lowering effects is significant during the morning and just misses the significance criterion in the afternoon, but the drug effect changes within the 20 seconds (i.e. does not run parallel to the zero line in Fig. 16). The highest diastolic blood pressure lowering effects in the morning can be seen between the 7th–11th second (by $- 7$ mm Hg) and during the last few seconds of the test (by $- 6$ to $- 11$ mm Hg), probably when peripheral vascular

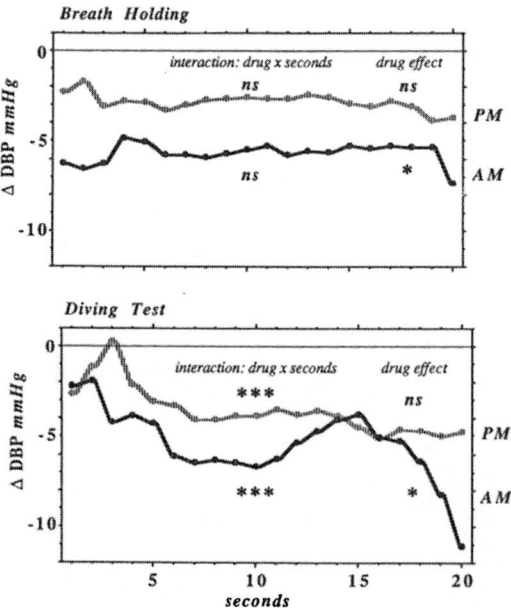

Fig. 16. Effect of Cilazapril (Cilazapril-placebo) on diastolic blood pressure during the breath holding and diving tests in the morning and afternoon laboratory test sessions (ns, non significant; *p < 0.05; ***p < 0.001)

resistance is increasing most. Slighter effects are found initially during the first few seconds and during the 14th–17th seconds. This indicates the interaction between the drug and time effect. In the afternoon the diastolic blood pressure lowering effect of the drug appears to be somewhat although not significantly, less than in the morning. Again, it is not the same throughout the 20 seconds of diving: it becomes somewhat more pronounced the longer the subjects are diving. When differences between the morning and afternoon course of the diastolic blood pressure lowering effect of the ACE-inhibitor are tested in analysis of variance (= interaction morning/afternoon × drug × 20 seconds) the 5% significance criterion is just missed (p = 0.072).

Figure 15c shows the heart rate during the breath holding and diving test in the morning and afternoon after Cilazapril and placebo medication. A significant drug effect can be seen only during the morning breath holding procedure. Here Cilazapril elevates heart rate by an average of 3.5 bpm (p = 0.049). However, a significant interaction (p = 0.013) between the drug and time effect indicates that this effect is not the same throughout the 20 seconds.

Cardiovascular Responses During the Diving Test when Compared to the Breath Holding Test

When the breath holding procedure is used as a "placebo diving test", by subtracting second-to-second blood pressure values obtained during this test from the corresponding diving test values, the cardiovascular changes stimulated by vasoconstriction while diving the face into cold water should come out more clearly. Thus, it can be further analysed how Cilazapril affects blood pressure differently throughout the 20 seconds of these test procedures. Entering these data into analyses of variance the results reveal highly significant time effects (i.e. 20 second intervals) in systolic and diastolic blood pressure as well as heart rate differences (p < 0.0001). No significant treatment effects can be seen in blood pressure but in heart rate differences. Drug and time effect interact significantly in diastolic blood pressure and heart rate differences. Moreover, significant carry over effects (p < 0.04) and significant interactions between carry over and time effects (p < 0.0001) can be seen in diastolic blood pressure differences both in the morning and afternoon test session. The same is also true for systolic blood pressure with the exception of the carry over effect in the morning test session which just misses the significance criterion (p = 0.073). These carry over effects point to differences between subjects who received placebo first and subjects who received Cilazapril first. Moreover, a significant interaction between the ACE-inhibitor and time effect can be seen in diastolic but not systolic blood pressure differences.

In Figure 17 the carry over effects of 20 second systolic and diastolic blood pressure differences are demonstrated by separating subjects who received placebo first and Cilazapril second (indicated by circles) from those having received Cilazapril first and placebo second (indicated by squares). The rises in systolic as well as diastolic blood pressure differences during these tests are more pronounced in the morning as well as the afternoon test session during both experimental days in the group which first received placebo. This might be due to

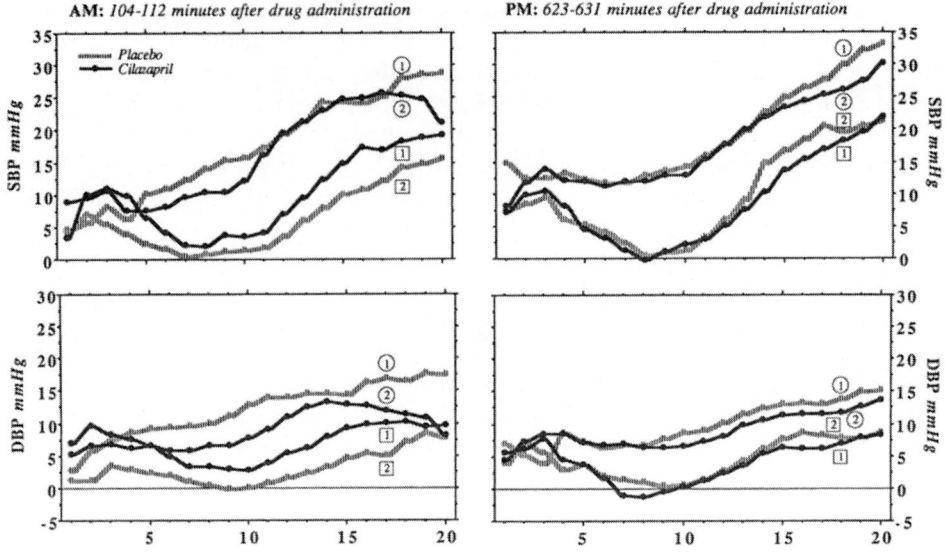

Fig. 17. Systolic and diastolic blood pressure differences *diving – breath holding test* in the morning and afternoon laboratory test sessions after placebo and Cilazapril medication separated for subjects beginning with placebo (*circles*) and Cilazapril medication (*squares*) on the first experimental day

bad luck in randomization of the two groups in this respect, i.e. both groups differ in this characteristic from the very beginning.

Figure 18 shows the effect of Cilazapril on 20 second systolic and diastolic blood pressure differences in the morning and afternoon test sessions. Values below zero indicate that Cilazapril lowers blood pressure more during the diving than during the breath holding test, whereas values above zero point to a stronger blood pressure lowering effect of this drug during the breath holding procedure. Although the courses of systolic and diastolic blood pressure look rather similar in Fig. 18, significant interactions between the drug and time effects are found only in diastolic blood pressure differences. This interaction is shown to be significant during both the morning (p = 0.0048) and afternoon test sessions (p = 0.0095). Moreover, this interaction interacts with the morning/afternoon test sessions significantly (p = 0.019) when both test sessions are introduced as an additional factor in analysis of variance. Again, this interaction is significant only in diastolic but not systolic blood pressure differences. The interaction indicates that the courses of morning and afternoon diastolic blood pressure differences in Figure 18 are different. During the first five seconds diastolic blood pressure is lowered less while diving than during the breath holding procedure in both the morning and afternoon test sessions, whereas from the 6th to the 20th second it is slightly more lowered while diving in the afternoon test session. During the morning test session, however, between the 12th and 16th second diastolic blood pressure is lowered more during the breath holding and after this time period it is more reduced during the diving test. This points to intricate drug effects on diastolic blood pressure

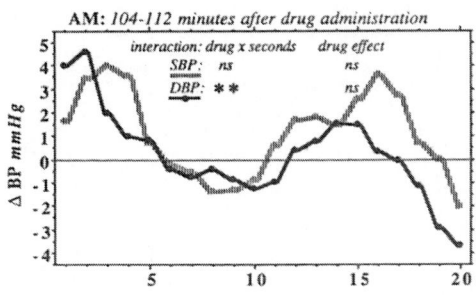

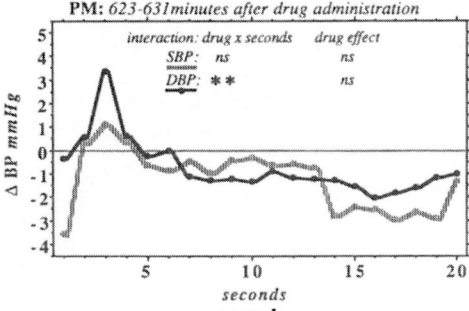

Fig. 18. Effect of Cilazapril (Cilazapril-placebo) on systolic and diastolic blood pressure differences *diving – breath holding test* in the morning and afternoon laboratory test sessions (*ns*, non significant; **p < 0.01)

reactivity which might change somewhat after drug administration during the passing of time. The reason why these interactions are significant only in diastolic but not systolic blood pressure differences is mainly because the variances, especially the error variances of systolic blood pressure are 3–4 times larger than those of diastolic blood pressure compared to a factor of about 2 for the variances explained by the design.

Heart rate differences show a significant drug effect in the morning (p = 0.046) and significant interactions between the drug and time effects in both morning (p = 0.014) and afternoon test sessions (p = 0.008) which are shown in Fig. 19. Again, values above and below zero indicate a heart rate above or below the heart rate during the breath holding procedure. There is no significant carry over effect or any significant interaction with a carry over effect. Cilazapril does not effect heart rate differences during the first 3 (AM) or 4 (PM) seconds but lowers these differences throughout the rest of the time by 2 to 5 bpm when compared to placebo. From about the 5th second the continuous decline of heart rate differences induced by the diving is preponed by 2–3 seconds through the ACE-inhibitor. Thus, when related to the breath holding test, Cilazapril might increase vagal activation and/or reduce sympathetic stimulation during the last 15 seconds of the morning as well as afternoon diving test.

Summarizing these results it has been shown that Cilazapril influences reliably blood pressure and heart rate reactivity in the diving test. This task is usually seen to stimulate a blood pressure rise by vasoconstriction, the mechanism which is acted upon by ACE-inhibitors. But we have also seen a probable beta-adrenergic stimulation (and/or vagal withdrawal) at the beginning of the diving test when it is compared to the breath holding procedure. This has been shown by second-to-

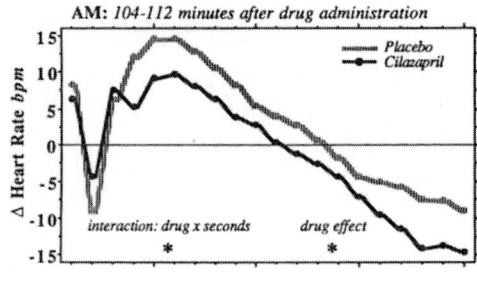

AM: *104-112 minutes after drug administration*

interaction: drug x seconds   drug effect
          *   *

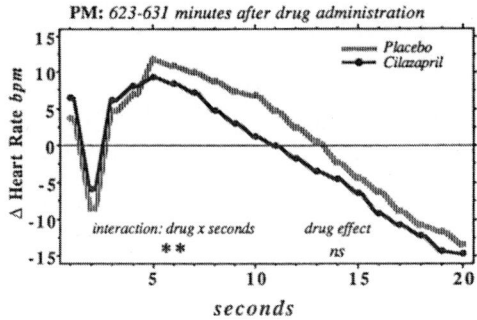

PM: *623-631 minutes after drug administration*

interaction: drug x seconds   drug effect
         **   ns

seconds

Fig. 19. Heart rate differences *diving – breath holding test* in the morning and afternoon laboratory test sessions after placebo and Cilazapril medication (*ns*, non significant; *p < 0.05; **p < 0.01)

second heart rate differences (diving minus breath holding test) exceeding the zero line in Figs. 14b and 19.

In the diving test this beta-adrenergic activation is continuously more and more withdrawn from the very beginning, and/or the vagal activation is stimulated. This, however, results in a heart rate below that seen during the breath holding test only in the last 8–9 seconds. It could be hypothesized that the initial probable beta-adrenergic stimulation during the diving test in our investigation might be caused by an activation starting before the actual diving and due to the subjects' knowing that they are just about to dive their face into ice water. The strong cold stimulus then activates an alpha-adrenergic stimulation resulting in vasoconstriction and a blood pressure rise, – but not before the 10th second. The continuous vagal stimulation and/or beta-adrenergic withdrawal, however, starts immediately (Figs. 14a, 15c), but compared to the breath holding test from an elevated beta-adrenergic level (Figs. 14b, 16). These hypotheses could, of course, only be further tested by systematic studies with autonomic blockade and continuous measures of haemodynamic variables.

The ACE-inhibitor Captopril has been shown to reduce heart rate during the diving test which has been attributed to an increased vagal activation (Sturani et al. 1982). We could not demonstrate such an effect with Cilazapril. However, when compared to the breath holding procedure heart rate is slightly but continuously and reliably lowered during the diving test by 2–5 bpm (Fig. 19). This effect can be shown to take place not only in the morning but also in a slightly more reduced way in the afternoon test session.

Cilazapril does not only lower diastolic blood pressure, but it also seems to influence the course of second-to-second diastolic blood pressure changes. This effect cannot be discovered if, as is usually done, averages of a whole test procedure lasting several seconds or minutes are subtracted from an average baseline. Such measures appear to be too crude for detecting the more intricate effects. Second-to-second or beat-to-beat analyses appear necessary for such effects to be seen. Why and how Cilazapril affects second-to-second diastolic blood pressure differently during the various phases of the diving test remains an open question to be answered through future investigations. It can be hypothesized that diastolic blood pressure is particularly reduced during such phases of the diving test when mainly total peripheral resistance is stimulated. This might also be a reason why diastolic blood pressure is not lowered immediately after commencing diving, as the major blood pressure rise probably due to vasoconstriction does not start in this test before the 10th second. However, it does not explain why in contrast to the diving test diastolic blood pressure is immediately lowered when holding the breath. These questions could further be investigated by analyzing the taped Portapres finger blood pressure wave form haemodynamically for beat-to-beat changes of relative measures of total peripheral resistance, stroke volume, and cardiac output using the pulse-contour method developed and adapted to Portapres/Finapres by Wesseling (Wesseling et al. 1983, 1992).

Discussion

Portapres, developed by TNO, Amsterdam, is the first portable prototype based on the volume-clamp method of Peñáz. Although still in an experimental state, this excellent device appears to open up a new dimension in human cardiovascular research. In contrast to the portable intermittent devices it adds the advantage of continuous blood pressure and heart rate recordings without the restrictions of invasive measurements. Portapres recordings include nearly all heartbeats during all occurring behaviors, thus giving a truer picture of blood pressure during everyday life. Moreover, multimodal assessment with Portapres enables for the first time a comprehensive investigation of the impact of behavioral and environmental factors on the human cardiovascular system in daily life with only minor restrictions necessitated by this measurement technique. It allows environmental and behavioral events to be related closely to beat-to-beat blood pressure, heart rate and even hemodynamic functions such as stroke volume, cardiac output and total peripheral resistance in everyday life to an as yet unexplored extent.

There are some minor restrictions, so far still limiting the application of Portapres to experimental studies. In its present state it is expensive in acquisition and use. The handling and control of the instrument needs some detailed understanding of its function. With its 3000 g Portapres is still heavier than modern intermittent devices. The hand used to measure finger blood pressure is somewhat restricted in its movements and use in daily life by the frontend box fixed on its back or on the wrist, and by the two finger cuffs. To avoid artefacts some additional precautions have to be introduced during measurements, further limiting free movement of the measured hand, especially while walking.

These restrictions are reflected by the subjects' estimations about how much they felt impeded by the measurements and device (Table 4). Around 50% felt mainly or very much impeded by the device during daily activities or felt

Table 4. Estimated impediments by Portapres measurements during 24 hour ambulatory monitoring in everyday life and other subjective estimations in percentages of altogether 32 experimental days of 16 healthy young male paid volunteers

	Totally/ Very much	Mainly	Rather	Somewhat	Not at all
Device impedes	25	21.9	21.9	31.2	–
Rucksack heavy	9.4	25	15.6	28.1	21.9
Hand impeded	25	37.5	21.9	15.6	–
Finger cuff uncomfortable	12.5	37.5	15.6	28.1	6.3
Noise unpleasant	–	3.1	15.6	50	31.3
Height correction uncomfortable	–	3.1	3.1	9.4	84.4
EMG disturbing	–	–	–	25	75
AC/DC switch disturbing	6.2	9.4	9.4	46.9	28.1
AC cable impedes	6.2	31.2	18.8	31.3	12.5
Diary documentation disturbing	9.4	18.7	31.3	31.2	9.4
Measurements unpleasant	–	28	15.7	43.8	12.5
Measurements interesting	21.9	21.9	31.2	21.9	3.1
Sleep refreshing	18.8	25	25	18.7	12.5
Environment reacts positively	3.1	34.4	34.4	18.7	9.4
Environment reacts negatively	–	9.4	9.4	31.2	50
Laboratory tests corresponds to everyday life	–	25	43.8	25	6.2
Diary mirrors emotions correctly	–	28.1	43.8	21.9	6.2
Day representative of others	–	25	34.4	34.4	6.2

uncomfortable with the finger cuffs. More than 60% reported that the measured hand was mainly or very much impeded. However, above half of the subjects thought the measurements were not at all or only somewhat unpleasant. Above 70% found them rather, mainly or very interesting and felt that the environment was reacting positively. 69% reported that their sleep was rather, mainly or very refreshing. The subjects felt least disturbed by the EMG and height correction system. None of the impediments stopped most of the subjects living a more or less usual day. Only 6.2% said that the day the measurements took place was not at all representative of others. Subjects walked around, climbed stairs, used their bicycles and cars, went to lectures, ate, drank, went to the toilet, cleaned their home, interacted with other people, were busy, angry and happy, met their girl friend and even had intercourse – forgetting about being measured by Portapres – i.e. they exhibited most of their usual daily activities.

Portapres appears to be a very useful tool for studying short and long-term effects of antihypertensive treatments in great detail. As nearly every heartbeat within the study time of up to 24 hours can be included in the analyses even small effects can be evaluated reliably. Only recordings at times when the measurement is switched from one finger to the other every half hour, which lasts about 20–30 seconds, as well as artefacts, have to be removed from data analyses. The Physiocal adjustments which check the setpoint on the pressure-volume diagram of the finger arteries and control for changes in vasoconstriction or vasodilatation, take place during continuous measurements on average once every minute. During these the systolic and diastolic blood pressure output signal is kept constant at the previous levels for just about 2 heartbeats, whereas the heart rate beat-to-beat signal continues. Containing so much information the 24 hour measurements with Portapres give a truer and more representative picture of blood pressure and heart rate during everyday behavior than intermittent devices can ever do. Therefore it might also be a better tool for evaluating the cardiovascular effects of antihypertensive treatments in daily life. But it must also be kept in mind that by better reflecting the impact of environmental, behavioral, and emotional factors on the cardiovascular system, Portapres measurements are, of course, sensitive to a great number of such behavioral and environmental confounding factors. This problem can be handled in different ways depending on the object of interest. Averages of the continuous measures over longer periods, for instance at 30 minute intervals as have been calculated in this investigation, will hide the influence of such behavioral factor if they occur at random at different times in different subjects. A greater number of subjects will also reduce such random behavioral chance effects. Such averages, however, will still show the effects of more synchronized factors, as can be seen in this study especially in the physical activity measure by the subjects coming to and leaving the laboratory at about the same time. Even the diurnal pattern of blood pressure might to some extent be due to masking, i.e. a consequence of more or less synchronized resting and sleeping at night (Baumgart et al. 1989; 1992, in this volume). Measuring cardiovascular variables together with major behavioral confounders such as physical activity is another way of controlling their effects.

This is the first study in which the effect of an antihypertensive medication is evaluated with 24 hour ambulatory continuous noninvasive blood pressure measurement in everyday life based on the volume-clamp method of Peñáz. Perhaps the best way is to study short and longterm effects of cardiovascular active drugs with Portapres during 24 hours in daily life in combination with measurements during standardized laboratory test procedures, during which major confounding variables can be controlled. Such a strategy, a macro- and micro-analysis, combines the advantages of both procedures. This was done in this investigation. The results support that the oral application of 2.5 mg of the ACE-inhibitor Cilazapril given to healthy young men once daily for one week has an acute lowering effect mainly on diastolic blood pressure, but not before 100 minutes after drug administration, which lasts for about 6 hours.

Moreover, in a detailed analysis of cardiovascular reactions on the basis of a second-to-second analysis in a highly standardized laboratory test session it was shown that Cilazapril affects diastolic blood pressure reactivity during the diving test. This effect lasts even longer than the blood pressure lowering one and can even be seen more than 10 hours after Cilazapril application. This is in contrast to what has been shown so far with other antihypertensive medications that lower blood pressure level effectively, but have not hitherto effected such blood pressure responses (Julius 1988; Rosenman and Ward 1988). Such investigations have not usually been done on a beat-to-beat or second-to-second basis with continuous blood pressure measurements. This, however, can now be done in a simple way with Portapres, which enables the mechanisms of cardiovascular reactivity to be studied in much greater detail.

Acknowledgements. We would like to thank Hoffmann-La Roche AG, Grenzach-Wyhlen, FRG, and the Verein zur Bekämpfung von Gefäßkrankheiten e.V. Engelskirchen, FRG, for supporting this investigation. We would also like to thank Ben DeWit, Gerard Langewouters, and Karel Wesseling, TNO Biomedical Instrumentation, Amsterdam, for their most helpful advice and painstaking assistance in our first steps in using Portapres.

References

Anastasiades P, Johnston DW (1990) A simple activity measure for use with ambulatory subjects. Psychophysiology 27, 1, p 87–93

Andren L, Hansson L (1980) Circulatory effects of stress in essential hypertension. Acta Med Scand 646:69–72

Baumgart P (1992) Impact of shifted sleeping and working phases on diurnal blood pressure rhythm. In: Schmidt TFH, Engel BT, Blümchen G (eds) Temporal variations of the cardiovascular system. Springer, Berlin Heidelberg New York, pp 318–323

Baumgart P, Walger P, Fuchs G, Dorst KG, Vetter H, Rahn KH (1989) Twenty-four-hour blood pressure is not dependent on endogenous circadian rhythm. J Hypertens 7:331–334

Fahrenberg J (1987) Zur psychophysiologischen Methodik: Konvergenz, Fraktionierung oder Synergismen. Diagnostica (Themenheft: Multimodale Diagnostik) 33/3:272–287

Fischli W, Hefti F, Clozel J-P (1989) Effects of acute and chronic cilazapril treatment in spontaneously hypertensive rats. Br J Clin Pharmacol 27:139S–9

Grizzle JE (1965) The two period change-over design and its use in clinical trials. Biometrics 21:467–480

Investigational Drug Brochure: Cilazapril (Ro 31-2848), third version, January 1989, data on file. F. Hoffmann-La Roche & Co. Ltd. Basel Switzerland

Imholz BPM, van Montfranz GA, Settels JJ, van der Hoeven GMA, Karemaker JM, Wieling (1988) Continuous, noninvasive blood pressure monitoring: Reliability of Finapres device during the Valsalva manoeuvre. Cardiovasc Res 22:390–397

Imholz BPM, Settels JJ, van den Meiracker AH, Wesseling KH, Wieling W (1990 a) Noninvasive beat-to-beat finger blood pressure measurement during orthostatic stress compared to intra-arterial pressure. Cardiovasc Res 24:214–221

Imholz BPM, van Montfrans G, Parati G, Villani A, Gropelli A, Langewouters G, Wesseling K, Mancia G, Wieling W (1990 b) First experience with Portapres: continuous noninvasive ambulatory finger blood pressure compared to intra-arterial blood pressure. J Hypertension 8, suppl 3, S 87

Imholz BPM (1991) Noninvasive Finger Arterial Pressure Waveform Registration: evaluation of Finapres™ and Portapres. MD Thesis of the University of Amsterdam, The Netherlands

Johnston DW, Anastasiades P, Wood C (1990a) The relationship between cardiovascular responses in the laboratory and in the field. Psychophysiology 27, 1, p 34–44

Johnston DW, Anastasiades P, Schmidt T, Steptoe A, Vögele C (1990b) The measurement of heart rate reactivity in real life and its relationship to reactions to laboratory stressors. Supplement to Psychophysiology, 27 Number 4A, pS 11

Julius S (1988) The blood pressure seeking properties of the central nervous system, Editorial Review. Journal of Hypertension 6:177–185

Langewouters GJ, de Wit B, van der Hoeven GMA, van Montfrans GA, Imholz BPM, Wieling W, Wesseling K (1990) Feasibility of continuous noninvasive 24 h ambulatory measurement of finger arterial blood pressure with Portapres. J Hypertension 8, suppl 3, S 88

Langewouters GJ, de Wit B, van der Hoeven GMA, Imholz BPM, Parati G, von Montfrans GA, Wesseling KH (1992) Feasibility of continuous noninvasive 24 h ambulatory finger blood pressure measurement with portapres: comparison with intra-arterial pressure. In: Schmidt TFH, Engel BT, Blümchen G (eds): Temporal variations of the cardiovascular system. Springer, Berlin Heidelberg New York London Paris Tokyo, pp 173–180

Ostle B (1969) Statistics in Research. The IOWA State University Press 1969 Ames

Parati G, Casadei R, Gropelli A, DiRienzo M, Mancia G (1989) Comparison of finger and intra-arterial blood pressure monitoring at rest and during laboratory testing. Hypertension 13, 647–655

Peñáz J (1973) Photoelectric measurement of blood pressure, volume and flow in the finger. In: Digest 10th int conf med biol engng. Dresden, p 104

Peñáz J, Voigt A, Teichmann W (1976) Beitrag zur fortlaufenden indirekten Blutdruckmessung. Zschr inn Med 31:1030–1033

Rosenman RH, Ward MW (1988) The changing concept of cardiovascular reactivity. Stress Medicine 4:241–251

Sanchez RA, Traballi CA, Barclay CA, Gilbert HB, Muscara M, Giannone C, Moledo LI (1988) Antihypertensive, Enzymatic, and Hormonal Activity of Cilazapril, a New Angiotensin-Converting Enzyme Inhibitor in Patients with Mild to Moderate Essential Hypertension. Journal of Cardiovascular Pharmacology 11:230–234

Schmidt TFH, Wittenhaus J, Steinmetz T, Piccolo P, Lüpsen H (1992) Twenty-Four Hour Ambulatory Noninvasive Continuous Finger Blood Pressure Measurement with Portapres – A New Tool in Cardiovascular Research. Journal of Cardiovascular Pharmacology 18 (Suppl. 11): S 256–284, in press

Stemmler G & Fahrenberg J (1989) Psychophysiological Assessment: Conceptual, Psychometric and Statistical Issues. In: Turpin G (ed.): Handbook of Clinical Psychology. pp 71–104

Sturani A, Chiarini C, Degli Esposti E et al. (1982) Heart rate control in hypertensive patients treated by captopril. Br J Clin Pharmacol 14:849–855

van Egeren L (1992) Effects of behavioral rhythms on blood pressure rhythms. In: Schmidt TFH, Engel BT, Blümchen G (eds): Temporal variations of the cardiovascular system. Springer, Berlin Heidelberg New York London Paris Tokyo, pp 283–296

Waterfall JF (1989) A review of the preclinical pharmacology of cilazapril, a new angiotensin-converting enzyme inhibitor. Br J Clin Pharmacol 27:139S–50

Wesseling KH, Sprangers RHL, Wieling W (1992) Peripheral resistance changes upon stand-up compared to those upon tilt-up and onset of cycling. Implication of the pulmonary reflex. In: Schmidt TFH, Engel BT, Blümchen G (eds): Temporal variations of the cardiovascular system. Springer, Berlin Heidelberg New York London Paris Tokyo, pp 220–239

Wesseling KH (1991) The FAST system User Manual. TNO Biomedical Instrumentation, Academic Medical Center, Amsterdam, The Netherlands

Wesseling KH, de Wit B, Weber JAP, Smith NT (1983) A simple device for the continuous measurement of cardiac output. Adv Cardiovasc Phys 5:16–52

Wesseling KH, Settels JJ, de Wit B (1986) The measurement of continuous finger arterial pressure noninvasively in stationary subjects. In: Schmidt TH, Dembroski TM, Blümchen G (eds): Biological and Psychological Factors in Cardiovascular Disease. Springer-Verlag Berlin Heidelberg New York London Paris Tokyo, p 355–375

Wesseling KH (1990) Finapres, continuous noninvasive finger arterial pressure based on the method of Peñáz. In: Meyer-Sabellek W, Anlauf M, Gotzen R, Steinfeld L (eds): Blood pressure measurement. Darmstadt: Steinkopff Verlag, 161–72

White WB, McCabe EJ, Hager WD, Schulman P (1988) The effects of the long-acting angiotensin-converting enzyme inhibitor cilazapril on casual, exercise, and ambulatory blood pressure. Clin Pharmacol Ther 44:173–178

ZAK (1982) Bioport – die Zukunft der Biosignal-Erforschung unter natürlichen Bedingungen. ZAK GmbH, Psychologische und physiologische Instrumente, D-8346 Simbach/Inn

Peripheral Resistance Changes upon Stand-up Compared to Those upon Tilt-up and Onset to Cycling: Implication of the Cardiopulmonary Reflex *

K. H. Wesseling, R. L. H. Sprangers, and W. Wieling

Introduction

The initial circulatory responses to stand-up from supine to an upright posture are complex and have proved difficult to analyze in terms of circulatory reflexes as it is difficult to record a sufficient number of relevant circulatory variables. With only the recording of pressure and heart rate an insufficient insight is gained. When previous studies showed that the initial hemodynamic responses to actively standing up from a supine position were very different from those to a similar but passive change in posture in tilted table experiments, it was hypothesized that the muscular effort of standing up caused hemodynamic responses in addition to those to passive postural changes [8, 9].

Therefore, the present study was designed such that the circulatory responses to changes in posture and to a burst of muscular exercise, as combined in the maneuver of stand-up from supine, could be studied separately in the same subject. Also, more hemodynamic variables were recorded by including beat-to-beat stroke volume, cardiac output, forearm blood flow, and total and forearm peripheral resistance changes to those of arterial pressure and heart rate. Analyzing the time course of the circulatory responses would test the hypothesis that rising from the supine is the superposition of the response to a change in posture with the subject passive on a tilted table and to a burst of exercise without a change in posture performed on a bicycle ergometer and might give clues to the mechanisms responsible.

Methods

Four healthy normotensive men of normal body weight, aged 28–37 years were trained to perform the three maneuvers of head-up tilt, onset to cycling, and stand-up from supine during inspiration, thereby avoiding Valsalva responses. Since the number of subjects is small we give individual results.

* This study was supported in part by the Dutch Heart Foundation.

Schmidt/Engel/Blümchen (Eds.)
Temporal Variations of the Cardiovascular System
© Springer-Verlag Berlin Heidelberg 1992

The maneuvers were as follows.

- *Tilt-up*. After 5 min of supine rest on a horizontal tilt table with foot support the subject was asked to inspire while being tilted head-up to 70° in 3 s. Subjects were trained to avoid straining of muscles during the maneuver. This was facilitated by limiting the tilt angle to avoid alarm reactions associated with a falling forward sensation. The gravitational stress at this tilt angle is 94% (sin 70°) of that at the vertical position.
- *Cycling*. After 2 min of quietly sitting on a Lode bicycle ergometer the subject was asked to inspire and abruptly bring the ergometer in motion for 3 s, then to return to motionless sitting. The ergometer was set at 50 W, but the effort to overcome the flywheel inertia of the ergometer was considerable, thus causing a forceful contraction of leg, abdominal, and back muscles. This maneuver allows the exercising of large muscle groups without postural changes or excitation of the vestibular system.
- *Stand-up*. After 5 min of supine rest the subject was asked to inspire while quickly rising to an erect posture and maintaining that position. The maneuver was done in about 3 s, with the concomitant forceful contraction of leg, abdominal, and back muscles lasting about 2 s. Here, both a change in posture and the exercising of large muscle groups take place.

The experiments were conducted in the morning, in random order, in a 23 °C air-conditioned room. After training each subject to perform the maneuvers while inspiring, each experiment was performed three times in succession to verify repeatability. All maneuvers started immediately after end-expiration. The time allowed between the experiments was sufficient to achieve a stable control state. The experimental protocol was approved by the hospital ethics committee.

Primary signals measured included an ECG, intrabrachial arterial pressure, and total forearm blood flow. The primary signals and a marker were recorded on a Bell and Howell model TI 4-channel FM instrumentation recorder for later evaluation. Intrabrachial arterial pressure was measured with a transducer fixed to the upper arm at heart level. Beat-to-beat mean pressure was computed from intrabrachial pressure. Changes in left ventricular stroke volume and cardiac output were derived from the pressure waveform using a Philips pulse contour cardiac output computing module. Age on the module's front panel was set at the 30–50 year position and the Z_{ao} calibration was set at 110. At this setting the instrument indicated 5 ± 0.5 l/min cardiac output under supine resting conditions in each of the four subjects. The overall precision of this method compared to dye dilution in 20 similar young adult humans was established at 13% under widely varying hemodynamic and pharmacological conditions [26, 33]. Its beat-to-beat precision compared to the electromagnetic flow probe in dogs is about 5% [31, 32]. These error figures include the errors of the reference methods. (See also "Appendix.") Changes in total peripheral resistance were computed on an Applied Dynamics 5 computer as the ratio of beat-to-beat mean pressure to beat-to-beat cardiac output. However, cardiac output measured at the aortic root may differ momentarily from total tissue perfusion due to the buffering capacity of the aortic Windkessel having a time constant of about 2 s. Therefore, during transients the time course of total peripheral resistance cannot be determined on a beat-to-beat basis from cardiac output. Hence, a five-beat running average algorithm was applied to the beat-to-beat total peripheral resistance values. This low pass filtered signal then reflects true total peripheral resistance changes at a heart rate near 1 Hz (60 bpm) quite closely.

Total forearm blood flow, including the flow to the hand, was measured in the right arm using a JSI Periflow ECG triggered venous occlusion plethysmograph, following a design developed by Barendsen et al. [5]. The occluding cuff was mounted just proximal of the elbow. A double stranded mercury-in-rubber strain gauge was placed approximately 6 cm distal to the elbow. The cuff was inflated quickly to 50 mm Hg, held for two heart beats, and released, producing a new flow measurement every third heart beat. The precision of the instrument in this mode is reported at 20%–25% [5], yielding noisy response curves. To reduce the noise we took the median of the three responses obtained in each subject, averaging again over the four subjects in this study, and this produced sufficiently clean responses. The right forearm was supported to keep it stable in height at approximately 10 cm above heart level during the maneuvers. The measurements were not reliable during stand-up. Forearm peripheral resistance was computed by dividing mean blood pressure by forearm blood flow at that instant.

The primary and the beat-to-beat derived signals were recorded on an 8-channel Gould-Brush model 200 strip chart recorder at a paper speed of 2 mm/s. The various computations were done in real time. Consequently, signals such as heart rate and cardiac output become available only when a beat has been completed and a new one begins. The digital pattern recognition algorithms require additional time and cause further delay in the outputs. Therefore, each derived signal has a certain delay and should be shifted back in time to line up properly with the primary signals. We have left the original measurements intact, but the necessary shift in time in each trace can be deduced easily from the comparison of features with those in the pressure wave pulsations.

Results

Detailed Description for One Subject

Figure 1 reproduces the responses obtained in subject SvZ showing the measurements for the maneuvers tilt-up, cycling, and stand-up. From above we note the intraarterially recorded pressure waveform, the beat-to-beat derived signals of mean pressure, stroke volume, and heart rate and the computed values of cardiac output, and total peripheral resistance (TPR), the latter both beat-to-beat and as a five-beat running average.

Tilt-up. On tilting to the upright position a reduction in stroke volume does not occur until after some six beats of normal stroke output. Then stroke volume gradually diminishes to reach a new stable level, reduced in this subject by 35%.

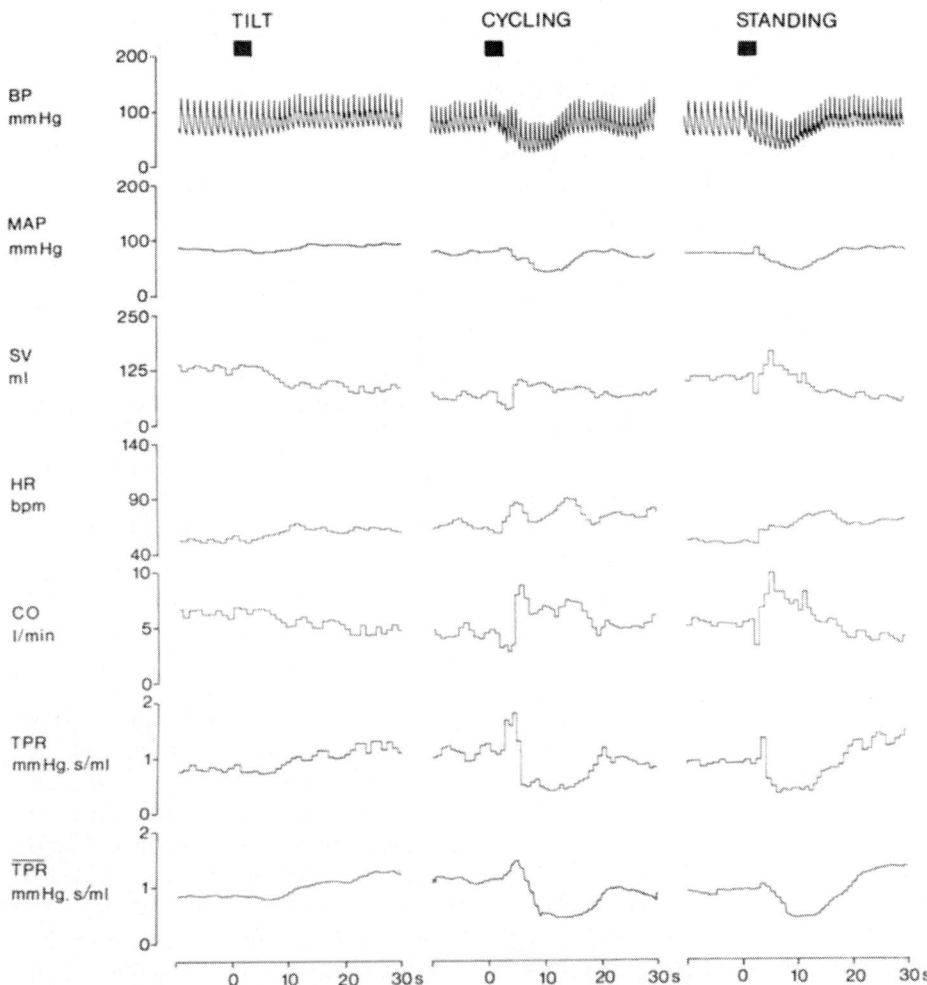

Fig. 1. Original measurement showing (*left to right*) the circulatory transients at tilt-up (*TILT*), cycling (*CYCLING*), and Stand-up (*STANDING*) in subject SvZ. *Upper traces*, the start and actual duration of each maneuver. the derived variables are delayed by one or two beats due to the real-time computations performed in the devices used. The onset of the maneuvers in these traces can, however, be seen clearly by comparison with features of the pressure pulsations. *BP*, Continuous intrabrachial; *MAP*, beat-to-beat mean arterial pressure; *SV*, stroke volume changes; *HR*, heart rate; *CO*, cardiac output changes; TPR, beat-to-beat and five-beat running average total peripheral resistance changes

Acceleration of the heart begins practically immediately. Vasoconstriction, increasing total peripheral resistance, begins after a delay of a few seconds. The modest increase in heart rate does not fully compensate for the decreased stroke volume. Therefore cardiac output decreases by about 25%. However, the simultaneous increase in TPR by about 50% results in a net mean arterial pressure rise of 12 mm Hg.

Cycling. Quietly sitting on the ergometer before the start of the maneuver, stroke volume was reduced from the supine control level in this subject by 45%. During cycling stroke volume was further reduced, and reduced arterial pulsations can be noted superposed on an elevated diastolic pressure. However, unlike Valsalva responses, the systolic pressure is not increased but continues to follow the normal systolic pressure modulations. At the end of the 3-s maneuver stroke volume increases a clear 40% over the resting level before the maneuver. This lasts another six to seven beats, after which stroke volume gradually decreases to reach steady levels at about preexercise levels. Heart rate increases almost immediately at the start of the maneuver. After the active 3 s of the maneuver mean blood pressure begins to fall at an approximate initial rate of 7 mm Hg/s. Total peripheral resistance reduces to less than 50% of control in 4 s after the start of the maneuver in the non-smoothed TPR trace, after 6 s in the smoothed trace. It remains stable to within 5%–10% over the next 10 s. After about 15 s peripheral resistance begins to rise. Heart rate increases further, and the increasing heart rate keeps cardiac output up during the initial 5 s of vasoconstriction that now takes place. This also has an immediate effect on blood pressure. It is only when blood pressure has returned to its preexercise level that heart rate and thereby cardiac output quickly begin to fall, preventing serious overshooting of the desired blood pressure level. Eventually, arterial pressure returns to normal some 20–30 s from the start of the maneuver.

Stand-up. During the maneuver of stand-up the change of the body long axis is approximately over the same angle as in tilt-up, and muscular exercise is approximately as severe as during the onset to cycling. We could therefore expect to observe almost their combined effects on the circulation. First note that the control levels for pressure and most derived variables are comparable for stand-up and tilt-up since subjects are initially in the supine position in both experiments, but not for cycling. The final levels of pressure and most derived variables 30 s after the start of the three maneuvers are also comparable. In all three cases the body axis is now almost vertical. The active part of stand-up is of shorter duration than that of cycling, and only the first beat in the stand-up maneuver has reduced stroke volume as against the first four in the maneuver of cycling in this subject. The time course of the changes in stroke volume from control after the initial beats in the maneuver of stand-up is an almost linear superposition of the stroke volume overshoot after cycling and the gradual linear decrease after tilt-up. Remarkably, the fall in TPR again reaches a level approximately 50% below control. However, although the TPR drops to the same level, the duration at that level is only 6 s, 4 s shorter than in cycling. Due to the short active period of the stand-up maneuver of only 2 s, it can be observed here how quickly peripheral resistance is reduced. It occurs in five beats or about 4 s.

Measurements in the Other Subjects

The original measurements of one maneuver obtained in each of the other three subjects are shown in Figs. 2, 3 and 4. Since repeatability within any one subject is

TILT

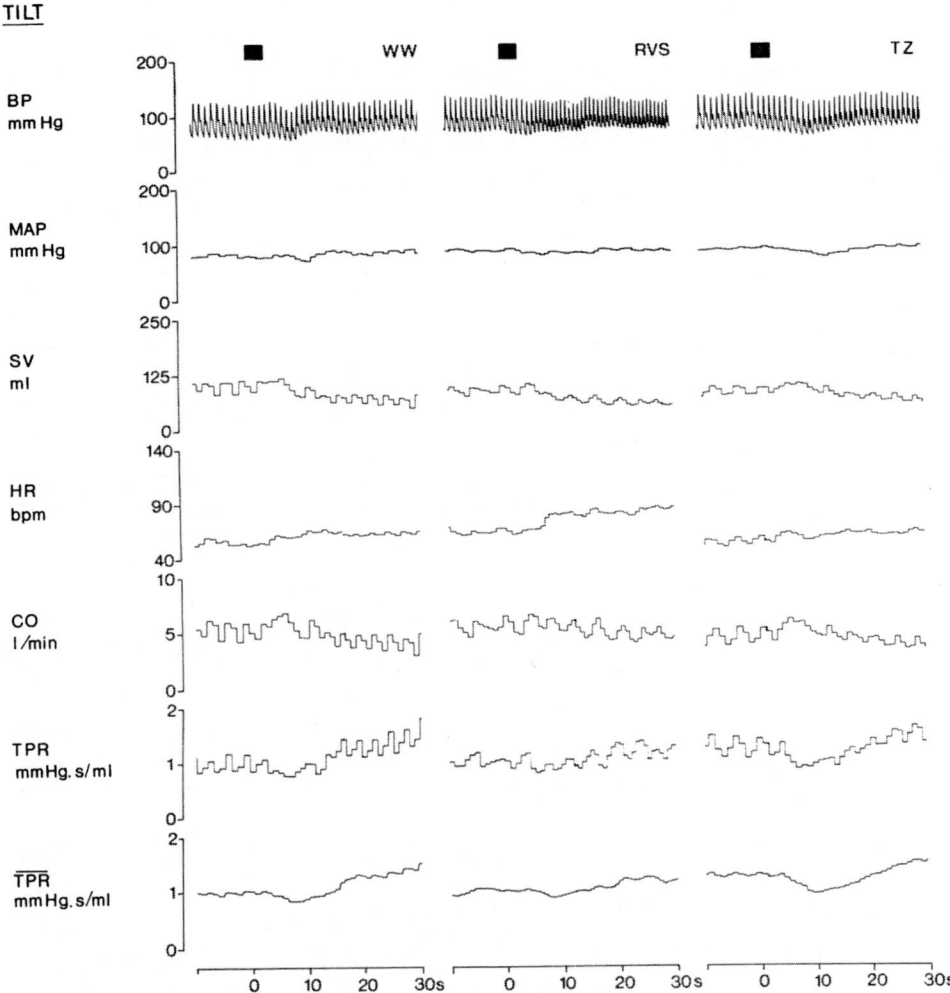

Fig. 2. Original measurements for the tilt-up maneuver obtained in the other three subjects WW, RVS, and TZ. Further as in Fig. 1

excellent, as demonstrated in Fig. 5, only the results of a single experiment for each maneuver are shown.

The responses to tilt-up are gradual in all four subjects with little difference among individuals. Apart from some differences in level and duration, the responses to cycling and stand-up are also comparable in the four subjects and in character identical.

Table 1 lists the median durations of the responses to cycling and stand-up and the control, valley, and end-level resistances in absolute numbers and in percentages from the individual supine control levels. Note that all standing end levels of peripheral resistance are higher than control, that all cycling, i.e., sitting control levels, are higher than supine, that all cycling end levels are lower than

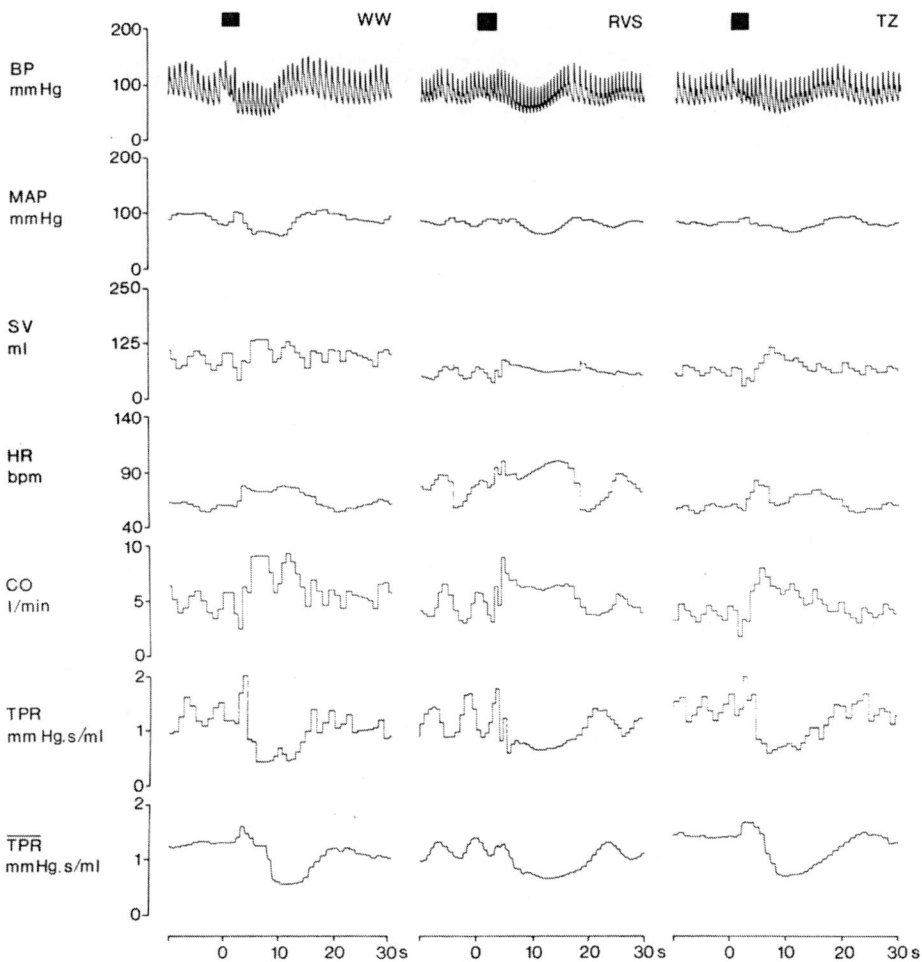

Fig. 3. Original measurements for the cycling maneuver obtained in the other three subjects WW, RVS, and TZ. Further as in Fig. 1

cycling control, and finally, remarkably, that valley levels are the same for each subject independent of maneuver although originating from higher levels in cycling than in stand-up.

Repeatability

Figure 5 summarizes repeatability in showing superimposed the three peripheral resistance curves obtained for each of the three maneuvers in the four subjects. It offers visual proof of repeatability.

STANDING

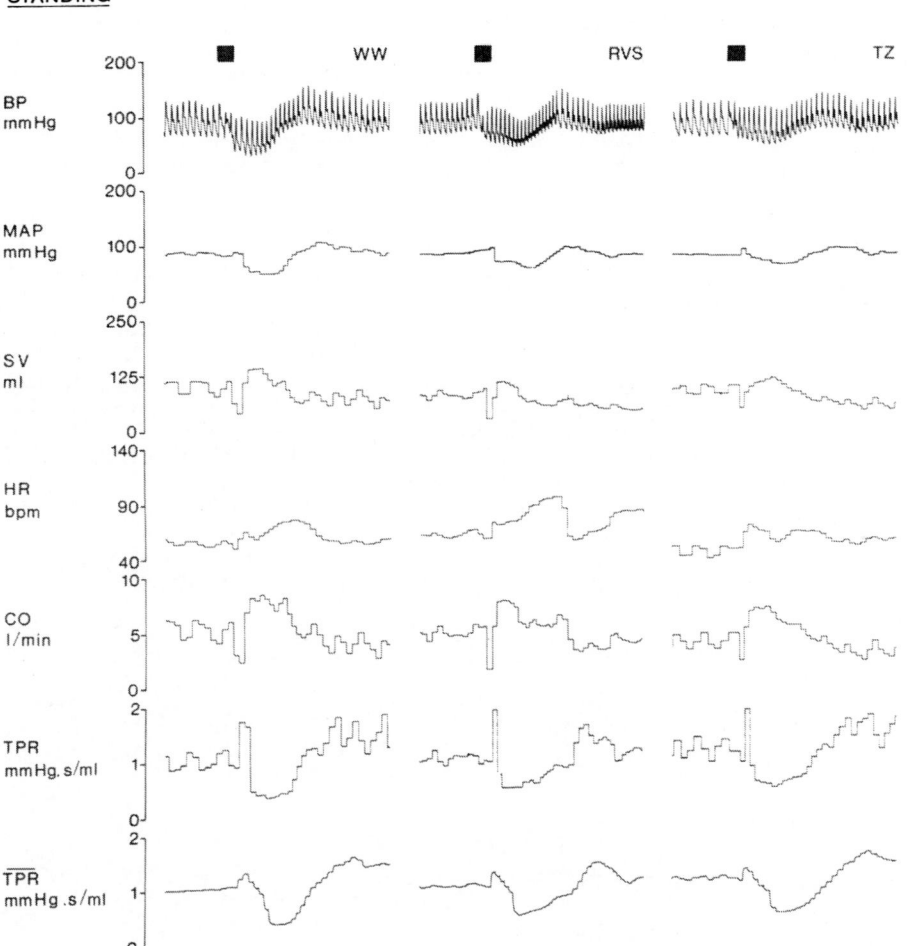

Fig. 4. Original measurements for the stand-up maneuver obtained in the other three subjects WW, RVS, and TZ. Further as in Fig. 1

Total and Forearm Peripheral Resistance

The forearm and smoothed TPR curves averaged over the four subjects are shown in Fig. 6. At tilt-up, both total and forearm peripheral resistances increase to reach levels about 25% above control after 30 s. However, forearm resistance reacts somewhat earlier and transiently shows an overshoot to about 80% above control. At cycling and stand-up, forearm resistance in none of the measurements showed the initial peak that could be seen in all of the measurements of TPR. After the maneuvers, both total and average forearm resistances drop to levels approximately 45% below control within a few seconds. However, the attainment

Table 1. Median values of the five-beat running average peripheral resistance responses to the maneuvers of cyclying and stand-up: absolute values and the percentage change from supine control before stand-up

Subject	Cycling				Stand-up			
	SvZ	WW	RvS	TZ	SvZ	WW	RvS	TZ
Time to valley	4	4	4	5	4	3	3	3
Time in valley	10	7	9	6	6	7	6	8
R_p control	1.18	1.29	1.25	1.57	1.04	1.25	1.18	1.50
R_p valley	0.57	0.68	0.71	0.86	0.57	0.64	0.68	0.86
R_p final	1.07	1.14	1.07	1.50	1.43	1.75	1.39	1.86
R_p control (%)	113	103	106	105	100	100	100	100
R_p valley (%)	55	54	60	57	55	51	58	57
R_p final (%)	103	91	91	100	137	140	118	124

Durations are in seconds. The absolute resistance values are in units of mmHg · s/ml. A cardiac output of 6 l/min (100 ml/s) at a mean pressure of 100 mmHg results in a resistance of 1 mmHg · s/ml.

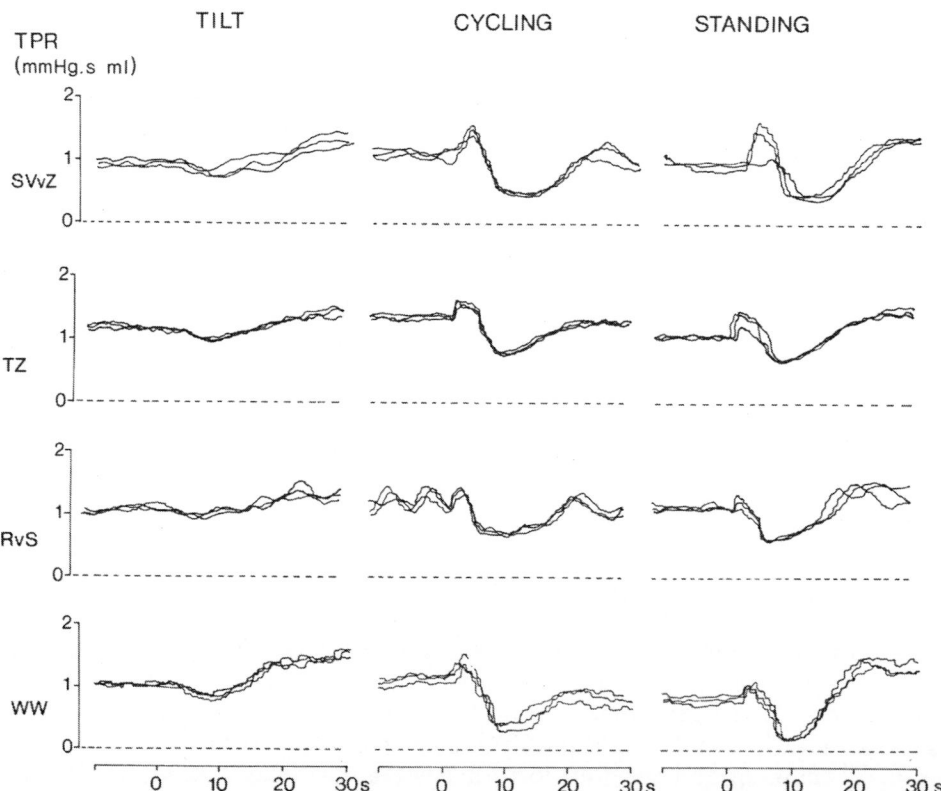

Fig. 5. The three superimposed registrations of the five-beat running average changes in total peripheral resistance for each maneuver and subject are shown here for visual verification of the intra- and inter-individual reproducibility of responses

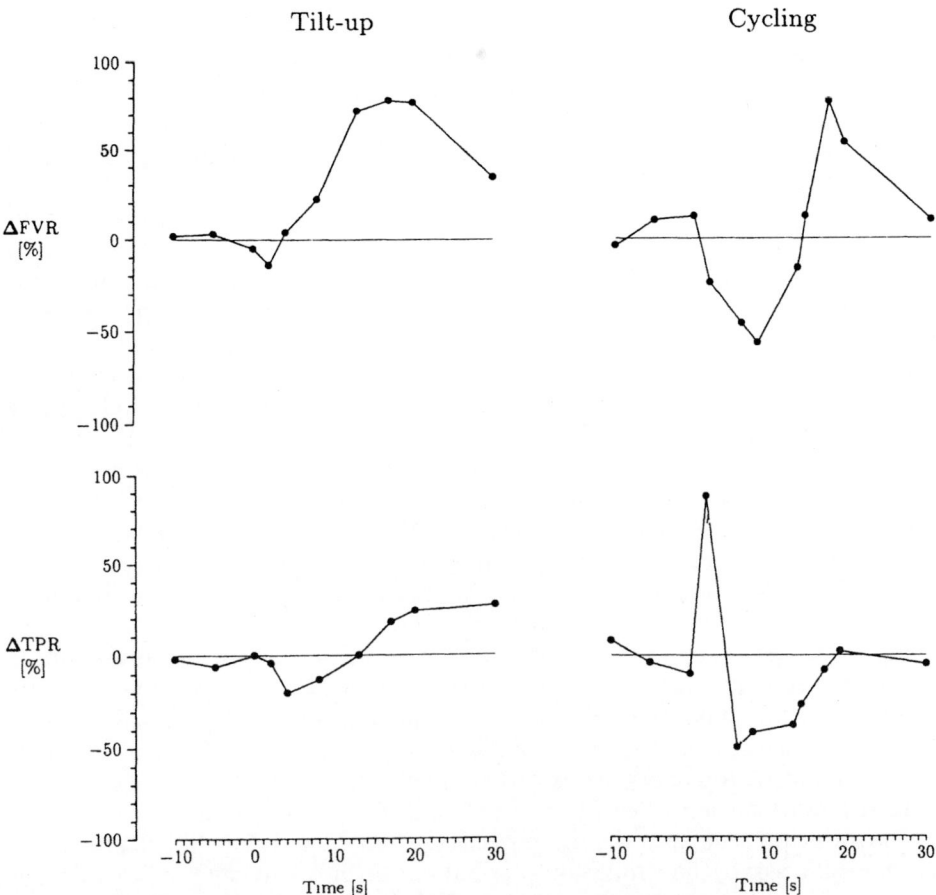

Fig. 6. Forearm (*FVR*) and total peripheral resistance (*TPR*) responses averaged over the four subjects in this study upon tilt-up and cycling. The individual responses to stand-up showed too much motion artifact to be useful. Values are plotted as percentage changes from control. The FVR and TPR responses are similar except for the overshoot in FVR

of the same percentage decrease as in TPR is fortuitous since the individual forearm blood flow patterns show substantial differences. Return to near control levels is after 30 s. However, before reaching end levels forearm resistance transiently overshoots the control level as it does after tilt-up, again by about 80% above control.

Discussion

We have presented beat-to-beat the initial circulatory responses to tilt-up, to cycling, and to stand-up. Given the small intra- and interindividual differences in the circulatory responses (Fig. 5) we restricted this first study to four subjects [27].

When comparing maneuvers, 70° head-up tilt in its gravitational effects is clearly not exactly identical to that of sitting on a bicycle ergometer or that of standing erect. Similarly, the muscle contractions in cycling and stand-up are not identical, although in both interventions large muscle groups are active. The point in this paper is that their effect on the propelling of blood to the thoracic compartments [13, 15, 17] is largely identical.

The methods used are traditional except for the flow measurements: for beat-to-beat cardiac output changes the use of a Philips pulse contour cardiac output computer (see "Appendix"), for forearm blood flow a JSI Periflow venous occlusion plethysmograph. The ECG-triggered Periflow venous occlusion plethysmograph provides a measurement every third heart beat. Compared to the more usual methods that record over many heart beats the Periflow trades precision for speed. Flow is measured as the increase in arm volume per heart period for one heart beat per measurement. The other two beats are used to empty the venous compartment of the forearm and to let pass the effect of cuff inflation on the plethysmogram. Actual cuff inflation and deflation are performed in less than 100 ms. As a result, fast changes in the circulation as studied here can be observed but with a certain amount of noise. By taking the median of three responses in each subject the noise is reduced while the resolution in the time domain is retained.

The differences between control and end-level cardiac output after the transition from the supine to the erect posture we observed with the pulse contour technique are comparable to those measured with direct oxygen Fick [6], dye dilution [28] and pulsed Doppler [17]. The same holds for the degree of peak-to-peak variability in resting stroke volume due to breathing [2]. The abrupt fall in stroke volume we found at the onset of cycling was also reported recently to occur at the onset of sustained leg exercise with a different technique [3].

The most spectacular of the responses is the abrupt and deep fall in TPR upon the maneuvers of cycling and stand-up, but not tilt-up. This can not be explained by excitation of the vestibular apparatus since cycling is without a change in body position but shows the response. It cannot be explained well by metabolic vasodilation since peripheral resistance also falls in the nonexercising forearm with the same high speed of response. A deep inspiration accompanied all maneuvers to avoid Valsalva effects. However, a deep inspiration in tilt-up caused no such drop in TPR or forearm resistance. A central command to withdraw vasoconstrictor tone to the muscles is a possible explanation, but it is remarkable that it seems undifferentiated since also affecting nonexercising forearm vessels [7] and thereby inefficient. In addition, central command has been shown only to increase blood pressure, not to decrease it [29], as is the case here.

There remain the baro- and cardiopulmonary reflexes. The vasoconstriction that is seen to develop in tilt-up can be caused by the baroreflex. In head-up tilted position the baroreceptors in the aortic arch and the carotid sinuses see a reduced blood pressure with respect to heart level, where blood pressure was measured, and vasoconstriction develops. In that case the final effect should be an increase in the blood pressure at heart level, and this is indeed clearly observed. However, at stand-up a similar position change occurs, and although the final effect is again an increase in blood pressure and peripheral resistance, and indeed of approximately equal magnitude, the initial effects are in the opposite direction and practically identical to those of cycling, not tilt-up. Thus these initial effects on peripheral resistance can not be caused by the baroreflex.

The exercising of leg, abdominal, and back muscles strongly compresses both arterial and venous compartments, forcing blood toward thorax [13, 15, 17], retrograde into the aorta, and antegrade into the vena cava, facilitated by a simultaneous deep inspiration causing negative intrathoracic pressure. Their effect is a strong and fast overfilling of the low-pressure cardiac and subsequent pulmonary compartments. Indeed, in contrast to tilt-up, both in cycling and stand-up there is a clear rise in stroke volume even though heart rate is increased. This suggests a substantial increase in left heart filling pressures which must be preceded by similar increases in right heart stroke volume and consequently preload or filling pressure. The cardiopulmonary stretch receptors then become excited, and their documented response is inhibition of the baroreflex [11, 20], withdrawing sympathetic tone and vasodilation [1, 12, 25]. The observed circulatory responses are in agreement with this description.

However, two aspects of the decrease in TPR require further scrutiny: the speed of the response and the amount decreased. The speed of the peripheral resistance response should be typical for sympathetic responses since vasoconstriction and dilation are largely sympathetically mediated. Sympathetic nervous control of peripheral resistance is relatively slow, showing a delay of 1–2 s and a total time to full response of about 6–8 s [10, 19, 24]. In the cycling and stand-up maneuvers the peripheral resistance drop reaches its deepest level in about five heart beats from the onset of the maneuver or in about 4–5 s, although the first part of that response is masked by the observed rise in resistance due to vascular compression by muscle contraction giving truly increased resistance and also, by causing retrograde flow, an apparent increased resistance. Although a 5-s response time is short for a sympathetic reflex, it should be noted that the input to the cardiopulmonary receptors is abrupt, and that these receptors react more strongly to abrupt than to gradual changes [23].

At the same time, and quite clearly, a valley is reached at which the resistance is stable for 6–10 s after cycling and 6–8 s after stand-up (Table 1). Also, to within 0.02 peripheral resistance units on average, the same valley level is reached for both maneuvers in each subject although the control levels before the maneuver differ by an average 0.08 units. It is as if total withdrawal of the existing sympathetic tone occurs lasting as long as the cardiopulmonary receptors are overstretched, i.e., as long as an increased stroke volume can be seen to exist. The hypothesis of total sympathetic withdrawal explains at once both the short time to full response and the maintenance of a valley level of resistance for such a long period of time, as well as the fact that the saturation level of peripheral resistance is the same for cycling and for stand-up within but not between subjects (Table 1).

Since pressures in the low pressure compartments were not measured, we must rely on other studies to document the pressure rises in the low pressure compartments guarded by the cardiopulmonary receptors. In a study by Grassi et al. [12] after passive leg raising a rise of only 1.5 mm Hg in central venous pressure is associated on average with a drop in forearm peripheral resistance of 30%. It is not clear from the literature that cardiopulmonary receptor stimulation alone is sufficient to cause TPR to drop by as much as 45%. Compared to the studies by

Grassi et al. and Vissing et al. [30], however, stimulation of the low-pressure receptors in our maneuvers must have been much stronger. Therefore, if these forearm resistance changes can be extrapolated to TPR, central command is not needed to explain our observations.

Cardiopulmonary receptors have been localized in the wall of the vena cava where it connects to the right atrium, in the walls of both atria, and in the vessels of the lung. The effect of stretching these receptors on heart rate have been controversial since they were first described by Bainbridge [4], with small increases or decreases reported. However, this controversy was clarified in a publication by Overbeck and Koepchen [23] which showed that the baroreflex and the cardiopulmonary reflex are competing controls, and that at a certain balance ratio between an arterial pressure rise decelerating the heart and a venous pressure rise accelerating the heart nothing happens to heart rate. However, when one pressure is changed while the other remains constant, a clear response is always seen to occur if control heart rate is low. In the responses discussed this can be seen at least in part as the initial heart rate increase to stand-up and to cycling. Initially, arterial pressure is constant or slightly raised, but the cardiopulmonary receptors are strongly stimulated, causing an immediate increase in rate. The remainder of the response amplitude could be caused by a further reflex, the muscle-heart reflex [14, 21]. In the later parts of the response the cardiopulmonary receptors are still excited to increase rate, and the baroreflex at reduced arterial pressure also increases rate so that an amplified and lasting cardiac acceleration is seen. Upon tilt-up only a moderate heart rate response is seen due to competing responses from the cardiopulmonary receptors subjected to decreased filling and baroreceptors subjected to decreased arterial pressure by being raised above heart level. In addition, there is hardly any muscle contraction to elicit a muscle-heart reflex.

Since the excitation of the cardiopulmonary receptors must unavoidably take place, and since all initial responses of peripheral resistance and heart rate are in accord with known actions of the reflex in direction and reasonable in magnitude, the cardiopulmonary reflex is the most likely candidate for explaining the abrupt fall in TPR upon cycling and stand-up described in this paper.

Acknowledgements. We would like to express our appreciation to Dr. J. T. Shepherd, Prof. L. N. Bouman, Prof. C. Borst, and Dr. J. M. Karemaker for critical suggestions and Mr. A. H. M. Jageneau and Mr. B. de Wit for technical assistance.

Appendix

Pulse contour methods have been studied since Otto Frank to compute cardiac stroke output from the arterial pressure pulse contour. A variety of formulas have been proposed [18].

The phenomenological basis of the pulse contour method used in this paper can be seen in Fig. 7. Here it is shown that the area under the electromagnetic flow curve, i.e., stroke volume, in a dog varies in the same manner as the area under the

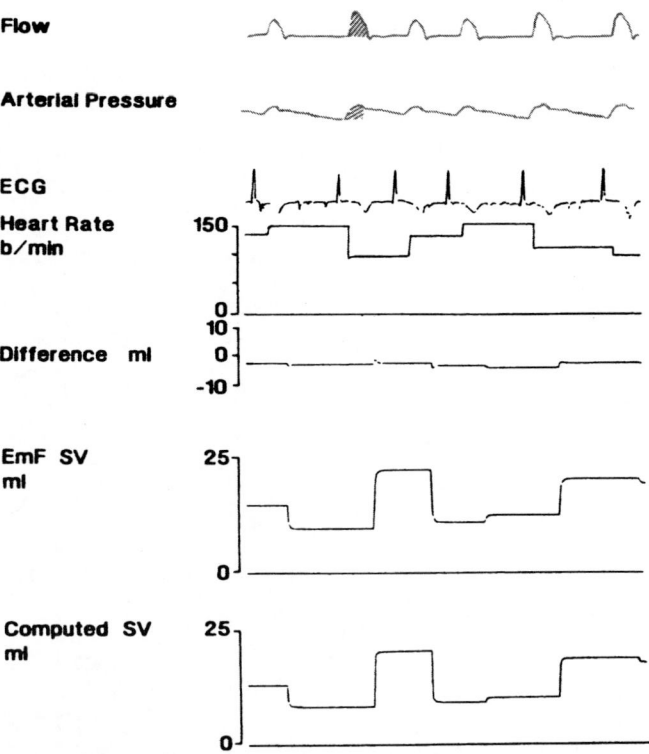

Fig. 7. Polygraph measurement in an anesthetized open-chest dog of continuous ascending aortic blood flow and pressure, ECG, beat-to-beat heart rate, difference in stroke volumes, stroke volume derived from the electromagnetic flow meter (EMF) and from the pressure waveform (computed) during a period of atrial fibrillation. Note the close tracking of both methods of stroke volume computation as stroke volume changes from beat-to-beat

aortic pressure pulse. Since the integral of flow over time has the dimension of volume (m^3) and the integral of pressure over time is an impulse (Pa. s) clearly the two quantities are not the same, but a dimensioned constant or calibration factor is needed to convert impulse to volume. The unit in which this calibrator is expressed is $m^3/Pa. s$, which is the unit of the inverse of an impedance. Numerically the calibrating impedance can be estimated from the tracing in Fig. 7. It is of the order of 6 MPa. s/m^3 whereas that of TPR is 100 MPa. s/m^3 or about 15 times as large. Obviously, therefore, peripheral resistance is not the calibrator.

The physical basis of this pulse contour formula, on the other hand, is the uniform transmission line as a model of the arterial system, in which pulsations propagate from the heart to the periphery. In this model pulsatile pressure and flow are related via the characteristic impedance, Z_0, of the transmission line. The Z_0 of an elastic tube filled with liquid, such as an aorta, is determined by the cross-sectional area of the tube, the density of the liquid, and the compliance of the tube per unit length. Obviously, this model for hemodynamics in the arterial system is too simple. An aorta is not uniform but tapered in cross-section. Also, its

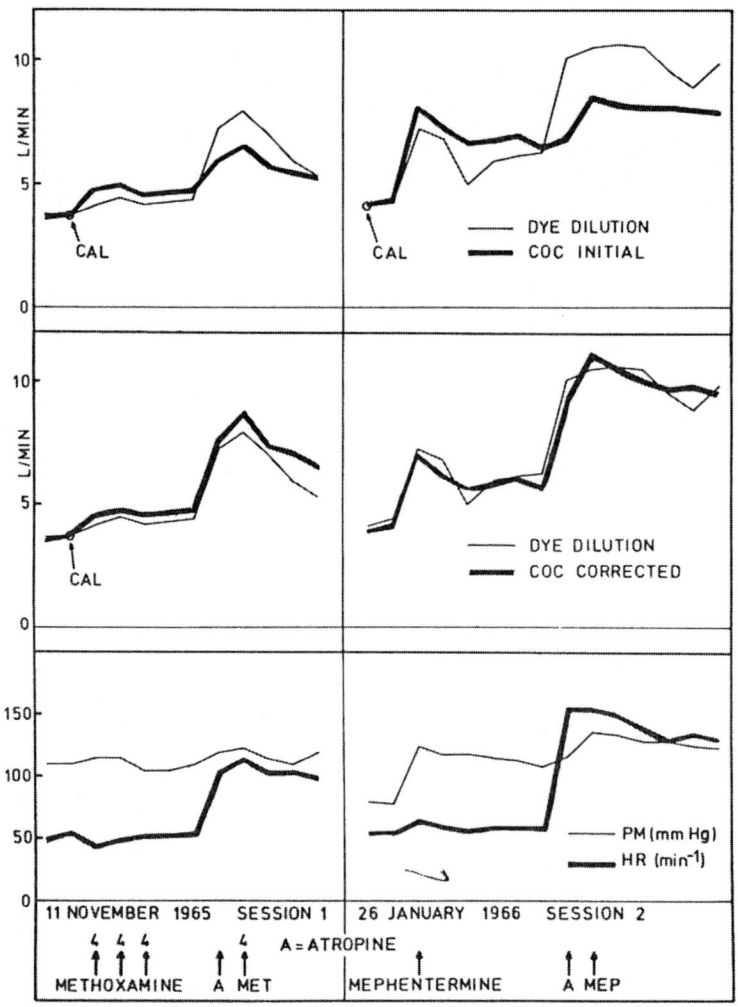

Fig. 8. Trend chart of cardiac output, blood pressure and heart rate in an awake volunteer subject during pharmacological interventions with methoxamine and mephentermine before and after atropine. The measurements were made on 2 different days separated by more than 2 months. *Upper two panels*, cardiogreen dye and pulse contour cardiac output measurements are compared. *Top panels* show uncorrected, *middle panels* corrected pulse contour outputs. Note the improvement in tracking when corrections are applied for the changes in blood pressure and heart rate induced by the injections of drugs. Application of the corrections also allowed the use on both days of the same calibration of the pulse contour method

compliance decreases toward the periphery. In combination this means that characteristic impedance is low at the aortic root but increases toward the periphery. This effect is somewhat moderated but not entirely abolished by the fact that, when pulses travel towards the periphery, they enter more and more side branches, thereby putting these impedances in parallel, somewhat lowering the otherwise more strongly increasing total impedance. Furthermore, both the aortic cross-section and the compliance are pressure dependent [16]. Cross-section increases and, in adults, compliance decreases with increasing pressure. These two effects compensate each other partially but not completely, and thus characteristic impedance increases moderately with increasing pressure.

As a result, the simple pulse contour formulas proved insufficiently precise in cases when certain vasoactive drugs were administered, in particular sympatho-mimetic amines. It was found later that drugs acted not through the direct modification of arterial characteristic impedance but indirectly through changes in pressure levels modifying characteristic impedance, and in heart rate changing the perceived net characteristic impedance due to taper. Since pressure level and rate are easily measured from the pressure waveform, it was possible to correct the simple pulse contour formula for changes in these quantities on the basis of arterial model studies [33].

The correctness of this approach was shown in a study [26] in which blood pressure, heart rate, stroke volume, and cardiac output were varied by pharmac-ological intervention. Figure 8 presents a result of this study. It shows that the uncorrected formula follows dye dilution cardiac output changes in direction but not always in magnitude when blood pressure or heart rate or both change. On the other hand, the corrected pulse contour formula follows the changes in cardiac output precisely. In this subject, measurements were done on two different dates. The calibrator, the subjects' arterial characteristic impedance, computed by equating the second pair of measurements, could be used unchanged on the 2nd day more than 2 months later. The value of the characteristic impedance in a subject thus appears rather constant in time.

It is concluded that the corrected pulse contour formula used in this paper follows changes in cardiac stroke output accurately on a beat-to-beat basis even when blood pressure or heart rate changes substantially. The evidence given here is only anecdotal. More information can be found in the references mentioned, where the method has been repeatedly shown to give precise cardiac output values under widely varying conditions in man [22, 31] and on arterial pulses recorded as far peripheral as the radial artery [26]. It is of unchanging precision when blood pressure and heart rate vary. In particular, the accuracy level of the method does not deteriorate when changes in peripheral resistance take place [33].

References

1. Abboud FM, Mark AL (1979) Cardiac baroreceptors in circulatory control in humans. In: Hainsworth R, Kidd C, Linden RJ (eds) Cardiac receptors. Cambridge University Press, Cambridge, pp 437–462
2. Adams J, Guz A, Hamilton RD, Innes JA, Murphy K (1986) Beat-by-beat changes in stroke volume during the respiratory cycle in conscious man. J Physiol (Lond) 371:128P
3. Adams L, Guz A, Innes JA, Murphy K (1987) The early circulatory and ventilatory response to voluntary and electrically induced exercise in man. J Physiol (Lond) 383:19–30
4. Bainbridge FA (1915) The influence of venous filling upon the rate of the heart. J Physiol (Lond) 50:65
5. Barendsen GJ, Venema H, van den Berg JW (1971) Semicontinuous blood flow measurement by triggered venous occlusion plethysmography. J Appl Physiol 31:288–291

6. Bevegård BS, Holmgren A, Jonsson B (1960) The effect of body position on the circulation at rest and during exercise, with special reference to the influence on the stroke volume. Acta Physiol Scand 49:279–298
7. Bevegård BS, Shepherd JT (1966) Reaction in man of resistance and capacity vessels in forearm and hand to leg exercise. J Appl Physiol 21:123–132
8. Borst C, Wieling W, van Brederode JFM, Hond A, de Rijk LG, Dunning AJ (1982) Mechanisms of initial heart rate response to postural change. Am J Physiol 243 (Heart Circ Physiol 12):H676–681
9. Borst C, van Brederode JFM, Wieling W, van Montfrans GA, Dunning AJ (1984) Mechanisms of initial blood pressure response to postural change. Clin Sci 67:321–327
10. Borst C, Karemaker JM (1983) Time delays in the human baroreceptor reflex. J Auton Nerv Syst 9:399–409
11. Edis AJ, Donald DE, Shepherd JT (1970) Cardiovascular reflexes from stretch of pulmonary vein-atrial junctions in the dog. Circ Res 27:1091–1100
12. Grassi G, Gavazzi C, Cesura AM, Picotti GB, Mancia G (1985) Changes in plasma catecholamines in response to reflex modulation of sympathetic vasoconstrictor tone by cardio-pulmonary receptors. Clin Sci 68:503–510
13. Guyton AC, Douglas BH, Langston JB, Richardson TQ (1962) Instantaneous increase in mean circulatory pressure and cardiac output at onset of muscular activity. Circ Res 11:431–441
14. Hollander AP, Bouman LN (1975) Cardiac acceleration in man elicited by a muscle-heart reflex. J Appl Physiol 38:272–278
15. Holmgren A (1956) Circulatory changes during muscular work in man with special reference to arterial and central venous pressures in the systemic circulation. Scand J Clin Lab Invest [Suppl] 24:1–97
16. Langewouters GJ, Wesseling KH, Goedhard WJA (1984) The static elastic properties of 45 human thoracic and 20 abdominal aortas in vitro and the parameters of a new model. J Biomech 17:425–435
17. Loeppky JA, Greene ER, Hoekenga DE, Caprihan A, Luft UC (1981) Beat-by-beat stroke volume assessment by pulsed Doppler in upright and supine exercise. J Appl Physiol 50:1173–1182
18. McDonald DA (1974) Blood flow in arteries. 2nd edn. Arnold, London, pp 420–445
19. Mancia G, Mark AL (1983) Arterial baroreflexes in humans. In: Shepherd JT, Abboud FM (eds) The cardiovascular system. Am Physiol Soc, Bethesda, pp 755–793 (Handbook of physiology, sect 2, vol III)
20. Mark AL, Mancia G (1983) Cardiopulmonary baroreflexes in humans. In: Shepherd JT, Abboud FM (eds) Peripheral circulation and organ blood flow. Am Physiol Soc, Bethesda, pp 795–813 (Handbook of physiology, sect 2, vol III, pt 2)
21. Mitchell JH, Schmidt RF (1983) Cardiovascular reflex control by afferent fibers from skeletal muscle receptors. In: Shepherd JT, Abboud FM (eds) Peripheral circulation and organ blood flow. Am Physiol Soc, Bethesda, pp 623–658 (Handbook of physiology, sect 2, vol III, pt 2)
22. Nichols WW (1973) Continuous cardiac output derived from the aortic pressure waveform: a review of current methods. Biomed Eng 8:376–379
23. Overbeck W, Koepchen HP (1956) Über die Wirkung von Druckänderungen im Gefäßsystem auf die Herzfrequenz bei schnellen Änderungen des Blutvolumens. Pflügers Arch 263:553–565
24. Pickering TG, Davies J (1973) Estimation of the conduction time of the baroreceptor-cardiac reflex in man. Cardiovasc Res 7:213–219
25. Roddie IC, Shepherd JT, Whelan RF (1957) Reflex changes in vasoconstrictor tone in human skeletal muscle in response to stimulation of receptors in a low-pressure area of the intra-thoracic vascular bed. J Physiol (Lond) 139:369–376
26. Smith NT, Wesseling KH, Weber JAP, de Wit B (1974) Preliminary evaluation of a pulse contour cardiac output computer in man. Feasibility of brachial or radial arterial pressures. Proc San Diego Biomed Symp 13:107–113
27. Sprangers RLH (1990) On the role of cardiopulmonary receptors at the onset of muscular exercise. Thesis, University of Amsterdam

28. Tuckman J, Shillingford J (1966) Effect of different degrees of tilt on cardiac output, heart rate, and blood pressure in normal man. Br Heart J 28:32–39
29. Victor RG, Pryor SL, Secher NH, Mitchell JH (1989) Effects of partial neuromuscular blockade on sympathetic nerve responses to static exercise in humans. Circ Res 65:468–476
30. Vissing SF, Scherrer U, Victor RG (1989) Relation between sympathetic outflow and vascular resistance in the calf during perturbations in central venous pressure. Circ Res 65:1710–1717
31. Wesseling KH, Smith NT, Nichols WW, Weber H, de Wit B, Beneken JEW (1974) Beat-to-beat cardiac output from the arterial pressure pulse contour. In: Feldman SA, Leigh JM, Spierdijk J (eds) Measurement anaesthesia. Leiden University Press, Leiden, pp 148–164
32. Wesseling KH, Smith NT, Nichols WW, de Wit B, Weber JAP (1974) A small, beat-to-beat cardiac output computer. Proc San Diego Biomed Symp 13:101–106
33. Wesseling KH, de Wit B, Weber JAP, Smith NT (1983) A simple device for the continuous measurement of cardiac output. Adv Cardiovasc Phys 5(II):16–52

Blood Pressure Control by Day Versus Night

J. Conway

Introduction

It has long been known that blood pressure and heart rate vary considerably throughout the day, and that they fall with sleep, at which time they both become less variable [1–4] (Fig. 1). Detailed analysis of changes with time have been made possible by intra-arterial monitoring, and these have suggested that the major fluctuation is due (in part at least) to an inherent diurnal rhythm. This has been supported by the fact that blood pressure tends to rise in the early morning before awakening [5]. However, without EEG monitoring the time of the change from sleep to wakefulness is difficult to determine accurately. Moreover, sleep induces a fall in blood pressure at whatever time of day it occurs. The classical studies required to differentiate between an inherent rhythm and one secondary to the sleep/activity cycle have not yet been carried out.

In studies directed at investigating blood pressure variability we have studied the waking process in some detail. After a period of adjustment to the laboratory surroundings subjects slept the night with brachial artery and venous catheters in position and a three-channel EEG record being made. During the night various measurements were made when the EEG confirmed that the patients were in a steady-sleep phase (stages 3 and 4). They were instructed to activate a signal when they awoke but to remain drowsy with eyes closed for a period of 30 min. The lights were then turned on, and they were asked to read a simple newspaper quietly; finally they were given a period of mental arithmetic. In this way the waking process was prolonged to permit physiological measurements to made.

Two observations became clear. First, blood pressure fell promptly with sleep, and a sustained rise was not observed unless the EEG pattern of sleep was disturbed. The fall in blood pressure with sleep was not so gradual as to suggest the presence of a cyclical process. If sleep occurred quickly, blood pressure fell abruptly, and the same applied to the awakening process (Fig. 2). Secondly, the blood pressure rise on awakening was not entirely due to the regaining of consciousness but was related to the level of mental activity. From Fig. 3 it can be seen that blood pressure and heart rate rose modestly as the subject passed from the sleep to the drowsy stage, and then it rose further as the patient was reading, and finally during mental arithmetic it reached its highest level.

Schmidt/Engel/Blümchen (Eds.)
Temporal Variations of the Cardiovascular System
© Springer-Verlag Berlin Heidelberg 1992

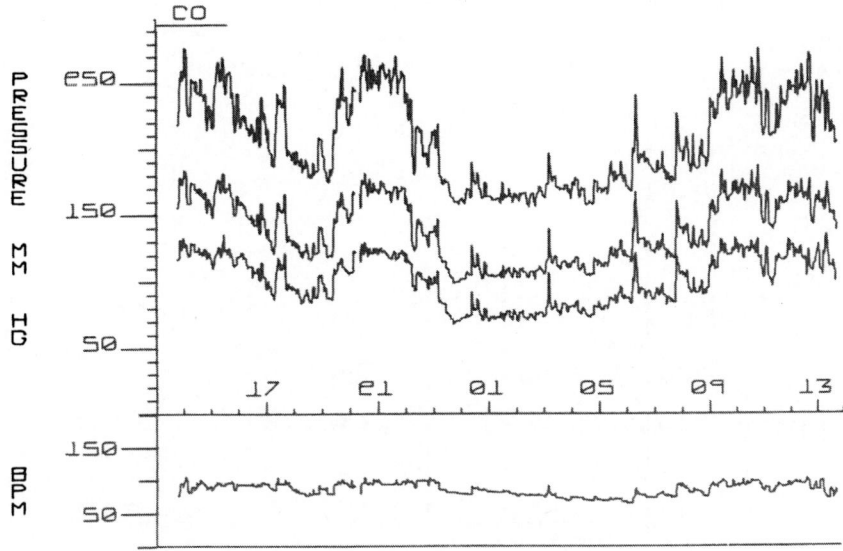

Fig. 1. Intra-arterial blood pressure record showing the diurnal rhythm and the variability in pressure

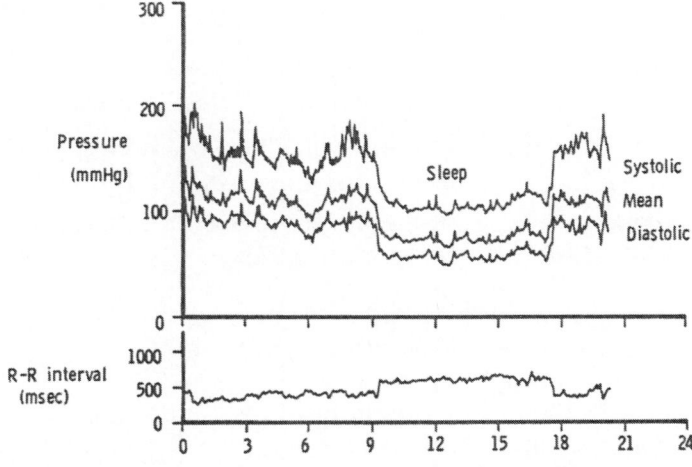

Fig. 2. Intra-arterial pressure record in a subject showing a rapid fall in pressure with sleep

A neurohumoral basis for these changes was also examined. With sleep plasma noradrenaline fell, as did that of adrenaline. The latter in fact fell to levels below the limits of detection (0.02 pmol/m) [6]. It is of interest to note that noradrenaline levels fluctuate with mental and physical activity, but there is no evidence for an inherent rhythm in the plasma level of this substance [7]. These changes indicate that sympathetic activity declines with sleep, and this has now been shown by power spectrum analysis of the heart period [8]. Sympathetic activity falls and vagal activity rises with sleep.

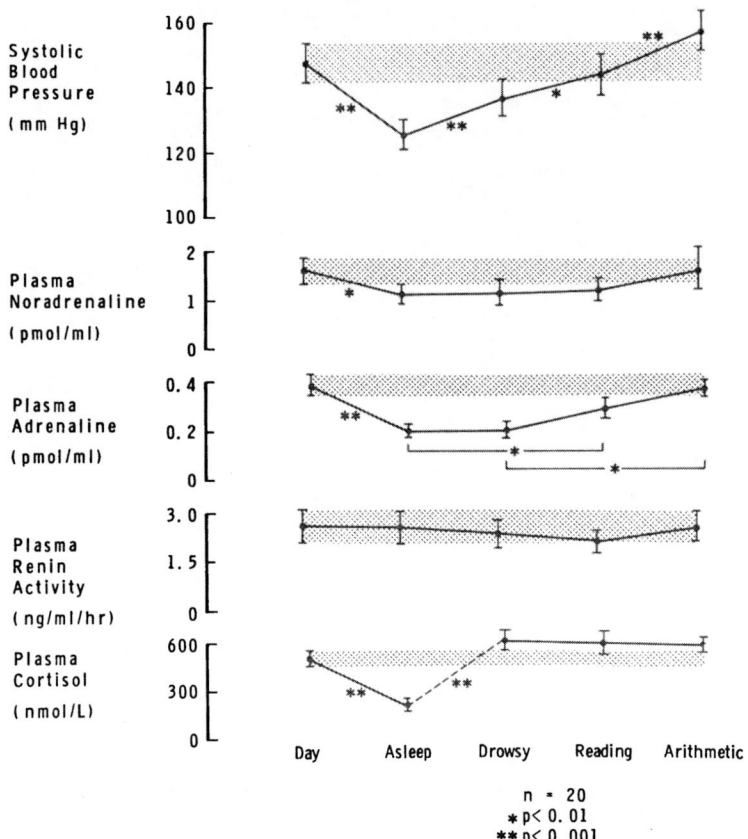

Fig. 3. Blood pressure and neurohumoral changes from sleep through the waking process and performing mental arithmetic

Control of Blood Pressure by Day

The magnitude of changes in blood pressure is greater during the day than is commonly appreciated. In a group of 140 patients we found the standard deviation of systolic blood pressure during the day to be about 17 mm Hg around a mean of about 150. This means that pressure oscillates in an irregular fashion by about 30% during the day. A degree of fluctuation in pressure is related to the sensitivity of the baroreflex. This reflex operates primarily by varying heart rate and stroke volume [9]. The heart therefore appears to play a dominant role in regulation of blood pressure during the day by adjusting cardiac output. Subjects in whom blood pressure is well regulated show considerable variation in heart rate during the day, and poor control of pressure is associated with a fairly fixed heart rate [6, 10] (Fig. 4).

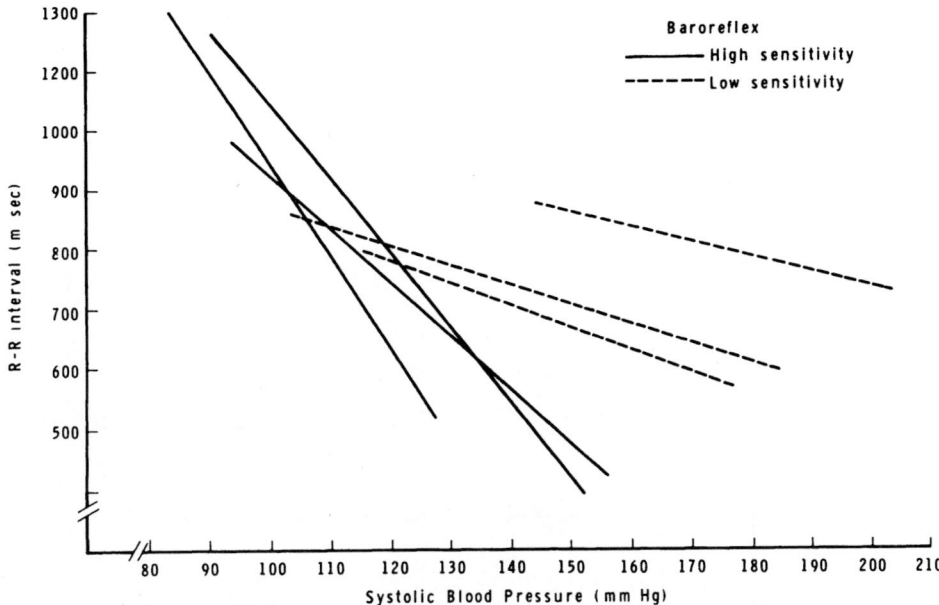

Fig. 4. Relationship between heart period and systolic blood pressure throughout the day in subjects with sensitive (*solid lines*) and insensitive baroreflexes (*broken lines*)

Blood Pressure at Night

At night blood pressure falls by approximately 20%, and its variability is reduced by about 50%. The same applies to heart rate. The fall in pressure is due to a combination of a reduction in cardiac output and peripheral resistance, as one would expect from the declining sympathetic activity and increase in vagal tone [11–13]. Some part of the decline in variability is induced by an increase in the activity of the baroreflex. Its sensitivity increases with sleep, and on awakening it declines more or less in parallel with the change in mental activity [14] (Fig. 5). It has also been shown in animal experiments that the reflex not only contributes to the fall in blood pressure but truly regulates it since it prevents undue reductions in blood pressure during sleep. Cats with deafferentation of the baroreflexes suffer severe falls in blood pressure periodically during the night [15]. There are large and transient increases in pressure during sleep, but these tend to be of brief duration and tend to be associated with external stimuli during light sleep and falls in pressure occurring with REM sleep [16].

Conclusion

The diurnal rhythm in blood pressure level appears to be related to the level of activity, and the possible contribution of an inherent rhythm has not been demonstrated. The baroreflexes play an important role in regulating pressure by

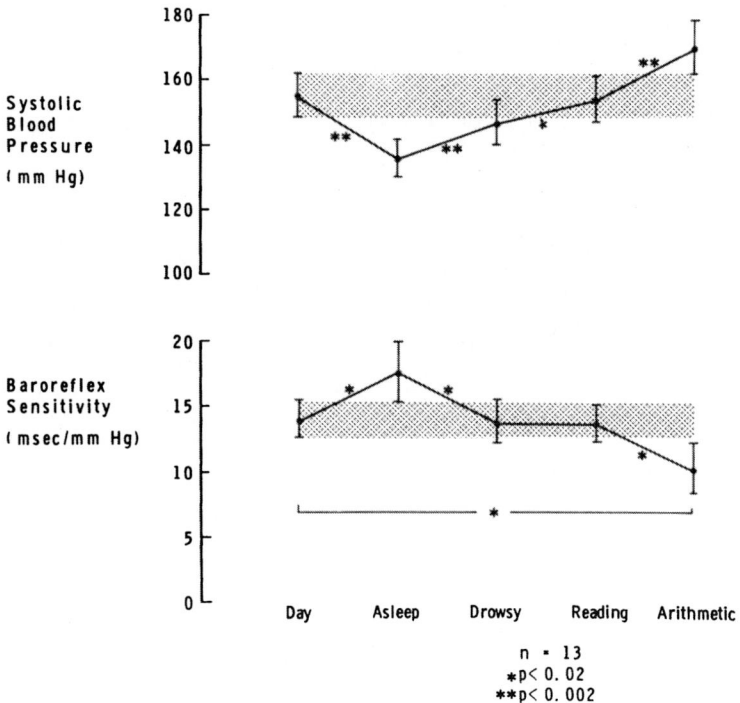

Fig. 5. Changes in sensitivity of the baroreflex during sleep and the stages of the waking process. (From [14] with permission)

regulating heart rate and cardiac output. With sleep the baroreflex becomes more sensitive, and this contributes to the greater stability in blood pressure at night.

References

1. Brooks H, Carroll JH (1912) A clinical study of the effects of sleep and rest on blood pressure. Arch Intern Med 10:97
2. Sayder T, Hobson JA, Morrison DF, Goldfrank F (1964) Changes in respiration, heart rate, and systolic pressure in human sleep. J Appl Physiol 19:417–421
3. Richardson DW, Honour AJ, Fenton GW, Stott FH, Pickering GW (1964) Variations in arterial pressure throughout the day and night. Clin Sci 26:445
4. Smyth HS, Sleight P, Pickering GW (1969) The reflex regulation of arterial pressure during sleep in man; a quantative method of assessing baroreflex sensitivity. Circ Res 24:109–121
5. Millar-Craig MW, Bishop CN, Raftery EB (1978) Circadian variation of blood pressure. Lancet I:796–797
6. Conway J, Boon N, Davies C, Jones JV, Sleight P (1984) Neural and humoral mechanisms involved in blood pressure variability. J Hypertens 2:203–208
7. Akerstedt T (1979) Altered sleep/wake patterns and circadian rhythms. Acta Physiol Scand [Suppl] 469:1–48
8. Furlan R, Gazzetti S, Crivellaro W, Dassi S, Tirelle M, Baselli G, Cerutti S, Lombardi F, Pagani M, Malliani (1990) Continuous 24-hour assessment of the neural regulation of systemic arterial pressure and RR variabilities in ambulant subjects. Circulation 81:537–547

9. Casadei B, Meyer T, Coats AJS, Murphy C, Conway J, Sleight P (1991) Baroreflex control of stroke volume in man (in press)
10. Mancia G, Parati G, Pomidossi G, Casadei R, Di Rienzo M, Zanchetti A (1985) Arterial baroreflexes and blood pressure and heart rate variabilities in humans. Hypertension 8:147–153
11. Bristow JD, Honour AJ, Pickering TG, Sleight P (1969) Cardiovascular and respiratory changes during sleep in normal and hypertensive subjects. Cardiovasc Res 3:476–485
12. Khatri IM, Freis ED (1967) Haemodynamics of sleep in hypertensive patients. Clin Res 15:451
13. Mancia G, Giorgio B, Adams OB, Zanchetti A (1970) Vasomotor regulation during sleep in the cat. Am J Physiol 220:1086–1093
14. Conway J, Boon N, Vann Jones, Sleight P (1983) Involvement of the baroreceptor reflexes in the changes in blood pressure with sleep and mental arousal. Hypertension 5:746–748
15. Kamazawa T, Baccelli G, Guazzi M, Mancia G, Zanchetti A (1969) Hemodynamic patterns during desynchronized sleep in intact cats and in cats with sinoaortic deafferentation. Circ Res 26:923–937
16. Jones JV, Sleight P, Smyth HS (1982) Haemodynamic changes during sleep in man. In: Ganten D, Pfaff D (eds) Current topics in hemoendocrinology: sleep. Springer, Berlin Heidelberg New York, pp 105–125

Dynamic Evaluation of Neural Cardiovascular Regulation Through the Analysis of Blood Pressure and Pulse Interval Variability over 24 Hours

G. Parati, M. Di Rienzo, S. Omboni, S. Trazzi, and G. Mancia

The mechanisms involved in neural cardiovascular regulation in humans have been traditionally studied using laboratory tests known to activate central and reflex influences on the heart and the peripheral circulation [1, 2]. Although valuable, these manoeuvres have important limitations, however [2, 3]. For example, their cardiovascular effects have a limited reproducibility. Furthermore, the effects of manoeuvres apparently involving similar neural mechanisms have a limited correlation. Finally, these manoeuvres interfere with the neural mechanisms under evaluation in the laboratory setting, and do not offer information on neural cardiovascular control in real life conditions.

Blood Pressure Variability and Neural Cardiovascular Regulation

Investigation of neural cardiovascular control under real life conditions has been made possible by the development of techniques for monitoring intra-arterial blood pressure and heart rate over 24 h in outpatients [4, 5]. This has shown that blood pressure undergoes marked spontaneous variations (Fig. 1) and has clarified some of the mechanisms responsible for this phenomenon [6–10]. These mechanisms are the mechanical factors associated with ventilation and probably some humoral factors, too. There is no doubt, however, that neural mechanisms both central and reflex innature [8], play a key role. The importance of central mechanisms has been shown by studies on the effects of behavior on blood pressure, which have documented that blood pressure may be markedly and persistently elevated by stress-elicited neural excitation and that, conversely, the reduction in sympathetic discharge taking place during sleep is associated with pronounced hypotension (Fig. 1). Overall blood pressure variability (as assessed by the standard deviation of each half hour of the recording time) is also greater during active wakefulness periods than during sleep, which also indicates the behavioral origin of this phenomenon (Fig. 2) [7, 11, 12].

The involvement of reflex influences in modulating blood pressure variability is suggested by studies in conscious animals, which show that section of the carotid sinus and the aortic nerves is accompanied by a pronounced increase in overall blood pressure variability [8, 13, 14] (Fig. 3). In man, evidence of reflex control of

Schmidt/Engel/Blümchen (Eds.)
Temporal Variations of the Cardiovascular System
© Springer-Verlag Berlin Heidelberg 1992

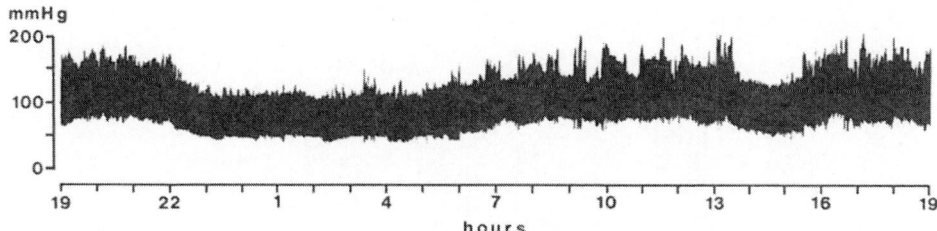

Fig. 1. Original intra-arterial blood pressure tracing obtained by ambulatory monitoring over 24 h. (From [6])

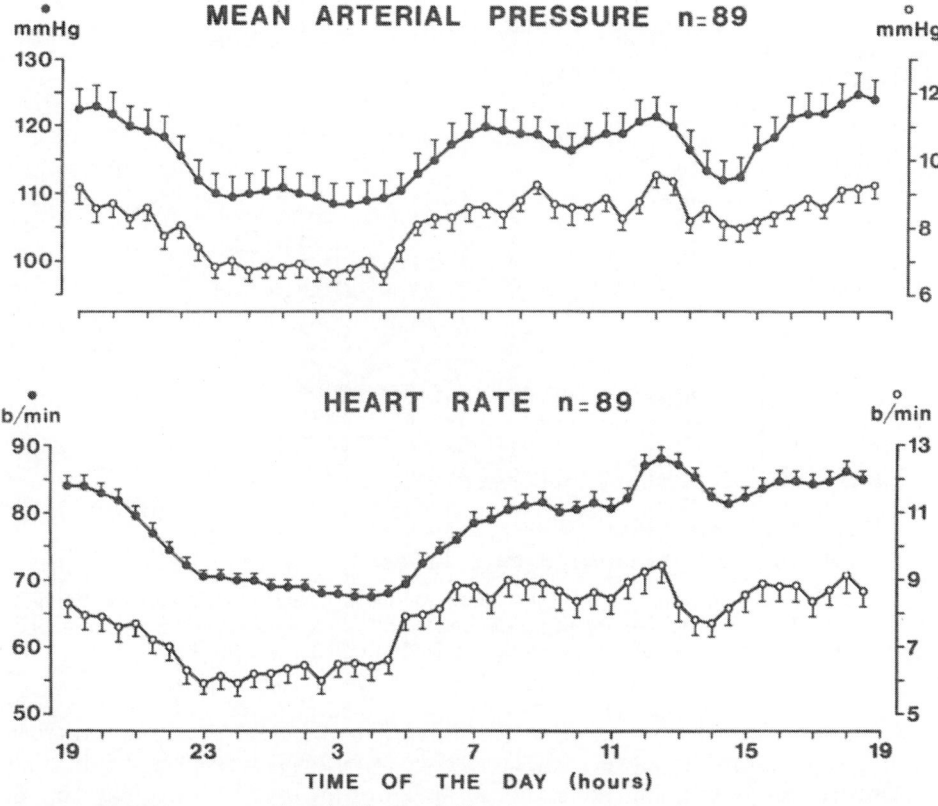

●—● means   ○—○ standard deviation

Fig. 2. Mean arterial pressure and heart rate average values and variabilities (standard deviations) separately obtained for each half-hour of a 24-h ambulatory recording. Data are shown as means ±SE for 89 subjects undergoing ambulatory intra-arterial blood pressure monitoring. The scales for the mean values are on the *left*, those for the standard deviations on the *right*. (From [7])

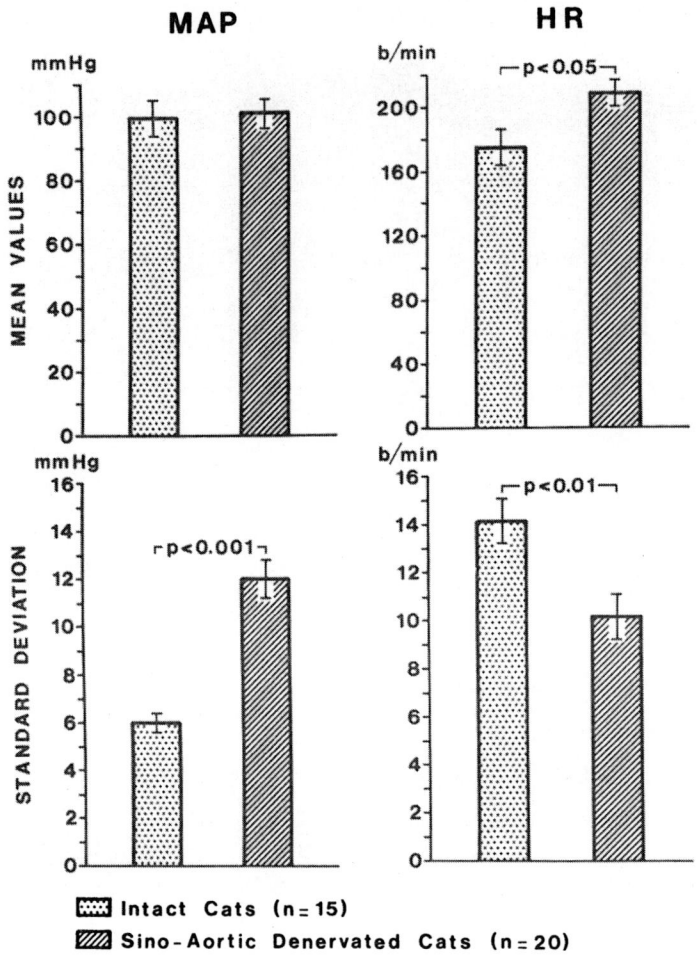

Fig. 3. Mean arterial pressure (*MAP*) and heart rate (*HR*) means and variabilites (standard deviation) in 15 cats with sino-aortic nerves intact and in 20 cats studied after sino-aortic denervation. Averages ±SE of a 3-h recording period are shown. (From [13])

blood pressure variability was obtained indirectly by the observation that there is an inverse relationship between baroreflex sensitivity, as assessed by traditional laboratory techniques, and the standard deviation of blood pressure [8, 15, 16] (Fig. 4). This means that an effective baroreflex is associated with a less pronounced blood pressure variability and vice versa. In contrast, heart rate variability is positively related to baroreflex sensitivity, suggesting that the arterial baroreflex buffers blood pressure variations at least in part through heart rate (and thus cardiac output) changes.

The cause-effect link between neural cardiovascular regulation and blood pressure and heart rate variability justifies a different experimental approach, i.e., analysis of different variability patterns as a tool to obtain information on the underlying neural mechanisms. Compared with the use of laboratory tests, this

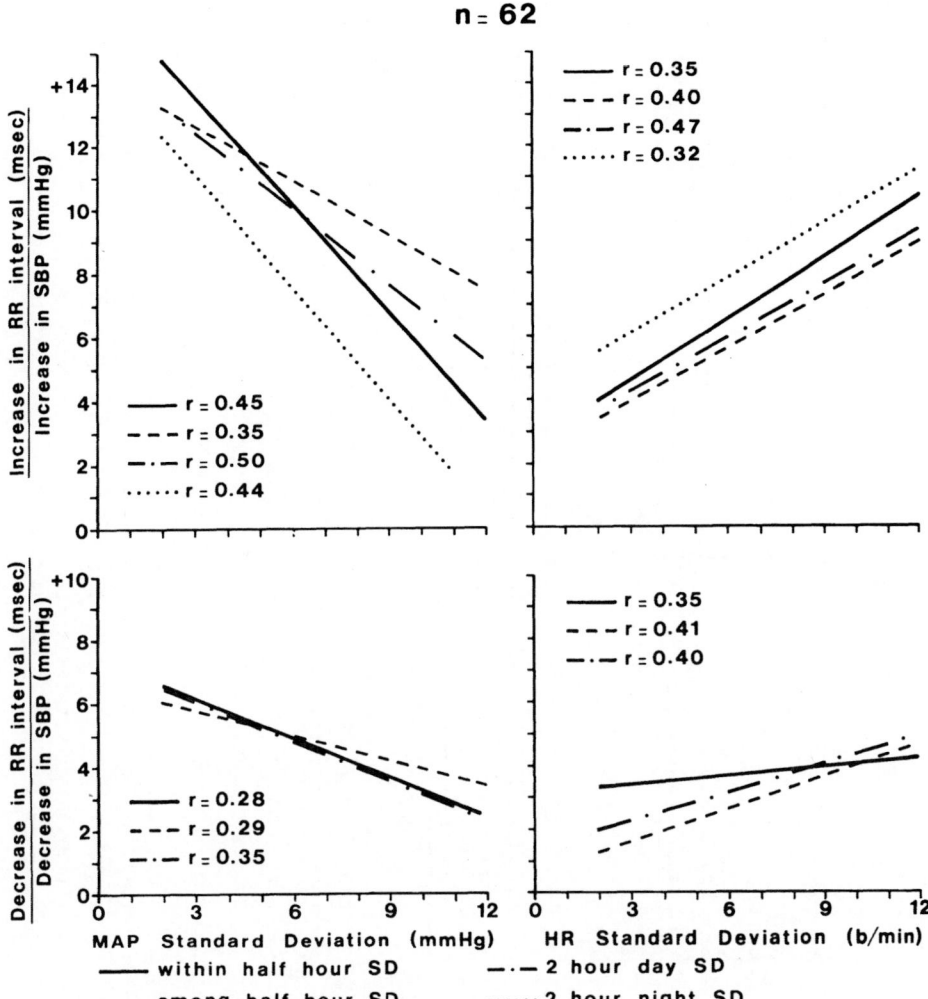

Fig. 4. Regression lines between mean arterial pressure (*MAP*) and heart rate (*HR*) standard deviations and baroreflex sensitivities as measured by the changes in RR interval induced by increasing and reducing systolic blood pressure (*SBP*) through phenylephrine and nitroglycerine injections. Only the regression lines that achieved statistical significance are drawn. (From [15])

approach has several advantages. Firstly, it does not interfere with the mechanisms under evaluation; second, it allows the evaluation to be obtained under everyday conditions, and, third, the dynamic features of neural cardiovascular control can be investigated.

In the next two sections, two components of blood pressure and heart rate variability will be addressed: first, the transient blood pressure and heart rate changes occurring over 24 h as analyzed in the time domain, and second, the rhythmic fluctuations occurring in different frequency bands which require the analysis to be carried out in the frequency domain.

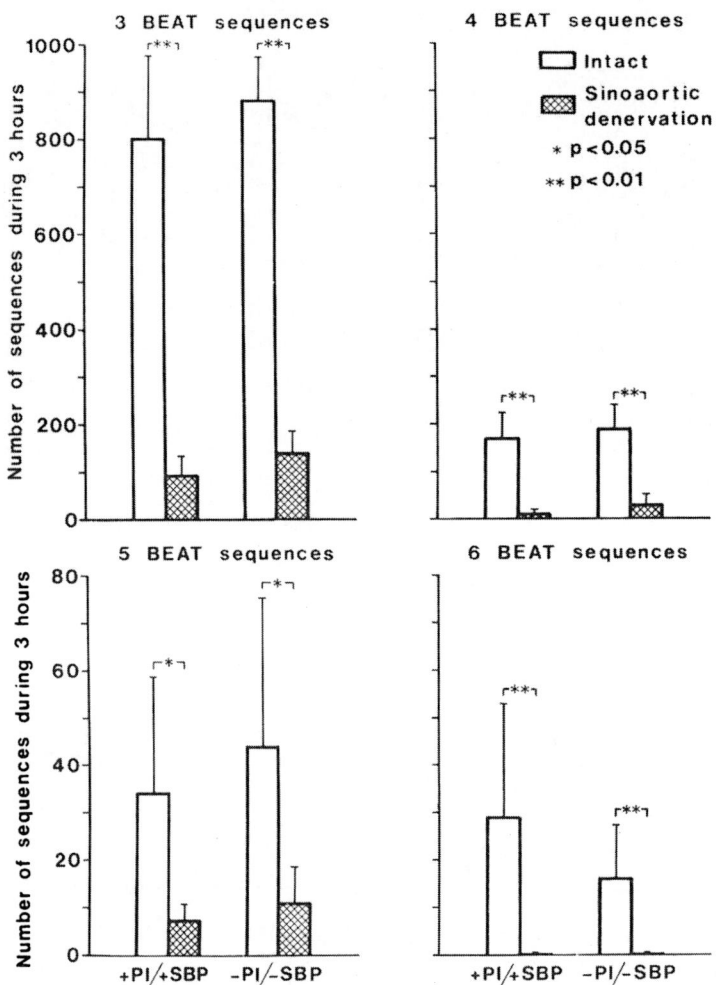

Fig. 5. Hypertension/bradycardia ($+SBP/+PI$) and hypotension/tachycardia ($-SBP/-PI$) sequences of 3-, 4-, 5- and 6-beat length before (intact) and after sino-aortic denervation. Data are shown as means $\pm$ SE of 10 cats. (From [17])

Transient Blood Pressure and Pulse Interval Changes: Sequence Analysis

An example of transient blood pressure and pulse interval (the reciprocal of heart rate) changes is represented by the sequences of consecutive heart beats characterized by spontaneously occurring and progressive (a) increases in blood pressure and lengthening in pulse interval, and (b) decreases in blood pressure and shortening in pulse interval [17]. These hypertension/bradycardia and hypotension/tachycardia sequences are similar to those obtained in the laboratory by i.v. bolus injections of phenylephrine and nitroglycerine, respectively, which are used

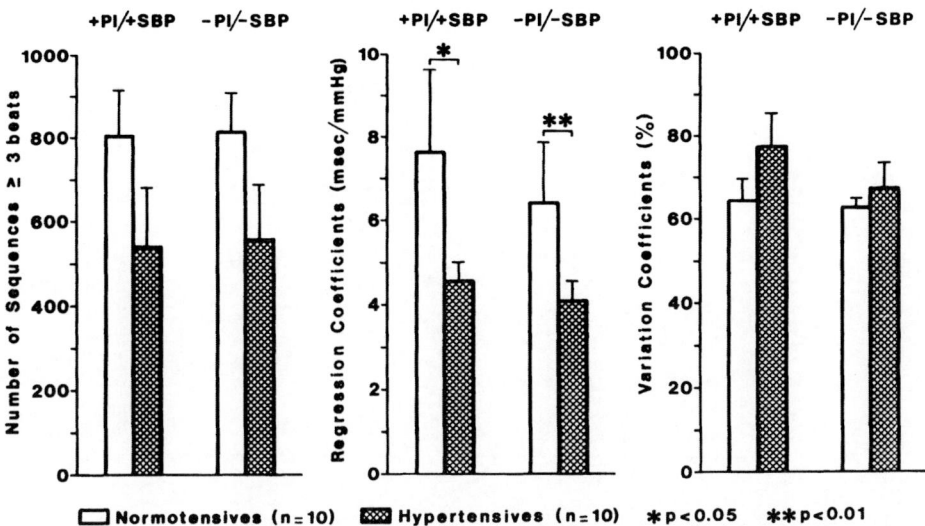

Fig. 6. Histograms illustrate the number of sequences characterized by a progressive increase ($+SBP/+PI$) or by a progressive reduction ($-SBP/-PI$) in pulse interval (PI) and systolic blood pressure (SBP) during 24 hours (*left panel*), their mean 24-h slopes (*central panel*) and the 24 h variation coefficient of this slope (*right panel*). Data are shown separately as means ±SE for 10 normotensive and 10 hypertensive subjects. (From [19])

to study the baroreceptor heart rate control [8, 18]. This control can be quantified by calculating the slope of the regression line between changes in systolic blood pressure and changes in pulse interval as an index of baroreflex sensitivity. As far as the spontaneous sequences are concerned, this is justified by the fact that in the experimental animal these sequences almost disappeared after sino-aortic denervation, leaving no doubt about their reflex nature (Fig. 5).

Sequence analysis has been applied to 24-h ambulatory intra-arterial blood pressure recordings obtained in humans [19]. As shown in Fig. 6, in both normotensive and hypertensive subjects the number of the hypertension/bradycardia and hypotension/tachycardia sequences was in the order of several hundreds over 24 h. Hypertensive subjects were characterized by a lower number of sequences than normotensive subjects, but the difference between the two groups was more evident for the slope of the sequences, i.e., for the sensitivity of the baroreflex, its reduction in hypertensive subjects confirming the well-known impairment of the baroreceptor-heart rate control in the chronically elevated blood pressure state [18]. The dynamic analysis of this phenomenon, however, allowed us to conclude that this is the case throughout the 24 h.

Figure 6 also shows that, rather than being stable, the slope of the sequences was highly variable within a given subject, the coefficient of variation ranging between 40% and 85%. This means that the sensitivity of the baroreceptor-heart rate reflex is continuously changing over 24 h. This is evident both in normotensive and in hypertensive subjects but, as shown in Fig. 7, the baroreflex sensitivity is modulated differently in the two groups. In normotensive subjects the sensitivity

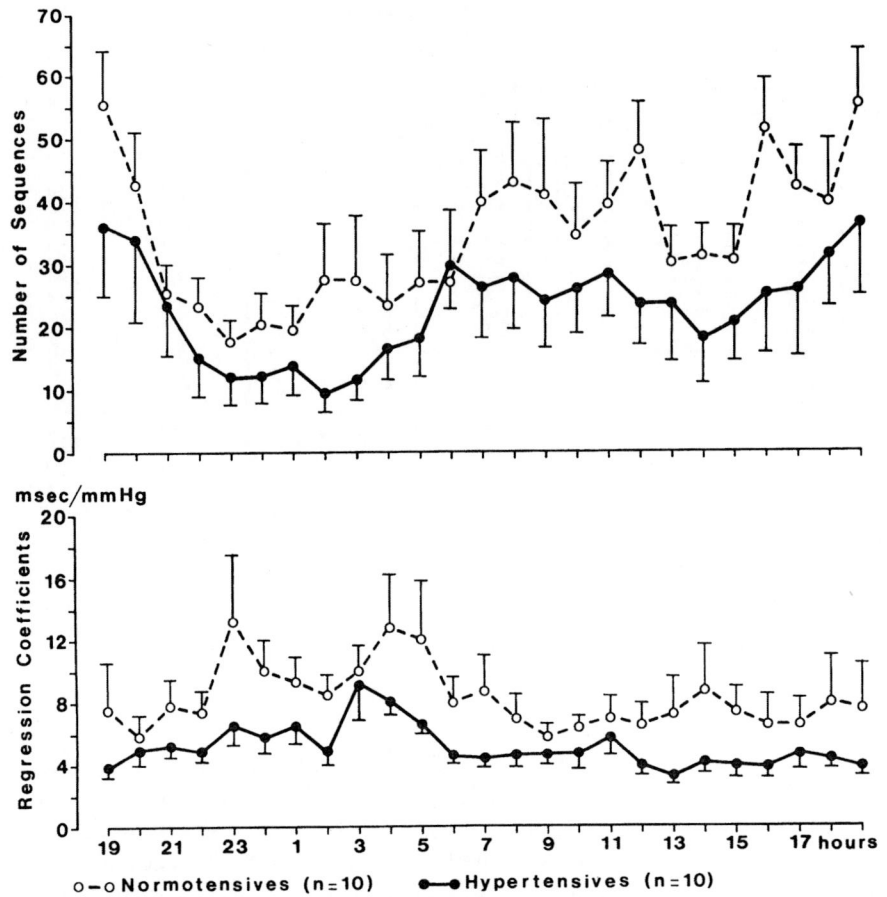

Fig. 7. Number and mean regression coefficient (slope) of +SBP/+PI sequences during each hour of the 24-h recording period. Data are shown separately as means ± SE for normotensive and hypertensive subjects. Sequences of different duration are pooled. (From [19])

is markedly increased during the night, while this is less evident in hypertensive patients.

Blood Pressure and Pulse Interval Changes in the Frequency Domain: Spectral Analysis

Another approach to investigating the relation between blood pressure and heart rate variability and neural control of circulation is based on spectral analysis of blood pressure and heart rate signals. This represents a means to quantify rhythmic blood pressure and heart rate fluctuations, the existence of which has been documented in studies carried out several years ago [20, 21]. These fluctuations have spectral powers which fall in different frequency bands. The bands most commonly addressed [21–24] are those between 0.5–0.14 Hz (high frequency,

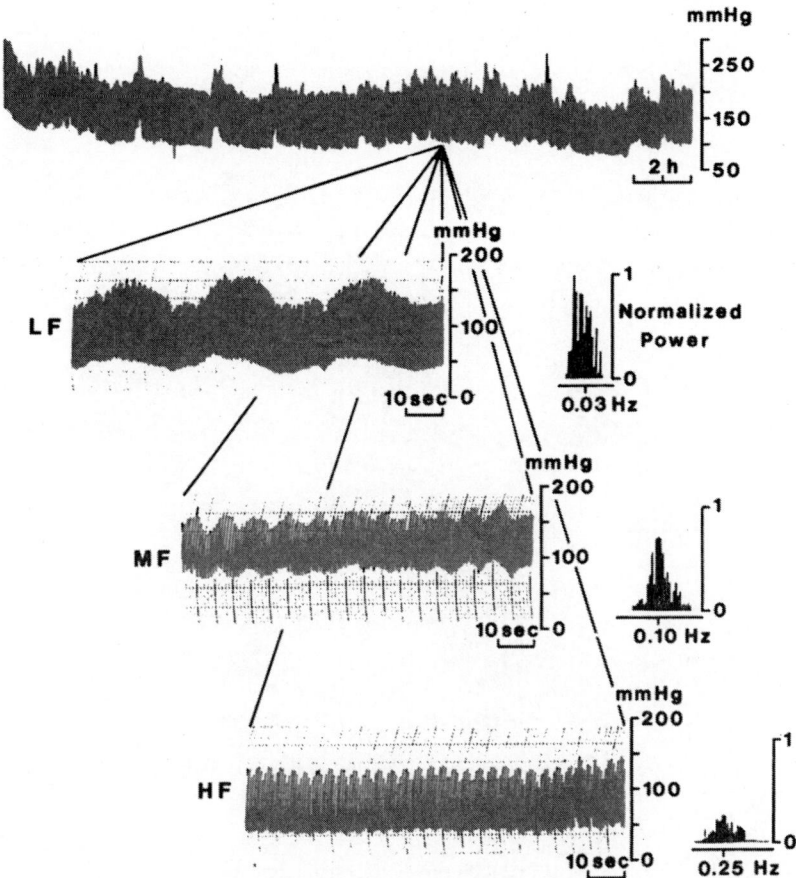

Fig. 8. Examples derived from original intra-arterial blood pressure tracings of so-called low-frequency (*LF*), mid-frequency (*MF*), and high-frequency (*HF*) blood pressure fluctuations

HF), 0.14–0.07 Hz (mid frequency, MF) and 0.07–0.025 Hz (low frequency, LF) (Fig. 8), although powers in the MF and LF bands are now pooled together and defined simply as LF powers by some investigators [25, 26].

What is the relationship between these spectral components of blood pressure and heart rate and neural cardiovascular control? Present evidence indicates that the HF powers of heart rate reflect parasympathetic modulation of the heart which is largely associated with respiratory activity. Although still under debate, it has also been suggested that MF and HF powers of heart rate and MF powers of blood pressure may reflect sympathetic modulation of the heart and peripheral resistance [25, 26].

Because these analyses were performed on short-lasting recordings obtained in the laboratory, the above-mentioned data do not provide information on the behaviour of these phenomena in real life conditions. In a recent study [27] we have extended the spectral analysis of blood pressure and heart rate to recordings

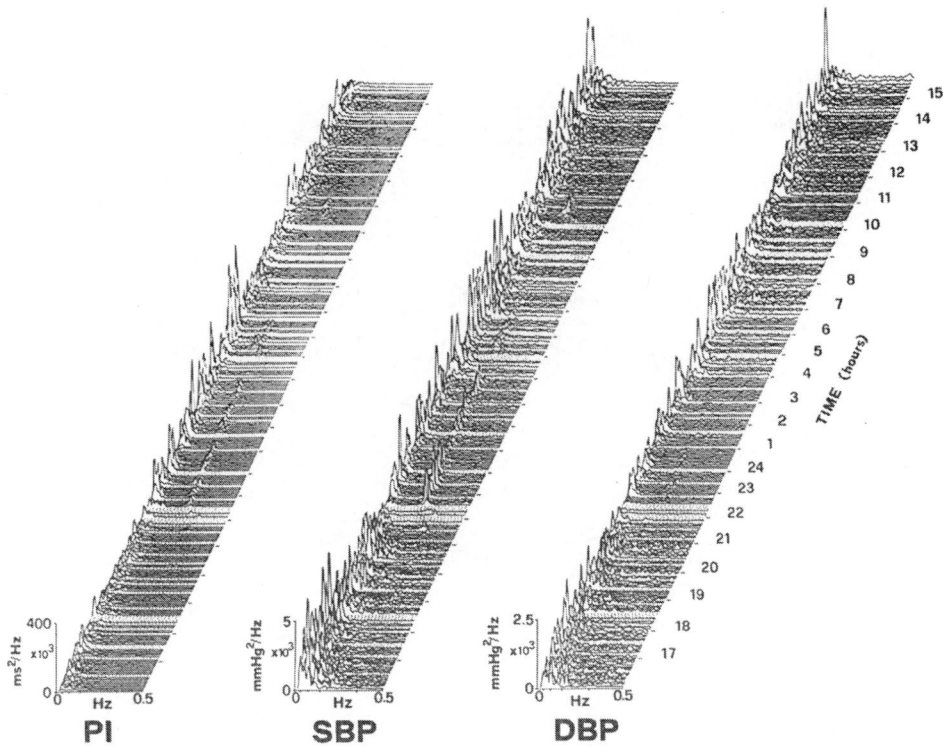

Fig. 9. Sequential power spectrum densities of low-, mid- and high-frequency fluctuations of pulse interval (*PI*), systolic blood pressure (*SBP*) and diastolic blood pressure (*DBP*) computed over consecutive segments of 256 beats throughout the 24-h period. Data are derived from a 24-h intra-arterial ambulatory blood pressure recording of a representative subject (B.E.). Dotted lines on each panel refer to segments in which power spectrum densities could not be estimated because of non-stationarities in the recorded signal. (From [27])

obtained intra-arterially in ambulant subjects over the 24 h. Spectral powers were computed by the Fast Fourier Transform (FFT) algorithm after splitting the 24-h recording into contiguous blocks of 256 beats and after removal of nonstationarities via an automatic procedure (Fig. 9). The powers of LF, MF and HF oscillations were all characterized by marked block-to-block changes. There were also systematic variations between the day and night, which consisted of a night-time reduction in MF powers of blood pressure and a night-time increase in LF and HF powers of pulse interval (Fig. 10). The hour-to-hour changes in spectral powers did not necessarily parallel the well-known day-night changes in overall variance of blood pressure and heart rate. Normotensive and hypertensive subjects were characterized by comparable directional changes in the hourly values of these blood pressure and heart rate spectral components [28] (Fig. 11).

Considering that the night is accompanied by an increase in vagal drive to the heart and a reduction in sympathetic drive to the systemic circulation, these data are compatible with a parasympathetic nature of the HF powers of heart rate and, to some extent, with a possible contribution of sympathetic influences to MF

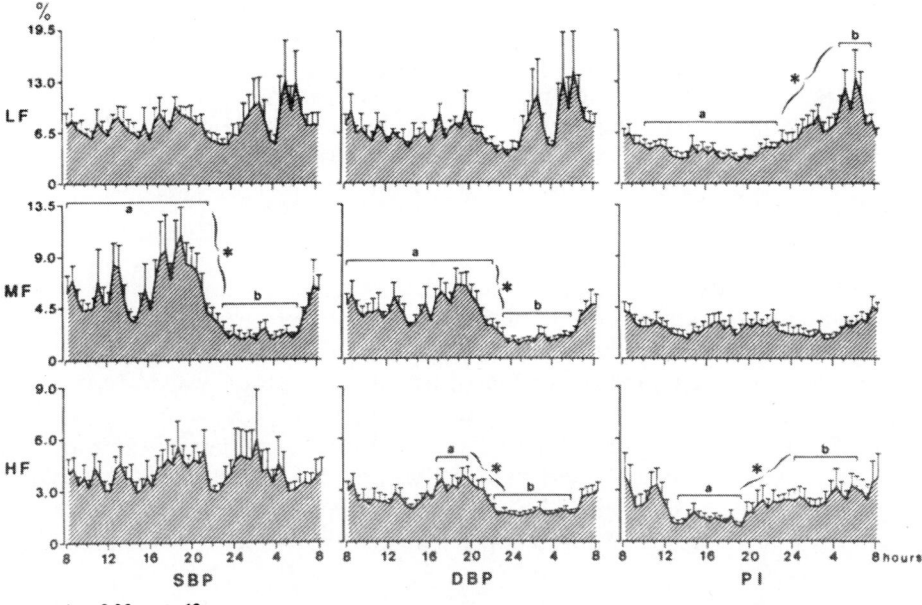

Fig. 10. Graphs showing low-*(LF)*, mid-*(MF)* and high-*(HF)* frequency powers of systolic blood pressure *(SBP)*, diastolic blood pressure *(DBP)* and pulse interval *(PI)* for seven normotensive subjects undergoing 24-h ambulatory intra-arterial blood pressure monitoring. Data are averaged for each half hour and shown as means ± SE. Powers are represented as a percentage of the 24-h variance. *Asterisk* shows statistical significance of differences between subperiods of day *(a)* and night *(b)*. Subperiod duration is indicated by *horizontal bars*. (From [28])

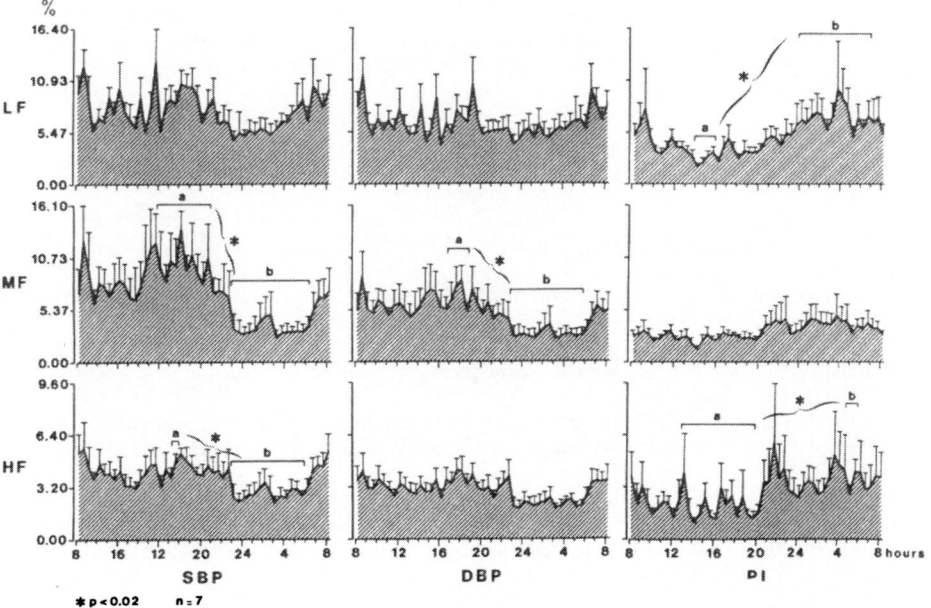

Fig. 11. Graphs showing LF, MF, and HF powers of SBP, DBP, and PI for ten hypertensive subjects. Key as for Fig. 10. (From [28])

powers of blood pressure. They do not support, however, a pure sympathetic nature of the LF blood pressure powers. Finally, these data show a pronounced spontaneous variability in blood pressure and heart rate powers. This emphasizes the need of caution in considering laboratory data as representative of everyday patterns.

Conclusions

Based on the above-mentioned evidence and considerations, the analysis of blood pressure and heart rate variability may represent a promising tool to investigate the factors involved in dynamic neural cardiovascular regulation. These studies can be made easier by a method which allows us to monitor beat-to-beat blood pressure noninvasively [29–32]. This method, which makes use of a small cuff wrapped around one or more fingers, may allow to avoid use of intra-arterial catheters, which were in the past the only way to continuously monitor blood pressure. It may thus extend 24-h ambulatory blood pressure monitoring to conditions where the intra-arterial approach is not regarded as a safe procedure [32].

References

1. Mancia G, Mark AL (1983) Arterial baroreflexes in humans. In: Shepherd JT, Abboud FM (eds) The cardiovascular system IV, vol 3. Peripheral circulation and organ blood flow, Part 2. American Physiological Society, Bethesda, pp 755–793 (Handbook of physiology, sect. 2)
2. Parati G, Pomidossi G, Ramirez AJ, Cesana B, Mancia G (1985) Variability of the haemodynamic responses to laboratory tests employed in assessment of neural cardiovascular regulation in man. Clin Sci 69:533–540
3. Parati G, Pomidossi G, Casadei R, Ravogli A, Groppelli A, Cesana B, Mancia G (1988) Comparison of the cardiovascular effects of different laboratory stressors and their relationship with blood pressure variability. J Hypertension 6:481–488
4. Bevan AT, Honour AJ, Stott FH (1969) Direct arterial pressure recording in unrestricted man. Clin Sci 36:329–345
5. Stott FD, Teny VG, Honour AJ (1976) Factors determining the design and construction of a portable pressure transducer system. Postgrad Med J 52 [Suppl. 7]:97–99
6. Mancia G (1990) Ambulatory blood pressure monitoring: research and clinical applications. Presidential Lecture. J Hypertension 8 [Suppl. 7]:S1–S13
7. Mancia G, Ferrari A, Gregorini L, Parati G, Pomidossi G, Bertinieri G, Grassi G, Di Rienzo M, Pedotti A, Zanchetti A (1983) Blood pressure and heart rate variabilities in normotensive and hypertensive human beings. Circ Res 53:96–104
8. Mancia G, Zanchetti A (1986) Blood pressure variability. In: Zanchetti A, Tarazi RC (eds) Handbook of hypertension, vol. 7. Elsevier, Amsterdam, pp 125–152
9. Mancia G, Bertinieri G, Cavallazzi A, Di Rienzo M, Parati G, Pomidossi G, Ramirez AJ, Zanchetti A (1985) Mechanisms of blood pressure variability in man. Clin Exp Hypertens 7:167–178
10. Floras JS, Hasson MH, Vann Jones J, Osikowska BA, Sever PS, Sleight P (1988) Factors influencing blood pressure and heart rate variability in hypertensive humans. Hypertension 11:273–281
11. Parati G, Pomidossi G, Mancia G (1986) Neural mechanisms in neural cardiovascular regulation. In: Schmidt TH, Dembroski TM, Blümchen G (eds) Biological and psychological factors in cardiovascular disease. Springer, Berlin Heidelberg New York, pp 379–388
12. Mancia G, Zanchetti A (1980) Cardiovascular regulation during sleep. In: Orem J, Barnes CD (eds) Physiology during sleep. Academic, New York, pp 1–50

13. Ramirez AJ, Bertinieri G, Belli L, Cavallazzi A, Di Rienzo M, Pedotti A, Mancia G (1985) Reflex control of blood pressure and heart rate by arterial baroreceptors and by cardiopulmonary receptors in the unanesthetized cat. J Hypertens 3:327–335

14. Cowley AW, Liard LF, Guyton AC (1973) Role of the baroreflex in daily control of arterial blood pressure and other variables in dogs. Circ Res 32:564–576

15. Mancia G, Parati G, Pomidossi G, Casadei R, Di Rienzo M, Zanchetti A (1986) Arterial baroreflexes and blood pressure and heart rate variabilities in humans. Hypertension 8:147–153

16. Conway J, Bonn N, Davies C, Vann Jones J, Sleight P (1984) Neural and humoral mechanisms involved in blood pressure variability. J Hypertens 2:203–208

17. Bertinieri G, Di Rienzo M, Cavallazzi A, Ferrari AU, Pedotti A, Mancia G (1988) Evaluation of baroreceptor reflex by blood pressure monitoring in unanesthetized cats. Am J Physiol 254 (Heart Circ Physiol 23):H377–H383

18. Smyth HS, Sleight P, Pickering GW (1969) Reflex regulation of arterial pressure during sleep in man: a quantitative method of assessing baroreflex sensitivity. Circ Res 74:109–121

19. Parati G, Di Rienzo M, Bertinieri G, Pedotti A, Zanchetti A, Mancia G (1988) Evaluation of baroreceptor-heart rate reflex by 24th intra-arterial blood pressure monitoring in humans. Hypertension 12:214–222

20. Hales S (1733) Statistical essays, vol. 2, Haemastaticks. Innys and Manly, London

21. Koepchen H-P (1984) History of studies and concepts of blood pressure waves. In: Miyakawa K, Koepchen H-P, Polosa C (eds) Mechanisms of blood pressure waves. Japan Science Society, Tokyo and Springer, Berlin Heidelberg New York, pp 3–23

22. Akselrod S, Gordon D, Uebel FA, Shannon DC, Barger AC, Cohen RJ (1981) Power spectrum analysis of heart rate fluctuations: a quantitative probe of beat to beat cardiovascular control. Science 213:220–223

23. Akselrod S, Gordon D, Ubel FA, Shannon DC, Barger AC, Cohen RJ (1985) Hemodynamic regulation: investigation by spectral analysis. Am J Physiol 249:H867–H875

24. DeBoer RW, Karemaker JM, van Montfrans GA (1986) Determination of baroreflex sensitivity by spectral analysis of spontaneous blood pressure and heart rate fluctuations in man. In: Lown B, Malliani A, Prosdocimi M (eds) Neural mechanisms and cardiovascular disease. Fidia Research Series. Liviana, Padua, pp 303–315

25. Pagani, M, Lombardi F, Guzzetti S, Rimoldi O, Furlan R, Pizzinelli P, Sandrone G, Malfatto G, Dell'Orto S, Piccaluga E, Turiel M, Baselli G, Cerutti S, Malliani A (1986) Power spectral analysis of heart rate and arterial pressure variabilities as a marker of sympato-vagal interaction in man and conscious dog. Circ Res 59:178–193

26. Rimoldi O, Pierini S, Ferrari A, Cerutti S, Pagani M, Malliani A (1990) Analysis of short-term oscillations of R-R and arterial pressure in conscious dogs. Am J Physiol 258 (Heart Circ Physiol 27):H967–H976

27. Di Rienzo M, Castiglioni P, Mancia G, Parati G, Pedotti A (1989) 24-h Sequential spectral analysis of arterial blood pressure and pulse interval in free-moving subjects. IEEE Transaction 36:1066–1075

28. Parati G, Castiglioni P, Di Rienzo M, Omboni S, Pedotti A, Mancia G (1990) Sequential spectral analysis of 24-hour blood pressure and pulse interval in humans. Hypertension 16:414–421

29. Peñáz J (1973) Photoelectric measurement of blood pressure, volume and flow in the finger. Conference Committee of the 10th International Conference on Medicine and Biological Engineering, Dresden, p 104

30. Wesseling KH, De Wit B, Settels JJ, Klaver WH (1982) On the indirect registration of finger blood pressure after Peñáz. Funkt Biol Med 1:245–250

31. Parati G, Casadei R, Groppelli A, Di Rienzo M, Mancia G (1989) Comparison of finger and intra-arterial blood pressure monitoring at rest and during laboratory testing. Hypertension 13:647–655

32. Imholz B, van Montfrans G, Parati G, Villani A, Groppelli A, Longewouters G, Wesseling K, Mancia G, Wieling W (1990) First experience with Portapres: continuous noninvasive ambulatory finger blood pressure compared to intra-brachial blood pressure. Proceedings of the 13th Scientific Meeting of International Society of Hypertension (ISH), Montreal, 1190:S87. J Hypertension [Suppl 3] 8:S87

Sources of Variability and Methodological Considerations in Ambulatory Blood Pressure *

M. D. Gellman, G. H. Ironson, N. Schneiderman, M. M. Llabre, and S. B. Spitzer

Introduction

The measurement of ambulatory blood pressure (ABP) has been of interest for some time. There are two compelling reasons for this focus on ABP. First, ABP is more representative than blood pressure (BP) taken in a single setting; second field measurements of BP have been related to subsequent hypertension (Rose et al. 1978), left ventricular hypertrophy (Devereux et al. 1983; Sokolow et al. 1966), hypertensive complications (Pickering et al. 1985), and morbidity and mortality (Perloff et al. 1983). More specifically, several studies have shown that ABP adds important information over and above office BP measurement in the relationship between BP and left ventricular hypertrophy (Devereux et al. 1983; Sokolow et al. 1966) and other hypertensive complications (Pickering et al. 1985).

Given the potential importance of ABP, our laboratory has been studying factors which may affect its level. These factors include within subject factors such as posture, place (i.e., home versus work), mood and social situation, and between subject factors such as race, hypertensive status, and individual differences in laboratory reactivity. A discussion of the relationship between each of these factors and ABP comprises the first part of this chapter.

While exploring the relationship between the above factors and ABP it was necessary to address several methodological issues raised by questions involved in the analyses. First, how many BP measurements need to be made in each setting for adequate reliability/generalizability? Second, what variables represent potential confounds in looking at the relationship between factors (such as place, home versus work) and ABP? For example, if people mostly stand at work and sit at home and standing is independently associated with BP, then any differences found between home and work ABP may be confounded with differences in posture. Method of measurement is another potential confound introduced when, for example, BP is measured in the office with a mercury sphygmomanometer whereas BP at work is measured with an ABP monitor. Results from the above studies will help to guide our third methodological question: What variables ought

* This work was supported by research grants HL 31648 and HL 36588 and by research training grant HL 07426 from the National Heart, Lung and Blood Institute of the NIH.

Schmidt/Engel/Blümchen (Eds.)
Temporal Variations of the Cardiovascular System
© Springer-Verlag Berlin Heidelberg 1992

to be included in ambulatory diaries? These three methodological questions comprise the second part of this chapter.

Factors Affecting ABP

Within-Subject Factors

It has been reported that posture influences BP: for example, BP while standing is greater than BP while sitting (Jorde and Williams 1986). In a study from our laboratory (Gellman et al. 1990b) posture was the most potent effect observed. In fact 33% and 47% of the within-subject variance in systolic BP and diastolic BP, respectively, could be explained by this factor. As noted in Table 1, as subjects' posture changed from lying down to sitting to standing, BP systematically increased by 14 mm Hg for systolic BP and 15 mm Hg for diastolic BP. This finding underscores the need to control for posture in the interpretation of ABP recording, and will be discussed in the methodology section later in this chapter.

Place (*Home versus Work*)

Place effects include BP measurements taken at home, at work, or at the clinic (Pickering et al. 1982; Harshfield et al. 1982; White 1986). As will be noted in the section on potential confounds, researchers must be cautious when making comparisons across settings within a study where the setting may be confounded with instrument or posture.

Table 1. Factors related to ABP

Factor	Levels	Systolic blood pressure (mmHg)		Diastolic blood pressure ((mmHg)	
		Mean	SD	Mean	SD
Posture[a]	Supine	119	16.8	70	12.6
	Sitting	127	17.2	81	12.6
	Standing	133	19.2	85	12.5
Place[a]	Home	127	18.6	79	13.2
	Work	131	18.6	83	11.6
Mood[a]	Neutral	128	18.5	81	13.1
	Positive	131	21.2	83	13.7
	Negative	132	20.6	83	15.0
Social situation[b]	Family	125	18.6	79	15.5
	Strangers	138	24.1	86	15.3
Measuring instrument[c]	Mercury sphygmomanometer	126	17.2	83	12.4
	Dinamap	131	16.4	82	13.0
	Spacelabs	121	18.4	80	14.4

SD, standard deviation.
[a] Gellman et al. 1990b.
[b] Results presented for seated posture only. Similar occured for standing BP. Spitzer et al. 1992.
[c] Llabre et al. 1988.

In the Gellman et al. (1990 b) study, the place effect explained 10 % and 15 % of the within subject variance in the systolic BP and diastolic BP, respectively, of seated subjects. This finding is consistent with findings from other studies (Pickering et al. 1982; White 1986). With respect to absolute levels (about 4 mm Hg), we found that BP was higher at work than at home (see Table 1), which is consistent with the reports of Clark et al. (1987) and Van Egeren and Madarasmi (1988).

Work Versus Nonwork Day Differences

A recent study from our laboratory (Gellman et al. 1990 a) examined the overall differences in ambulatory BP and heart rate monitoring across work and nonwork days during waking hours. We restricted the examination to the differences in BP and heart rate when controlling for posture by making comparisons to when the subjects were either sitting or standing. Participants in the study were 52 healthy men and women aged 25–54. They wore the Suntech Accutracker ABP monitor from morning till bedtime. On one of the days, the subjects left the clinic and went to work and then home; on the other day, after leaving the clinic, the subjects participated in leisure activities. Diary cards were filled out by the subjects to indicate their activities.

Our results indicated significant BP differences between the 2 days. When comparison were made controlling for posture we found statistically significant differences only for BP readings taken while the subjects were in the sitting position. The patterns of BP and heart rate across the 2 days were highly correlated. The BP readings were significantly higher on the work day, but there were no differences in heart rate across the 2 days, suggesting that the subjects maintained a similar activity level across the 2 days. The BP results suggest that the work day contributes to an elevation of BP that lasts throughout the day, not just when the subjects are at work. Comparisons made while the subjects were in the standing position showed differences that approached significance, however, due to the large amount of variability they were not found to be significant.

Mood Effects

Emotional state or mood has been examined by James et al. (1986), Southard et al. (1986), and Sokolow et al. (1970) as well as by our research group. Some of these studies of the effect of mood on BP have provided partially contradictory results. The studies that have examined this variable have all shown that negative mood ratings are associated with higher BP. However positive moods were either not significantly associated with BP ("patient, interested, energetic") (Southard et al. 1986) or were associated with lower BP ("happiness") (James et al. 1986). None of these studies, however, included a sufficiently full range of moods (positive, neutral, and negative) in combination with a large enough sample to permit a completely within-subject comparison that also could adjust for posture. In our studies we found that *both* positive and negative moods affect BP equally. The effect, however, was small (6 % and 8 %, respectively, when subjects were sitting). The relationship between contentment and lowered BP has also been found by

Sokolow and colleagues (1970). Previous research had suggested that it was primarily the negative moods that were associated with increases in BP (James et al. 1986; Southard et al. 1986; Sokolow et al. 1970). James and co-workers (1986) assessed their subjects' degree of happiness, sadness, anger, or anxiety based on a 10-point scale. Southard and co-workers (1986) had their subjects monitor their moods during daily activities with a form that included 11 affective states ratings and 5 perception-of-the-environment ratings on Likert-type scales. Sokolow and co-workers used a mood ratings form that included adjectives describing anxiety, depression, alertness, hostility, time pressure, and contentment. Our findings are based on the subjects informing us about their mood for each BP reading by answering on the diary card whether they were neutral (content), positive (happy and smiling), or negative (tense, annoyed, upset, and angry). Our finding may have been due to our distinction between neutral and positive moods compared with other studies.

Social Situation Effects

The degree to which BP varies across everyday social situations may have important consequences for the interpretation of BP levels assessed in clinical settings. It has been suggested that the social situation encountered when diagnostic levels of BP are being assessed in the clinic may play a role in "white coat hypertension" (Pickering et al. 1988). "White coat hypertension" refers to the situation in which BP reaches hypertensive levels only when the patient is in a clinic as opposed to in other settings. Pickering and colleagues found patients with white coat hypertension were more likely to be female, of younger age, to weigh less, and to have a shorter duration of hypertension than other patients. Additionally, this phenomenon was most pronounced when patients were confronted by a physician as opposed to a nurse or technician.

In a study conducted by Long and colleagues (1982), half of a group of normotensive college students were randomly selected to sit quietly in a room with an experimenter who was dressed in a casual manner and who described himself as a graduate student working as a research assistant; the other half of the subjects sat with the same experimenter who was dressed neatly in a white laboratory jacket and who identified himself as an internist. The average mean arterial BP was somewhat higher for the "high status" condition than for the "equal status" condition. Larger differences were observed, however, for subjects who read aloud to the "high status" experimenter as compared to the "equal status" experimenter. This suggests that the effect of social situations on BP levels is dependent upon the relative status of the persons involved. Differences in social situations may also underlie other cardiovascular phenomena that have been reported. For instance, Lynch (1985) has suggested that the significantly higher death rates from hypertension among black Americans and the economically disadvantaged may in part be due to those persons having to relate interpersonally in a world where virtually everyone else is perceived to be of higher status.

A study was conducted in our laboratory (Spitzer et al. 1992) which examined the relationships between various naturally occurring social situations and BP levels in black and white, male and female, normotensive and mild to moderate hypertensive subjects. Given our previous knowledge of the strong influence of posture, it was controlled for when comparing BP levels across varying social situations. Our results indicated that social situation accounted for a substantial proportion of the within-subject variance of seated BP levels (37%). The highest levels of BP were found when subjects were with strangers, and the lowest levels were found when subjects were with family (see Table 1). The two main findings of the study are a significant effect of social situation on BP and an exaggerated effect of social situation for mild to moderate hypertensives as compared with normotensives.

Constitutional Between-Subject Factors

Race

Blacks have a much higher prevalence of hypertension than whites (Roberts and Rowland 1981). Despite this, very few studies have examined how environmental factors may relate to ABP differences between blacks and whites. Our group (Gellman et al. 1990 b) investigated differences between BP at home and at work separately by race and found that differences between BP at home and at work were greater for whites than for blacks.

More specifically, whites decreased their BP more than blacks as they moved from work to home. This finding is particularly interesting because both groups revealed comparable BP levels at work. One possible interpretation of these results might be that the black subjects in our study did not "unwind" as well as the white subjects after the work day, perhaps because the socioeconomic stressors that they faced were more pervasive (Harburg et al. 1973). Previous research has also indicated that black subjects exhibit slower BP recovery than white subjects after performing some behavioral laboratory tasks (Anderson et al. 1989; Light et al. 1986), which in turn might be related to variables such as inhibited sodium excretion (Grim et al. 1984).

Our laboratory has also investigated racial differences in the prediction of ABP from performance on laboratory tasks (Ironson et al. 1989). For blacks, but not whites, the cold pressor task added significantly to the prediction of ABP over baseline BP. In addition reactivity during the cold pressor task predicted ABP (diastolic) for blacks at work ($r = 0.73$) significantly greater than the correlation for whites ($r = 0.40$). These findings together with the observation that the cold pressor task tends to elicit alpha-adrenergic activity (Baughman and Green 1981) lead us to hypothesize that differences in alpha-adrenergic mediation of BP may exist between blacks and whites. Further investigation of these mechanisms (total peripheral resistance versus cardiac output differences in reactivity in blacks and whites) are now underway.

Hypertensive Status

As was true with race, very few studies have examined how environmental factors may relate to ABP differences between hypertensives and normotensives. The main question of interest in this context is whether hypertensives respond to a given environmental stressor with a larger increase in BP than normotensives do. Evidence from the laboratory suggests that hypertensives have greater BP responses than normotensives to such varied tasks as mental arithmetic, other cognitive tasks, stressful interviews, and video games (see Schneiderman et al. 1987, for a review) as well as increased reactivity to a more naturalistic task such as talking (Lynch et al. 1981). Evidence from our ambulatory studies, in which we found larger systolic BP differences (Gellman et al. 1990 b) between home and work for mild hypertensives (10 mm Hg) than for normotensives (3 mm Hg), and larger systolic BP differences (Spitzer et al. 1992) between social situation for mild-moderate hypertensives (10 mm Hg family verus friends; 21 mm Hg family versus strangers) than for normotensives (5 mm Hg family versus friends; 6 mm Hg family versus strangers) supports the extension of increased reactivity for hypertensives from the laboratory to the ambulatory setting.

Laboratory Reactivity

Given the potential usefulness of ABP measurement, as noted in the introduction, the relationships among one-time clinic or laboratory measurement, laboratory responses to provocative laboratory challenges, and ABP responses in various situations (e.g., home versus work) deserve study. Two major questions arise: can laboratory tasks elicit increases in BP comparable to those seen in ambulatory settings? Is an individual's responses to provocative laboratory challenges related to ABP responses beyond the relationship found between initial baseline measurements and ABP? Thus, the possibility exists that just as dynamic tests in other areas of medicine have provided important additional information over static measurements, e.g., oral glucose tolerance test for glycemic control or exercise stress test for assessing electrocardiographic (ECG) abnormalities, standardized psychophysiologic challenges in the laboratory may provide useful new information, particularly if they are related to ABP measurements. Furthermore, the laboratory assessment of reactivity to provocative challenges offers the possibility of comprehensive assessment under conditions of precise stimulus control of those hemodynamic and hormonal factors that may be influencing BP regulation.

The first question examining whether the reactivity increases in BP found under laboratory conditions were as great as those found in more naturalistic settings during ABP was affirmatively answered by a study done in our laboratory (Ironson et al. 1989). Increases in systolic BP (over baseline) during tasks were + 11 (interview), + 14 (video game), + 34 (exercise), and + 10 mm Hg (cold pressor) compared with increases during ABP of + 4 (home), and + 10 mm Hg (work). For diastolic BP the increases during tasks were + 10 (interview), + 11 (video game), + 30 (exercise), and + 10 mm Hg (cold pressor) respectively, compared with + 4 and + 11 mm Hg for ABP. Thus, laboratory tasks were able to elicit increases comparable to or greater than those elicited during ABP measurement.

The second question, whether individual differences in reactivity provided information over and above baseline differences in predicting ABP was also a major focus of this study (Ironson et al. 1989) and was also answered affirmatively. A number of tasks, especially the interview, added a significant proportion of variance to the prediction of work BP over and above baseline although the additional variance was small ($3\% - 7\%$). Other tasks such as the cold pressor task and the video game were significant predictors in certain subpopulations (blacks and females, respectively). It is interesting to note that tasks correlating highest with ABP (interview and video game) involved more emotional than physical stress, and that both alpha-adrenergic (cold pressor) and beta-adrenergic (video game) tasks have a significant association with ABP.

Although reactivity tasks did provide useful information, the baseline played a pre-eminent role in predicting ABP. In the Ironson et al. (1989) study, the baseline accounted for as much as $36\% - 59\%$ of the variance in ABP.

Finally, although the amount of variance accounted for by the reactivity tasks was low, the data provided by the responses to these tasks were intriguing. As noted above, the finding that the cold pressor test predicted diastolic BP significantly better for blacks than for whites suggested that further exploration into differential mechanisms for BP regulation in blacks and whites (e.g., alpha-adrenergic versus beta-adrenergic sensitivity) would be useful.

In a recently completed but as yet unpublished study from our laboratory, healthy, normotensive white women ($n = 10$) and men ($n = 10$), aged $22 - 54$ years old served as subjects. Heart rate, BP, and several impedance-derived parameters were measured during three tasks: a videotaped speech task containing a preparation component and a speaking component; a mirror star tracing task; and a foot cold pressor task.

The behavioral stressors elicited comparable increases in systolic BP, diastolic BP, and heart rate. Although there were no significant differences between men and women on any cardiovascular measure, the stressors were differentiated by the underlying variables that supported the BP increases. Specifically, during the preparation period of the speech task, during which the subjects were planning their speech, the elevation of BP appears to have resulted from an increase in cardiac output ($\dot{Q}$). The augmentation of BP during the ensuing talk period of the task resulted in significant increases in both $\dot{Q}$ and total peripheral resistance (TPR) compared with baseline. The rise in systolic BP and diastolic BP during both the mirror star tracing and cold pressor tasks appears to have resulted from the significant increases that occur in TPR.

Changes in TPR and $\dot{Q}$ observed during the preparation and speaking components of the speech task were significantly related to ABP measurements obtained during waking hours on 2 separate days. Basically, changes in TPR observed during the speech task were positively correlated with ABP, whereas, changes in $\dot{Q}$ observed during this task were negatively correlated with ABP. Thus, those individuals showing the greatest TPR response during the speech task had the highest ABP, whereas those showing the greatest $\dot{Q}$ response during the same task had the lowest ABP.

Methodological Considerations

Reliability: How Many BP Measurements Are Enough?

The issue of BP reliability is complicated because a variety of variables can influence the values obtained. Most studies of BP reliability have considered only one source of variation at a time. An extension of reliability theory, known as generalizability theory, permits the determination of the number of measurements needed to ensure high reliability over a wide variety of conditions (Cronbach et al. 1972). Our group (Llabre et al. 1988) has applied the principles of generalizability theory to BP measurements taken under various designs in order to consider multiple sources of variation. First, the generalizability of blood pressure measurements across measurement devices was assessed. Analyses using three instruments (mercury sphygmamanometer, Dinamap monitor, and Spacelabs ambulatory monitor) indicated that at least one replication with each of two instruments may be necessary when one wishes to generalize to any instrument. This finding suggests that instrumentation is a source of BP measurement variance which must be taken into consideration.

Next, generalizability across time was considered. Llabre et al. (1988) showed that only one reading may be necessary whenever generalizations are restricted to a short time interval during the same day in the laboratory. When generalizations across days are intended, the results indicated that a single reading from each of 2 or 3 days or two readings from each of 2 days would yield generalizable systolic BP measurements. With diastolic BP, however, the readings from more than 3 days seem to be required. The random variability observed across days is not surprising and has been reported in the literature (Pickering et al. 1985). Also, systolic BP readings are more reliable than diastolic BP readings. This pattern was also observed by Rosner and Polk (1979) who recommended that BP screening programs rely on two replications from each of three visits. The lower values observed in the Llabre et al. (1988) data may be due to sampling fluctuations and to the racial composition of their sample which included black and white men and women.

If the setting of the universe of generalization is shifted to the home and the workplace, coefficients decrease considerably, reflecting a higher level of within-subject variability in these settings than in the laboratory. Llabre et al. (1988) results showed that at least six replications of systolic BP are needed at home and at work, and six to ten diastolic BP readings may be required from work and home, respectively, in order to ensure acceptable levels of generalizability.

These results underscore the need for multiple measurements of BP in multiple settings and may help explain why ambulatory readings have proved superior to casual measurements in predicting target organ damage. Ambulatory monitoring devices should prove very useful to the understanding of the factors responsible for this setting variability.

Potentially Confounding Variables

Potentially confounding variables are variables which may be systematically associated with a variable of interest and may mask the true relationship between the variable of interest and ABP. For example, if the variable of interest is place (home versus work), then posture could be a potential confound in examining the home versus work ABP difference, if, for example, people spend more time sitting at home than they do at work. In this section we discuss posture, instrumentation, activity level, and time of day as potential confounds. It should be noted that some of these variables are independent variables as well as potential confounds, and their possible influence in both these ways needs to be kept in mind in analyzing factors influencing ABP.

Posture

As noted above posture has a strong, significant effect on ABP, accounting for 33%–47% of the variance in BP or a 4–5 mm Hg difference from sitting to standing. As also noted above, an observed finding of differences in BP between settings (of 4 mm Hg) might possibly have been completely explained by differences in posture if people sat at home and stood at work. Because of this, subsequent analyses of the effect of environmental factors were controlled by holding it constant under two conditions: sitting and standing. We found significant effects of place and mood when subjects were sitting, but not standing. These findings suggest that the increased BP needed to sustain subjects in a standing as opposed to a sitting posture overrides the effects of place and mood. At the same time it should be recognized that posture and activity effects are not necessarily independent of one another, and that people tend to do different things while standing as opposed to sitting.

Instruments

As noted many studies compare BP across settings, i.e., home, work, and clinic. This introduces other possible sources of variation that may confound a "true difference" between BP in various settings. For example if BP in the clinic is measured by manual sphygmomanometer and BP at home by an ABP device the difference between the clinical and home BP may be due to either instrument or setting.

The introduction of automatic detection devices removes observer bias as a variable, but raises other issues concerning the reliability and validity of the automated readings. For this reason it is important to compare measurements made with automatic devices against a known standard.

In our work we compared measurements made simultaneously using a mercury sphygmomanometer, an automatic Dinamap monitor and a Spacelabs ambulatory monitor (Ironson et al. 1989). Correlation coefficients between the means of three BP measurements for each instrument ranged from 0.88 to 0.95. The correlation show substantial agreement in ordering subjects. Correlations of this size also indicate that for many purposes measurements using different instruments are likely to be linearly related.

However, mean BP levels for the three instruments, presented in Table 1, were quite different in some cases. While the differences between the mercury sphygmomanometer measurements and each of the automatic instruments was only about 5 mm Hg for systolic BP, the differences obtained between the Dinamap and the Spacelabs automatic measurements averaged 10 mm Hg. Thus, it would be inappropriate to conclude, for example, that a decrease in systolic BP of 10 mm Hg obtained between the laboratory (using a Dinamap) and the home (using a Spacelabs automatic monitor) reflected a "true" difference in BP.

The issues of validity and comparability are important ones, which can usually be handled by making comparisons across instruments and adjusting values. Ideally, such measurements should be made across a range of values that can easily be changed by taking BP in the sitting position after having the subject rest while seated, move from supine to standing to sitting, and be seated immediately after mild exercise. This can be used to show that the differences obtained across instruments remain constant across a range of BP values.

Other Potentially Confounding Variables

Two other potentially confounding variables are activity level and time of day. For example, competing hypotheses about the higher BP observed during work days versus nonwork days might include greater activity at work, greater stress at work, more interaction with strangers at work, or a variety of other plausible explanations. To investigate activity as a possible confounding factor, we used heart rates as a measure of activity level. There were no differences between work and nonwork days in heart rate (Gellman et al. 1990a) suggesting that higher BP on work days is due to a factor other than activity level. In a similar analysis (Spitzer et al. 1992) there were no differences in activity levels as measured by heart rate between social situations, e.g., interacting with family versus interacting with strangers, therefore, suggesting higher BP when interacting with strangers was due to a factor other than activity level.

In addition to the objective measure of heart rate, we incorporated into our diary a subjective item where the subject circles one of (a) busy, (b) inactive or (c) other, to indicate their activity level at any given time point (see Fig. 1). In addition to a general activity level, certain specific activities such as talking or walking have also been related to BP (Pickering 1988). Because of this we included certain specific activities in our current diary as well (see "Diary Entries" below).

Time of day also represents another potentially confounding variable. Blood pressure has a diurnal pattern, being highest in the morning and lowest at night (Pickering 1988). In our research, we have noted this variation as well, accounting for roughly a 10-mm Hg difference in BP (Gellman et al. 1990a). A major question that arises from this observation is whether the diurnal variation is intrinsic or is due to differences in activity during the course of the day. Work done by Pickering (1988) and studies of immobilized orthopedic patients (Athassaniadis et al. 1969) and hospitalized patients (Young et al. 1983) suggests activity to be a more powerful predictor of BP than time of day.

Diary Entries

In any study relating activities to ABP one needs a method for recording activities. Our group has developed, based upon our experiences in several studies, the diary

Table 2. Example of a diary card

Time: _____ ☐ AM ☐ PM

1. Place (circle one)

  a. job
  b. home
  c. clinic
  d. other ____

2. Activity level (circle one)

  a. busy
  b. inactive
  c. other ____

3. Posture (circle one)

  a. lying down
  b. sitting down
  c. standing

4. Mood (circle one)

Was your mood
  a. very good
  b. good
  c. neutral
  d. bad
  e. very bad

5. Stress level (circle one)

Were you
  a. relaxed
  b. tense
  c. stressed

6. Physical activity

Were you	Yes
... relaxing	☐
... napping?	☐
... talking?	☐
... moving around?	☐
... exercising?	☐
... eating?	☐
... concentrating?	☐

7. Consumption

Since the previous reading, did you ...	Yes
... smoke?	☐
... have alcohol?	☐
... have caffeine?	☐
(soda, tea, coffee, chocolate)	

Comments:

---

format pictured in Table 2. At a minimum a diary should include the variables of interest which one wishes to relate to ABP, and potential confounding variables. Some variables, e.g., activity level, may function as both. Variables of interest have most commonly included place (home, work, clinic), activities, mood, and social situation. Potential confounds, some of which were mentioned above, include posture, time of day, activity level, specific activities, e.g., eating, sleeping, relaxing, exercising, and talking, and exogenous substances, e.g., caffeine and alcohol. A more complete review of questions to include in diaries, together with several examples, may be found in Chesney and Ironson (1989). Information should also be collected, though not necessarily through the diary, on the measuring instrument used, medications taken, and heart rate corresponding to each BP measurement.

Another issue of importance in ambulatory monitoring is getting subject compliance in filling out diaries. To maximize compliance we give subjects the stack of cards in a pouch (with a pencil) which can be attached to a belt; the diary is kept short (one card), comprehensive instructions are given, and finally subjects are paid upon successful completion.

Conclusion

As interest in the clinical usefulness of ABP and heart rate monitoring increases, attention needs to be focused on the sources of BP and heart rate variability. In this chapter we have reviewed both the content and methodological findings of our research group.

Content findings based upon within-subject factors suggest that posture has a potent effect on BP. Other within-subject factors significantly affecting BP include place, mood, and social situation. In analyses of between-subject factors such as race and hypertensive status, intriguing results were found. For race, BP in blacks remains higher at home after work than in whites, suggesting a failure to unwind. In addition a stronger relationship between BP reactivity and the cold pressor and diastolic ABP at work for blacks has led to an investigation of differential mechanisms for BP regulation in blacks versus whites. Our results for hypertensive status support the extension of increased BP reactivity in the laboratory to the ambulatory setting. Finally, studies of the relationship between laboratory reactivity and ABP suggest that, although task reactivity does add a significant amount to the prediction of ABP, it is small compared with the prediction of ABP from a well-measured baseline alone.

Methodological findings emphasized the importance of getting enough measurements in various settings in order to obtain adequate reliability/generalizability in ABP studies. A discussion of potential confounds suggest that, in addition to content variables of interest, attention must be paid to, and data collected on diaries or other format on posture, BP instrument used, time of day, activity level, specific activities, and the use of exogenous substances.

Interest in ABP measurement is likely to continue to increase, particularly because ambulatory readings have proved superior to casual measurements in predicting target organ damage. Ambulatory monitoring devices have proven useful in our understanding of the factors responsible for this variability. It is hoped that inclusion of content variables of interest, subject variables of interest, and attention to methodological considerations such as obtaining a careful baseline, getting enough measurements in each setting for adequate reliability, and paying attention to potential confounds will improve our understanding of variables that affect ABP.

References

Anderson NB, Lane JD, Taguchi F, Williams RB, Houseworth SJ (1989) Race, parental history of hypertension, and patterns of cardiovascular reactivity in women. Psychophysiology 26:39–47

Athassaniadis D, Drayer GJ, Honour AJ, Cranston WJ (1969) Variability of automatic blood pressure measurements over 24 hour period. Clin Sci 36:147–156

Baughman KL, Green BM (1981) Clinical diagnostic manual for the house officer. Williams and Wilkins, Baltimore

Chesney MA, Ironson G (1989) Diaries in ambulatory monitoring. In: Schneiderman N, Weiss S, Kaufmann P (eds) Handbook of research methods in cardiovascular behavioral medicine. Plenum, New York

Clark LA, Denby L, Pregibon D, Harshfield GA, Pickering TG, Blank S, Laragh JH (1987) A quantitative analysis of the effects of activity and time of day on the diurnal variations of blood pressure. J Chronic Dis 40:671–681

Cronbach LJ, Glaser GC, Nanda H, Rajaratnam N (1972) The dependability of behavioral measurements. Wiley, New York

Devereux RB, Pickering TG, Harshfield GA, Kleinert HD, Denby L, Clark L, Pregibon D, Jason M, Kleiner B, Borer JS, Laragh JH (1983) Left ventricular hypertrophy in patients with hypertension: Importance of blood pressure response to regularly occurring stress. Circulation 68:470

Gellman M, Massie C, Spitzer S, Llabre M, Schneiderman N (1990a) Repeatability of ambulatory blood pressure and heart rate over days: does activity make a difference? First international congress of behavioral medicine, vol 1 (abstract 387), Uppsala, Sweden, June 1990

Gellman M, Spitzer S, Ironson G, Llabre M, Saab P, Pasin R, Weidler D, Schneiderman N (1990b) Posture, place and mood effects on ambulatory monitoring. Psychophysiology 27:541–555

Grim C, Luft F, Weinberger M, Miller J, Rose R, Christian J (1984) Genetic, familial, and racial influences on blood pressure control systems in man. Aust N Z J Med 14:453–457

Harburg E, Erfurt JC, Hauenstein LS, Chaps C, Schull WJ, Schork MA (1973) Socio-ecological stress, suppressed hostility, skin color, and black-white male blood pressure: Detroit. Psychosomatic Medicine 35:276–283

Harshfield GA, Pickering TG, Kleiner HD, Blank S, Laragh JH (1982) Situational variations of blood pressure in ambulatory hypertensive patients. Psychosom Med 44:237–245

Ironson GH, Gellman MD, Spitzer SB, Llabre MM, Pasin RD, Weidler DJ, Schneiderman N (1989) Predicting home and work blood pressure measurements from resting baselines and laboratory reactivity in black and white Americans. Psychophysiology 26:174–184

James GD, Yee LS, Harshfield GA, Blank SG, Pickering TG (1986) The influence of happiness, anger and anxiety on the blood pressure of borderline hypertensives. Psychosom Med 48:502–508

Jorde LP, Williams RR (1986) Innovative blood pressure measurements yield information not reflected by sitting measurements. Hypertension 8:252–257

Light K, Sherwood A, Obrist P, James S, Strogatz D, Willis P (1986) Biobehavioral aspects of hypertension in blacks: current findings. Symposium conducted at the meeting of the American Psychological Association, Washington, DC

Long J, Lynch J, Machinan N, Thomas S, Malinow K (1982) The effect of status on blood pressure during verbal communication. J Behav Med 5:165–172

Llabre MM, Ironson GH, Spitzer SB, Gellman MD, Weidler DJ, Schneiderman N (1988) How many blood pressure measurements are enough? An application of generalizability theory to the study of blood pressure reliability. Psychophysiology 25:97–106

Lynch J (1985) The language of the heart. Basic Books, New York

Lynch JJ, Long JM, Thomas SA, Malinow KL, Katcher AH (1981) The effects of talking on the blood pressure of hypertensive and normotensive individual. Psychol Med 43:25–33

Perloff D, Sokolow M, Cowan R (1983) The prognostic value of ambulatory blood pressures. JAMA 249:2793–2798

Pickering T, James G, Boddie C, Harshfield G, Blank S, Laragh J (1988) How common is white coat hypertension? JAMA 259:225–228

Pickering TG (1988) The study of blood pressure in everyday life. In: Elbert T, Langosch A, Steptoe A, Vaitl D (eds) Behavioral medicine in cardiovascular disorders. Wiley, New York

Pickering TG, Harshfield GA, Kleinert HD, Blank S, Laragh JH (1982) Blood pressure during normal daily activities, sleep and exercise. Comparison of values in normal and hypertensive subjects. JAMA 247:992–996

Pickering TG, Harshfield GA, Devereux RB, Laragh JH (1985) What is the role of ambulatory blood pressure monitoring in the management of hypertensive patients? Hypertension 7:171–177

Roberts J, Rowland M (1981) Vital and health statistics (Series II, No. 221). Hypertension in adults 25–74 years of age: United States, 1971–1975 (DHEW Publication No. PHS 81-1671). U.S. Government Printing Offfice, Washington, DC

Rose R, Jenkins C, Hurst M (1978) Air traffic controller health change study. Boston University School of Medicine

Rosner B, Polk BF (1979) The implications of blood pressure variability for clinical and screening purposes. J Chronic Dis 32:451–461

Schneiderman N, Ironson GH, McCabe P (1987) Physiology of behavior and blood pressure regulation in humans. In: Julins S, Bassett DR (eds) Handbook of hypertension: behavioral factors in hypertension, vol 9. Elsevier, New York

Sokolow M, Werdegar D, Kain H, Hinman A (1966) Relationships between level of blood pressure measured casually and by portable recorder and severity of complications in essential hypertension. Circulation 34:279–298

Sokolow M, Werdegar D, Perloff D, Cowan R, Brenenstuhl H (1970) Preliminary studies relating recorded blood pressures to daily life events in patients with essential hypertension. Biblio Psychia 144:164–189

Southard DR, Coates TJ, Kolodner K, Parter C, Padgett NE, Kennedy HL (1986) Relationship between mood and blood pressure in the natural environment: an adolescent population. Health Psy 5:469–480

Spitzer SB, Llabre MM, Ironson GH, Gellman MD, Schneiderman N (1992) The influence of social situations on ambulatory blood pressure in mild-moderate hypertensives and normotensives. Psychosom Med 54:79–86

Van Egeren LF, Madarasmi S (1988) A computer-assisted diary (CAD) for ambulatory blood pressure monitoring. Am J Hyper 1:179S–185S

White WB (1986) Assessment of patients with office hypertension by 24-hour noninvasive ambulatory blood pressure monitoring. Arch Intern Med 146:2196–2199

Young MA, Rowland DB, Sta Vard TH, Watson RDS, Littler WA (1983) Effect of environment on blood pressure: Home versus hospital. Br Med J 286:1235–1236

Factors Associated with Differences in the Diurnal Variation of Blood Pressure in Humans

G. A. Harshfield

Diurnal Variation of Blood Pressure

Previous studies using both invasive and noninvasive ambulatory blood pressure (ABP) recorders have demonstrated a diurnal rhythm of BP, with higher BP levels during waking hours and lower ones during sleep [1, 2]. The diurnal rhythm of BP has been described in both hypertensive [3–8] and normotensive [9–11] populations, with hypertensives having higher levels but similar patterns of BP as normotensives. Older persons also have higher levels but similar patterns of BP as young persons [12–14], and men have higher levels but similar patterns to women [13–15].

The factor(s) responsible for ABP patterns has yet to be identified. One hypothesis is that the level and changes in BP throughout the 24 h are regulated by the sympathetic nervous system (SNS) in response to changes in physical and psychological demands. Four lines of research support this hypothesis. First, Littler and his colleagues [16] examined ABP patterns adjusted for the time of awakening and found that BP increases at this time. Second, Rowlands and colleagues [17] studied the ABP patterns of six hypertensive patients on 2 consecutive days who were matched for activity level. They found similar patterns across the 2 days, with similar changes in response to periods of activity and inactivity.

The third series of studies in support of the SNS hypothesis are the studies by our group at Cornell [5, 11]. We examined differences in BP between the clinic, work, and home environments. BP was higher in the clinic and at work, periods associated with stress, with a decline in BP from work to home and a further decline from home to sleep. However, not all individuals displayed this pattern. In another study we found that 34% of essential hypertensive patients had their highest BP levels in the clinic, 56% at work, and 8% at home [18]. We have also compared the effects of time of day versus 21 different activities on the changes in BP from the clinic BP over the course of 24 h [19]. Time of day accounted for 33% of the variance of the changes in BP while activity accounted for 40%. The combination of time and activity accounted for only an additional 1% of the variance over and above activity alone. In another study, we examined differences in BP associated with changes in emotional states, including happiness, anger, and

Schmidt/Engel/Blümchen (Eds.)
Temporal Variations of the Cardiovascular System
© Springer-Verlag Berlin Heidelberg 1992

anxiety [20]. Each of the states was associated with significant increases in BP, with similar and higher levels during periods of anxiety and anger relative to periods of happiness.

The fourth line of research in support of the SNS hypothesis comes from studies which have examined ABP patterns in shift workers. In one study, Sundberg [21] monitored the ABP patterns of seven shift workers on 3 consecutive days as they changed from a day shift to a night shift. These subjects had a normal ABP pattern on the 1st day but a totally reversed pattern by the 3rd day, with higher BP levels at night during the work hours. A second study by Baumgart [22] on 15 shift workers employed a similar methodology and found similar results, with comparable 24-h averages and similar levels of work and sleep BP on the 2 days, despite the shift change. A third study by Chau also employing this methodology in 15 subjects also found comparable results [23].

The study by Chau [23] also provided evidence for an internal diurnal rhythm of BP independent of activity. Chau and colleagues isolated periods of high and low BP independent of periods of work and rest and found that BP during the low-pressure span was lower when the subjects worked in the afternoon relative to the other two shifts. The work of Raftery and colleagues provides the major source of support for this hypothesis [2]. According to these investigators, BP reaches a peak during midmorning, with a second peak in the early evening and a nadir at 03:00 hours [4]. BP then rises from the nadir until the time before awakening. They have demonstrated this pattern in both hypertensive and normotensive individuals. In addition, they found that the pattern is similar during an active day and a day of bedrest [24]. Furthermore, these investigators demonstrated that antihypertensive therapy reduces the level of BP throughout the 24 h but does not influence the rhythm per se [4]. Finally, although it was intially suggested that the diurnal rhythm was an artifact of the examination of grouped data, in contrast to the data by Littler and colleagues, reanalysis of the data based on the time of awakening did not alter the results [2].

Diurnal Rhythms in Clinical Populations

The diurnal rhythm of BP is different in a number of clinical populations with different etiologies. These are summarized in Table 1. Littler and Honour [25] compared the ABP patterns of three patients before and after the removal of a pheochromocytoma. Prior to the removal of the pheochromocytoma, in two of the three cases BP did not fall at night, and in the third case the nocturnal decline in BP was small. After removal of the pheochromocytoma, two patients had normal nocturnal BP, while that of a third remained elevated at night. However, these results were not confirmed in a study by Imai et al. [26], on eight patients with a pheochromocytoma. These patients had similar nocturnal declines in BP as patients with untreated essential hypertension. Redman et al. [27] examined BP changes in three patients with severe preeclampsia, four with mild uncomplicated hypertension, and six who were primigravid. BP levels were recorded in the hospital at 10-min intervals with an arteriosonde and hourly intervals calculated. The preeclamptic patients increased their BP between the hours of midnight and 04:00 hours relative to levels recorded between noon and 18:00 hours, while the

Table 1. Studies reporting clinical conditions associated with blunted nocturnal decline of blood pressure

Diagnosis/condition	BP	Reference
Pheochromocytoma ($n = 4$)		
Presurgery	↑	[25]
Postsurgery	↓	[25]
Pheochromocytoma ($n = 8$)	↓	[26]
Preeclampsia ($n = 10$)	↑	[27]
Uncomplicated hypertension ($n = 4$)	↓	[27]
Primigravida ($n = 6$)	↓	[27]
Autonomic failure ($n = 6$)	↑	[28]
Elderly		
without complications ($n = 14$)	↓	[29]
with complications ($n = 7$)	↑	[29]
Cardiac transplantation ($n = 55$)	↑	[30]
Diabetes with neuropathy ($n = 10$)	↑	[30]
Secondary hypertension ($n = 20$); variety of diagnosis combined)	↑	[31, 32]
Primary aldosteronism ($n = 11$)	↑	[33]
Primary aldosteronism postsurgery	↓	[33]
Renovascular hypertension ($n = 15$)	↓	[33]
Renovascular hypertension postsurgery	↓	[33]
Cushing's syndrome ($n = 15$)	↑	[34]
Primary aldosteronism ($n = 13$)	↓	[34]

other patients all had lower levels at night relative to the day. Mann et al. [28] examined the ABP patterns of six patients with autonomic failure. These patients had the highest BP during the night and the lowest in the morning hours. In addition, confinement to bedrest did not alter this pattern in four subjects who continued to wear the recorder for an additional 24 h. Kobrin et al. [29] performed ABP recordings in 21 elderly patients with established hypertension. The authors observed two different patterns, with 14 of the patients having significant drops in BP from awake to asleep states. Systolic BP (SBP) of the other seven subjects increased to clinic levels during sleep, and diastolic BP (DBP) remained at awake levels. These seven subjects were also characterized by a greater degree of cardiovascular complications relative to the patients who had significant decreases in BP at night, including atherosclerotic impairment. Reeves et al. [30] compared the ABP patterns of patients who underwent heart transplantation with patterns of diabetic and hypertensive patients. Almost half of the heart transplant patients had higher BP levels at night than during the day, while all of the hypertensive patients had a 10 % decline in BP. The average decrease in BP at night was similar for the heart transplant and diabetic patients. Baumgart and colleagues [31, 32] measured ABP patterns in 80 patients with a variety of forms of secondary hypertension and in 26 normotensive patients with chronic renal disease. Both of these grups displayed reduced variability in BP, characterized primarily by a diminished drop in BP at night. Tanaka et al. [33] examined the ABP patterns of 11 subjects with primary aldosteronism and found a rise in BP

Table 2. Additional PB load imposed by blunted nocturnal decline in blood pressure

Duration			Years at Age		
Hours/day		*Days/year*	*20 years*	*40 years*	*60 years*
4	=	61	=	3.3	6.6	9.9
6	=	91	=	5.0	10.0	15.0
8	=	122	=	6.6	13.2	19.8

during the late evening hours. The adrenal adenoma was extirpated in six of these subjects, which resulted in a flattening out of the ABP pattern. These investigators also examined the rhythms of 15 patients with renovascular hypertension. These patients had a normal ABP pattern, which was not altered in eight patients who received surgical treatment. Finally, Imai et al. [34] examined the ABP patterns of patients with primary aldosteronism and Cushing's syndrome. These investigators did not find an altered BP pattern in patients with primary aldosteronism; however, patients with Cushing's syndrome did not have a nocturnal decline in BP.

Blunted Nocturnal Decline in BP in Healthy Populations

O'Brien [35] pointed out that the identification of healthy individuals or populations who do not have a normal decline in BP at night may be particularly important because it exposes them to additional BP load over the course of the 24 h. This is demonstrated in Table 2, which compares the additional strain resulting from 4, 6, or 8 h of awake levels of BP at night by ages 20, 40, and 60. For example, an individual who is exposed to an additional 4 h of awake levels of BP each night is exposed to an additional 61 days per year, which results in an additional 3.3 years by age 20. In comparison, an individual who is exposed to an additional 8 h each night is exposed to an additional 122 days per year, which results in an additional 19.8 years by age 60!

Racial Differences in ABP Patterns

We have conducted a series of studies over the past several years to identify healthy individuals who have a blunted nocturnal declines in BP and to identify the factors associated with this pattern. Our major finding to date has been the discovery of racial differences in ABP patterns, with blacks showing a blunted nocturnal decline in BP. Our first study [13] examined the ABP patterns of 60 healthy, normotensive black adults. As shown in the upper section of Fig. 1, SBP and DBP remained at awake levels well into the nighttime hours, not dropping until about 02:00 hours, well after the subjects went to sleep. A further examination of this pattern by location/activity in the lower section of Fig. 1 showed a significantly different pattern than we previously observed in white subjects [5, 11]. Although BP declined from work to home, and from home to sleep, these declines were not significant. These results were the first to our knowledge to demonstrate a blunted

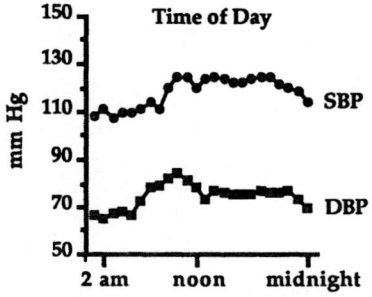

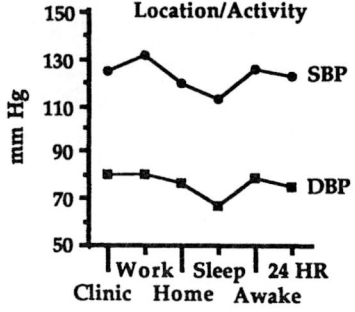

Fig. 1. Systolic (*SBP*) and diastolic (*DBP*) blood pressure of black adults as a function of time and location/activity

nocturnal decline in BP in a healthy population, but one which is at a high risk for the development of hypertension as well as cardiovascular and renal disease [36].

Our second study extended these findings to a an adolescent population [37]. The ABP recordings of a biracial sample of healthy, normotensive male and female adolescent (9–18 years of age) were divided into periods of awake and asleep. As shown in the upper section of Fig. 2, black and white children had similar BP levels while awake, with males having higher levels of SBP and comparable levels of DBP relative to females. The patterns while the children were asleep, however, were quite different. As shown in the lower section of Fig. 2, black males had higher levels of SBP than white males, white females, or black females. In addition, black adolescents as a group had higher levels of DBP at night than white adolescents.

Our results on racial differences in ABP patterns have now been confirmed in preliminary studies from other laboratories. These studies are summarized in Table 3. Murphy [38] compared the ABP patterns of 44 black and 37 white adults under evaluation for borderline essential hypertension. The average daytime BP levels of the black and white adults were equivalent, but the black adults had a significantly smaller decline in BP during sleep. Murphy also reported that the nighttime BP in blacks was associated with greater left ventricular hypertrophy [39]. In a another study, James examined racial differences in ABP patterns in 27 black and 83 white women [40]. Despite similar levels of awake BP, the black women had higher levels BP at night.

Several studies, however, have not reported racial differences in ABP patterns. These studies are also summarized in Table 3. The common denominator of these

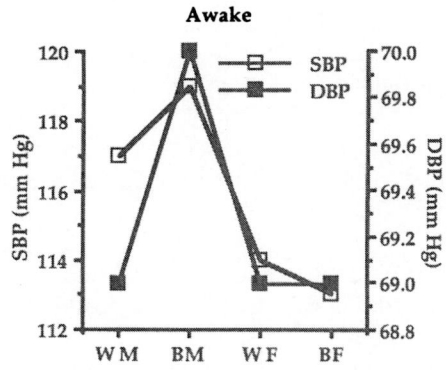

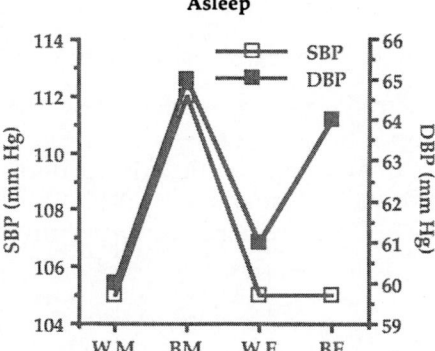

Fig. 2. Systolic (*SBP*) and diastolic (*DBP*) blood pressure of white male (*WM*), black male (*BM*), white female (*WF*), and black female (*BF*) adolescents while awake and asleep

Table 3. Studies examining racial differencies in the decline in blood pressure at night

Subject characteristics	BP	Reference
American normotensive black adults ($n = 60$)	↑	[13]
American black adolescents ($n = 107$)	↑	[37]
American white adolescents ($n = 92$)	↓	[37]
American black adult ($n = 44$)	↑	[38]
White hypertensive adults ($n = 37$)	↓	[38]
American black women ($n = 27]$	↑	[40]
American white women ($n = 83$)	↓	[40]
Jamacian blacks in England ($n = 16$)	↓	[41]
British white hypertensives ($n = 16$)	↓	[41]
African blacks in Africa ($n = 18$)	↓	[42]
American blacks in America ($n = 18$)	↑	[42]
Normotensive African born blacks in America ($n = 21]$	↓	[43]
Normotensive Barbadian blacks in Barbados ($n = 40$)	↓	[44]

studies is the measurement of ABP patterns in blacks who are not American. The first study by Rowlands and his colleagues [41] found similar ABP patterns in 16 British white adults and 16 Jamaican-born black adults living in the United Kingdom. The second study by Murphy [42] compared the ABP patterns of 18 American blacks and 18 African blacks. The American blacks had a blunted nocturnal decline in BP while the African blacks had a normal nocturnal decline in BP. The third and fourth studies were by Grim's group, examining ABP patterns in 21 normotensive blacks of African origin living in America [43] and 40 normotensive blacks in Barbados [44]. Both of these groups had normal nocturnal declines in BP. Based on the results of these studies, it is reasonable to hypothesize that black Americans either inherit some factor or are exposed to some environmental factor which results in a blunted nocturnal decline in BP, perhaps placing then at a greater risk for the development of hypertension [45].

Electrolyte Intake and Racial Differences in ABP Patterns

Electrolyte intake, as reflected by 24-h urinary excretions, is one factor which we have found to be associated with racial differences in ABP patterns [46]. In a recent study we compared the ABP patterns of black and white adolescents based on their sodium excretion ($U_{Na}V$), potassium excretion (U_KV), and the ratio of $U_{Na}V$ to U_KV. ABP patterns were again divided into those of awake and asleep periods.

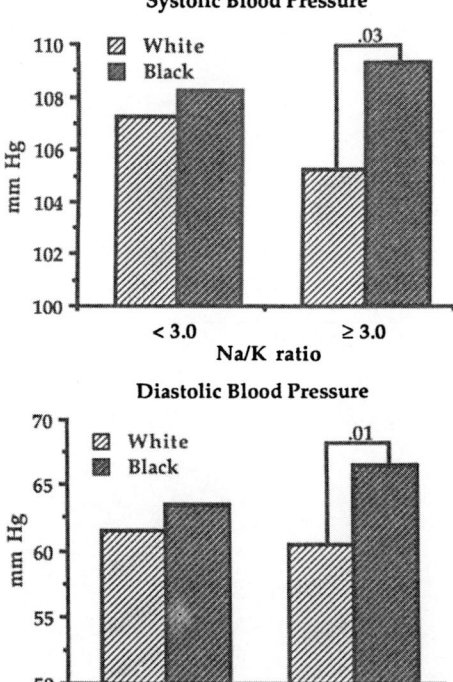

Fig. 3. Systolic and diastolic blood pressure of white and black adolescents as a function of the ratio of sodium to potassium excretion

Black and white adolescents with a $U_{Na}V$ under 150 mEq/24 h had similar SBP as white adolescents both while awake and while asleep. However, black adolescents with a $U_{Na}V$ of at least 150 mEq/24 h had higher SBP than white adolescents both while awake and while asleep, and higher DBP while asleep. Black and white adolescents with a U_KV of at least 30 mEq/24 h had similar SBP and DBP both while awake and while asleep. However, black adolescents with a U_KV under 30 mEq/24 h had higher SBP and DBP than white adolescents while asleep, despite similar levels of BP while awake. Finally, black and white adolescents had similar levels of awake BP independent of the ratio of $U_{Na}V$ to U_KV. Sleep BP provided a very different picture. As shown in Fig. 3, black and white adolescents with a ratio of $U_{Na}V$ to U_KV under 3.0 had similar levels of both SBP and DBP as white adolescents. However, black adolescents with a $U_{Na}V$ to U_KV ratio of at least 3.0 had higher SBP and DBP than white adolescents with similar ratios.

Renin-Angiotensin-Aldosterone System and ABP Patterns

The renin-angiotensin-aldosterone system is a another factor which is related to differences in ABP patterns [47]. We developed a renin-sodium nomogram for normotensive children and adolescents and categorized the children as low, intermediate, or high, based on the nomogram. We then compared the casual BP and ABP patterns of subjects classified by the nomogram. As shown in Fig. 4, the

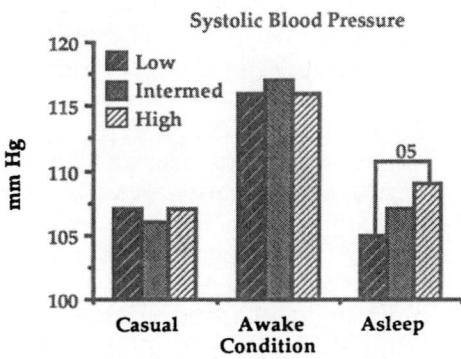

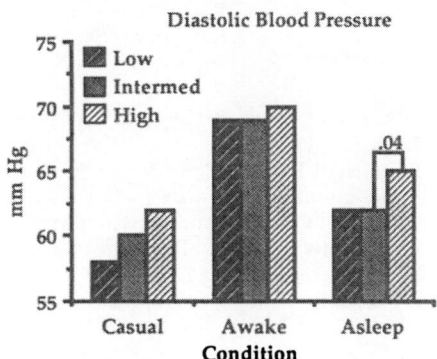

Fig. 4. Systolic and diastolic blood pressures of adolescents characterized by low, intermediate, and high plasma renin activity referenced to sodium excretion

three groups had comparable levels of casual and awake BP. High-renin subjects, however, had a smaller decline in SBP with sleep than low-renin subjects, and higher DBP during sleep than intermediate-renin subjects. In addition, the high-renin subjects also had greater variability in DBP during sleep than either low-renin or intermediate-renin subjects.

Summary and Conclusions

In summary, a diurnal rhythm of BP has been identified which follows the wake/sleep cycle, with higher BP levels during the day and lower levels at night. However, several clinical populations have been identified who have different ABP patterns. These patients have either elevated or comparable levels of BP at night relative to BP during the day. In addition, recent studies from our laboratory and others have identified two other groups with blunted nocturnal declines in BP. The first group is black Americans, in whom the blunted nocturnal decline is related to the level of electrolyte intake. The second group is normotensive adolescents with high levels of plasma renin activity relative to sodium intake.

What are the underlying mechanisms responsible for the diurnal rhythm of BP? The answer to this question is as varied and complex as the question of BP regulation itself. The studies of clinical populations with different patterns indicate that disturbances in SNS activity, hormonal function, and volume regulation can all lead to altered diurnal patterns. The studies on normotensive and uncomplicated essential hypertensive subjects indicate that ABP patterns also differ in healthy populations based on the long-term mechanism(s) which are regulating their BP. Furthermore, these studies demonstrate that both diet and stress can influence the pattern.

Further research is needed to continue to identify factors associated with differences in ABP patterns and to determine the clinical significance of different patterns. In addition, research is needed to examine concomitant changes in BP and its regulatory systems to directly determine the mechanisms responsible for changes over extended periods, such as while at work and during sleep. Finally, the functioning of these systems need to be compared across groups who are characterized by different ABP patterns.

References

1. Bevan AT, Honor AJ, Stott F (1969) Direct arterial pressure reading in unrestricted man. Clin Sci 36:329–344
2. Raftery EB (1990) The direct intra-arterial method for ambulatory blood pressure recording: present status and future applications. In: Meyer-Sabellek W, Anlauf M, Gotzen R, Steinfeld L (eds) Blood pressure measurements: new techniques in automatic and 24-hour indirect monitoring. Steinkopff, Darmstadt, pp 111–119
3. Littler WA, Honour AJ, Sleight P, Stott FD (1972) Continuous recording of direct arterial pressure and electrocardiogram in unrestricted man. Br Med J 3:76–78
4. Millar-Craig MW, Mann S, Balasubramanian V, Raftery EB (1978) Blood pressure circadian rhythm in essential hypertension. Clin Sci Mol Med 55:391 s–393 s

5. Harshfield GA, Pickering TG, Kleinert HD, Blank S, Laragh JH (1982) Situational variations of blood pressure in ambulatory hypertensive patients. Psychosom Med 44:237–245

6. Mancia G, Parati G, Pomidossi G, DiRienzo M (1985) Validity and usefulness of non-invasive ambulatory blood pressure monitoring. J Hypertens 3 [Suppl 2]: S 5–S 11

7. Palatini P, Sperti G, Mormino P, Di Marco A, Bastanzetti M, Pessina AC (1985) Reliability of indirect blood pressure monitoring for the evaluation of hypertension. Clin Exp Hypertens [A] 7 (2, 3): 437–443

8. Parati G, Pomidossi G, Casadei R, Malsapina D, Colombo A, Ravogli A, Guiseppe M (1985) Ambulatory blood pressure monitoring does not interfere with the hemodynamic effects of sleep. J Hypertens 3 [Suppl 2]: S 107–S 109

9. Drayer JIM, Weber MA, Hoeger WJ (1985) Whole-day monitoring in ambulatory normotensive men. Arch Intern Med 145:271–274

10. Weber MA, Drayer JIM, Nakamura DK, Wyle F (1984) The circadian blood pressure pattern in ambulatory normal subjects. Am J Cardiol 54:115–119

11. Pickering TG, Harshfield GA, Kleinert HD, Blank S, Laragh JH (1982) Comparisons of blood pressure during normal daily activities, sleep, and exercise in normal and hypertensive subjects. JAMA 247:992–996

12. Drayer JIM, Weber MA, DeYoung JL, Wyle FA (1982) Circadian blood pressure patterns in ambulatory hypertensive patients. Am J Med 73:493–499

13. Harshfield GA, Hwang C, Grim CE (1990) Circadian variation of blood pressure in blacks: influence of age, gender and activity. J Hum Hypertens 4:43–47

14. De Guademaris R, Mallion JM, Battistella P, Battistella B, Siche JP, Blatier JF, Francois M (1987) Ambulatory blood pressure and variability by age and sex in 200 normotensive subjects: reference population values. J Hypertens 5 [Suppl]: S 429–S 430

15. James GD, Yee LS, Harshfield GA, Pickering TG (1988) Sex differences in factors affecting daily variation of blood pressure. Soc. Sci Med 26(10):1019–1023

16. Floras JS, Jones V, Johnston JA, Brooks DE, Hassan MO, Sleight P (1978) Arousal and the circadian rhythm of blood pressure. Clin Sci Mol Med 55:395 s–397 s

17. Rowlands DB, Stallard TJ, Watson RDS, Littler WA (1980) The influence of physical activity on arterial pressure during ambulatory recordings in man. Clin Sci 58:115–117

18. Harshfield GA, Pickering TG, Blank SG, Laragh JH (1986) How well do casual blood pressures reflect ambulatory blood pressures? In: Germano G (ed) Blood pressure recording in the clinical management of hypertension. Pozzi, Rome, pp 50–54

19. Clark LA, Denby L, Pregibon D, Harshfield GA, Pickering TG, Blank S, Laragh JH (1987) The effects of activity and time of day on the diurnal variations of blood pressure. J Chronic Dis 40:671–681

20. James GD, Yee LS, Harshfield GA, Blank SG, Pickering TG (1986) The influence of happiness, anger, and anxiety on the blood pressure of borderline hypertensive. Psychosom Med 48(7):502–508

21. Sundberg S, Kohvakka A, Gordin A (1988) Rapid reversal of circadian blood pressure rhythm in shift workers. J Hypertens 6:393–396

22. Baumgart P, Walger P, Fuchs G, Dorst KG, Vetter H, Rahn KH (1989) Twenty-four-hour blood pressure is not dependent on endogenous circadian rhythm. J Hypertens 7:331–334

23. Chau NP, Mallion JM, Gaudemaris Rd, Ruche E, Siche JP, Pelen O, Mathern G (1989) Twenty-four-hour ambulatory blood pressure in shift workers. Circulation 80:341–347

24. Mann S, Millar-Craig MW, Melville DI, Balasubrqamanian V, Raftery EB (1979) Physical activity and the circadian rhythm of blood pressure. Clin Sci 57:291 s–294 s

25. Littler WA, Honour AJ (1974) Direct arterial pressure, heart rate, and electrocardiogram in unrestricted patients before and after removal of a phaeochromocyoma. Q J Med 43:441–449

26. Imai Y, Abe K, Miura Y, Nihei M, Sasaki S, Minami N, Munaka M, Taira N, Sekino H, Yamakoshi K, Yoshinaga K (1988) Hypertensive episodes and circadian fluctuations of blood pressure in patients with phaeochromocytoma: studies by longterm blood pressure monitoring based on a volume-oscillometric method. J Hypertens 6:9–15

27. Redman CWG, Beilin LJ, Bonnar J (1976) Reversed diurnal blood pressure rhythm in hypertensive pregnancies. Clin Sci Mol Med 51:687 s–689 s

28. Mann S, Altman DG, Raftery EB, Bannister R (1983) Circadian variation of blood pressure in autonomic failure. Circulation 68:477–483
29. Kobrin I, Oigman W, Kumar A, Ventura HO, Messerli FH, Frohlich ED, Dunn FG (1984) Diurnal variation of blood pressure in elderly patients with essential hypertension. J Am Geriatr Soc 32:896–899
30. Reeves RA, Shapiro AP, Thompson ME, Johnson AM (1986) Loss of nocturnal decline in blood pressure after cardiac transplantation. Circulation 73:401–408
31. Hany S, Baumgart P, Frielingsdorf J, Vetter H, Vetter W (1987) Circadian blood pressure variability in secondary and essential hypertension. J Hypertens 5 [Suppl]: S 487–S 489
32. Baumgart P, Walger P, Dorst KG, Eiff Mv, Rahn KH, Vetter H: Can secondary hypertension be identified by twenty-four-hour ambulatory pressure monitoring? J Hypertens [Suppl 3]: S 25–S 28
33. Tanaka T, Natsume T, Shibata H, Nozawa K, Kojima S, Tsuchiya M, Ashida T, Ikeda M (1983) Circadian rhythm of blood pressure in primary aldosteronism and renovascular hypertension: analysis by the cosinor method. Jpn Circ J 47:788–794
34. Imai Y, Abe K, Sasaki S, Minami N, Nihei M, Munakata M, Murakami O, Matsue K, Sekino H, Miura Y, Yoshinga K (1988) Altered circadian blood pressure rhythm in patients with Cushing's syndrome. Hypertension 12:11–19
35. Obrien E, Sheridan J, O'Malley K (1988) Dippers and non-dippers. Lancet ii:397
36. United States Department of Health and Human Services (1986) Report of the Secretary's Task Force on Black and Minority Health IV: cardiovascular and cerebrovascular disease (part 1)
37. Harshfield GA, Alpert BS, Willey ES, Somes GW, Murphy JK, Dupaul LM (1989) Race and gender influence ambulatory blood pressure patterns of adolescents. Hypertension 14:598–603
38. Murphy MB, Nelson KS, Elliott WJ (1988) Racial differences in diurnal blood pressure profile. Am J Hypertens 1 (A):55
39. Murphy MB, Lang RL, Nelson KS, Bednarz J, Elliott WJ (1990) Diurnal blood pressure differences are associated with inter-racial differences in cardiac hypertrophy. J Hum Hypertens 4:194
40. James GD (1990) The independent effects of race and stress on the diurnal variation of blood pressure in women. Am J Hypertens 3 (5, 2):33 A
41. Rowlands DB, DeGiovanni J, McLeay RAB, Watson RDS, Stallard TJ, Littler WA (1982) Cardiovascular responses in black and white hypertensives. Hypertension 4:817–820
42. Murphy MB, Tiegar S, Sareli P, Neumann A, Fumo MA, Borow KM, Lang RM (1990) Circadian variation in blood pressure in African blacks and American blacks. Am J Hypertens 3 (2):37 A
43. Egbunike AC, Wilson TW, Grim CE (1990) 24 hour blood pressure patterns of African born blacks living in US differ from US born blacks. [Procedings of the International Society of Hypertension in Blacks] Long Beach, p 20
44. Wilson TW, Grim CM, Wilson DM, Garrett SS, Nicholson GD, Fraser HS, Hassel TA, Grim CE (1990) Barbadian blacks and US blacks differ in 24 hour blood pressure patterns. [Procedings of the International Society of Hypertension in Blacks] Long Beach, p 65
45. Grim CE, Wilson TW, Nicholson GD, Hassell TA, Fraser HS, Grim CE, Wilson DM (1990) Blood pressure in blacks: twin studies in Barbados. Hypertension 15:803–809
46. Harshfield GA, Alpert BS, Pulliam DA, Willey ES, Somes GW, Stapleton BF (1991) Sodium, potassium excretion and racial differences in nocturnal blood pressure (to be published)
47. Harshfield GA, Pulliam DA, Alpert BS, Stapleton FB, Willey ES, Somes GW (1991) Renin-sodium profiles influence ambulatory blood pressure patterns in children and adolescents. Pediat (in press)

Effects of Behavioral Rhythms on Blood Pressure Rhythms

L. F. Van Egeren

Introduction

The walls that once separated the laboratory from "real life" are being pierced by new noninvasive devices for monitoring blood pressure while people go about their normal daily routine. Many investigations of the sources of blood pressure variability which were once impossible have recently become feasible. Blood pressure has a predictable daily rhythm. After reaching a nadir around 0200 or 0300 h, it rises slowly during the remainder of the sleep period and more markedly when the person awakens and begins to move about [1, 2]. Nested like Chinese boxes inside the larger diurnal rhythm, shorter cycles – 3-s respiratory waves, 10-s Mayer waves, and perhaps 90-min ultradian waves – may contribute additional sources of blood pressure variability [3].

Behavior also has a predictable daily rhythm. Alternating cycles of sleep and wakefulness, hunger and satiety, work and play, interaction and solitude, and effort and rest create a definite temporal order or "schedule", which imposes its demands on the circulatory system for blood flow to active tissues. When the demands cannot be met by shifting blood from inactive tissues, cardiac output must increase, usually accompanied by a rise in blood pressure.

Behavior-Pressure Integration

To what extent is the blood pressure schedule imposed by the behavioral schedule? The answer to this question will likely vary according to whether the person is emotional or unemotional, inwardly attentive (introversive) or outwardly attentive (extraversive), or physically fit or unfit. When attention is directed inward, skeletal muscle appears to vasodilate, whereas it vasoconstricts when it is directed outward [4]. During emotion and exercise, commands from the central nervous system can cause the baroreflex to significantly alter its regulation of blood pressure [5].

To further complicate matters, the behavior-pressure coupling is affected by influences that radiate outward from medullary cardiomotor centers to the neocortex and the limbic system via the ascending reticular system (reviewed

Schmidt/Engel/Blümchen (Eds.)
Temporal Variations of the Cardiovascular System
© Springer-Verlag Berlin Heidelberg 1992

briefly below). Via this "centrifugal" route, changes in pressure can influence behavior. This pressure-behavior pathway is worth noting, even though the present focus is on "centripetal" effects, in which behavior influences pressure.

Voluntary, goal-directed behaviors integrate mental (neocortical), emotional (limbic), and physical (extrapyramidal) aspects of motor activity into a unified pattern. It is difficult to determine how these separate aspects of behavior affect blood pressure. The present focus will be the integrated behavior itself (labeled "activity"), its physical dimension (labeled "motility"), and its emotional dimension (limited to a measure of "stress"). Motility will be measured as gross body movement. It represents the level or *intensity* of behavior. The person's specific "activity" such as walking, talking, or driving a car represents the type or *direction* of behavior, in contrast to its intensity. These two aspects of behavior, intensity and direction, overlap, but also are distinguishable. A person may perform an activity at different levels of pace, movement, and energy cost. Conversely, the same amount of energy and movement may be invested in radically different types of behavior.

Some Questions

Is the diurnal rhythm in blood pressure imposed *externally* by the schedule of routine activities, or *internally* by a biological clock? Of what importance to the scheduling of blood pressure is the physical aspect of behavior, by contrast to its mental and emotional aspects? In addition to these, there are a number of subsidiary questions. How much variation in blood pressure remains after removing that due to behavior? How does the relationship of behavior to blood pressure vary with time of day? How much do people differ in the dependency of blood pressure on activity?

Recent Past Studies

Effects of Pressure on Behavior

That visceral processes, including functions of the heart, influence human emotion and behavior is an ancient idea woven into the traditional mythology and folklore of many cultures. Do scientific data provide any support for this traditional view? Some findings suggest that changes in arterial pressure, operating through baroreceptor reflexes, can affect behavior directly. Stimulation of the carotid sinus nerve can suppress cerebral activation and psychomotor performance [6]. When sufficiently intense, such stimulation can even put an animal to sleep [7]. Pressure-induced cerebral and behavioral suppression appears to affect humans as well as animals. Patients with hypertension sometimes suffer subtle but measurable mental and psychomotor impairments. Such impairments have been reversed by drugs which lower blood pressure without passing through the blood-brain barrier to influence brain function directly [8].

Effects of Behavior on Pressure

Simultaneous recordings of pressure and behavior have revealed their close connection in everyday life [3, 9, 10]. A wide range of behaviors have been investigated such as walking, talking, driving a car, attending meetings, desk work, household chores, watching television, relaxing, reading, eating, drinking caffeinated or alcoholic beverages, sexual intercourse, micturation, defecation, and smoking cigarettes. All these activities have a measurable effect on arterial pressure. Measured against sleep, the size of the effect varies from 5–7 mm Hg for relaxation, 10–15 mm Hg for watching television, desk work, and reading, and 20–30 mm Hg for diving a car and walking, to even greater pressure elevations for vigorous exercise and sexual intercourse [11]. The sleep-wakefulness cycle has a marked predictable effect on the blood pressure in healthy subjects, typically falling 15–20 mm Hg at night and rising a comparable amount in the morning, with the rise beginning during the last half of the sleep period [12].

Personal traits and the workplace environment may alter the behavioral effects on blood pressure. Twenty-four hour monitoring has produced different pressure and heart rate results for hostile-impatient Type A people, compared with more relaxed Type B people. Systolic pressures were found to be more variable during sleep, but less variable during work [13], while diastolic pressures were more variable during the 24-h period and elevated while walking, talking, and drinking either an alcoholic or a caffeinated beverage [14]. Higher heart rates were found at home and at work [15].

High levels of job strain, defined as the combination of high psychological demand and low decision latitude, has been linked to elevated workplace diastolic pressure and greater left ventricular cardiac mass [16]. We recently observed significantly higher systolic pressures and heart rates at the workplace in university employees who had a high level of job strain than in employees who had a low level.

What portion of 24-h blood pressure variance can be attributed to changes in activity during the course of an ordinary day? To obtain an answer for hypertension patients, Clark et al. [17] regressed ambulatory pressures on 15 everyday activities (most of those listed above, plus sleep). After covariance adjustment for the blood pressure reading in the clinic, the activities accounted for 41% of systolic and 36% of diastolic variance. We monitored a similar set of 16 activities and blood pressure, but in normotensive subjects [18]. To sharpen the focus on the acute effects of transient activities, intersubject variance was more completely removed by adjusting individual readings for the person's average pressure during the entire 24-h period. The 16 activities accounted for 21% of systolic variance. Roughly one-fifth of the waxing and waning of systolic pressure about the 24-h average could be attributed to the person's specific activity at the time of the reading.

Gross Body Motility

New electronic sensors for measuring gross body movement around the clock provide moment-by-moment quantitative estimates of the intensity of a person's behavioral activity that are related to energy cost [19]. The devices, which are about the size of a wrist watch, do not interfere with the person's normal routine and require little cooperation by the subject. The devices record dynamic (isotonic), not static (isometric), aspects of behavior. For many research purposes, this limitation is not critical when subjects do little lifting or pushing of heavy objects.

Gross human motion is difficult to define and quantify. The mechanics of displacement and rotation of the body are complex, and different motion sensors capture this information with varying degrees of success [20]. People differ greatly in motility, even while performing the same task [21]. To be useful, motility monitors must be capable of distinguishing common everyday activities, have low energy costs, and be insensitive to electrical noise over a wide range of home and work environments. The best motility monitors available today incorporate significant advances in sensor design over earlier mechanical recorders.

Electronic motility sensors have been used to study manic-depressive adults [22], hyperactive children [23], sleep disorders [24], hypnotic [25] and antidepressant [22] drugs, patients recovering from myocardial infarction [26], and motion-and-temperature circadian or diurnal rhythms [27]. We recently reported similar 24-h rhythms in body motility and blood pressure [28].

Our Current Studies

The gross body motility, 16 specific activities, and the blood pressure of healthy normotensive university employees (administrators, managers, technicians, and secretaries) were monitored on 1 work day (37 subjects) or on 2 work days a month apart (45 subjects). The age range was 20–64 years; 44 employees were women. A SpaceLabs 90202 monitor recorded the employee's blood pressure every 30 min during the day (0600–0000 hours) and every 60 min during the night (0000–0600 hours). The procedure for preparing subjects, checking the accuracy of the recorder, and editing readings for artifacts has been described elsewhere [14].

A Precision Control Design (PCD) actigraph worn on the wrist, or on the wrist and at the waist, recorded body motility continuously. The actigraph recorded either the frequency or the amplitude of body movements and stored cumulative values for each minute. Unless otherwise noted, the movement frequency (counts) of the wrist will be reported. Details on the PCD actigraph appear elsewhere [20, 28].

Employees reported to the laboratory at 0800 hours and were instructed to follow their normal daily routine when they left. Immediately after each blood pressure reading, employees recorded the time, their body posture (sitting, standing, reclining), their location (work, home, car, other), their activity, and their mood state, by marking boxes on a computer-readable diary card described previously [18]. The 16 specific activities monitored were walking, driving a car, eating, drinking a caffeinated or an alcoholic beverage, cigarette smoking, talking on the telephone, watching television, working, household chores, talking, attending a meeting, desk work, reading, relaxing, and sleeping. Three activities that had very low frequencies (cigarette smoking, drinking an alcoholic beverage, relaxing) and one that was highly redundant (working) were dropped from some analyses, reducing the number of activities to 12. Mood ratings for anger, emotional tension, and the feeling of being rushed were summed to estimate the employee's level of "stress" at each blood pressure reading. Stress scores for readings during sleep were set at zero.

Wrist movements and waist movements were highly interdependent ($r = 0.76$; mean instrasubject correlation). Movement at each site reflected whole body motility as well as movement specific to the site.

Not surprisingly, body motility, the specific activity performed, and body posture were all highly interdependent. The multiple correlation between wrist movement and 12 activities computed for all blood pressure readings of all 82 subjects ($n = 4954$) was $r = 0.69$. The multiple correlation between wrist movement and body posture was $r = 0.64$. The canonical correlation between body posture and the 12 activities was $r = 0.80$.

Mean wrist movement frequency for each of sixteen activities is shown in Fig. 1. Greatest wrist movement occurred while driving a car (290 counts per minute), walking (255), doing household chores (237), and working (210). The least movement occurred while watching television (122), relaxing (74), and sleeping (24). Large standard deviations shown in the figure reveal that different employees performed the same activity with different degrees of pace or intensity.

Some motility counts while driving a car were imparted by the motion of the car itself. Monitors mounted on the dash and the seat of the car recorded between 100 and 250 counts per minute. Car motion interacted with wrist motion to produce resultant displacements of the wrist monitor. The contribution of car motion to wrist monitor counts was probably substantial.

Blood pressure, heart rate, and wrist movement diurnal rhythms for the employees who were monitored on 2 work days appear in Fig. 2. The wrist values

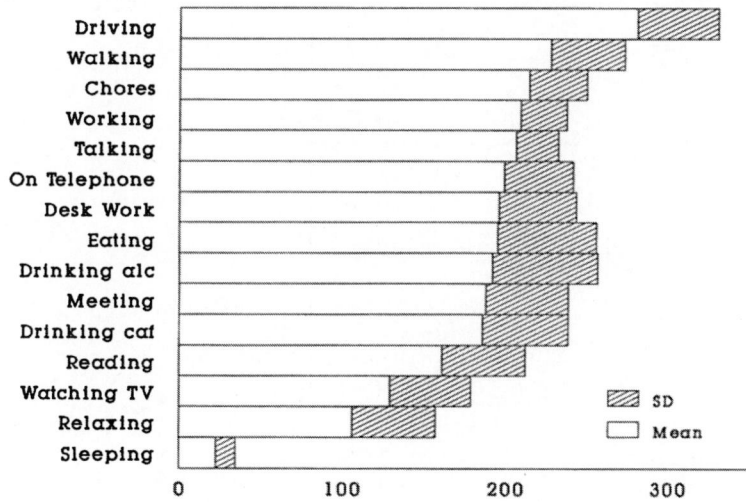

Fig. 1. Mean and standard deviation of wrist movement frequency for each of 16 common activities

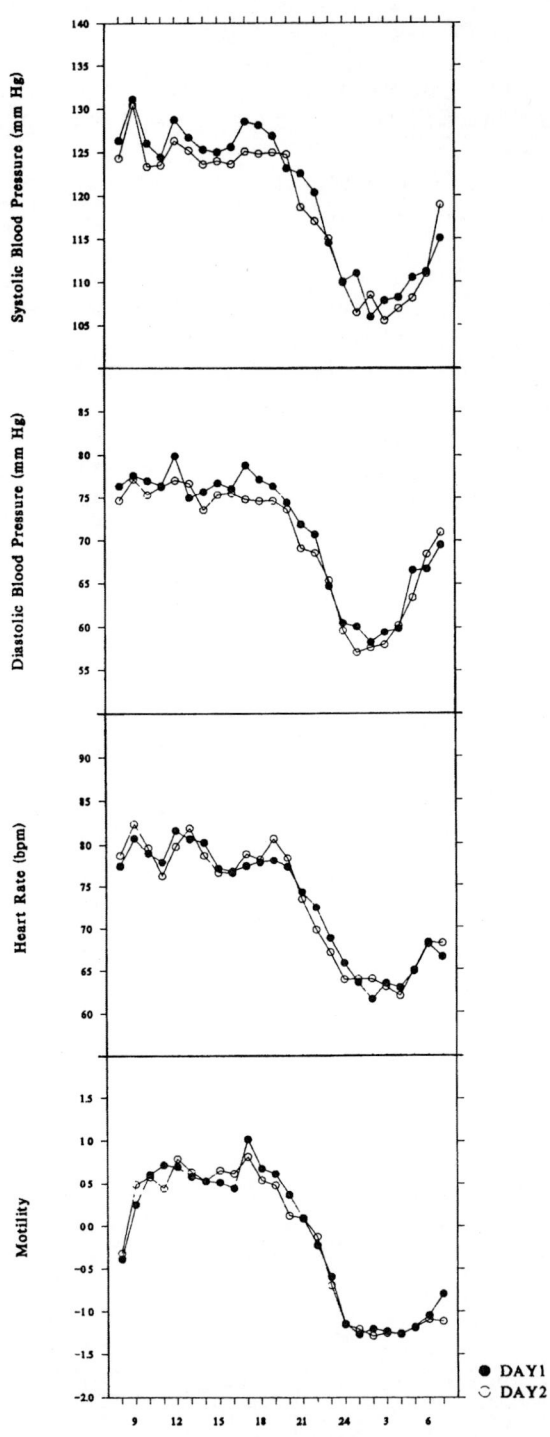

Fig. 2. 24-h blood pressure, heart rate, and wrist movement (motility) curves on 2 days of monitoring. Each data point is a 1-h average

● DAY1
○ DAY2

Time of Day (hours)

given are averages for the 10 min prior to cuff inflations. The four rhythms were highly reproducible over a 1-month interval. The daily blood pressure curve has a nadir around 0200 or 0300 hours and a rapid rise upon awakening, as reported by others [1, 2].

Figure 2 represents averages for the 1-h intervals preceding the hour plotted. For example, the 0800 hour values represent the average of all readings obtained between 0700 hours and 0800 hours. The 0800 hours motility values are probably artificially low. Some employees removed the monitor to shower in the morning. During this time the monitor was stationary. With the exception of the 0800 hours values, the daily blood pressure and heart rate curves agree closely with the wrist motility curve. All curves have a similar form.

One interpretation of the above results is that the blood pressure and heart rate temporal patterns were imposed *externally* by demands on the circulation made by the skeletal motor system. Causation would presumably move from the physical environment (cycle of night and day) to behavioral adaptation (cycle of sleep and wakefulness), to the cardiovascular system (metabolically supportive cycle of blood circulation). A necessary caveat is that correlational data of this kind lack controls that are necessary to move beyond plausibility to proof. The possibility of *internal* sources of temporal order, imposed on both the circulatory and the skeletal motor systems, cannot be ruled out.

The high reproducibility of the wrist movement curve suggests that employees did not alter their gross body activity as an adaptation to wearing the blood pressure monitor. For example, there is no evidence that the employees because of unfamiliarity with the monitoring procedure restricted their movement on the first day of monitoring. Such information is needed to evaluate the *representativeness* of blood pressure values obtained on a single monitoring day.

The significant interdependence between body motility, the specific activity performed, and body posture complicates the interpretation of results. It is never clear whether a particular variable is influencing blood pressure on its own, or is acting as a proxy for some other variable upon which it is dependent. To attempt to clarify the results, the *independent* dimensions extant in the motility-activity-posture system were determined by principal components analysis. The components were extracted from the intercorrelations among 12 activities, wrist movement, and a stress score (defined above), which was added as a measure of the level of emotionality at the time of each blood pressure reading. To better focus on intrasubject variability, the motility values and stress ratings were standardized (centered at 0, scaled to a standard deviation of 1.0) within each employee separately by the transformation $z = (X - M)/SD$, where M and SD were the employee's own mean and standard deviation for the variable x (stress value or motility value). Following their extraction, principal components were rotated to a varimax criterion. The component loadings for six components with eigenvalues greater than 1.0 appear in Table 1. The two largest components also appear in Figs. 3 and 4.

The largest component of the system of motility-activity-posture-emotionality variables is a pattern of general activation associated with wakefulness. Simply being awake has a large weight or "loading" (0.71) on this component. As "sitting" has a much larger loading than "standing", 0.62 versus 0.21, the component was

Table 1. Rotated component loadings of variables [a]

Variables	Components					
	1	2	3	4	5	6
Stress	80	18	09	23	20	17
Awake	71	16	10	07	08	18
Motility	69	31	−00	−06	−06	−17
Sitting	62	−52	22	17	27	16
Driving	53	−33	−19	−43	−23	−33
Standing	21	86	−16	08	−02	−02
Walking	12	68	01	−01	02	−09
Desk work	20	−16	68	36	−01	−23
Reading	10	−03	63	−08	19	18
On telephone	12	−06	00	77	−12	−10
Drinking caffeinated beverage	02	05	12	05	69	−17
Eating	11	−03	04	−20	61	12
Watching	08	−15	00	−04	−06	85
Chores	11	33	07	−12	−05	30
Talking	43	11	−46	43	26	10
Meeting	09	−18	−36	17	41	−05

[a] Decimal points omitted.

labeled "upper body activity". Other important elements include high levels of stress and of wrist motion.

The second largest component is bipolar (Table 1). The positive pole, represented by positively loading variables, is primarily a composite of standing, walking, doing household chores, and greater than average wrist movement. The negative pole is primarily a composite of sitting, driving, and attending a meeting. This component appears to represent primarily "lower body activity", which was independent of upper body activity.

The two largest patterns of behavioral variability accounted for 18% and 13% of the total variance of the 16 variables, respectively. The four remaining smaller patterns represent primarily one or two dominant (high-loading) variables. Component three, defined primarily by reading and desk work, represents variability in motility, activity, posture, and emotionality associated with reading at home and at work. Component four (talking in general, talking specifically on the telephone) was labeled "talking on the telephone", as talking on the telephone clearly was the highest loading variable (Table 1). Component five (eating, drinking caffeinated beverage) was labeled "eating". Component six was labeled "watching television." Altogether, the six components accounted for 61% of the total variance of the 16 variables.

Behavioral component scores were computed for every blood pressure reading of all subjects who were monitored on 2 work days. Plots of the averaged 24-h curves for each component indicated the following: The diurnal curves of upper body activity and lower body activity were similar to each other, as well as to the curves shown in Fig. 1. Upper body activity was highly reproducible from one work day to the next; lower body activity was not.

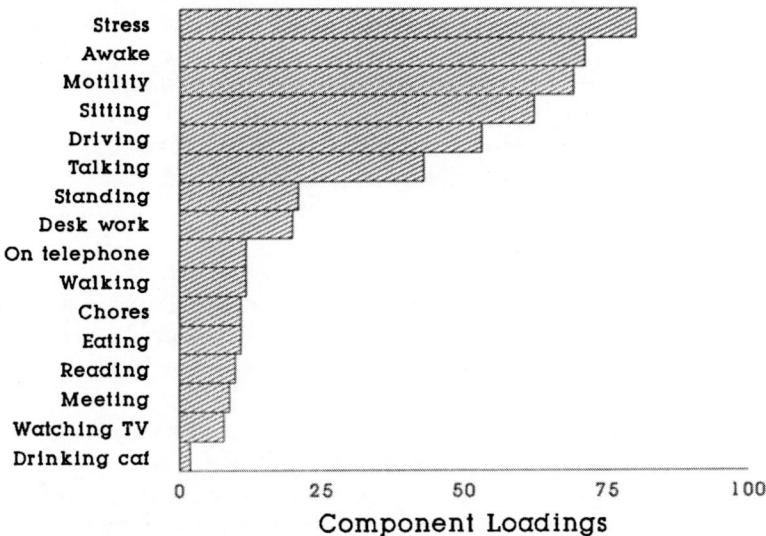

Fig. 3. Component loadings (weights) for the largest principal component of 16 motility, activity, posture, and stress variables (upper body activity 18%)

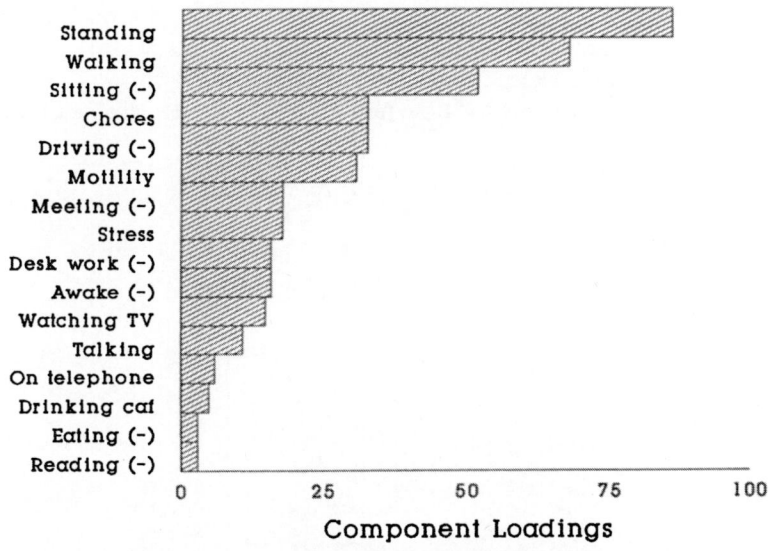

Fig. 4. Component loadings (weights) for the second largest principal component of 16 motility, activity, posture, and stress variables (lower body activity 13%)

The diurnal curves for the four smaller behavioral components were highly reproducible. The "eating" component peaked sharply at 1200 hours and 1800 hours (noon and evening meals), with moderate elevations at the early and middle parts of the morning and afternoon, presumably reflecting snacking. "Watching television", component six, rose rapidly at 1800 hours, peaked at 2000 hours and returned to a very low value by 2400 hours. Component four, "talking on the telephone", was high during the morning and afternoon hours, low in the evening, and very low at mealtimes. "Reading" was high during morning, afternoon, and evening hours, and very low at mealtimes. As would be expected, all four curves were generally very low and quite flat between 2400 hours and 0600 hours (during sleep), although "reading" and "watching television" began a slow rise around 0500 hours, revealing some early morning behavior in those areas.

To explore how the relationship between blood pressure and behavior varied with the time of day, the 24-h period was divided into six blocks of 4 h each, beginning at 0000 hours. Employees' blood pressure readings and behavior component scores were pooled and intercorrelated within each time block separately. The percent of variance accounted for by each of the six behavior components during each time period is shown in Fig. 5.

The predictive power, i.e., the percent of variance accounted for by the six behavioral components, varied greatly with time of day: 23% of diastolic variance during time period one (0000–0400 hours), 35% (0400–0800 hours), 7% (0800–1200 hours), 9% (1200–1600 hours and 1600–2000 hours), and 30% for the last time period (2000–2400 hours). The pattern of results was much the same for systolic pressure, except that the percentage of variance accounted for by the behavioral components for time periods one, two, and six was somewhat smaller.

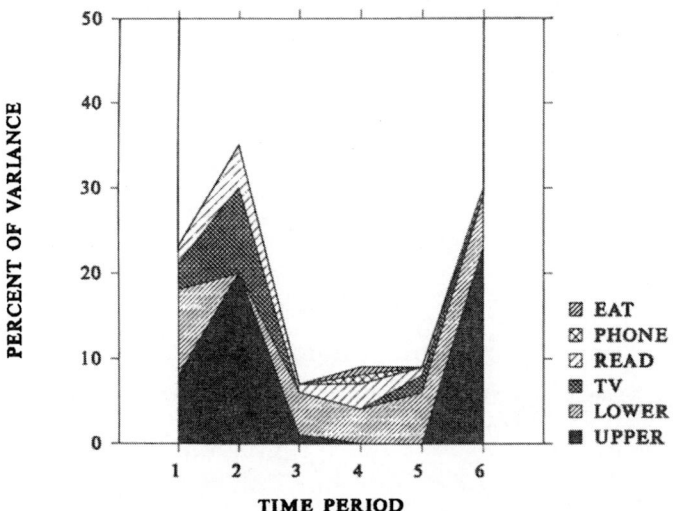

Fig. 5. Percentage of variance of diastolic blood pressure accounted for by each of six behavioral components (eating, talking on the telephone, reading, watching television, lower body activity, upper body activity) during each of six 4-h time periods from 0000–0400 hours (period 1) to 2000–2400 hours (period 6)

Clearly, the impact of behavior on blood pressure was very specific to the time of day. Time periods one, two, and six – when the impact was the greatest – included observations surrounding the sleep-wakefulness cycle. Employees went to bed either early (period six) or late (period one); everyone awakened and got out of bed during period two. Employees were on the job during time periods three and four, and were usually at home, and awake, throughout period five.

Figure 5 illustrates the powerful influence of the alternation of activity and inactivity associated with the sleep-wakefulness cycle. Component behaviors (Table 1) accounted for a much higher percent of diastolic pressure variability during the time periods when employees went to bed or awakened (23%, 35%, and 30%) than the time periods when they were awake and active throughout (7%, 9%, and 9%).

Upper body activity and lower body activity influenced diastolic pressure at different times of the day (Fig. 5). Lower body activity was a more important influence on the job and at home in the early evening, and a less important influence during the time period when employees awakened (0400–0800 hours) and many employees went to bed (2000–2400 hours).

With few exceptions, the employees had sedentary jobs requiring upper body movement, which was occasionally punctuated by lower body activity (usually walking). The intermittency of the walking and greater constancy of upper body activity in highly structured sedentary work routines may account for the slightly greater influence of lower body, as against upper body, activity in diastolic pressure at the workplace.

Variability in watching television and reading had a significant influence on variability in diastolic pressure during early morning hours (0400–0800 hours). This may reflect the influence on blood pressure of the pace of early morning activities prior to leaving home for work. Some employees may have greeted the new day with a spurt of activity, while others eased into it more gradually by reading the morning newspaper or watching television. Differences in early morning activation levels would be expected to affect variability in blood pressure.

The sedentariness of early morning activities such as reading and watching television may also help explain why upper body activity had a greater influence on blood pressure than lower body activity during the 0400–0800 hours time period. Variability in sedentary behaviors would permit considerable intra- and inter-employee variability in upper body, but not lower body, movement, which would tend to influence blood pressure levels.

Any attempts to explain the results illustrated in Fig. 5 must at this point remain speculative and questionable. The figure, however, shows beyond question that the influence of behavior on blood pressure had a *structure*. It was not random, it was not constant temporally, and it was not the same for all components of behavior at any point in time.

Given the linkage of blood pressure to behavior, it is of interest to determine what variability and periodicity in blood pressure remains after removing the influence of behavior. What intrinsic temporal order and inherent instability remains after blood pressure has been "scrubbed free" of external influences? We would like to remove the effects of changes in posture (cerebellar effects), physical motility (extrapyramidal effects), the type of voluntary, skilled activity (neocortical effects), and stress (limbic effects) that occurred during the course of a routine day in order to see what remains of blood pressure rhythmicity due to the operation of intrinsic, lower-level (brain stem, baroreceptor, vascular, etc.) mechanisms and sources of control.

In order to focus directly on the 24-h organization of blood pressure, differences between employees in level of pressure were set aside by analyzing standardized blood pressures, that is, blood pressure readings were so transformed that each employee's readings had a mean of zero and a standard deviation of one. Standardized pressures were regressed on the 16 behavioral (motility, activity, posture, stress) variables described above. The multiple correlations were 0.63 (diastolic pressure) and 0.57 (systolic pressure). Regression results (coefficients) were used to compute residual blood pressures, that is, the parts of blood pressure readings that remained after removing arithmetically the parts attributable to the behavioral variables. Residual blood pressures were pooled in 1-h intervals and averaged. The averaged residual diastolic pressure curves for the 2 days of monitoring appear in Fig. 6.

The nonrhythmic nature of the curves is clear. Results were similar for systolic pressure (not shown in Fig. 6). Removing behavioral influences by arithmetic means eliminated virtually all rhythmicity in blood pressure. Considerable moment-to-moment variability in blood pressure still remained after stripping

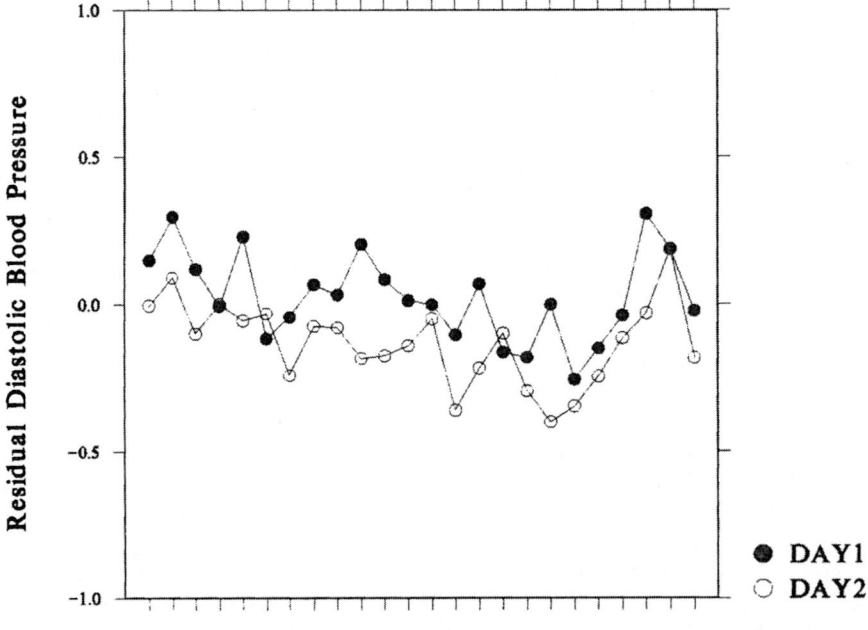

Fig. 6. 24-h diastolic blood pressure curve following removal of the influence of 16 behavioral variables. Each data point is a 1-h average

away the behavioral influences – 60% (diastolic) and 67% (systolic) of the original variability – but this variability was no longer rhythmic.

Conclusions

It appears that much, if not all, of the diurnal rhythmicity in blood pressure was imposed externally by the schedule of motility and activity, posture, and emotion that is deeply rooted in the normal routine of daily living. The magnitude of relationship of blood pressure to behavior varied greatly with time of day, and was linked primarily to the sleep-wakefulness cycle. The schedule of meals and of activities apart from sleep appeared to contribute comparatively little to blood pressure variability. Arithmetic removal of behavioral influences left considerable variability, but no rhythmicity, remaining in the blood pressure readings.

Whether the causation of blood pressure rhythmicity truly arises in the behavioral (neocortical-limbic, extrapyramidal-cerebellar) system or in other sources that impose cyclic order on blood pressure and behavior simultaneously cannot be decided solely by the experimentally uncontrolled statistical approaches used. The present results are suggestive, but by no means definitive.

References

1. Cheung D, Gasster J, Weber M (1989) Assessing duration of antihypertensive effects with whole-day blood pressure monitoring. Arch Int Med 149:2021–2025
2. Verdecchia P, Schillaci G, Guerreri M, Gatteschi C, Benemio G, Boldrini F, Porcellati C (1990) Circadian blood pressure changes and left ventricular hypertrophy in essential hypertension. Circulation 81(2):528–536
3. Pickering TG (1990) Physiological aspects of noninvasive ambulatory blood pressure monitoring. News Physiol Sci 5:176–179
4. Williams RB (1986) Patterns in reactivity and stress. In: Matthews K, Weiss S, Detre T, Dembroski T, Falkner B, Manuck S, Williams R (eds) Handbook of stress, reactivity, and cardiovascular disease. Wiley, New York
5. Stephenson R (1984) Modification of reflex regulation of blood pressure by behavior. Ann Rev Physiol 46:133–142
6. Sandman C, Walker B, Berka C (1982) Influence of afferent cardiovascular feedback on behavior and the cortical evoked potential. In: Cacioppo J, Petty R (eds) Perspectives in cardiovascular psychophysiology. Guilford, New York
7. Koch E (1932) Die Irradiation der pressoreceptorischen Kreislaufreflexe. Klin Wochensch 11:225–227
8. Miller R, Shapiro A, King H, Ginchereau E, Hosutt J (1984) Effect of antihypertensive treatment on the behavioral consequences of elevated blood pressure. Hypertension 6:202–208
9. Pickering TG (1989) Ambulatory monitoring: applications and limitations. In: Schneiderman N, Weiss S, Kaufmann P (eds) Handbook of research methods in cardiovascular behavioral medicine. Plenum, New York
10. Pickering TG, Harshfield GA, Kleinert H, Blank S, Laragh J (1982) Blood pressure during normal daily activities, sleep, and exercise. JAMA 247(7):992–996
11. Littler W, Honour A, Sleight P (1974) Direct arterial pressure, heart rate, and electrocardiogram during human coitus. J Reprod Fertil 40:321–331
12. Millar-Craig M, Bishop C, Raftery E (1978) Circadian variation in blood pressure. Lancet i:795–798

13. Schneider R, Julius S, Karunas R (1989) Ambulatory blood pressure monitoring and laboratory reactivity in Type A behavior and components. Psychosom Med 51:290–305
14. Van Egeren LF, Sparrow AW (1990) Ambulatory monitoring to assess real-life cardiovascular reactivity in Type A and Type B subjects. Psychosom Med 52:297–306
15. Van Egeren LF (1988) Repeated measurements of ambulatory blood pressure. J Hypertens 6(9):753–755
16. Schnall P, Pieper C, Schwartz J, Karasek R, Schlussel Y, Devereux R, Ganau A, Alderman M, Warren K, Pickering T (1990) The relationship between 'job strain,' workplace diastolic blood pressure, and left ventricular mass index. JAMA 263(14):1929–1935
17. Clark L, Denby L, Pregibon D, Harshfield G, Pickering T, Blank S, Laragh J (1987) A quantitative analysis of the effects of activity and time of day on the diurnal variations of blood pressure. J Chron Dis 40:671–681
18. Van Egeren LF, Madarasmi S (1988) A computer-assisted diary (CAD) for ambulatory blood pressure monitoring. Am J Hypertens 1:179s–185s
19. Meijer G, Westerterp K, Koper H, Ten Hoor F (1989) Assessment of energy expenditure by recording heart rate and body acceleration. Med Sci Sports Exerc 21(3):343–347
20. Redmond D, Hegge F (1985) Observations on the design and specification of a wrist-worn human activity monitoring system. Behav Res Meth Inst Comput 17(6):659–669
21. Montoye H, Washburn R, Servais S, Ertl A, Webster J, Nagle F (1983) Estimation of energy expenditure by a portable accelerometer. Med Sci Sports Exerc 15:403–407
22. Kupfer D, Weiss B, Foster F, Detre T, Delgado J, McPartland R (1976) Psychomotor activity in affective states. Arch Gen Psychiatry 30:765–768
23. Porrino L, Rapoport J, Behar D, Sceery W, Ismond D, Bunney W (1983) A naturalistic assessment of the motor activity of hyperactive boys. Arch Gen Psychiatry 40:681–687
24. Mullaney D, Kripke D, Messin S (1980) Wrist-actigraphic estimation of sleep time. Sleep 3(1):83–92
25. Corwley T, Hydinger-Macdonald M (1979) Bedtime flurazepam and the human circadian rhythm of spontaneous motility. Psychopharmacology 62:157–161
26. Fentem P, Fitton D, Hampton J (1976) Long-term recording of activity patterns. Postgrad Med J 52:163–166
27. Broughton R, Stampi C, Dunham W, Rivers M (1990) Ambulant monitoring of sleep-wake state, core body temperature and body movement. In: Miles L, Broughton R (eds) Medical monitoring in the home and work environment. Raven, New York
28. Van Egeren LF (1990) Computer-based monitoring of physical activity. In: Miles L, Broughton R (eds) Medical monitoring in the home and work environment. Raven, New York

The Relationship Between Self-Reported Emotional Strain and Ambulatory Blood Pressure and Heart Rate

H. Schächinger, W. Langewitz, H. Rüddel, and W. Schulte

Introduction

Experimental psychosocial stress has been identified as causing disease in certain animal populations [1], and it is now widely accepted that adverse stress also contributes to cardiovascular morbidity in humans [2]. Part of this contribution may be explained by stress-induced alterations in established cardiovascular risk factors [3]. Epidemiologic surveys, for example, have documented that cardio-vascular risk factors are elevated after natural disasters [4, 5]. However, most of the evidence about pathophysiological stress effects is derived from laboratory studies. It is well established that blood pressure increases in response to mental stress [6]. Even short-term increases in blood pressure (BP) may contribute to chronic BP elevation by structural vascular changes and subsequently increasing total peripheral resistance [7]. Presumably BP or factors associated closely to BP changes have some trophic effects on the vascular wall, thereby increasing BP reactivity, and, as a self-perpetuating process, this leads to reduced internal vascular diameters and enhanced vascular resistance [8]. Taking this into account, a pathogenetic significance of stress for onset and maintenance of arterial hypertension might be suggested, and patients should be encouraged to avoid stressful situations if possible.

Such a strategy assumes the subject's capability of identifying properly corresponding stressful events; however, there is no general agreement on what exactly should be considered as a stressful event. Sokolow and coworkers instructed 50 patients to report their mood and affect on a checklist at each ambulatory BP measurement [9]. The checklist allowed the assessment of contentent, alertness, anxiety, time pressure, depression, and hostility. Their data showed an association of higher BP values with higher scores in some psycholog-ical variables. However, intraindividual correlation analyses showed that a positive correlation between cardiovascular parameters and alertness was by no means present in all subjects. A significant positive correlation was found only in a few patients (most did not show a significant positive association or even showed a negative correlation). However, as until now no data on test-retest analysis have been published, it is not yet clear whether the intraindividual correlation coefficients reflects individual characteristics or depends on random influences.

Schmidt/Engel/Blümchen (Eds.)
Temporal Variations of the Cardiovascular System
© Springer-Verlag Berlin Heidelberg 1992

Our aim was therefore to study whether BP and heart rate (HR) are truly related to self-reported emotional strain, and whether such relations are stable individual characteristics.

Methods

Two groups of subjects were investigated. Group 1 consisted of 85 normotensive adult volunteers with a mean age of 37 ± 6 years. None of the subjects suffered from any cardiovascular disease. Subjects were examined for 11 working hours during daytime and were instructed to behave as on a normal working day. Thus, subjects were not asked to restrict themself to any protocol. The second study was performed in 87 children, 48 boys and 39 girls aged from 12 to 15 years. Monitorings were performed during school time and during the afternoon; children were asked to behave as on a normal day. Thus again, no restriction to any protocol was intended. The second investigation was based on a subsample of the study population examined in the Bonn Kinderstudie, a survey initiated by von Eiff. The BP monitorings have been carried out in 1985.

Cardiovascular hemodynamics were recorded with the Physioport system [10]. This device is based on the auscultatory technique. Korotkoff sounds were registered by a microphone placed under the cuff over the brachial artery. The system was attached by a well-trained nurse. At the beginning of the monitoring period a calibration measurement was performed with standard auscultatory blood pressure measurement techniques. If differences were detectable, the sensitivity of the microphone was changed. If differences in obtained values persisted, the microphone was reattached. An ECG was performed at the same time. The Physioport system uses an inbuilt program to indicate artifacts. Only those acoustical phenomena that fulfill specific frequency characteristics and occur during a certain time period after the R-wave trigger are accepted as possible Korotkoff sounds.

In the adult subjects a further channel of the Physioport system was used to mark their actual level of stress by pushing numbered buttons on a special marker device every time BP measurements were taken. The scale ranged from 1, totally relaxed, up to 5, extremely stressed. In children the indication of perceived stress was achieved by an additional questionnaire. A four-point scale from 1, not stressed at all, to 4, very stressed and upset, was employed. As only few children occasionally admitted to feeling very stressed and upset (2.8% of all readings) we converted the four-point scale to a three-point scale by recording 4 as 3. The children performed the monitoring three times. The interval between consecutive measurements was 4 months. A total of 235 BP and HR profiles were collected in children. Every time BP was measured, the children were asked to mark their emotional strain in the questionnaire. However, the children did this properly in approximately only 65% of all occasions.

In both parts of the study BP measurements were made automatically at intervals of random length (mean 15 min). At the end of the monitoring period a further calibration measurement was performed by standard auscultatory method to identify possible shifts in measurement accuracy. Before data were transmitted to an IBM mainframe computer for further statistical analyses, all data were checked by hand to eliminate outliers.

Data analyses were based on two different approaches separately for both groups of subjects. The dependence of hemodynamic parameters on subjective stress was analyzed by an one-way ANOVA design using the pooled data of each group ($n = 1634$ for adults, $n = 4747$ for children). In a second approach Pearson correlation coefficients between perceived level of stress and cardiovascular parameters were calculated for each subject.

A separate retest analysis was performed to determine reproducibility of these intraindividual correlation coefficients in both groups. BP was monitored again in 21 adult subjects after 3 weeks. As the correlation coefficients were not normally distributed in the adult sample, we analyzed test-retest reproducibility of whether the association between hemodynamic parameters and perceived level of stress was positive or negative using the χ^2 test. For children the intraindividual correlation coefficients between cardiovascular parameters and perceived stress levels appeared to be normally distributed. Therefore we performed Pearson correlation analyses to test for reproducibility of the correlation coefficients. All statistical analyses were performed on an IBM 3081 mainframe computer of the University of Bonn (FRG) using SAS routines [11].

Results

A significant dependence of systolic BP ($F = 25.5$, $p < 0.0001$), diastolic BP ($F = 40.4$, $p < 0.0001$), and HR ($F = 24.9$, $p < 0.0001$) on level of perceived stress was detected in adult subjects (see Fig. 1). BP and HR readings tend to be significantly higher, the higher subjects scored their emotional strain. In children, although less pronounced, a significant positive association between level of

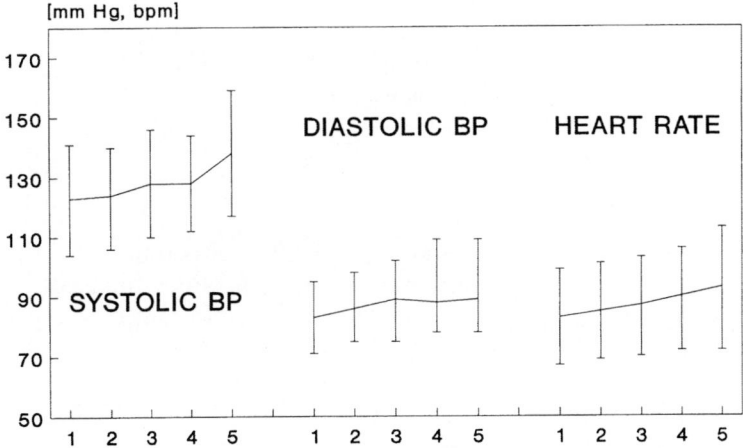

Fig. 1. Dependence of hemodynamic parameters on emotional strain in pooled data from adult subjects. Scale: 1, relaxed; 5, stressed

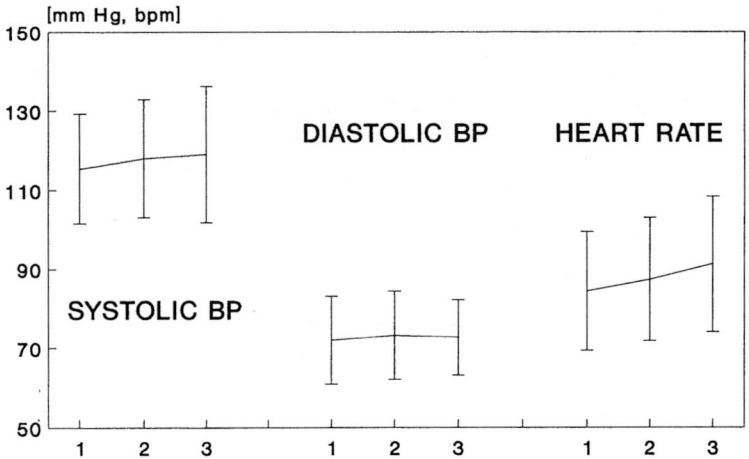

Fig. 2. Dependence of hemodynamic parameters on emotional strain in pooled data from children. Scale: 1, relaxed; 3, relaxed

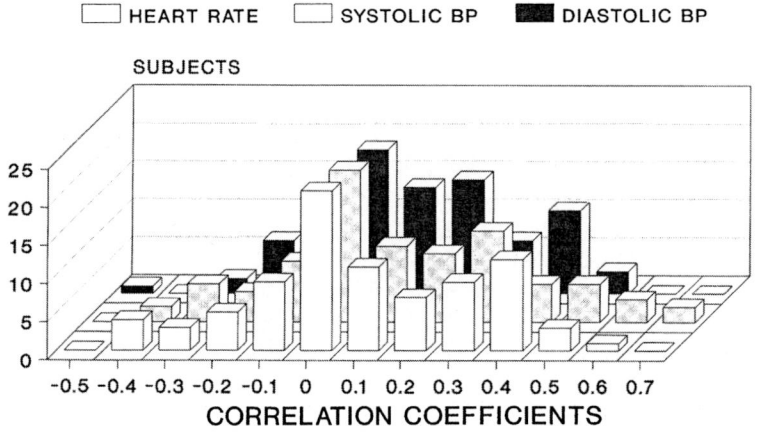

Fig. 3. Frequency distribution of individual correlation coefficients between hemodynamic parameters and perceived level of stress in adult subjects ($n = 85$)

perceived stress and systolic BP ($F = 4.7$, $p < 0.01$), diastolic BP ($F = 11.4$, $p < 0.0001$), and HR ($F = 49.9$, $p < 0.0001$) was found (see Fig. 2).

Figure 3 presents the distributions of the intraindividual correlation coefficients between heart rate, systolic and diastolic BP, and perceived level of stress for adult subjects. Although more subjects tended to have a positive correlation between stress and cardiovascular parameters, a remarkable number showed no intraindividual correlation or even an inverse association between perceived stress and BP or HR. We found that only 29% of the adult subjects showed a positive correlation greater than $r = 0.30$ between systolic BP, 25% between diastolic BP, and 32% between HR and perceived stress levels.

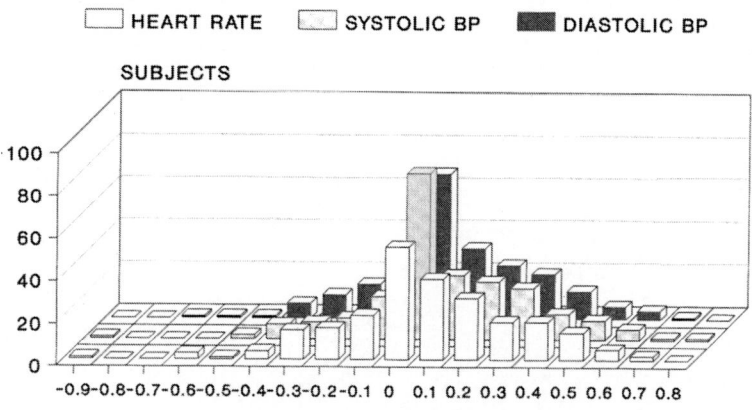

Fig. 4. Frequency distribution of individual correlation coefficients between hemodynamic parameters and perceived level of stress in ambulatory profiles ($n = 235$) obtained in children (two repeated measures)

Table 1. Reproducibility of correlation patterns (frequencies) between hemodynamic parameters and perceived level of stress (21 adult subjects)

Retest	Negative correlation	Positive correlation
Negative correlation 1st examination		
sBP/stress	5	5
dBP/stress	3	7
HR/stress	4	6
Positive correlation 1st examination		
sBP/stress	1	10
dBP/stress	5	6
HR/stress	6	5

Retest analysis sBP/stress: $\chi^2 = 4.3$, $p < 0.04$.
Retest analysis dBP/stress: $\chi^2 = 0.5$, $p < 0.47$.
Retest analysis HR/stress: $\chi^2 = 0.4$, $p < 0.51$.

Among the children group it was also found that BP and HR were not significantly related to perceived stress levels in all subjects. In some of the children BP and HR was even negatively related to the perceived level of stress (Fig. 4). It was found that the correlation between emotional strain and systolic BP, diastolic BP, and HR was greater than $r = 0.30$ in 22%, 19%, and 24% of the children, respectively.

In 21 adult subjects we considered whether a positive relationship between perceived level of stress and hemodynamic parameters was detectable during a second examination. For diastolic BP and HR no stability of the relationship to perceived stress could be demonstrated (Table 1). However, the association of

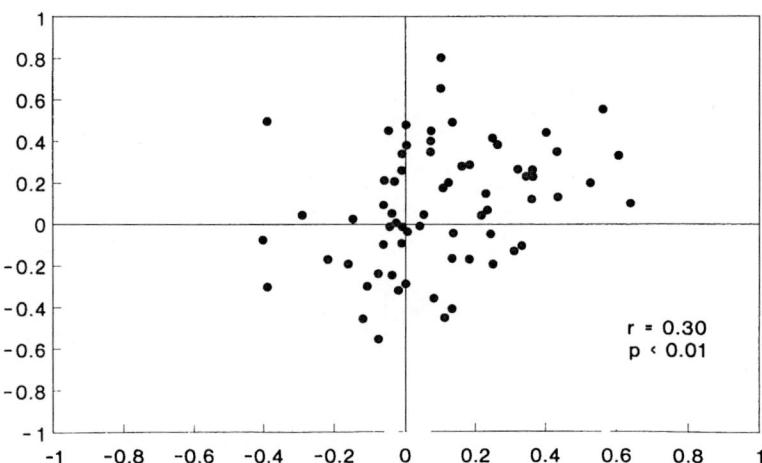

Fig. 5. Test-retest stability of individual correlation coefficients between systolic BP and perceived level of stress in children

systolic BP and stress seemed to be somewhat reproducible in adults (Table 1). Retest analyses revealed significant but poor reproducibility of intraindividual correlation coefficients between systolic BP and emotional strain ($\chi^2 = 4.4$, $n = 21$, $p = 0.04$). In children we found a significant test-retest correlation ($r = 0.30$, $n = 68$, $p < 0.01$) for the dependence of stress and systolic BP (see Fig. 5). The dependence of stress and diastolic BP was not reproducible nor was the dependence of HR and perceived level of stress.

Discussion

The relationship of perceived emotional strain and ambulatory recorded BP and HR was investigated in 85 adults and 87 children who were tested three times. We demonstrated a discrepancy between findings derived by intragroup and intraindividual analyses. In the adult subjects we found a substantially varying relationship between cardiovascular parameters and perceived level of stress. This relationship was often even negative. Also in children we demonstrated that intraindividual correlations between hemodynamic parameters and perceived stress levels could vary substantially among subjects.

A retest performed in 21 adult subjects indicated significant but low test-retest stability of whether the association between stress level and systolic BP was positive or negative. In children correlation analyses between first and second monitorings revealed some reproducibility for the correlation coefficients between systolic BP and perceived level of stress. Analyses based on pooled data repeatedly revealed associations of elevated BP and HR with high perceived level of stress [12, 13]. Analyses based on intraindividual designs have been performed less frequently. Our results corroborate those of Sokolow et al. who found a positive correlation between alertness and BP only in a subgroup of patients [9]. Other authors have found the same result for ambulatory HR [14]. The intraindividual analyses provides more reliable information.

However, one should take into consideration some methodological problems. The perception of stress must not necessarily be accompanied by changes in physiological variables of all systems. Furthermore, increases in BP or HR are not always related to changing psychological parameters. In fact, other behavioral factors such as level of activity, smoking, eating, or body position are also determinants of BP and HR and perhaps of greater importance [15]. This suggests that the low specificity of perceived stress in explaining alterations in BP and HR may be due to overwhelming influences of additional behavioral factors in some subjects. However, some fundamental methodological problems must be discussed when psychological items are assessed during ambulatory BP and HR monitoring. A simple questionnaire as employed in this study, although easy to communicate, allows only poor insight in the complex human emotional state. However, because psychological items are assessed approximately every 15 min, a simple approach elicits the compliance of patients who may become upset working with a more time-consuming questionnaire. Accordingly, Sokolow and coworker's sophisticated approach differentiates between certain psychological items; however, being a time-consuming procedure, it determines patient's behavior so that the assessed measures hardly refer to normal daily life conditions. Small scaling might produce too little variance; however, large scales tend to be skewed and not normally distributed. Rüddel et al. (unpublished data) found that scales from 1 to 100 applied to determine perceived stress did not relate to hemoynamic parameters assessed during 24-h ambulatory BP monitoring.

No data are yet available on whether the correlation between perceived stress level and cardiovascular parameters depends on mainly random influences. Here we point out that there is only a low test-retest stability in associations between perceived stress levels and systolic BP, indicating influences of nonreproducible measurement irregularities. However, the lack of consistency in these correlation patterns, at least in a subgroup of patients, emphasizes the great variability of BP, psychological factors, and their individual relationships.

These results indicate that determination of emotional strain as well as the individual impact of emotional strain on hemodynamic variables must be incorporated into research strategies dealing with dependence of ambulatory BP on behavioral factors. As has been pointed out here, subjects differ in terms of correlation coefficients, and it cannot be assumed that regression slopes are homogeneous for all subjects. Thus, it must be emphasized that pooling hemodynamic data and psychological data over a whole group and performing covariance analyses for adjustment of emotional states must be avoided. Furthermore, these results demonstrate that perception of stress differs tremendously among subjects. It is assumed that correct indication of emotional strain probably needs special cognitive and behavioral training in at least a subgroup of subjects. These findings have implications for behavioral strategies to lower blood pressure.

References

1. Schneiderman N (1987) Psychophysiologic factors in atherogenesis and coronary artery disease. Circulation 76 [Suppl I]:41–47
2. Buell JC, Eliot RS (1980) Psychosocial and behavioral influences in the pathogenesis of acquired cardiovascular disease. Am Heart J 100:723–740
3. McKinney ME, Witte H (1985) Dietary habits and blood chemistry levels of the stress-prone individual: the hot reactor. Compr Ther 11:21–28
4. Trevisan M, Celentano E, Meucci C, Farinaro E, Jossa F, Krogh V, Giumetti D, Panico S, Scottoni A, Mancini M (1986) Short-term effect of natural disaster on coronary heart disease risk factors. Arteriosclerosis 6:491–494
5. Byrne DG (1981) Type A behavior, life-events and myocardial infarction: independent or related risk factors? Br J Med Psychol 54:371–377
6. Krantz DS, Manuck SB (1984) Acute psychophysiologic reactivity and risk of cardiovascular disease: a review and methodologic critique. Psychol Bull 96:435–464
7. Lever AF (1986) Slow pressor mechanisms in hypertension: a role for hypertrophy of resistance vessels? J Hypertens 4:515–524
8. Folkow B (1978) Cardiovascular structural adaptation: its role in the inhibition and maintenance of primary hypertension. Clin Sci 55:3s–22s
9. Sokolow M, Werdegar D, Perloff DB, Cowan RM, Brennenstuhl H (1970) Preliminary studies relating portable recorded blood pressure to daily life events in patients with essential hypertension. Bibl Psychiatr 144:164–189
10. Langewitz W, Dähnert A, Rüddel H (1987) On the validity of a new, portable blood pressure measurement device (Physioport). Med Welt 38:816–821
11. SAS Institute: SAS user's guide: statistics, 5th edn., SAS Institute, Cary
12. Langewitz W, Rüddel H, von Eiff AW (1987) Influence of perceived level of stress upon ambulatory blood pressure, heart rate, and respiratory frequency. J Clin Hypertens 3:743–748
13. Schmieder R, Rüddel H, Langewitz W, Neuss J, Wagner O, von Eiff AW (1985) The influence of monotherapy with oxprenolol and nitrendipine on ambulatory blood pressure in hypertensives. Clin Exp Hypertens 3:445–454
14. Johnston DW, Anastasiades P (1990) The relationship between heart rate and mood in real life. J Psychosom Res 34:21–27
15. van Egeren LF, Madarasmi S (1988) A computer-assisted diary (CAD) for ambulatory blood pressure monitoring. Am J Hypertens 1:179S–185S

The Effect of Occupational and Domestic Stress on the Diurnal Rhythm of Blood Pressure

T. G. Pickering, W. Gerin, G. D. James, C. Pieper, Y. L. Schlussel, and P. L. Schnall

It has been known for many years that blood pressure is not a fixed entity but varies as a function both of the time of day and of changes in physical and mental activity. The development of noninvasive ambulatory blood pressure monitoring has made it possible to begin to sort out the effects of these different influences on blood pressure. In this paper we discuss its applications in the evaluation of the influence of occupational and domestic stress on blood pressure.

The Role of Ambulatory Monitoring

The technique of noninvasive ambulatory blood pressure monitoring enables measurements to be made every 15 min throughout the day and night and hence to give a better estimate of the overall level of blood pressure and its variations than can be achieved with more traditional methods. It is customary to have the subjects keep a diary describing their location, activities, and mood at the times of each reading, so that the blood pressure can be related to changes of physical and mental activity.

This type of analysis has shown that there is a marked variability of blood pressure throughout the day and night [1, 2]. The highest values of both the absolute level and the short-term variability occur between 6:00 A.M. and noon and the lowest at night [2]. The level of physical activity is a major determinant of blood pressure, and higher values tend to be seen when subjects are in the upright position than when they are sitting or lying. However, the currently available noninvasive monitors cannot provide accurate readings during exercise which is any more vigorous than quiet walking.

Some of the major sources of blood pressure variability are illustrated schematically in Fig. 1. There are a number of rhythmical variations with different time courses, ranging from respiratory variations at one extreme to seasonal variations at the other. Diurnal variations come into this category. These may be modified by physical and mental activity on the one hand, and by random variations on the other. Short-term variability cannot be evaluated by noninvasive intermittent ambulatory monitoring, and it is unclear to what extent ultradian rhythms (with a periodicity of 90 min) affect blood pressure in man.

Schmidt/Engel/Blümchen (Eds.)
Temporal Variations of the Cardiovascular System
© Springer-Verlag Berlin Heidelberg 1992

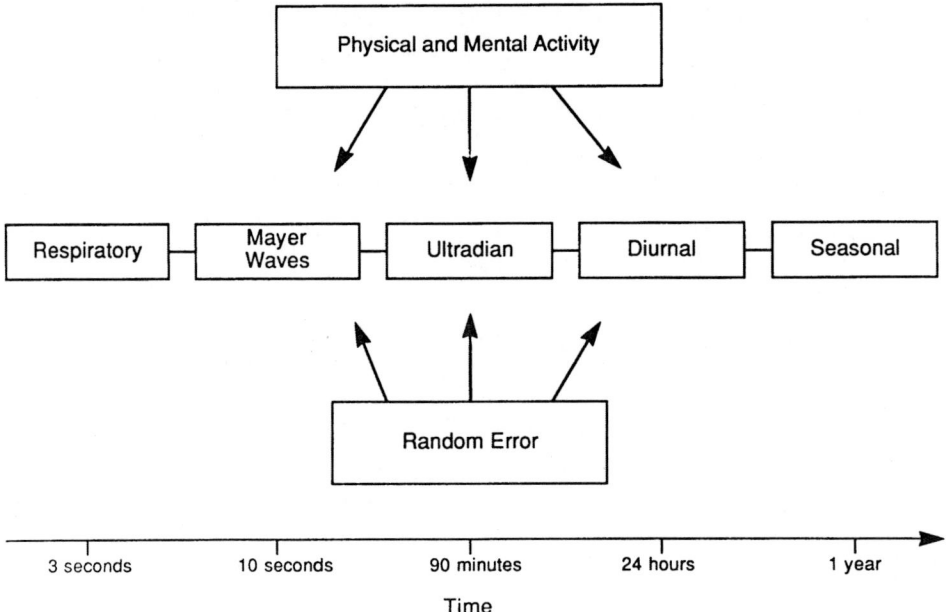

Fig. 1. The major sources of blood pressure variability, with time courses ranging from a few seconds to a year

Our discussion focuses on diurnal variations and on the extent to which these are influenced by changes of physical and mental activity.

While the association of activity and blood pressure recorded during ambulatory monitoring has yielded much useful information, one of the problems is that there is a high degree of multicollinearity among the different activities. Thus, when the influence of postural change on ambulatory pressure is analyzed, it may be concluded that the upright posture results in a significant increase of both systolic and diastolic pressure [3] although it is clear from laboratory studies that postural change by itself causes a negligible change in systolic pressure [4]. The different results can be explained by the activities that are associated with different postures in free-living people. Thus, most of the time during which people are lying down is spent asleep, and while standing they are usually either working or walking. Two other problems are that serial measurements of blood pressure are not independent, and that different stimuli may interact with each other. This was illustrated in a study by Freestone and Ramsay, who showed that either smoking a cigarette or drinking a cup of coffee raised blood pressure for about 15 min, but when they were combined there was a much larger increase, which was still present after 1.5 h [5].

Despite these limitations, it has been shown that both physical and mental activities raise blood pressure. The former are easier to evaluate, particularly with the use of automated activity monitors, described by Van Egeren elsewhere in this volume. Changes in mood are also associated with blood pressure changes. The largest increases are seen with anger and anxiety, although happiness is also associated with slightly higher pressures than emotional neutrality [6]. The contribution of these to the overall level of blood pressure is relatively slight, however, because most people are in a relatively neutral mood for most of the day. We have observed some interesting gender differences in these factors. The effects of anger on blood pressure tend to be more pronounced in men, while anxiety has a bigger effect in women [7]. The setting in which these emotions are experienced may also be a factor: in men, anger expressed while at work appears to be associated with a bigger increase of pressure than at home [7].

Is There a Circadian Rhythm of Blood Pressure?

The diurnal rhythmicity of blood pressure has been recognized for many years, although there has been dispute as to whether it is a truly endogenous circadian rhythm or merely follows the cycle of rest and activity.

Blood pressure changes are closely linked to the level of arousal. During the 1st h of sleep there is a progressive fall, which usually shows its maximal decrease of about 20% 2 h after sleep onset [8–10] and coincides with the deepest stages of slow wave sleep. Later in the night, when dreaming or rapid eye movement (REM) sleep occurs, the pressure tends to be higher, and it shows a further increase on waking up.

There is some confusion in the literature about the "early morning rise of blood pressure." Some authors, particularly Raftery's group in the United Kingdom, have maintained that there is a progressive rise in pressure starting at 3:00 A.M., and that this may contribute to the increased incidence of cardiovascular morbid events that occurs in the early morning hours [11] While there is a tendency for blood pressure to rise a small amount between 3:00 A.M. and 6:00 A.M., it is relatively modest compared to the sharp rise that occurs on waking and can be explained by the generally lighter level of sleep. It is also to some extent an artifact of individual variations in the time of waking, such that when the average blood pressure of several subjects is plotted against the time of waking rather than against the time of day, it is much less pronounced [12, 13], as shown in Fig. 2, which is taken from a study performed by Floras et al. [13].

In the past few years several different lines of evidence have overwhelmingly supported the view that the diurnal rhythm of blood pressure is largely determined by the cycle of rest and activity. These may be summarized as follows. First, studies of shift workers have shown that the blood pressure profile changes immediately on switching from a day shift to a night shift, while heart rate takes several days [14–16]. This work is reviewed elsewhere in this volume by Baumgart. Second, patients studied during 24 h of bed rest show a greatly diminished variation of blood pressure in comparison to free-living individuals. This was first shown by Athanassiadis et al. [17], who monitored blood pressure noninvasively for 24 h in patients in an orthopedic ward who were immobilized in plaster casts. In this situation blood pressure did not show a sinusoidal diurnal pattern but remained relatively constant during the day and decreased during sleep. Somewhat similar observations were made by Mann et al. [19], who studied patients on 2 consecutive days. During 1 day, while on bed rest, the diurnal profile of blood

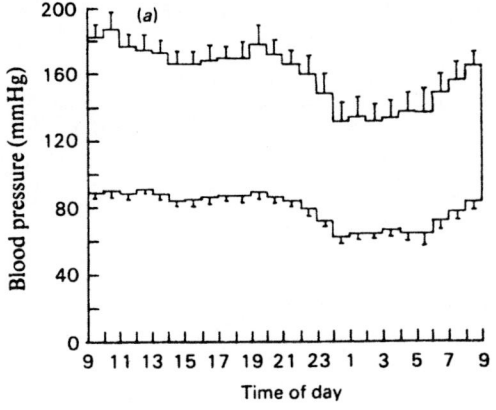

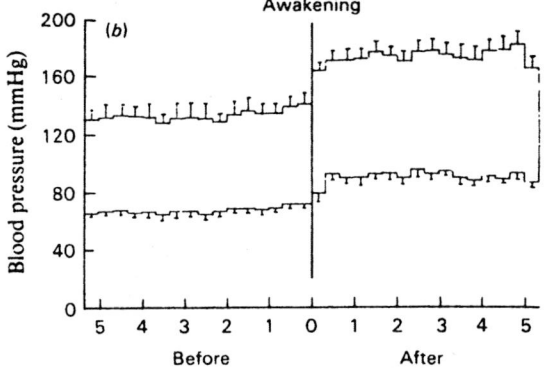

Fig. 2. Diurnal rhythm of blood pressure evaluated by continuous intra-arterial monitoring in hypertensive patients. *Above*, data plotted by time of day; note the apparently gradual increase in blood pressure during the early morning hours. *Below*, the same data plotted according to the time of awakening; the increase in blood pressure is now abrupt. (From [13])

pressure was flatter than on the other, when they were physically active. Third, when we analyzed the effects of 16 commonly occurring daily activities (including sleep) and time of day on the diurnal blood pressure profile, we concluded that most of the diurnal variation could be explained on the basis of the activities, and that time of day was not an important determinant [19].

Patients with hypertension show a generally similar diurnal profile to normotensive subjects, with some increase in the absolute level of blood pressure variability but a relatively minor difference when this is expressed in relative terms [20, 21]. Thus, the fall of blood pressure during sleep is about 20% in both normotensive and hypertensive individuals [8]. The most consistent change is an upward resetting of the diurnal profile to a higher overall level of pressure.

Although most hypertensives do show the normal nocturnal fall in blood pressure (the "dippers"), there are some in whom the pressure remains relatively high (the "nondippers") [22]. There is some disagreement as to whether patients with left ventricular hypertrophy (LVH) are more likely to be nondippers. Raftery

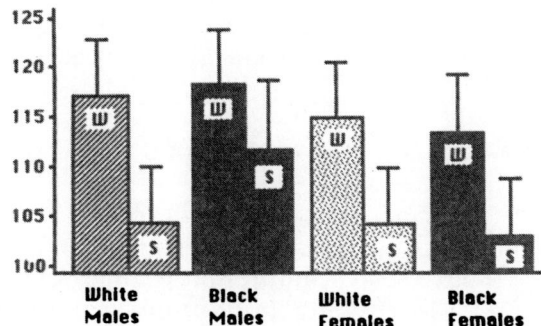

Fig. 3. Mean systolic blood pressure for white and black, male and female adolescents while awake (*W*) and asleep (*S*). (From [27])

has reported that the diurnal pattern is similar in patients with and without LVH [23]. Verdecchia et al. looked at the question to other way round and compared dippers and nondippers; LVH was more prevalent in the nondippers [24].

The finding is of considerable interest because it raises the possibility that the diurnal rhythm of blood pressure may be of pathological significance. Thus, it could be argued that the overall "blood pressure load" on the heart and circulation is increased if the pressure remains elevated during the night. Blacks are commonly nondippers (Fig. 3), for reasons which are probably environmental rather than genetic, and it is conceivable that this is related to the increased prevalence of hypertension among them [25–27].

Problems in Relating Stress and Cardiovascular Disease

The idea that stress is important in the development of hypertension and heart disease is popular but also very difficult to confirm. One of the problems is that both conditions take years to develop, and psychosocial factors which may be sources of chronic stress are unlikely to remain constant. Epidemiological cross-sectional studies have shown that different occupations may be associated with significant differences in the incidence of coronary heart disease, but it has been very difficult to identify the factor responsible for these differences. The two principle candidates as sources of chronic stress are occupational and domestic. Although it is fashionable to state that one's job is highly stressful, occupational issues are not necessarily paramount for the average American worker. In a national survey, only 38% of respondents rated an interesting job as extremely important, while 74% gave this rating for a happy marriage [28]. In a study of women employed in clerical and technical jobs, 55% rated their jobs as more stressful than their home life, while for 45% it was the other way around [29].

Given the problems in relating stress to chronic disease, it has been argued by Kasl that there is a need for more objective outcome measures to establish the effects of stress on health [30]. Clearly, measurement of blood pressure changes during everyday life comes into this category. Another trend has been to emphasize the subjective element, that is, the importance of individual differences in the perception of stressors, which is achieved by self-report measures.

The Influence of Occupational Stress on Blood Pressure

For most employed people a typical day can be broken down into three periods of approximately 8 h each, corresponding to time spent at work, at home, and asleep. We observed that blood pressure tends to be highest while at work [31], as shown in Fig. 4. This is seen even in people with sedentary jobs and is unlikely to be explained solely by differences in physical activity; we originally attributed the phenomenon to the influence of psychosocial factors [31]. In support of this, we observed in another study of employed women that higher levels of blood pressure at work are likely to occur in women who rate their jobs as stressful [32].

In a subsequent study, Gellman et al. also observed an overall difference between work and home pressures, but when they analyzed the situational differences separately for different postures (standing versus sitting), the work pressure was not significantly different from the home pressure while standing, although it was still higher while sitting [3]. This observation makes an important point, namely that the subtle effects of psychosocial factors on blood pressure may be swamped by the effects of changes in physical activity. Gellman et al. also found that change of posture was a major determinant of the overall variance of blood pressure. This, however, may be another example of multicollinearity, since the overall level of physical activity is likely to be higher when people are upright than when they are sitting, and it may be these activities which are responsible for the higher pressures, rather than posture per se.

The possibility that the higher pressure at work is due to the time of day should also be considered, however, since most studies have been done on people who work during the day and are at home during the evening. We have shown that this explanation is invalid, however, because when the same subjects are studied on

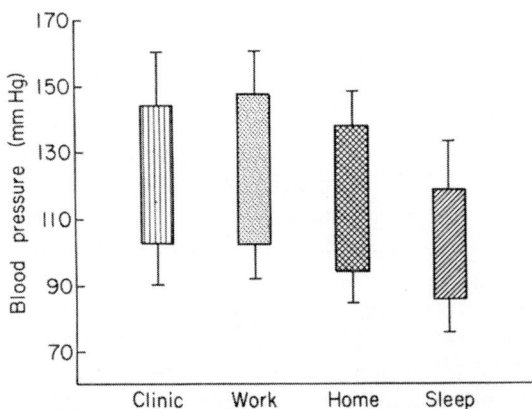

Fig. 4. Mean systolic (*upper limit of bars*) and diastolic (*lower limit of bars*) in hypertensive patients measured in different situations by ambulatory monitoring. (From [31])

2 workdays and 1 nonwork day the higher pressures during the earlier part of the day is no longer seen if the subjects are at home all day [33], as shown in Fig. 5. This is in contrast to the pattern of heart rate, which is higher during the day than in the evening regardless of whether the subject goes to work or stays at home all day. Similar conclusions can be drawn from studies of shift workers.

An interesting finding of our study comparing a workday and a nonworkday was that in some individuals the blood pressure remained elevated in the evening after they had returned home from work, suggesting the existence of a "carry-over effect" of work to home. This too was not observed for heart rate.

Whether or not the higher blood pressure observed during work contributes to the development of hypertension or heart disease is an interesting question. Support for the view may come from our observation that the correlation between ambulatory blood pressure and LVH is closer when blood pressure is measured on a work day [34]. LVH is thought to reflect the cumulative effects of blood pressure on the heart and is itself a potent and independent risk factor for cardiovascular morbidity, as has now been demonstrated by our own and other groups [35, 36].

In order to investigate the association between occupational stress and blood pressure more closely we used a questionnaire developed by Karasek and Theorell called the Job Content Survey [37, 38]. This gives a self-rating of job strain on two orthogonal scales – psychological demand (a measure of the intensity of the work) and decision latitude (a measure of the perceived level of control of the job). Subjects who score high on psychological demand and low on decision latitude are classified as having high-strain jobs. Our reason for using this was that it had been shown in studies conducted both in Sweden and the United States to predict coronary heart disease symptoms and morbidity [37–39]. We used a case-control study design in which the cases were 87 hypertensive subjects and the controls 128 normotensives [40]. Subjects were recruited from seven different worksites in order to encompass a wide range of job titles, which we hoped would include subjects in both high- and low-strain jobs. Our hypothesis was that cases would be more likely to be employed in high-strain jobs. This was in fact confirmed, with a

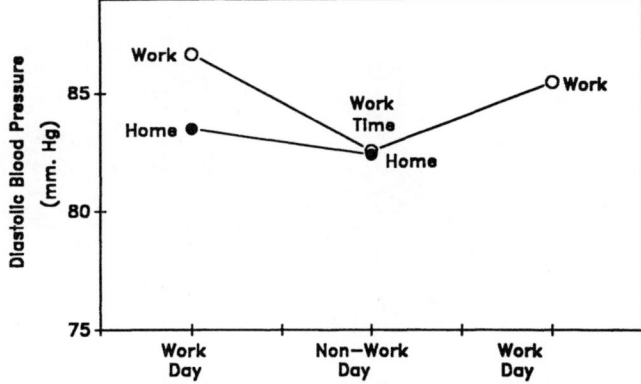

Fig. 5. Comparison of diastolic blood pressure measured on 2 workdays interspersed by a nonworkday, showing that the higher pressure during work is not attributable to the time of day

highly significant odds ratio ranging from 1.2 to 5.2, depending on the age of the subjects (Fig. 6). Furthermore, this relationship was independent of other factors known to influence blood pressure, such as education, sodium and alcohol intake, and body mass index.

We also measured left ventricular mass in these subjects and found an association with job strain, but only in the younger men (aged 30–40 years). This was surprising, because the association between blood pressure and job strain was more marked in the older subjects. A possible explanation for the lack of any significant relationship between LV mass and job strain in the older subjects is that older subjects with increased LV mass may have been excluded from the study because their hypertension was more severe. The suggestion that job strain may affect LV mass before it affects blood pressure is intriguing, although at first sight unlikely. Two pieces of evidence are consistent with it, however. First, in a prospective study of normotensive individuals the best predictor or future hypertension was an increased LV mass [41], and, second, intermittent elevations of blood pressure produced by thigh compression in dogs can increase LV mass before there is any change in the basal level of pressure [42]. It must be admitted that in this latter example there is no tendency for the basal level of pressure to change.

We had expected that the biggest difference in ambulatory blood pressure between the high- and low-strain subjects would be during the hours of work, so

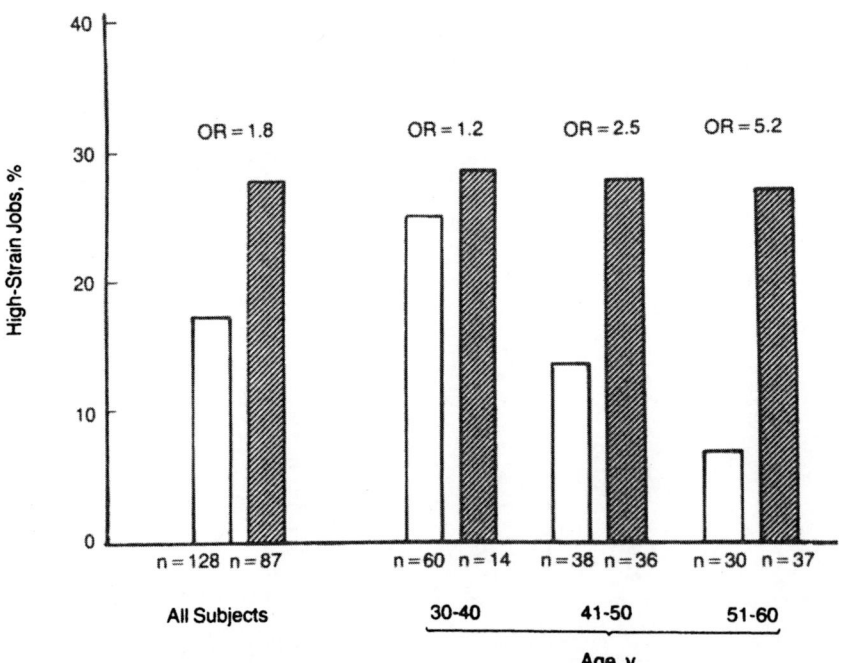

Fig. 6. Percentages of subjects in high-strain jobs in a study relating job strain and hypertension. *Open bars*, normotensives; *hatched bars*, hypertensives. *OR*, Odds ratio of hypertensives being in high strain jobs. (From [40])

that it came as a surprise to find that the difference was equally marked during the home and sleep periods [43]. In other words, the subjects in high-strain jobs showed a sustained elevation of their diurnal profile of blood pressure which, as we have seen earlier, characterizes patients with sustained hypertension. While it is difficult to infer a direct causal relationship from such cross-sectional data, our findings are at least consistent with the hypothesis that chronic exposure to low-grade occupational stress may be a contributory factor in the development of sustained hypertension.

The Influence of Domestic Stress on Blood Pressure

When men return home from work in the evening, their workday is typically at an end, but for employed women the distinction between work and leisure time is much less distinct since they often must care for their husbands and children in the evening. In a study of normotensive women employed in clerical and technical jobs in a large teaching hospital who were studied with ambulatory blood pressure monitoring on a working day we asked them to rate whether their home or work time was more stressful on the day of the recording [32]. Women who rated their work period as being more stressful had a quite different diurnal blood pressure profile than those who said thei time at home was more stressful, with significantly higher pressures occurring during the working hours but with no difference during the home and sleep periods. When we compared married women with childen who rated their time at home as being more stressful than their work time with single women who rated their jobs as more stressful, an even more striking difference in the diurnal blood pressure profile was evident. The single women had higher pressures until about 6:00 P.M., after which the married women's pressures were significantly higher (Fig. 7).

A somewhat similar study has been performed by Frankenhaeuser et al. in white-collar employees of the Volvo automobile company in Sweden [44]. They

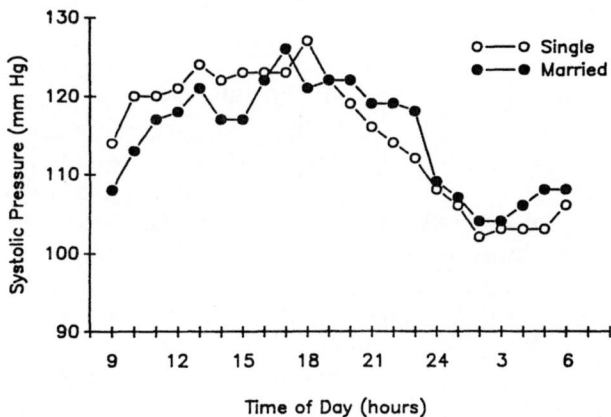

Fig. 7. Diurnal profile of systolic blood pressure in working women who are single and childless (n = 43), or married with children (n = 12)

studied four groups of men and women managers and clerical workers. Subjects measured their own blood pressure once an hour using a semiautomated device for a 12-h period, and they also kept timed urine collections for measurement of catecholamine and cortisol excretion. They were monitored both on a workday and a nonworkday. For all four groups blood pressure was higher on the workday and tended to be highest in the morning. After work the male managers' blood pressure dropped, while the female managers' pressure showed no change. Urinary epinephrine excretion was higher on the workday than on the nonwork-day. Both epinephrine and norepinephrine excretion were generally lower in the evening, which may be partly a result of the normal diurnal rhythm, but in the female managers the norepinephrine levels actually rose when they went home. It was suggested that this inability to unwind in the evening reflected the heavy workload experienced by these women, who had a unique combination of occupational and domestic responsibilities.

Conclusions

In normal persons there is a marked diurnal rhythm of blood pressure, with higher levels occurring during the morning hours and lowest levels at night. It has been debated to what extent this rhythm reflects a truly independent or circadian rhythm, as opposed to being determined by the cycle of physical activity and arousal. Most of the evidence favors the latter view, as shown by studies of subjects maintained on bed rest and of shift workers.

Ambulatory blood pressure monitoring provides an ideal method for evaluating the factors influencing this rhythm, by having subjects keep diaries of their physical and mental activities, which can be related to the corresponding blood pressure readings. The roles of subtle psychosocial factors such as occupational and domestic stress can also be investigated in principle, although in practice it may be difficult to decide which particular factor is responsible for a given change in blood pressure. This is in part because many of the independent variables covary; for example, periods of mental stress may be accompanied by increased physical activity, and it is uncertain what is the duration of the effect of a particular stimulus on blood pressure.

Blood pressure tends to be highest at work in the majority of subjects, and there is some evidence that occupational stress may contribute to this. Domestic stress may also influence the diurnal profile of blood pressure. Thus, in single women with stressful jobs the pressure is higher during the working hours than in the evening, while in married women with children the opposite may be true.

These considerations are of potential significance to the development and manifestation of cardiovascular disease for two reasons. First, there is a growing body of evidence which indicates that the majority of cardiovascular morbid events, including myocardial infarction, sudden cardiac death, and stroke, are more likely to occur in the morning hours (between 6:00 A.M. and noon) than at other times of day [45]. This period corresponds with the peak level of a number of manifestations of sympathetic nervous activity, including blood pressure, and it has been proposed that such surges of autonomic arousal act at "triggers" in susceptible patients and initiate a morbid event [45].

A second possible consequence of effects of chronic exposure to environmental stressors is to promote the development of hypertension and coronary heart disease. Our observations of an association between job strain and hypertension are consistent with this possibility. Sustained hypertension is characterized by an upward resetting of the diurnal profile of blood pressure, with some increase of short-term variability, which is what we observed in our subjects employed in high-strain jobs. However, we must be cautious in inferring a direct causal relationship between job strain and hypertension at the present time because this association is based on cross-sectional rather than prospective studies.

References

1. Bevan AT, Honour AJ, Stott FH (1969) Direct arterial pressure recording in unrestricted man. Clin Sci 36:329–344
2. Mancia G, Ferrari A, Gregorini L, Parati G, Pomidossi G, Bertinier G, Grassi G, Di Rienzo M, Pedotti A, Zanchetti A (1983) Blood pressure and heart rate variabilities in normotensive and hypertensive human beings. Circ Res 53:96–104
3. Gellman M, Spitzer S, Ironson G, Llabre M, Saab P, De Carlo RP, Weidler DJ, Schneiderman N (1990) Posture, place and mood effects on ambulatory blood pressure. Psychophysiology 27:544–551
4. Zachariah PK, Sheps SG, Moore AG (1991) Office blood pressures in supine, sitting, and standing positions: correlations with ambulatory blood pressure. Int J Cardiol (in press)
5. Freestone S, Ramsay LE (1982) Effect of coffee and cigarette smoking on the blood pressure of untreated and diuretic-treated hypertensive patients. Am J Med 73:348–353
6. James GD, Yee LS, Harshfield GA, Blank SG, Pickering TG (1986) The influence of happiness, anger, and anxiety on the blood pressure of borderline hypertensives. Psychosom Med 48:502–508
7. James GD, Yee LS, Harshfield GA, Pickering TG (1988) Sex differences in factors affecting the daily variation of blood pressure. Soc Sci Med 26:1019–1023
8. Snyder F, Hobson JA, Morrison DF et al. (1964) Changes in respirations, heart rate, and systolic blood pressure in human sleep. J Appl Physiol 19:417–422
9. Littler WA, Honour AJ, Carter RD, Sleight P (1975) Sleep and blood pressure. Br Med J 3:346–348
10. Bristow JD, Honour AJ, Pickering TG, Sleight P (1969) Cardiovascular and respiratory changes during sleep in normal and hypertensive subjects. Cardiovasc Res 3:476–485
11. Millar-Craig MW, Bishop CN, Raftery EB (1978) Circadian variation of blood pressure. Lancet 1:795–797
12. Littler WA, Watson RDS (1978) Circadian variation in blood pressure. Lancet 1:995–996
13. Floras JS, Jones JV, Johnston JA, Brooks DE, Hassan MO, Sleight P (1978) Arousal and the circadian rhythm of blood pressure. Clin Sci Mol Med 55:395S–397S
14. Sundberg S, Kohvakka A, Gordin A (1988) Rapid reversal of circadian blood pressure rhythm in shift workers. J Hypertens 6:393–396
15. Baumgart P, Walger P, Fuchs G, Dorst KG, Vetter H, Rahm KH (1989) Twenty-four-hour blood pressure is not dependent on endogenous circadian rhythm. J Hypertens 7:331–334
16. Chau HP, Mallion JP, de Gaudemaris R, Ruche E, Siche JP, Pelen O, Mathern G (1989) Twenty-four-hour ambulatory blood pressure in shift workers. Circulation 80:341–347
17. Athanassiadis D, Draper GJ, Honour AJ, Cranston WI (1969) Variability of automatic blood pressure measurements over 24 hour periods. Clin Sci 36:147–156
18. Mann S, Millar-Craig MW, Melville DI, Balasubramanian V, Raftery EB (1979) Physical activity and the circadian rhythm of blood pressure. Clin Sci 57:291S–294S
19. Clark LA, Denby L, Pregibon D, Harshfield GA, Pickering TG, Blank S, Laragh JH (1987) A quantitative analysis of the effects of activity and time of day on the diurnal variations of blood pressure. J Chronic Dis 40:671–681

20. Pickering TG, Harshfield GA, Kleinert HD, Blank S, Laragh JH (1982) Blood pressure during normal daily activities, sleep, and exercise. Comparison of values in normal and hypertensive subjects. JAMA 247:992–996
21. Messerli FH, Glade LB, Ventura HO, Dreslinski GR, Suarez DH, MacPhee AA, Aristimuno GG, Cole FE, Frohlich ED (1982) Diurnal variations of cardiac rhythm, arterial pressure, and urinary catecholamines in borderline and established essential hypertension. Am Heart J 104:109–113
22. Pickering TG (1990) The clinical significance of diurnal blood pressure variations: dippers and nondippers. Circulation 81:700–702
23. Raftery EB (1984) Understanding hypertension. The contribution of direct ambulatory blood pressure monitoring. In: Weber MA, Drayer JIM (eds) Ambulatory blood pressure monitoring. Steinkopff, Darmstadt, pp 105–106
24. Verdecchia P, Schillaci G, Guerreri M, Gatteschi C, Benemia G, Boldrini F, Porcellati C (1990) Circadian blood pressure changes and left ventricular hypertrophy in essential hypertension. Circulation 81:528–536
25. Murphy MB, Nielson KS, Elliott WJ (1988) Racial differences in diurnal blood pressure profile. Am J Hypertens 1:55A
26. Wilson TW, Grim CM, Wilson DM, Carrett SS, Nicholson GD, Fraser HS, Hassell TA, Grim TE (1990) 24 hour blood pressure patterns in Barbadian blacks differ from US blacks. Circulation 8:726
27. Harshfield GA, Alpert BS, Willey ES, Somes GW, Murphy JK, Dupaul LM (1989) Race and gender influence ambulatory blood pressure patterns of adolescents. Hypertension 14:598–603
28. Campbell A, Converse PE, Rodgers WL (1976) The quality of American life. Russell Sage Foundation, New York
29. James GD, Moucha OP, Pickering TG (1990) The normal hourly variation of blood pressure in women: average patterns and the effects of work stress. Am J Hypertens 3:31A
30. Kasl SV Epidemiological contributions to the study of work stress. In: Cooper CL, Payne R (eds) Stress at work. Wiley, New York, pp 3–47
31. Harshfield GA, Pickering TG, Kleinert HD, Blank S, Laragh JH (1982) Situational variations of blood pressure in ambulatory hypertensive patients. Psychosom Med 44:237–245
32. James GD, Cates EM, Pickering TG, Laragh JH (1989) Parity and perceived job stress elevate blood pressure in young normotensive working women. Am J Hypertens 2:637–639
33. Pieper C, Schnall PL, Warren K, Pickering TG (1991) Comparison of ambulatory blood pressure and heart rate on a work day and a non-work day: evidence of a "carry-over effect" (to be published)
34. Devereux RB, Pickering TG, Harshfield GA, Kleinert HD, Denby L, Clark L, Pregibon D, Jason MN, Kleiner B, Borer JS, Laragh JH (1983) Left ventricular hypertrophy in patients with hypertension: importance of blood pressure response to regularly recurring stress. Circulation 68:479–476
35. Casale PN, Devereux RB, Milner M, Zullo G, Harshfield GA, Pickering TG, Laragh JH (1986) Value of echocardiographic measurement of left ventricular mass in predicting cardiovascular morbid events in hypertensive men. Ann Int Med 105:173–178
36. Levy D, Garrison RJ, Savage DD, Kannel WB, Castelli WP (1989) Left ventricular mass and incidence of coronary heart disease in an elderly cohort. The Framingham Heart Study. Ann Intern Med 110:101–107
37. Karasek R, Baker D, Marxer F, Ahlbohm A, Theorell T (1981) Job decision latitude, job demands, and cardiovascular disease: a prospective study of Swedish men. Am J Public Health 75:694–705
38. Alfredsson L, Karasek R, Theorell T (1982) Myocardial infarction risk and psychosocial work environment: an analysis of the male Swedish working force. Soc Sci Med 16:463–467
39. Karasek RA, Theorell T, Schwartz JE, Schnall PL, Pieper CF, Michela JL (1988) Job characteristics in relation to the prevalence of myocardial infarction in the US Health Examination Survey (HES) and the Health and Nutrition Examination Survey (HANES). Am J Public Health 78:910–918

40. Schnall PL, Pieper C, Karasek RA, Schwartz JE, Pickering TG (1990) The relationship between job strain and diastolic blood pressure and left ventricular mass index: results of a case control study. JAMA 263:1929–1935
41. De Simone G, Devereux RB, Roman MJ, Schlussel Y, Alderman MH, Laragh JH (1991) Echocardiographic left ventricular mass and electrolyte intake predict subsequent hypertension in initially normotensive adults. Ann Intern Med 114:202–209
42. Julius S, Li L, Brant D, Krause L, Buda AJ (1989) Neurogenic pressor episodes fail to cause hypertension, but do induce cardiac hypertrophy. Hypertension 13:422–429
43. Schnall PL, Pieper C, Schwartz JE, Karasek R, Schlussel YR, Devereux RB, Warren K, Pickering TG (1992) The relationship between job strain, alcohol, and ambulatory blood pressure. Hypertension (in press)
44. Frankenhaueser M, Lundberg U, Fredrikson M, Melin B, Tuomisto M, Myrsten A-L (1989) Stress on and off the job as related to sex and occupational status in white-collar workers. J Org Behav 10:321–346
45. Muller JE, Tofler GH, Stone PH (1989) Circadian variation and triggers of onset of acute cardiovascular disease. Circulation 70:733–743

Impact of Shifted Sleeping and Working Phases on Diurnal Blood Pressure Rhythm

P. Baumgart

The 24-h blood pressure rhythm is usually characterized by higher levels during daytime and lower levels at night. This rhythm is frequently altered in certain diseases [1–5] and hence has gained clinical interest. A number of bioparameters such as body temperature and plasma cortisol levels are largely dependent on an internal clock in their circadian rhythm. Circadian 24-h body temperature after a transmeridian flight adapts only with considerable delay to the new sleep-wakefulness cycle [6]; sleep deprivation does not significantly affect the circadian rhythm of cortisol levels [7]. In animals, the blood pressure rhythm closely follows the sleep-wakefullness cycle. In nocturnal animals, such as rats, it is high during activity at night and lower during the daytime resting period [8, 9]. Many physiological parameters exhibit a so-called free-running rhythm in animals when they are kept in constant darkness or in constant light [10, 11]. Whether the blood pressure continues following sleep and activities in animals during deprivation from external time triggers has yet to be established.

Since 24-h ambulatory blood pressure monitoring (ABPM) by portable recorders has become feasible, the characteristics of 24-h blood pressure variations can be assessed noninvasively in man. Clark et al. investigated the impact of time triggers on 24-h blood pressure rhythm in normal time schedules [12]. Covariance analysis of the effects of activity and time of day on diurnal blood pressure variations gave no evidence for an important circadian rhythm. After allowing for the effects of activity on blood pressure, where sleep was one of the activities, there was no significant diurnal variation of blood pressure.

The impact of internal or external time triggers on diurnal blood pressure rhythm in man can be evaluated by the resistance against shifts of activity and sleep such as in slowly rotated shift work and in flight across time zones. We investigated the resistance of 24-h blood pressure rhythm by ABPM in shift workers [13]. Seventeen workers at a chemical factory, having a weekly-rotated three-shift schedule underwent 24-h ABPM during the morning shift and during the night shift on Fridays (after 5 days of adjustment to the respective schedule). Blood pressure was measured every 30 min by oscillometric recorders (SpaceLabs 90202, Redmont, WA, USA). The morning shift lasted from 6 A.M. to 2 P.M., the night shift from 10 P.M. to 6 A.M. The group 24-h blood pressure profiles are presented in Fig. 1. In the morning shift as in the night shift, blood pressure was

Schmidt/Engel/Blümchen (Eds.)
Temporal Variations of the Cardiovascular System
© Springer-Verlag Berlin Heidelberg 1992

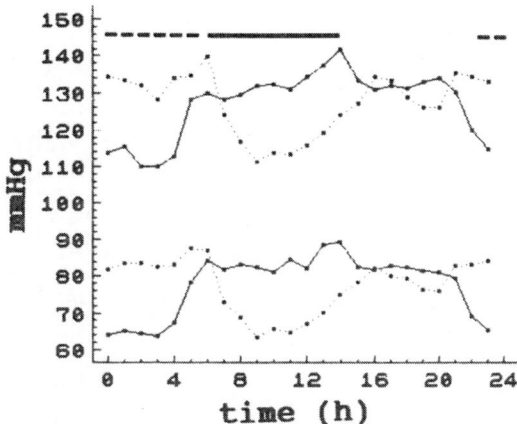

Fig. 1. Hourly mean systolic and diastolic blood pressure of 17 shift workers during daytime work (————), and nighttime work (-----)

Table 1. Average blood pressure (mmHg) of 17 shift workers in 24-h and in various time segments. Mean values (±SEM) during morning and night shifts

	Morning shift	Night shift
24 h	127.6±2.1/78.4±1.5	127.6±1.4/77.9±1.2
8 A.M.–8 P.M.	133.4±2.2/83.8±1.7	122.2±1.5/72.8±1.1
8 P.M.–8 A.M.	121.3±2.2/72.5±1.5	132.5±1.7/82.6±1.5
Sleep	112.5±1.9/64.4±1.6	114.1±1.5/65.3±1.4
Work	132.4±2.3/83.8±1.7	133.3±1.7/83.8±1.6

substantially lower during sleep and higher at work. Diurnal fluctuations had comparable amplitudes in both shifts.

During both shifts the 24-h mean values during sleep and at work were almost identical (Table 1). In the night shift, mean nighttime values were equal to the daytime values in the morning shift; daytime blood pressure of the night shift corresponded to the nighttime blood pressure of the morning shift. The phase difference between the two 24-h blood pressure curves was assessed by cross-correlation analysis. The resulting phase difference was exactly 8 h – corresponding to the lag of 8 h between the two working periods (Fig. 2).

To study whether the reentrainment had occurred immediately or gradually over the 5 days, ABPM was repeated in five subjects again on day 1 (Monday) of the night shift. Figure 3 indicates that there were no major differences between the 24-h blood pressure curves of day 1 and day 5 after shift rotation. Hence, the adaptation of the 24-h blood pressure rhythm occurred immediately.

The 24-h heart rate profiles also followed the 24-h blood pressure characteristics after shift rotation. Regardless of the working shift, heart rate levels were low during sleeping periods and high at work (Fig. 4). As with the 24-h blood pressure curves, the 24-h heart rate profiles were also almost completely reversed on day 1 after shift rotation (Fig. 5).

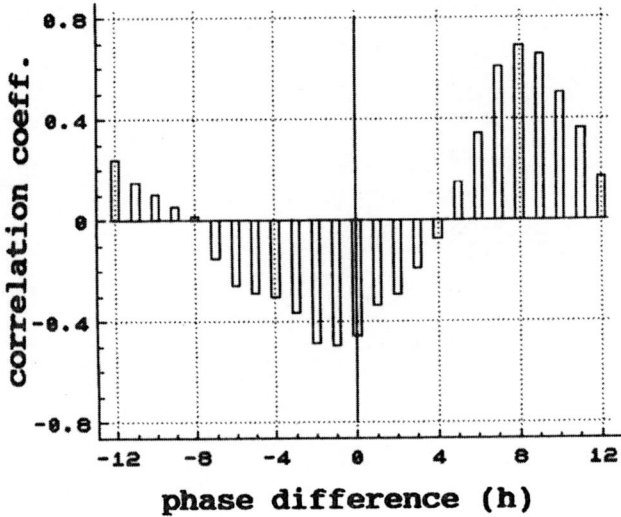

Fig. 2. Cross-correlation coefficients between systolic 24-h blood pressure profiles of the morning and night shift. The phase difference at maximal correlation (8 h) corresponds to the lag between the two working periods

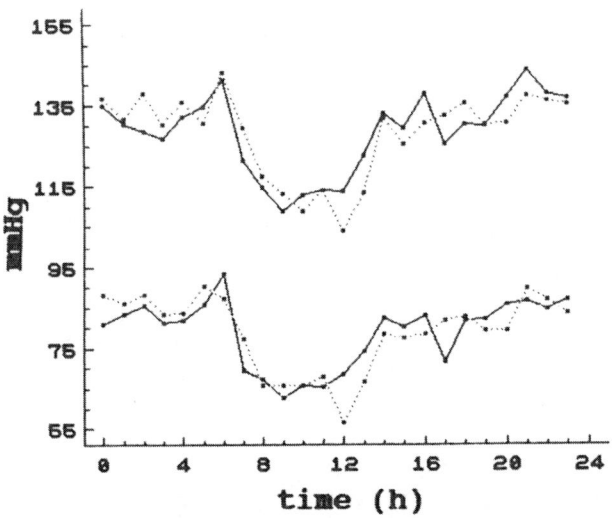

Fig. 3. Hourly mean systolic and diastolic blood pressure of five shift workers during the 1st (——) and 5th (·····) days of the night-shift week

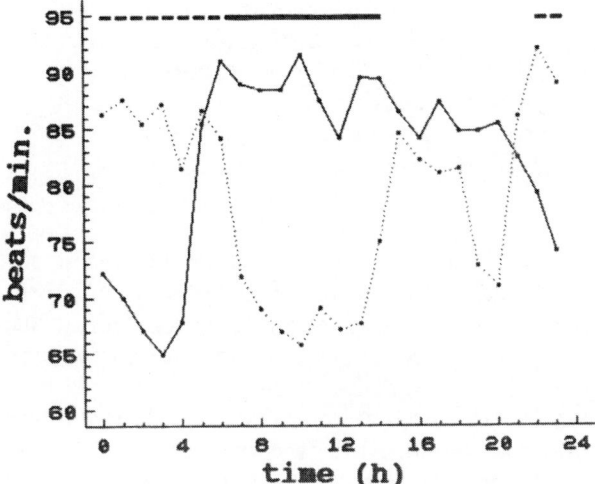

Fig. 4. Hourly mean heart rate of 17 shift workers during daytime work (———), and night-time work (– – – –). Working periods see Fig. 1

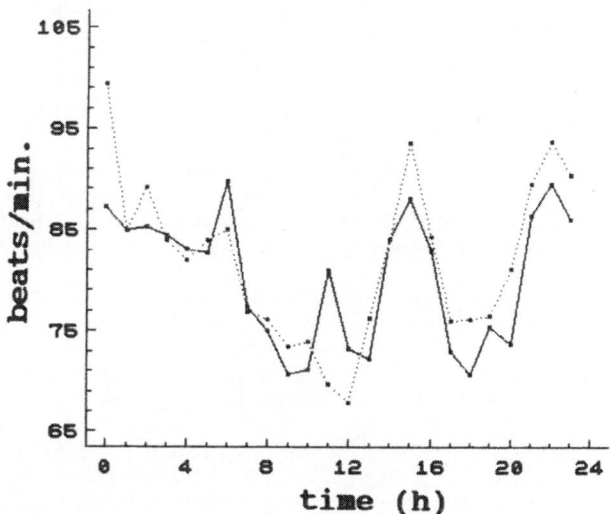

Fig. 5. Hourly mean heart rate of five workers during the 1st (———) and 5th (·····) days of the night-shift week. Working periods see Fig. 1

Similar investigations of 24-h blood pressure in shift workers were performed by Sundberg et al. [14]. Also in this study there was an immediate and complete reversal of the 24-h blood pressure curve after shift rotation closely following sleep and activities. Heart rate was also reversed, although less pronounced than blood pressure.

Another investigation of 24-h ABPM in shift workers was reported by Chau et al. [15]. Here 24-h blood pressure was assessed during the morning shift, afternoon shift, and night shift. In all three shifts, high blood pressure coincided with the working periods, and low blood pressure occurred during sleep. However, time-microscopic examination of 24-h blood pressure rhythm by Fourier analysis revealed some evidence for internal regulation which is not apparent from gross evaluation of the 24-h blood pressure curve. Similar results were reported by Halberg et al., applying cosinor analysis to 24-h blood pressure profiles of shift workers [16]. Also after transmeridian flights blood pressure rhythm exhibited rapid adjustment, which was incomplete at time series analysis [17, 18].

Summarizing the results from the various experiments, it can be concluded that the 24-h blood pressure curve is almost completely and immediately reversed after shifting of activity and sleeping periods. Influences of internal rhythm can only be detected by mathematical time-microscopic analysis. This strongly suggests that the circadian blood pressure rhythm is largely dependent on external time triggers whereas an internal clock may only play a minor role for 24-h blood pressure regulation.

References

1. Baumgart P (1989) 24 h-Blutdruck bei primärer und sekundärer Hypertonie. Herz 14: 246–250
2. Imai Y, Abe K, Sasaki S, Minami N, Niehi M, Munakata M, Murakami O, Matsue K, Sekino H, Miura Y, Yoshinaga K (1988) Altered circadian blood pressure rhythm in patients with Cushing's syndrome. Hypertension 12:11–19
3. Isaksson H, Svanborg E (1992) Obstructive sleep apnea syndrome in male hypertensives, refractory to drug therapy. Nocturnal automatic blood pressure measurements – an aid to diagnosis? Clin Exp Hypertens [A] (in press)
4. Middeke M, Mika E, Schreiber MA, Beck B, Wächter B, Holzgreve H (1989) Ambulante indirekte Blutdrucklangzeitmessung bei primärer und sekundärer Hypertonie. Klin Wochenschr 67:713–716
5. Schrader J, Person C, Pfertner U, Buhr-Schinner H, Schoel G, Warneke G, Haupt A, Scheler F (1989) Fehlender nächtlicher Blutdruckabfall in der 24-Stunden Blutdruckmessung: Hinweis auf eine sekundäre Hypertonie. Klin Wochenschr 67:659–665
6. Gander PH, Graeber RC, Anderson HT, Lauber JK (1989) Adjustment of sleep and the circadian temperature rhythm after flights across nine time zones. Aviat Space Environ Med 60:733–743
7. Moldofsky H, Lue FA, Davidson JR, Girczynski R (1989) Effects of sleep deprivation on human immune functions. FASEB J 3:1972–1977
8. Smith TL, Coleman TG, Stanek KA, Murphy WR (1987) Hemodynamic monitoring for 24 h in unanesthetized rats. Am J Physiol 253:H1335–H1341
9. Munakata M, Imai Y, Minami N, Sasaki S, Icijyo T, Yoshizawa M, Sekino H, Abe K, Yoshinaga K (1990) Cosinor analysis of changes in circadian blood pressure rhythm with aging in spontaneously hypertensive rats. Tohoku J Exp Med 161:55–64
10. Rusak B, Zucker I (1979) Neural regulation of circadian rhythms. Physiol Rev 59:449–526
11. Turek FW (1985) Circadian neural rhythms in mammals. Annu Rev Physiol 47:49–64

12. Clark LA, Denby L, Pregibon D, Harshfield GA, Pickering TG, Blank S, Laragh JH (1987) A quantitative analysis of the effects of activity and of time of day on the diurnal variations of blood pressure. J Chronic Dis 40:671–681
13. Baumgart P, Walger P, Fuchs G, von Eiff M, Rahn KH (1989) Diurnal variations of blood pressure in shift workers during day and night shifts. Int Arch Occup Environ Health 61:463–466
14. Sundberg S, Kohvakka A, Gordin A (1988) Rapid reversal of circadian blood pressure rhythm in shift workers. J Hypertens 6:292–296
15. Chau NP, Mallion JM, de Gaudemaris R, Ruche E, Siche JP, Pelen O, Mathern G (1989) Twenty-four-hour ambulatory blood pressure in shift workers. Circulation 80:341–347
16. Halberg JU, Halberg E, Cornelissen G, Hillman D, Sanchez de la Pena S, Wu JY, Otto S, Halberg F (1990) Chronobiologically deviant blood pressure in shift working police on metropolitan street duty. Prog Clin Biol Res 341 B:281–290
17. Cornelissen G (1988) Incomplete though very rapid circadian cardivascular adjustment after a transmeridian flight. J Minn Acad Sci 53:18
18. Pangerl A, März W, Halberg F (1986) Rapid but not abrupt transmeridian adjustment of circadian acrophase of systolic blood pressure. J Minn Acad Sci 51:15–16

How and How Often Should Blood Pressure Be Measured for Optimum Hypertension Control?

S. Eckert, H. Mannebach, H. Ohlmeier, J. Volmar, and U. Gleichmann

Introduction

The technique of 24-h indirect ambulatory blood pressure monitoring (ABPM) is gaining importance in the diagnosis and therapy of arterial hypertension. Devices with different measuring methods (auscultatory, oscillometric, or both) and individual choice of measuring intervals are available. The devices of the newest generation allow about 80 readings of systolic and diastolic values. At least 80 readings in 24 h are recommended in the Berlin Consensus Document of 1990. Mean systolic and diastolic pressure values during day- and nighttime and the number of readings above normal levels (WHO criteria) are calculated. The newly offered devices are light in weight, the pump is soft, the handling is easy, but the equipment is still expensive.

Blood pressure self-measurement (BP-SM) has also become very popular. This is important for lifelong control of hypertension and for the compliance of patients. Various studies confirm that blood pressure values taken by nurses, by automated devices, or measured by the patient himself are generally lower than those measured by the physician [1–3]. Values measured by the patients themselves correlate better with 24-h blood pressure readings than office blood pressure [4, 5]. Comparing ABPM with casual blood pressure readings, Brunner [2], Mancia [3], and Magometschnigg [6] showed that at least 40% of the patients are overtreated due to casual measurements.

Blood pressure can be measured continuously and discontinuously. Continuous methods using the volume clamp method of Peñáz [7] and the physiocal method of Wesseling [8] provide a beat-to-beat analysis and detection of short-term changes in blood pressure. The method of invasive blood pressure measurement in humans via intra-arterial brachial catheter (Oxford system [9, 10]) has not become common due to the risk of bleeding, infection and nerve lesion. The development of the portable noninvasive blood pressure recorder (Portapres) makes it possible to investigate blood pressure regulation during sleep and regular activities. Blood pressure can be measured discontinuously with the Doppler and piezo technique. Neither technique is very common. The sphygmomanometric and, in the past 3 years, the oscillometric techniques have become the most widely used procedures for discontinuous measurements of arterial blood pressure in daily routine.

Schmidt/Engel/Blümchen (Eds.)
Temporal Variations of the Cardiovascular System
© Springer-Verlag Berlin Heidelberg 1992

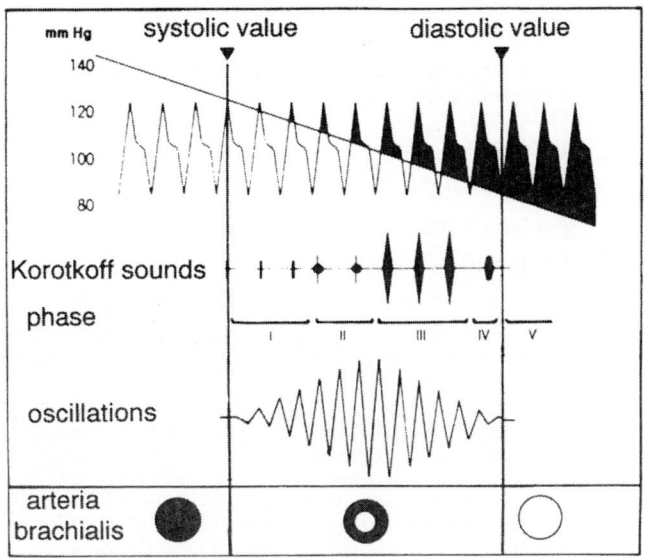

Fig. 1. Blood pressure measurements: invasive and noninvasive measurement by Korotkoff sounds or oscillations during deflating of an occluded cuff

Von Recklinghausen [11] introduced the oscillometric method in 1940. This method has been strongly criticized in the past because pulse pressure may be influenced by cardiac output, peripheral resistance, and stiffness of the artery [12, 13]. The accuracy of this method was recently improved after computer-assisted calculation was introduced in the 1980s. Arterial pulse waves are transmitted via the cuff. The cuff is inflated up to a pressure of 30 mm Hg above the systolic blood pressure and then slowly deflated at 2–3 mm Hg/s to a pressure below diastolic blood pressure [14]. While the cuff is being deflated, the first detectable oscillations establish the systolic value of blood pressure, whereas the last detectable oscillations establish the diastolic value (Fig. 1).

The main goal of our study was do determine whether more than two blood BP-SM readings during daytime enable us to optimize hypertension control. First, we verified the accuracy of some of the newly offered automatic devices used for BP-SM (first study). Then we determined the frequency of readings for an optimum hypertension control (second study). Finally we established whether repeated BP-SM is sufficient for therapeutic decision making (third study).

Methods

First Study. In 253 patients the blood pressure was measured simultaneously by invasive and noninvasive methods (devices 1–6, Table 1) following diagnostic heart catheterization (supine position, stable hemodynamics, pigtail catheter placed in the ascending aorta). Of the 253 patients 72 were women (aged 23–73, with an upper arm circumference of 21–29 cm) and 153 men (aged 43–70, with an

Table 1. Tested devices for BP-SM on the upper arm and on the left index finger

	Device	Method	Technique
1	Bosch-272	Sphygmomanometric	Semiautomatic
2	Roland digital automatic	Sphygmomanometric	Fully automatic
3	Hestia Visomat OZ 1	Oscillometric	Semiautomatic
4	Boso oscillomat	Oscillometric	Fully automatic
Auto-inflate digital blood pressure monitor			
5	Luminoscope	Oscillometric	Fully automatic
6	Omron	Oscillometric	Fully automatic

Table 2. Testing of automatic blood pressure systems: correlation of non-invasive/invasive and auscultatory/oscillometric values (total 1212 measurements in 253 patients)

	Device	Method	Systolic	Diastolic	n
1	Bosch-272	Sphygmomanometric/invasive	0.90	0.70	39
2	Roland digital automatic	Sphygmomanometric/invasive	0.89	0.83	36
3a	Hestia Visomat OZ 1	Oscillometric/invasive	0.80	0.69	55
3b	Hestia Visomat OZ 1	Korotkoff/invasive	0.84	0.69	55
3c	Hestia Visomat OZ 1	Korotkoff/oscillometric	0.96	0.89	55
4	Boso Oscillomat	Oscillometric/invasive	0.84	0.77	73
5	Luminoscope	Oscillometric/invasive	0.85	0.61	25
6	Omron	Oscillometric/invasive	0.56	0.39	25
Range (mm Hg)			96–207	43–100	

upper arm circumference of 25–31 cm). A total of 506 invasive measurements were carried out on these patients. The results of invasive (mean value of four cycles) and noninvasive readings were compared (Table 2). With the boso-oscillomat, the data of 14 measurements can be stored at any time and printed out afterwards. The process can be repeated as often as required. With the Visomat, blood pressure can also be measured auscultatorily at the same time, which allowed us to compare three different techniques. We tested these simultaneously in the same set of 55 patients. With the autoinflate digital blood pressure monitor BP-SM can be performed easily on the left index finger. Persons with thin and cold fingers may have problems. In the case of ten women with anorexia nervosa and cold fingers measurements with the Luminoscope were impossible.

Second Study. In this study 50 patients with treated arterial hypertension of mild to severe degree were included. There were 18 women and 32 men aged 21–84 years. All patients underwent ABPM with the Space-Labs 90207. The measurements were carried out every 20 min from 6 A.M. to 10 P.M. The mean number of readings per patient was 41 ± 3.5 (Table 4). To find out the optimum number of readings for therapeutic decisions we subdivided the data obtained with ABPM into three periods. Thereafter we randomly selected four, three, two, and one reading, respectively, out of each period. We then compared the therapeutic decisions of two cardiologists whether to change or to continue with the present therapy based on the stepwise reduced data as compared with the full data.

Third Study. To determine whether repeated BP-SM is feasible and sufficient for therapeutic decisions, 15 patients with treated arterial hypertension underwent blood pressure monitoring during daytime with Space-Labs 90207. The patients were also asked to measure their blood pressure with the boso-oscillomat in 1-h intervals on the other arm (12 ± 2 measurements were analyzed). The difference in blood pressure values between the left and right upper arms was below 10 mm Hg. After a short instruction all patients were able to perform blood pressure self-measurements with the fully automated device on their own and without any problems. The data obtained with both systems were analyzed in a blind test by three cardiologists experienced in analyzing blood pressure profiles. Their decisions whether to change or maintain the present therapy were compared.

Results

First Study. High correlations were found between invasive measurements and both the sphygmomanometric and oscillometric methods concerning systolic values and weaker correlations concerning diastolic values (devices 1–4, Table 1; correlation coefficients, Table 2). There is a very high correlation between the measurements for the oscillometric and the auscultatory methods; the correlation coefficient for systolic values was 0.96 and for diastolic values was 0.89. The differences between the mean systolic and diastolic values measured by the oscillometric systems used on the upper arm and those measured invasively show that by the oscillometric method there is a tendency to slight underestimation of the systolic and overestimation of the diastolic values of blood pressure (Table 3).

Table 3. Differences between the mean systolic and diastolic values measured invasively by Boso oscillomat (oscillometric I) and Hestia Visomat (oscillometric II)

Method	n	Indirect [b]	Invasive [c]	Difference
		Systolic BP (mmHg)		
Oscillometric I	73	133 ± 21	138 ± 24	−5
Oscillometric II [a]	55	132 ± 20	138 ± 25	−6
Korotkoff [a]	55	132 ± 21	138 ± 25	−6
		Diastolic BP (mmHg)		
Oscillometric I	73	78 ± 11	76 ± 10	+2
Oscillometric II [a]	55	76 ± 11	75 ± 10	+1
Korotkoff [a]	55	79 ± 10	75 ± 10	+4

[a] Measured simultaneously in the same patients.
[b] Coefficient of variation 15.8% – 15.9% for Systolic BP and 17.3% – 18.1% for Diastolic BP.
[c] Coefficient of variation 12.6% – 14.5% for Systolic BP and 13.1% – 13.3% for Diastolic BP.

Table 4. How often should blood pressure be measured? Full data set (41 ± 3.5 readings) during daytime (6 A.M. – 10 P.M.) and stepwise data by random selection of 12, 9, 6 and 3 readings

Period of the day					Number of selected values			
06:07	110	74	85	41				
06:27	99	60	77	49				
06:47	95	71	79	73				
07:07	98	75	83	56				
07:27	96	68	79	47				
07:47	97	63	74	45				
09:30	111	70	83	52				
09:47	107	69	80	49	4	3	2	1
10:07	104	75	83	47				
10:27	112	73	88	46				
10:47	106	72	82	46				
11:07	109	75	86	44				
11:27	117	74	91	48				
11:47	111	77	88	45				
12:10	127	92	99	50				
12:27	119	73	82	59				
12:47	105	75	86	65				
13:07	101	62	71	52				
13:27	105	66	84	50				
13:47	111	61	72	52				
14:27	130	90	100	56				
14:47	109	76	88	53	4	3	2	1
15:27	119	76	87	54				
15:47	108	75	86	50				
16:10	111	75	87	63				
16:27	111	76	90	50				
16:47	127	83	101	56				
17:07	125	84	93	54				
17:27	122	76	91	47				
17:47	127	81	96	48				
18:07	111	76	87	61				
18:27	108	62	82	70				
18:47	110	62	76	65				
19:07	113	64	77	61				
19:27	103	68	81	79	4	3	2	1
19:47	106	61	73	55				
20:07	104	65	77	54				
20:27	106	66	79	55				
20:49	96	68	76	74				
21:07	103	63	75	47				
21:37	103	61	75	47				
21:37	109	63	77	46				
	41 ± 3.5				12	9	6	3

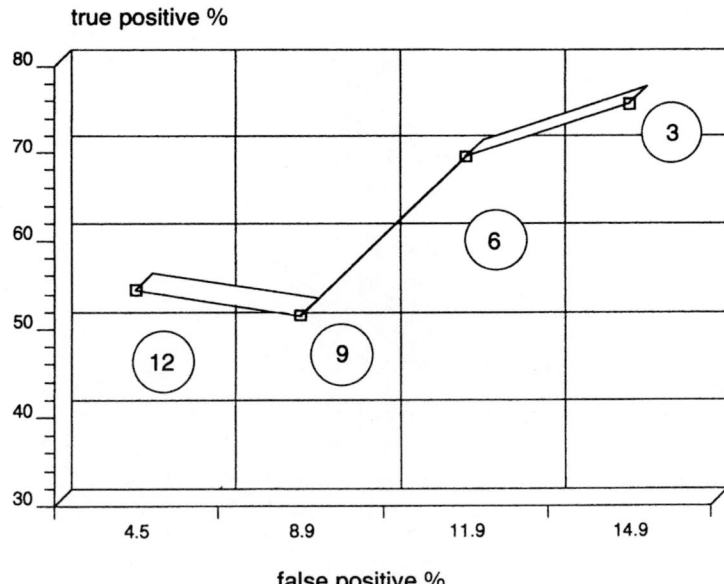

Fig. 2. How often should blood pressure be measured? Receiver operator characteristic curve: therapeutic decisions whether to change or to continue with therapy taken by two cardiologists. *Numbers in circles*, number of selected values from the full data set of 41 ± 3.5 readings (*n* = 50)

Second Study. With full data set, therapy was changed in 33%. The overall agreement in therapeutic decisions with reduced data sets ranged from 78% to 82%. The receiver-operator characteristic curve showed that the best corresponding decisions were made using six readings with 70% true-positive and 12% false-positive changes as compared with decisions based on the full set of data (Fig. 2). True positive means agreement and false positive disagreement of therapeutic decision.

Third Study. In 80% of all cases therapeutic decisions based on ABPM and repeated BP-SM were identical. We found agreement between the two methods in decision making in 80%. In 66% of different decisions change of therapy was based on single and short-term increases in blood pressure registered with ABPM.

Discussion

We can recommend the electronic devices for BP-SM using the sphygmomanometric and oscillometric method on the upper arm tested in our study. Oscillometric devices are easy to handle and may have some advantages over those devices using the sphygmomanometric method.

Using the Finapres system Veermann and coworkers [15] showed that while manually inflating the cuff for BP-SM there was a transient rise in blood pressure due to muscle activity. They found a rise in systolic blood pressure of 13 and

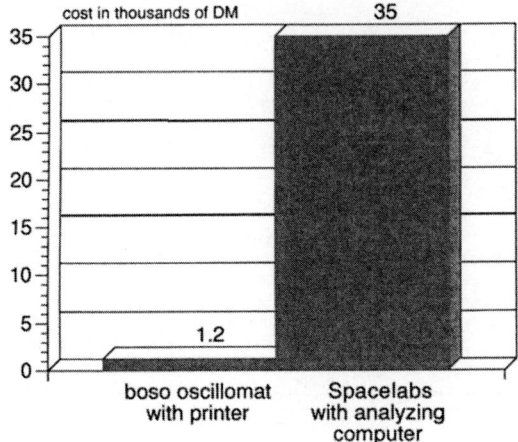

Fig. 3. Comparison of list prices for boso oscillomat and Spacelabs 90207 (two devices each)

12 mm Hg (hypertensive and normotensive subjects, respectively). The systolic blood pressure took an average of 7 s and at most 21 s to return to baseline level after stopping cuff inflation. To be certain that the blood pressure is measured correctly, we therefore recommend a fully automatic device for BP-SM. The equipment for ABPM is still expensive. Figure 3 shows the cost (list prices) for two devices: the boso-oscillomat with a storage capacity of 14 measurements and printer, each at DM 600 and the Space-Labs system with analyzing computer, about DM 13,000 for the computer and about DM 11,000 for each device.

We have shown that repeated BP-SM is useful for controlling treated arterial hypertension. The majority of the indications for 24-h blood pressure monitoring among patients staying in our clinic in 1989 for diagnosis and treatment of various cardiovascular diseases was for controlling treated arterial hypertension (80%), diagnosis of arterial hypertension (14%), and discriminating primary from secondary arterial hypertension (6%). The total number was 715, 17% of all patients. We recommend ABPM mostly for clinical questions and research.

Conclusions

Fully automatic devices for BP-SM using the oscillometric method on the upper arm are highly recommendable because of their simple handling and the reliable technique. For the time being BP-SM on the finger using the oscillometric method can not be generally recommended as an alternative to BP-SM on the upper arm. Optimum control of hypertension by self-measurement should be based on about six readings during daytime. Because of the lower cost, this represents an alternative to the established blood pressure monitoring, unless nocturnal blood pressure measurements are necessary. In our opinion the main indication for repeated BP-SM is the control of treated arterial hypertension. Of course it is not appropriate for differentiation of primary and secondary arterial hypertension, nor for exertional arterial hypertension or for observation of day and night variation. Further studies will have to show whether repeated BP-SM is appropriate for controlling borderline hypertension and for screening of arterial hypertension.

References

1. Mancia G et al. (1983) Effects of blood pressure measurement by the doctor on patients blood pressure and heart rate. Lancet 2:695–697
2. Brunner H (1987) Selbstmessung und 24-Stunden-Blutdruckprofile als Grundlage für epidemiologische Schlußfolgerungen. In: Magometschnigg D (ed) Blutdruckselbstkontrolle. Uhlen, Vienna, p 384
3. Mancia G (1987) Bewertung der Hypertonie mit Hilfe des Belastungsblutdruckes, des 24-Stunden-Blutdruckprofils und der Blutdruckselbstmessung. In: Magometschnigg D (ed) Blutdruckselbstkontrolle. Uhlen, Vienna, p 63
4. Perloff D, Sokolow M (1978) The representative blood pressure: usefulness of office, basal, home and ambulatory readings. Cardiovasc Med 3(6):655
5. Floras JS et al. (1981) Cuff and ambulatory blood pressure in subjects with essential hypertension. Lancet 2:107
6. Magometschnigg D (1989) Clinical relevance of casual blood pressure readings versus self-measurement. In: Meyer-Sabellek W et al. (eds) Blood pressure measurements. Steinkopff, Darmstadt
7. Peñáz J (1973) Photoelectrical measurement of blood pressure, volume and flow in the finger. Digest of the 10th international conference on medical and biological engineering, Dresden, p 104
8. Wesseling KH (1988) Finapres-Kontinuierliche, nichtinvasive arterielle Blutdruckmessung am Finger nach der Methode von Peñáz. In: Meyer-Sabellek W, Gotzen R (eds) Indirekte 24-Stunden-Blutdruckmessung. Steinkopff, Darmstadt
9. Bevan AT et al. (1966) Portable recorder for continuous arterial pressure measurement in man. J Physiol (Lond) 186:3
10. Millar-Craig MW (1978) A new system for reading ambulatory blood pressure in man. Med Biol Eng Comput 16:727
11. von Recklinghausen H (1940) Blutdruckmessung und Kreislauf in den Arterien des Menschen. Steinkopff, Dresden
12. Forster FK (1987) Oscillometric determination of diastolic, mean and systolic blood pressure – a numerical model. J Biomech Eng 108:359–364
13. Friesen RH, Lictor JL (1981) Indirect measurement of blood pressure in neonates and infants utilizing an automatic noninvasive oscillometric monitor. Anesth Analg 60:742–745
14. Frohlich ED et al. (1988) Report of a special task force appointed by the Steering Committee, American Heart Association: Recommendations for human blood pressure determination by sphygmomanometers. Hypertension 11:209A–222A
15. Veerman DP et al. (1990) Effects of cuff inflation on self-recorded blood pressure. Lancet 335:451–453

Sleep-Related Breathing Disorders and Nocturnal Hypertension

J. Mayer and J. H. Peter

Introduction

For a long time, the investigation and description of diseases was related to changes which could be observed and measured during the day. In recent years there has been an increasing awareness that pathological states also occur during the night. These escape detection by usual methods and require techniques of investigation which can also be used in sleep. Since the 1970s sleep-related disturbances of breathing (in particular sleep apnea) have been increasingly explored on the basis of this approach.

The obstructive sleep apnea syndrome is characterized by a complete or incomplete obstruction of the pharynx. In partial obstruction, there is continuous obstructive snoring. In complete obstruction (occlusion), there is obstructive apnea with intermittent (mostly loud) snoring, especially during the hyperventilation terminating the apnea. The difference between these two forms of snoring is quantitative rather than qualitative. Continuous nonobstructive or primary snoring which (like obstructive snoring) is caused by vibration of the soft palate and the lateral wall of the pharynx, is to be distinguished from snoring caused by partial obstruction. By definition, this form of snoring has no effects on blood gases or hemodynamics. Accordingly, it is to be rated as rather harmless in most cases [12]. A more precise differentiation of the various forms of snoring and their pathophysiological classification is being investigated in studies currently in progress.

Acute alterations of blood pressure correlated with individual phases of apnea are observed in polysomnographic measurements. As a rule, the following blood pressure profile is found: a fall at the beginning of the phase of apnea, a plateau with a slight fall or even a rise during the apneic phase, and an overshoot rise of blood pressure during the hyperventilation terminating the apnea. During the latter phase, rises of systolic blood pressure to more than 300 mm Hg have been observed. The blood pressure values reached during an obstructive apnea are indeed still underestimated, since the transmural pressure must be considered because of the highly negative intrathoracic pressure fluctuations, so that the endinspiratory values are in fact about 10% higher than those measured in the periphery [24]. This results from the calibration of the values measured intra-

Schmidt/Engel/Blümchen (Eds.)
Temporal Variations of the Cardiovascular System
© Springer-Verlag Berlin Heidelberg 1992

arterially against the atmospheric pressure at the level of the right atrium and not against the esophageal pressure, which has the actual intrathoracic pressure as reference value. The same also applies in principle to the blood pressure in obstructive snoring. We were able to show that the blood pressure rises during 2- to 10-min phases of obstructive snoring and sometimes reaches higher values than in obstructive apnea [14, 18].

Various factors are discussed as causes for the effects on the blood pressure profile, including biochemical, autonomic, and mechanical changes induced by the apnea. These comprise hypoxemia and hypercapnia, endocrine mechanisms such as activation of catecholamine, and the renin-angiotensin-aldosterone system. They also include effects on the production of atrial natriuretic factor and further effects on the sympathetic system caused by the central nervous arousal reactions associated with the apnea as well as the disturbed sleep structure. Finally, the effects on blood pressure may also be caused by mechanical factors, leading to variations in intrathoracic pressure and thus to alterations in the hemodynamics of the systemic and pulmonary circulation resulting from repeated Müller maneuvers during apnea [3, 22]. The specific individual role of all these factors has not yet been established at present.

It is to be suspected that in the course of time the mechanisms described (which lead to an appreciable variability in blood pressure during sleep) also give rise to an increase in blood pressure values during the day. This is indicated by the results of numerous epidemiological studies. It has been described that the frequency of sleep apnea in patients with arterial hypertension is up to 50%, whereas arterial hypertension is found in up to 90% of patients with sleep apnea [4, 8–10, 20, 21, 25]. With a prevalence of sleep apnea between 1% and 10%, a large number of patients is affected [6, 11, 16, 25, 27]. In addition, a large number of patients with obstructive sleep apnea and only mild hypertension or indeed normal values of blood pressure by day display appreciable rises in arterial blood pressure at night during sleep. The cardiovascular risk of this group of patients is increased. In order to attain an effective therapy, the underlying disorder of nocturnal breathing should be considered.

For the therapy of the sleep apnea syndrome, we have developed a graduated schedule which is oriented to the degree of severity of the breathing disorder [23]. General measures such as regularization of the sleep/wake cycle, attainment of normal weight, avoidance of central sedatives, relaxants, and respiratory depressants (e.g., alcohol and also tranquilizers and hypnotics) are of primary importance. In mild to moderate sleep apnea, pharmacotherapy takes second place. Low-dose theophylline preparations (serum levels 5–10 µg/ml) are given to treat apnea [15].

Breathing by nasal continuous positive airway pressure (nCPAP) has become established as the therapy of choice in recent years in severe sleep apnea [28]. Tracheostomy, which was formerly used efficiently in treatment, has been replaced by nCPAP respiration (apart from a few exceptional cases). Other surgical measures such as uvulo-palato-pharyngoplasty (UPPP) are subject to dispute since they have a less than 50% rate of success, and it is not possible to predict the result of therapy with certainty since irreversible side effects may be caused in some cases by the clearance of pharyngeal tissue, and other methods may no longer be successfully applied [5]. A study by He et al. demonstrated that the mortality in sleep apnea is raised, and that this raised risk is abolished by nCPAP therapy but not by UPPP [7].

The treatment of sleep apnea is nowadays based mainly on pharmacotherapeutic and mechanical methods besides general treatment measures. The effects of nCPAP therapy and the effects of an antihypertensive drug therapy in patients with sleep apnea and arterial hypertension are described below.

nCPAP Therapy in Sleep Apnea and Arterial Hypertension

In a study comprising 20 men with sleep apnea [apnea index 61 (range 50–79) phases of apnea per hour of sleep], the effect of nCPAP therapy was investigated after 3 days of treatment [17]. Eighteen of the 20 patients had arterial hypertension with diastolic blood pressure values in excess of 95 mm Hg measured at three separate times with the method of Riva Rocci. Fifteen patients had NYHA stages 1 or 2 heart failure (New York Heart Association). Four patients displayed coronary heart disease. Any medication with antihypertensive action was discontinued at least 1 week before the measurements. The polysomnographic measurements in the sleep laboratory registered the breathing activity via one induction-plethysmographic belt in the region of the thorax and another in the region of the abdomen (Respitrace system) as well as via a nasal thermistor. The transcutaneous oxygen saturation was also measured (Ohmeda). To classify the sleep stages, two standard recordings of EEG, EMG, and EOG were taken and evaluated in accordance with the criteria of Rechtschaffen and Kales [26]. The cardiovascular parameters were registered by means of long-term ECG, and intra-arterial blood pressure was measured by means of a catheter in the brachial artery via a pressure transducer (Statham) and processed beat-to-beat with a mainframe computer.

After 2 nights of baseline measurement, the patients were adapted to nCPAP therapy during a further 2 nights. One night was then measured under nCPAP therapy observing the same conditions as those for the baseline measurement.

Without therapy, the highest systolic and diastolic blood pressure values were found during REM sleep. However, a statistically significant difference was not found between the values measured in the waking phase (30 min before falling asleep and 30 min after waking up) and the values during non-REM and REM sleep. Under nCPAP therapy, a reduction in blood pressure was found during all sleep and waking phases. It is noteworthy that the blood pressure values during the sleep phases (non-REM and REM sleep) were lower than during the waking phase. The blood pressure profile during baseline is comparable to the profiles such as are also found in secondary hypertension. A restoration of the physiological profile of nocturnal blood pressure was thus found under therapy, besides the normalization of the absolute values.

Long-Term Results Under nCPAP Therapy

In accordance with the same design as that specified above, 12 men with sleep apnea (apnea index over 30 per hour) and arterial hypertension (diastolic blood pressure in the sitting position over 95 mm Hg at three different times of measurement) were investigated after 6 months of nCPAP therapy [13]. For clinical data see Table 1. In addition to the invasive measurement of blood pressure during the night, a noninvasive measurement of blood pressure with the method of Riva Rocci was carried out in the sitting position during the day at 8 A.M., 12 A.M., and 4 P.M. All patients showed clinical symptoms of heart failure (NYHA 1 or 2) but showed no enlargement of the heart and no restriction of pump function in the echocardiogram. According to clinical criteria and the exercise ECG, none of the patients had coronary heart disease. Two patients displayed latent pulmonary hypertension. In cases of ongoing antihypertensive medication, the therapy was discontinued at least 1 week before the baseline measurements and during the entire 6 months of nCPAP therapy. Only patients who regularly used their nCPAP instrument during the therapy phase were included in the study.

The apnea index was lowered from 58 (46–73) to 2 (0–7) apneas per hour ($p < 0.01$). The indirect noninvasively measured rise in blood pressure by day showed a fall in the systolic values from 169.3 (range 151–180) mm Hg to 138.3 (range 123–144) mm Hg ($p < 0.01$) under nCPAP therapy. The diastolic values fell from 104.1 (range 97–116) mm Hg to 87.1 (range 70–95) ($p < 0.01$). The values measured invasively during the night also showed a fall in the values for systole from 147.1 (± 1.5) mm Hg to 126.4 (± 1.5) mm Hg ($p < 0.001$) and for diastole from 81.6 (± 0.8) mm Hg to 69.4 (± 0.7) mm Hg ($p < 0.001$). The difference between the higher indirectly measured and lower invasively measured values is attributable mainly to the differences between the technique and time of measurement (day as opposed to night).

With regard to the analysis of blood pressure in relation to the stage of sleep, the baseline measurements showed the same quality of results as that obtained in the short-term study. Under therapy, lowering of blood pressure was found to normalize again during the waking phase and in the non-REM and REM stages of sleep with restoration of the physiological profile of blood pressure at night

Table 1. Clinical data without therapy and after 6 months of nCPAP therapy ($n = 12$)

	No therapy	nCPAP	p
Age (years)	50 (38–64)		
Weight (kg)	89 (74–110)	89 (77–110)	n.s.
BMI (kg/m²)	29.3 (25.4–38.5)	29.3 (25.0–38.5)	n.s.
AI (n/h)	58 (46–73)	2 (0–7)	$p < 0.01$

BMI, Body mass index; AI, apnea index.

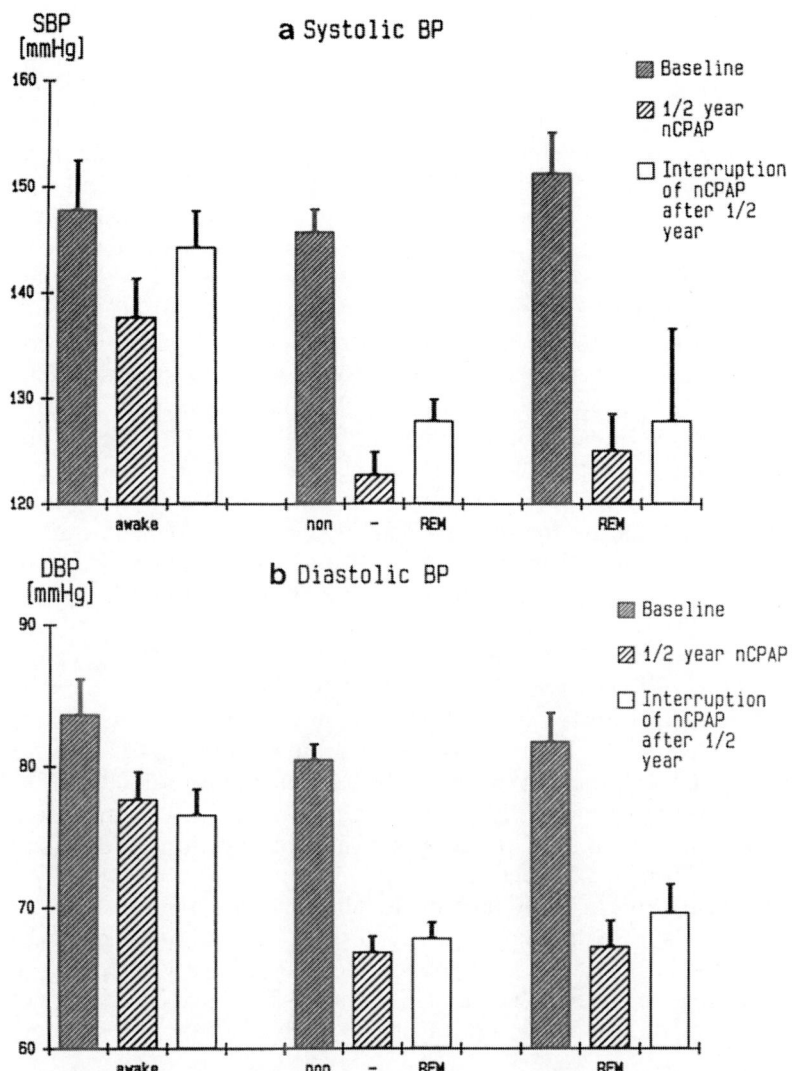

Fig. 1. Systolic (**a**) and diastolic (**b**) blood pressure during waking and sleep (stages non-REM and REM sleep) without therapy on baseline, after 6 months of nCPAP therapy and after interruption of nCPAP. Mean values and 95% confidence intervals

(Fig. 1). In addition, the variability of blood pressure was determined. It was calculated over the range of the measurement values in consecutive 10-min intervals for the entire measurement night. Without therapy, the variability during non-REM and REM sleep was higher than during the waking phase. On the other hand, it was lower than during the waking phase in both stages of sleep under therapy (Fig. 2).

For the first time, we were able to demonstrate that nCPAP therapy leads not only to normalization of the nocturnal breathing pattern but also to normaliza-

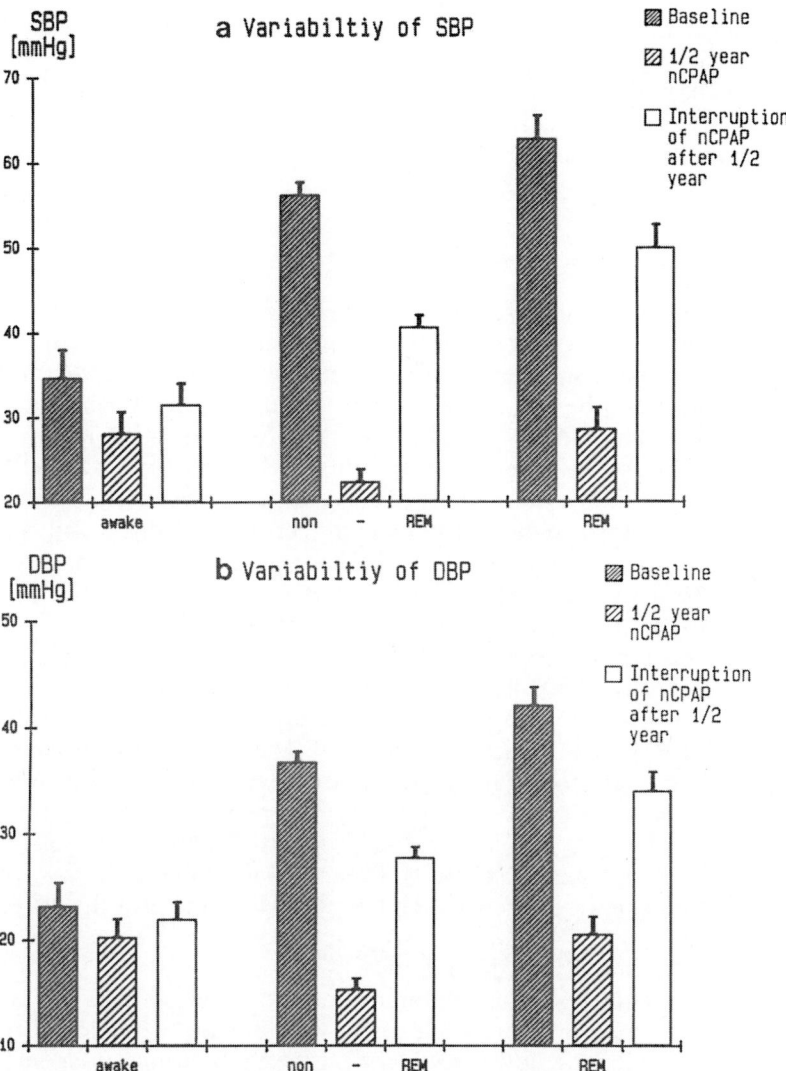

Fig. 2. Variability of systolic (**a**) and diastolic (**b**) blood pressure during waking and sleep (stages non-REM and REM sleep) without therapy on baseline, after 6 months of nCPAP therapy, and after interruption of nCPAP. Mean values and 95% confidence intervals

tion of arterial hypertension in sleep apnea both during the day and at night in the short and the long term.

Furthermore, the same 12 patients in whom the measurements specified above were carried out were also investigated in the sleep laboratory for 1 night without nCPAP. In these measurements, a rise in apnea index and blood pressure was again found. The apnea index of 52 (20–78) apneas per hour did not differ from the initial measurements. Indeed, it was higher in some patients. The values for blood pressure were higher than under therapy but did not reach the initial values.

By comparison, there was a greater increase in variability (Figs. 1, 2). This suggests that the increase in blood pressure in sleep apnea results from the raised variability during the night. It is to be assumed that the full picture of sleep apnea is attained again only a few days after interrupting successful treatment when compensation of hemodynamic conditions and normalization of the sleep structure is abolished.

Pharmacotherapy of Arterial Hypertension in Sleep Apnea

Whereas nCPAP therapy is the agent of choice for patients with pronounced sleep apnea, there are a large number of patients with still slight to moderately pronounced sleep apnea who also often show arterial hypertension at an early stage. Pharmacotherapy is the most important treatment measure for this group of patients. The therapy should not intensify the existing nocturnal breathing disorder and the disturbed sleep structure or the symptoms by day. These include in particular a restricted capacity to concentrate and reduced functional efficiency as well as intolerance of monotony with increased tiredness and tendency to fall asleep during the day. In addition, it is important that the cardiovascular diseases associated with sleep apnea such as heart failure, arrhythmias, and pulmonary hypertension are not exacerbated by the medication.

On the basis of these postulations, we carried out a randomized double-blind study on 12 men with sleep apnea (apnea index over 10 per hour) and arterial hypertension (diastolic blood pressure over 95 mm Hg in the sitting position at three different times of measurement) [19]. The polysomnographic measurements in the sleep laboratory during the night were carried out in accordance with the method described above. In addition, a continuous invasive measurement of blood pressure was carried out over 24 h with the Oxford system, which can be used under out-patient conditions. The mean age of the patients was 50 years (33–69). The body mass index was 32.6 kg/m^2 (24.9–40.6). For the distribution of the clinical data within the two therapy groups see Table 2. There was no statistically significant difference in these data.

In accordance with the randomization plan, the patients received either the beta-blocker metoprolol (1 × 100 mg/day) or the newly developed ACE inhibitor cilazapril (1 × 2.5 mg/day) for 8 days after the baseline measurements. Cilazapril is a structurally new ACE inhibitor prodrug which is rapidly converted into its active form cilazaprilate (recommended dose 2.5–5 mg/day, bioavailability >65%, effective half-life 9 h, renal elimination 91%).

Table 2. Clinical data

	Total (n = 12)		Metoprolol (n = 6)		Cilazapril (n = 6)	
Age (years)	50	(33–69)	52	(33–69)	48	(41–60)
Height (cm)	178	(158–192)	179	(172–192)	176	(158–185)
Weight (kg)	104	(78–136)	106	(90–132)	103	(78–136)
Broca index	134	(101–164)	134	(125–145)	135	(101–164)
BMI (kg/m^2)	32.6	(24.9–40.6)	32.0	(30.9–33.6)	33.2	(24.9–40.6)

Table 3. Results for noninvasively measured blood pressure during the day

	Metoprolol		Cilazapril	
	Baseline	Therapy	Baseline	Therapy
SBP	171	152 [a]	156	133 [a]
(mm Hg)	(143–190)	(126–167)	(130–210)	(112–163)
DBP	108	93 [a]	100	83 [a]
(mm Hg)	(98–1277	(85–102)	(95–108)	(60–100)
TST	382	341	381	368
(min)	(359–425)	(297–383)	(370–405)	(265–434)
REM	19	12	17	20
(%)	(17–23)	(6–22)	(10–22)	(10–29)
AI	45	34 [a]	54	40 [a]
(n/h)	(15–91)	(2–57)	(21–84)	(8–72)

SBP, Systolic blood pressure; DBP, diastolic blood pressure; TST, total sleep time; REM, proportion of REM sleep; AI, apnea index.
[a] $p < 0.01$.

No directional changes were shown in clinical test parameters or the analysis of pulmonary function before and after therapy. The sleep profile did not show any alteration in the total sleeping time or in the ratio of REM to non-REM sleep in the two therapy groups. In the cilazapril group, a tendency for the REM sleep to increase was seen. The average number of apnea phases per hour of sleep (the apnea index) was lowered under both substances. As expected, the values of blood pressure measured noninvasively were lowered under the two agents both systolically and diastolically (Table 3). The values measured invasively were lowered by both substances during the 24-h period. Differences were shown in comparison of the values measured during the day (6 A.M.–8 P.M.) and the values during the night (8 P.M.–6 A.M.). In the daytime, metoprolol showed only a tendency to lower diastolic values, whereas cilazapril lowered the blood pressure both by day and during the night (Fig. 3). In an analysis of the stages of sleep, blood pressure was found to be lowered under cilazapril both during non-REM and during REM sleep, whereas under metoprolol the blood pressure values were just as high during REM sleep as they were without therapy (Fig. 4).

Discussion

Correlations between snoring and arterial hypertension have been known for a long time from epidemiological studies. In recent years, it has become established that there are different forms of snoring, as made evident by the increasing elucidation of the obstructive sleep-related disorders of breathing (in particular the obstructive sleep apnea syndrome). One form (primary snoring) has only little or no effect on hemodynamics and is probably more a factor of noise stress for the environment than a cause of disease for the sleeping person. However, the forms of obstruction of the upper airways such as occur in obstructive sleep apnea

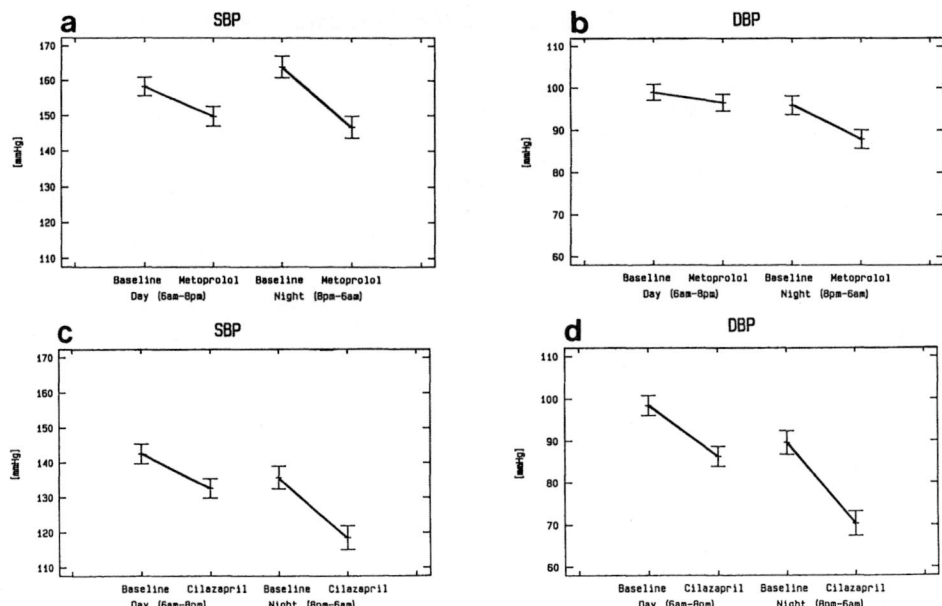

Fig. 3a–d. Comparison of 24-h continuously measured blood pressure for day (6 A.M.–8 P.M.) and night (8 P.M.–6 A.M.). **a, b** Metoprolol group. **c, d** Cilazapril group. **a, c** Systolic blood pressure (*SBP*). **b, d** Diastolic blood pressure (*DBP*). Mean values and 95% confidence intervals. Beat-to-beat analysis with averaging every 20 min

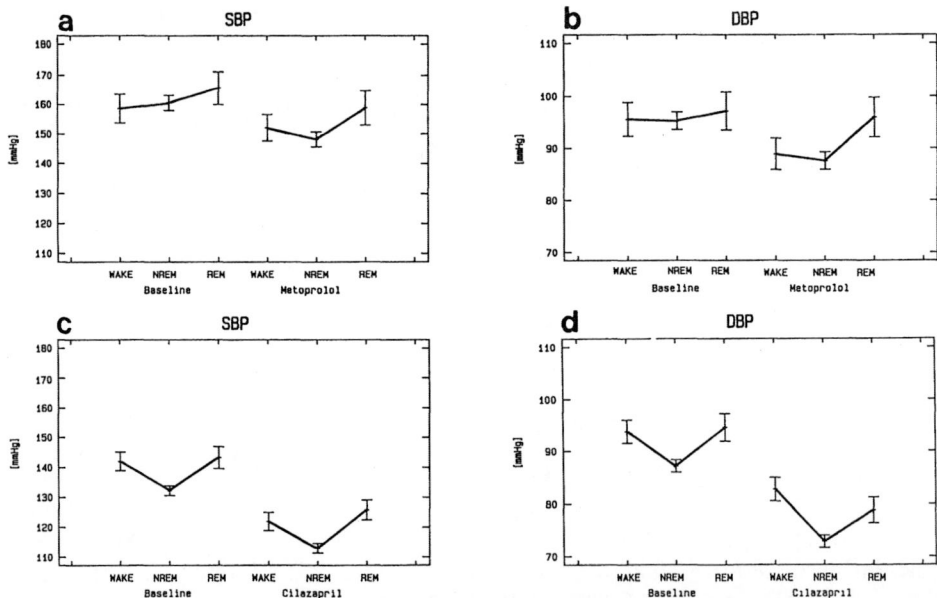

Fig. 4a–d. Comparison of continuously measured blood pressure. Sleep stage correlated and during waking. **a, b** Metoprolol group. **c, d** Cilazapril group. **a, c** Systolic blood pressure (*SBP*). **b, d** Diastolic blood pressure (*DBP*). Mean values and 95% confidence intervals. Beat-to-beat analysis with averaging every 5 min

syndrome in the form of obstructive continuous snoring or apneic intermittent snoring are to be discriminated from primary snoring.

It could be shown that these forms are accompanied by a lowering of oxygen saturation and an increase in blood pressure. The most important indicator for the causal correlation between these forms of snoring and arterial hypertension is the reversibility of the raised blood pressure value when the nocturnal breathing disorder is treated on its own. This was shown for the first time by Coccagna, who found normalization of the previously raised blood pressure values in successful tracheostoma treatment of patients with obstructive sleep apnea [1, 2]. In our investigations on patients with sleep apnea who underwent nCPAP therapy, we were able to show that this form of therapy also leads to a normalization of blood pressure. Furthermore, an increase in the apnea symptoms and blood pressure values occurs after discontinuation of therapy. Moreover, differences could be shown in antihypertensive drug treatment of patients with sleep apnea and hypertension. No effect on the raised blood pressure values was found during REM sleep under treatment with the beta-blocker metoprolol, whereas there was a lowering of the raised pressure values both by day and in the night during all stages of sleep with the ACE inhibitor cilazapril. At the same time, there was a lowering of the number of apneas under therapy. Since there was no alteration in the sleep duration or in the ratio of non-REM to REM sleep, this result is most likely a nonspecific effect of the antihypertensive medication. However, it must be mentioned that an exacerbation of the apnea symptoms must be expected in administration of some other antihypertensives, especially those manifesting sedative effects on the central nervous system. In an ongoing study we are investigating to what extent placebo effects or effects of hospitalization (stress reduction) played a role. The reasons for the differences in the effect on the blood pressure characteristics cannot be definitely established at present.

Irrespective of this, however, it is to be emphasized that the blood pressure characteristics were more favorably affected in the sleep apnea patients by administration of the ACE inhibitor. The results also show that it is not sufficient to know that a drug lowers blood pressure during the day; it is probably even more important to know the effects of each antihypertensive agent on the nocturnal blood pressure time course which is not subject to the arbitrary stress factors during the day. Furthermore, in view of the large number of patients with sleep-related breathing disorders and nonturnal arterial hypertension, the effect of antihypertensive therapy on obstructive snoring and nocturnal apnea must be considered as well as the presence of sleep-related breathing disorders in the differential diagnosis of arterial hypertension.

References

1. Coccagna G, Cirignotta F, Lugaresi E (1991) Changes in general circulation in sleep apnea syndrome. In: Peter JH, Penzel T, Podszus T, von Wichert P (eds) Sleep and health risk. Springer, Berlin Heidelberg New York, pp 300–309
2. Coccagna G, Mantovani M, Brignani F, Parchi C, Lugaresi E (1972) Tracheostomy in hypersomnia with periodic breathing. Bull Physiopathol Respir 8:1217–1227

3. Ehlenz K, Peter JH, Dugi K, Firle K, Goubeaud R (1991) Changes in volume and pressure regulating hormone system during nCPAP therapy in patients with obstructive sleep apnea syndrome. In: Peter JH, Penzel T, Podszus T, von Wichert P (eds) Sleep and health risk. Springer, Berlin Heidelberg New York, pp 518–531
4. Fletcher EC, DeBehuke RD, Lovoi MS, Gorin A (1985) Undiagnosed sleep apnea in patients with essential hypertension. Ann Intern Med 103:190–195
5. Guilleminault C, Riley RW, Powell NB (1989) Surgical treatment of obstructive sleep apnea. In: Kryger MH, Roth T, Dement WC (eds) Principles and practice of sleep medicine. Saunders, Philadelphia, pp 571–583
6. Guilleminault C (1983) Natural history, cardiac impact, and long-term follow-up of sleep apnea syndrome. In: Guilleminault C, Lugaresi E (eds) Sleep/wake disorders. Raven, New York, pp 107–125
7. He J, Kryger MH, Zorick FJ, Conwway V, Roth T (1988) Mortality and apnea index in obstructive sleep apnea. Chest 94:9–14
8. Kales A, Bixler EO, Cadieux RJ, Schneck DW, Shaw LC, Loke TW, Vela-Bueno A, Soldatos CR (1984) Sleep apnoea in a hypertensive population. Lancet 3:1005–1008
9. Koskenvuo M, Kaprio J, Partinen M, Langinvainio H, Sarna S, Heikkilä K (1985) Snoring as a risk factor for hypertension and angina pectoris. Lancet 1:893–896
10. Lavie P, Ben-Yosef R, Rubin A (1984) Prevalence of sleep apnea syndrome among patients with essential hypertension. Am Heart J 108:373–376
11. Lavie P, Sleep apnea in industrial workers. In: Guilleminault C, Lugaresi E (eds) Sleep wake disorders. Raven, New York, pp 853–856
12. Lugaresi E, Cirignotta F, Montagna P (1989) Snoring: pathogenetic, clinical, and therapeutic aspects. In: Kryger MH, Roth T, Dement WC (eds) Principles and practice of sleep medicine. Saunders, Philadelphia, pp 494–500
13. Mayer J, Becker H, Brandenburg U, Penzel T, Peter JH, von Wichert P (1991) Blood pressure and sleep apnea. Results of long-term nasal continuous positive airway pressure therapy. Cardiology 79:84–92
14. Mayer J, Brandenburg U, Krzyzanek E, Peter JH, Weichler U, von Wichert P (1991) Increase in blood pressure due to continuous obstructive snoring. Pneumologie 45:306–308
15. Mayer J, Fuchs E, Hügens M, Penzel T, Peter JH, Podszus T, von Wichert P (1984) Long-term theophylline therapy of sleep apnea-syndrome. Am Rev Respir Dis 129 [Suppl II]: A 252
16. Mayer J, Himmelmann H, Köhler U, Penzel T, Peter JH, Podszus T, von Wichert P, Zahorka M (1986) The prevalence of essential hypertension and sleep apnea in industrial workers. Bull Eur Physiopathol Respir 22 [Suppl 8]: 59
17. Mayer J, Becker H, Penzel T, Weichler U, Peter JH, Wichert P (1989) Sleep apnea induced changes in blood pressure and heart rate. In: Horne J (ed) Sleep'88. Fischer, Stuttgart, pp 270–272
18. Mayer J (1991) Sleep related breathing disorders and arterial hypertension. In: Peter JH, Penzel T, Podszus T, von Wichert P (eds) Sleep and health risk. Springer, Berlin Heidelberg New York, pp 310–318
19. Mayer J, Weichler U, Herres-Mayer B, Schneider H, Marx U, Peter JH (1990) Influence of metoprolol and cilazapril on blood pressure and on sleep apnea activity. J Cardiovasc Pharmacol 16:952–961
20. Peter JH, Bolm-Audorff U, Becker E, Eble R, Fuchs E, Meinzer K, Penzel T, von Wichert P (1983) Schlafapnoe und essentielle Hypertonie. Verh Dtsch Ges Inn Med 89:1132–1135
21. Peter JH, Fuchs E, Köhler U, Mayer J, Penzel T, Podszus T, Siegrist J, Wichert P (1986) Studies in the prevalence of sleep apnea activity: evaluation of ambulatory screening results. Eur J Respir Dis 69 [Suppl 146]:451–458
22. Peter JH (1990) Sleep apnea and cardiovascular diseases. In: Guilleminault C, Partinen M (eds) Obstructive sleep apnea syndrome: clinical research and treatment. Raven, New York, pp 81–98
23. Peter JH, Weiss W, Mayer G et al. (1990) Empfehlungen zur Diagnostik, Therapie und Langzeitbetreuung von Patienten mit Schlafapnoe. Med Klin (in press) 86:46–50
24. Peter JH (1990) Transmural arterial blood pressure in obstructive sleep apnea. Sleep Res 19:267

25. Peter JH (1988) Modes of selection: epidemiology of sleep apnea. In: Levi-Valensi P, Duron B (eds) Sleep disorders and respiration. Colloque INSERM. Libbey Eurotext, Paris, 168:135–150
26. Rechtschaffen A, Kales A (1968) A manual of standardized terminology, techniques and scoring system for sleep stages of human subjects. US Government Printing Office, Washington DC (Public Health Service Publication 204)
27. Schmidt-Nowara W, Jennum P (1990) Epidemiology of sleep apnea. In: Guilleminault C, Partinen M (eds) Obstructive sleep apnea syndrome: clinical research and treatment. Raven, New York, pp 1–8
28. Sullivan CE, Issa FG, Berthon-Jones M, Eves L (1981) Reversal of obstructive sleep apnoea by continuous positive airway pressure therapy. Lancet 1:862–865

Seasonal and Environmental Temperature Effects on Arterial Blood Pressure

S. Giaconi and S. Ghione

Arterial blood pressure is not a fixed variable but rather fluctuates continuously over short and long periods [1]. Seasonal variations represent a source of long-term blood pressure variability which is well known to many hypertensive patients (who spontaneously decrease their antihypertensive medications during the summer) and to many doctors (who observe that patients in the borderline to mild hypertensive range often need pharmacological treatment only in winter). The aim of the present paper is to summarize the relatively few published reports in this field and to discuss briefly the possible causes and mechanisms of seasonally related blood pressure changes and some of their implications.

Table 1 gives a brief outline of the studies on the effects of the season (or environmental temperature) on arterial blood pressure. A first observation is that we were able to find relatively few pertinent data in this field. In general, two different approaches were used. One was more clinically oriented and implied a longitudinal follow-up of relatively few subjects with measurements repeated over a prolonged time; the other was more epidemiologically oriented and was based on the transversal comparison of blood pressure measurements obtained in large numbers of subjects in different periods of the year. The latter studies concerned the evaluation of constitutional, environmental, or methodological determinants of blood pressure where the effect of environmental temperature on blood pressure represented only one aspect of a more general study.

Rose [2] was, to our knowledge, the first to report on the seasonally dependent variability of blood pressure. In 1961 he analyzed repeated blood pressure measurements in 56 men with coronary heart disease and found a clear seasonal trend for blood pressure with highest and lowest values, respectively, in spring and in late summer. These differences were about 4 mm Hg for both systolic and diastolic blood pressure. Somewhat greater seasonal variations of blood pressure (of about 9 mm Hg) were reported by Hata [3] in small groups of patients with borderline and established essential hypertension. Interestingly, no seasonal effect was observed in normotensives. Hata attributed this phenomenon to increased sympathetic nervous activity as assessed by catecholamine levels. Heller [4] in the UK Heart Disease Prevention Project found a marked effect of room temperature on blood pressure with higher room temperatures strongly associated with lower blood pressure irrespective of whether measurements were obtained in summer or

Schmidt/Engel/Blümchen (Eds.)
Temporal Variations of the Cardiovascular System
© Springer-Verlag Berlin Heidelberg 1992

Table 1. Studies on temperature-dependent BP variation

Authors	n	Subjects	Place	BP	Temperature	Aim of study
Clinical (longitudinal)						
Rose [2]	56	Men with CHD	UK	Standard	No information	Ad hoc
Hata [3]	34	NT (14), HT (20)	Japan	Standard	In-, outdoor	Ad hoc
Giaconi [11]	22	Borderline	Italy	BP monit.	In-, outdoor	Ad hoc
Epidemiological (transversal)						
Heller [4]	8 397	40–59 years, men	UK	Random zero	Indoor	Prevention trial
Prineas [5]	9 977	6–9 years, children	USA	Random zero	Indoor	Minneapolis Study
Brennan [6]	17 282	HT 90–109 mmHg	UK	Random zero	Outdoor	MRC trial
de Swiet [8]	1 307	4–5 years, children	UK	various	Indoor	Brompton Study
Jenner [9]	1 037	9 years, children	Australia	Dynamap	Outdoor	Long-term longitudinal
Knuiman [10]	1 023	8–9 years, boys	Europe	Random zero	In-, outdoor	Electrolyte excretion

winter. He also reported that the standardization for room temperature largely removed a seasonal effect on blood pressure. Effects of room temperature on blood pressure were also found in public school children by Prineas [5]; colder indoor temperatures were associated with higher systolic but, surprisingly, with lower diastolic blood pressure.

Brennan [6] analyzed a large set of data collected for the MRC trial for mild hypertension and for each age, sex, and treatment group; systolic and diastolic pressures were higher in winter than in summer. On average, a 20 °C difference of maximum daily temperature corresponded to a variation of approximately 5 and 3 mmHg, respectively. This effect was stronger in thin and older subjects than in obese and younger subjects. He further pointed out that the seasonal effects on arterial blood pressure could, at least in part, account for the higher winter mortality from ischemic heart disease and stroke [7]. On the other hand, de Swiet [8] in the Brompton study found only small seasonal effects and no consistent relationship with room temperature in children, even if slight increases of 3–4 mmHg were observed for indoor temperatures less than 15 °C. Jenner [9] in another study on constitutional and environmental determinants of blood pressure in 9-year-old Australian children found a significant negative relationship between blood pressure and maximum outdoor temperature on the measurement day (with falls of about 5–7 mmHg for a rise of 10 °C). Similar results were found by Knuiman [10] in a study on the relationship between blood pressure and electrolyte excretion.

We also recently performed a study [11] on 22 patients in the high normal to mild hypertensive range by repeating an ambulatory blood pressure monitoring and a series of cardiovascular reactivity tests after an interval of 6 months, i.e., once in a cold and once in a warm period of the year, or vice versa. The different order of the evaluations was chosen to exclude the possible familiarization effect of repeated measurements. Blood pressure was measured under casual conditions, during handgrip, mental arithmetic test, and submaximal multistage bicycle exercise and serially during the following 24 h with a noninvasive ambulatory blood pressure recorder. Daily outdoor maximum and indoor laboratory temperatures were also obtained. In the cold season in both groups significantly higher values (on the average by 5–10 mm Hg) were obtained for mean diastolic daytime blood pressure but not for nighttime measurements. For the other parameters a trend toward higher values in the cold season was observed in both groups, although statistical significance was not obtained in all instances. In addition, highly significant correlations were found between the differences of the average daytime ambulatory blood pressures and the corresponding changes in daily maximum outdoor temperatures, suggesting that seasonal influences could also be detected in small-scale studies, especially when integrated evaluations by ambulatory monitoring are employed, and that these effects were limited to the daytime period.

The data briefly mentioned above cannot be easily summarized in a single, clear-cut message, and a number of questions remain open, for example, on the role of outdoor versus indoor ambient temperature, of blood pressure status, age, constitutional determinants, and on the possible different effects of systolic and diastolic blood pressure. Despite these uncertainties, which arise mainly from the difficulty in comparing studies with widely different design, we feel not unjustified in concluding that major evidence has been provided for an association between environmental temperature (or seasonal variations) and blood pressure. In Table 2 we have tried to quantify this association as observed in the various studies. For some of them we had to estimate these parameters from the original authors' data, since they were not explicitly reported. From this table one can see that, if one excludes the contrasting data of Prineas on diastolic blood pressure, a systolic and diastolic blood pressure variation of about 7 mm Hg can be predicted for temperature differences of 20 °C. It is interesting to observe that a greater temperature effect on blood pressure was found when maximum outdoor temperature on the examination day was used, as in the study of Jenner's and of our group, or when mean outside temperature was evaluated, as in Knujman's study. Relatively smaller blood pressure variations were observed in the studies of Hata and Brennan, but we must consider that in these two cases the assessment of temperature was less accurate; in the first case mean monthly temperatures were used, and in the second in relating blood pressure readings to temperature measurements data from three cities were arbitrarily extended by the authors to the other clinics geographically related to these.

Several questions remain open regarding the causes and mechanisms of seasonal variations of blood pressure.

As suggested by Brennan, seasonally related blood pressure changes may reflect the acute response to ambient temperature, perhaps mediated by a sympathetic

Table 2. Environmental temperature and arterial blood pressure

		Systolic BP		Diastolic BP			
		Slope[a]	Δ BP for Δ 20 C°	Slope[a]	Δ BP for Δ 20 C°		
Heller [4][b]	In			−0.35	− 7.0		
Prineas [5][b]	In	−0.15	− 3.0	0.26	5.2		
Hata [3][b]	Out	−0.28	− 5.6	−0.28	− 5.6		
Brennan [6][b]	Out	−0.27	− 5.4	−0.15	− 3.0		
Jenner [9]	Out	−0.55	−11.0	−0.65	−13.0		
Knuiman [10]	Out	N.S.		−0.42	− 8.4		
Giaconi [11]	Out	−0.49	− 9.8	−0.39	− 7.8		
Mean		−0.35	− 6.96	−0.28	− 5.66	−0.37[c]	−7.47[c]
SD		0.17	3.33	0.28	5.67	0.17[c]	3.32[c]

In/Out, in/outdoors;
[a] mmHg/C°;
[b] Estimated values since not originally reported in the papers.
[c] Mean and SD excluding the outlying values of Prineas [5].

reflex initiated by skin cooling. However, in several studies [2, 3, 9, 11] indoor measurements were made in the cold period and in (presumably) comfortably warm rooms, and in our study patients spent at least 20 min in a waiting room before starting blood pressure measurements. It is therefore plausible that long-acting mechanism(s) rather than an acute effect should account for the temperature-dependent blood pressure changes. In any case, further studies are needed to assess the time course of this acclimatization and its role.

Hata's data strongly suggest an important role of the adrenergic system in the colder months. In fact, he observed that plasma norepinephrine in hypertensives and urinary norepinephrine excretion in both controls and hypertensives were higher in winter than in summer. However, the seasonal differences in blood pressure did not correlate with changes in catecholamines, and while this factor could be responsible for the increases of blood pressure in winter in hypertensives, in spite of similar increases of sympathetic tone (as assessed by urinary catecholamine), no blood pressure variations were found in normotensive controls.

Other data also suggest a possible involvement of the adrenergic system. An increased urinary excretion of total metanephrines has been reported in winter [12], and, as observed in our study, seasonal differences of blood pressure were absent for nighttime measurements. This finding may simply reflect smaller differences in temperatures experienced by the sleeping subjects, but since it is well known that sleep is associated with a pronounced reduction in sympathetic tone [13], one may speculate that the lack of seasonal effects on nighttime blood pressure might in some way reflect a role of the adrenergic system in mediating the seasonal changes of arterial blood pressure. Our finding of a steeper increase in heart rate during bicycle exercise in the cold period and the recent report of Izzo [14] of a trend in winter toward peaks not only of blood pressure but also of plasma norepinephrine and systemic vascular resistance may indicate an increase in

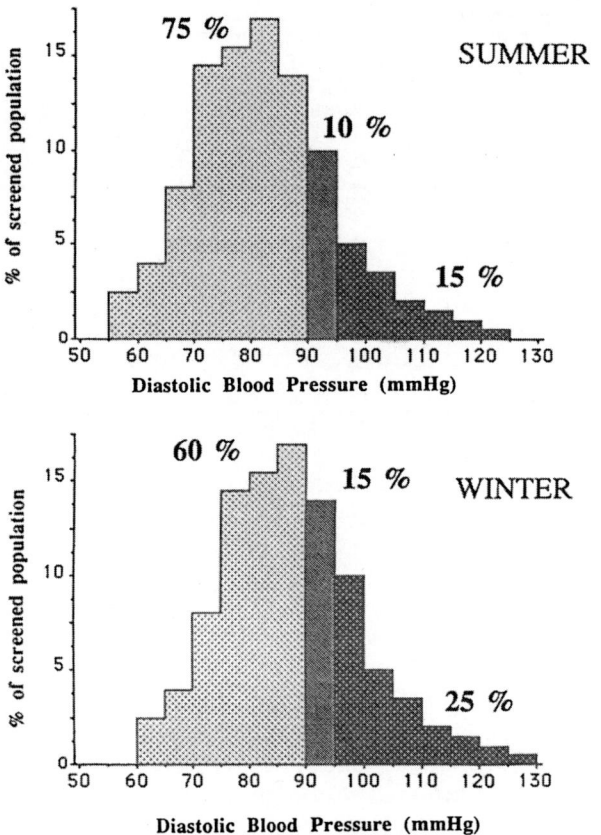

Fig. 1. Example of the possible effect of seasonal variations on estimation of the prevalence of hypertension in a population according to the frequency distribution of diastolic blood pressure. The assumption was made that an equal shift of 5 mm Hg occurs in diastolic blood pressure for the entire population between summer and winter. In the figure the frequency distribution of diastolic blood pressure obtained in the HDFP study [18] has been arbitrarly referred to summer period

sympathetic nervous activity with colder temperatures. Finally, it is interesting to observe that in the MRC study reported by Brennan the patients under propranolol treatment exhibited seasonally dependent blood pressure changes similar to those under diuretic treatment or placebo. This finding, the observation of a lack of seasonal influences on heart rate, and the previously mentioned report on an effect on vascular resistances would suggest an alpha-mediated mechanism underlying this phenomenon.

Other factors may also play a role but are poorly studied. Differences in sodium balance could exert a role, as suggested by the observation of Hata of an increased sodium excretion in winter. Endocrinological mechanisms may be of importance; in fact, seasonal variations of thyroidal and adrenal cortical activity in humans have been described [15, 16]. On the other hand, no significant differences in plasma renin activity and plasma aldosterone were found [3].

Another question still open is whether and to what extent factors other than ambient temperature could account for seasonal variations of blood pressure. One might well conceive that one of the numerous seasonal changes in lifestyle, such as changes in dietary habits (e.g., salt, alcohol, meat) or in physical activity, may be of some importance. Finally, one cannot exclude the role of psychological mechanisms, as indirectly suggested by the well-known seasonal pattern of several psychiatric and psychosomatic disorders.

A final question concerns the relevance of seasonally related blood pressure changes. Two different aspects may be considered; one concerns the management of the individual hypertensive patient, the other the design and interpretation of studies on hypertension. As regards the first aspect one may consider especially the subjects in the upper normal to mild hypertensive range, who are by far the majority [17] of the patients seeking medical advice for arterial hypertension and represent a clinical problem especially for what concerns the decision to start a pharmacological treatment. As seasonal variation per se can determine blood pressure differences of 5–7 mm Hg, one must emphasize the necessity of long-term follow-up for a correct evaluation of these patients. Furthermore the temperature- (or season-) dependent blood pressure variation could account, as suggested by Brennan, for the higher cardiovascular mortality observed in colder periods [7]; in fact there is no evidence to our knowledge that other risk factors for cardiovascular disease show such consistent seasonal differences.

This phenomenon should be considered also in the design and analysis of (intervention) studies on arterial hypertension (as a nonnegligeable confounding factor). The magnitude of this effect is exemplified in Fig. 1. If one takes 90 mm Hg as a fixed cut-off point for arterial hypertension (borderline and established hypertension) and assumes that variations of environmental temperature of 20 °C would shift the diastolic blood pressure distribution in a given population by 5–10 mm Hg, then according to the season during which the determinations are made, one could expect that the estimated prevalence of arterial hypertension could change as high as between 25% and 40%.

References

1. Pickering TG (1990) Diurnal rhythms and other sources of blood pressure variability in normal and hypertensive subject. Hypertension 2:1397–1406
2. Rose G (1961) Seasonal variation in blood pressure in man. Nature 189:235
3. Hata T, Ogihara T, Maruyama A, Mikami H, Nakamaru M, Naka T, Kumahara Y, Nugent CA (1982) The seasonal variation of blood pressure in patients with essential hypertension. Clin Exp Hypertens [A] 4:341–354
4. Heller RF, Rose G, Tunstall-Pedoe HD, Christie DGS (1978) Blood pressure measurement in the United Kingdom Heart Disease Prevention Project. J Epidemiol Community Health 32:235–238
5. Prineas RJ, Gillum RF, Horibe H, Hannan PJ, Stat M (1980) The Minneapolis Children's Blood Pressure Study. I. Standards of measurement for children's blood pressure. Hypertension 2 [Suppl I]:I18–I18
6. Brennan PJ, Greenberg G, Miall WE, Thompson SG (1982) Seasonal variation in arterial blood pressure. Br Med J 285:919–923
7. Rose G (1966) Cold weather and ischaemic heart disease. Br J Prev Soc Med 20:97–100

8. de Swiet M, Fayers PM, Shineboume EA (1984) Blood pressure in four- and five-year-old children: the effects of environment and other factors in its measurement. J Hypertens 2:501–505

9. Jenner AD, English DR, Vandongen R, Beilin LJ, Armstrong BK, Dunbar D (1987) Environmental temperature and blood pressure in 9-year-old Australian children. J Hypertens 5:683–686

10. Knuiman JT, Hautvast JGAJ, Zwiauer KFM et al. (1988) Blood pressure and excretion of sodium, potassium, calcium and magnesium in 8- and 9-year old boys from 19 European centres. Eur J Clin Nutr 42:847–855

11. Giaconi S, Ghione S, Palombo C et al. (1989) Seasonal influences on blood pressure in high normal to mild hypertensive range. Hypertension 14:22–27

12. Yamamoto T, Doi K, Takeuchi Y, Baba M, Tanaka M (1976) Seasonal variation of urinary excretion of total metanephrines. Clin Chim Acta 68:241–244

13. Richards AM, Nicholls MG, Espiner EA, Ikram H, Cullens M, Hinton D (1986) Diurnal patterns of blood pressure, heart rate and vasoactive hormones in normal man. Clin Exp Hypertens [A] 8:153–166

14. Izzo JL, Larrabee PS, Sander E, Kallay MC (1989) Hemodynamics of seasonal adaptation. (abs. N 1328) Am J Hypertens 2:82A

15. Nagata H, Izumiyama T, Kamata K (1976) An increase of plasma triiodothyronine concentration in man in a cold environment. J Clin Endocrinol Metab 43:1153–1156

16. Watanabe G (1964) Seasonal variation of adrenal cortex activity. Arch Environ Health 9:122–126

17. Hypertension prevalence and status of awareness, treatment, and control in the United States (1985) Final report of the Subcommittee on Definition and Prevalence of the 1984 Joint National Committee. Hypertension 7:457–468

18. The Hypertension Detection and Follow-up Cooperative Group (1978) Mild hypertensives in the hypertension detection and follow-up program. In: Mild hypertension: to treat or not to treat. Ann NY Acad Sci 304:254–266

Age-Dependent Variation of Diurnal Blood Pressure Profile in Normotensive Subjects *

G. Prager, R. Prager, and P. Klein

Introduction

Knowledge of the normal blood pressure range is of the greatest interest for pathophysiological, clinical, therapeutic, and epidemiological purposes. Studies carried out to investigate age-dependent diurnal blood pressure profile have led to conflicting results [1–8]. This is probably due partly to the nonuniform numbers and sex distribution within the individual age decades and partly to the unbalanced age stratification. The aim of the current study is to investigate the age- and sex-dependent 24-h blood pressure profile, with the distribution of age and sex perfectly balanced within the individual age decades.

Subjects and Methods

A total of 120 healthy subjects were selected, in each age decade there were 20 subjects, exactly half of them men and half women. The following checks were carried out on all patients: medical history, physical examination, 12-lead resting ECG, bicycle tolerance test, chest X-ray, and routine laboratory screening. All subjects had normal cardiothoracic ratio and normal echocardiographic dimensions.

The main criterion for inclusion in the study was resting blood pressure below 140/90 mm Hg, recorded supine at approximately 8 or 9 A.M. in a quiet room by trained study nurses as follows: 5 min reclining, 2 min standing, 5 min reclining, 2 min standing. Resting blood pressure was calculated from the two periods reclining. Once this criterion had been met, 24-h blood pressure monitoring was carried out using Spacelabs 90202; the measurements were made every 30 min. A diary was kept by each patient to record all his activities as well as the beginning and end of the sleeping phase.

---

* Preliminary results published in *Journal of Hypertension* (suppl 3 abstracts), vol. 8 (1990), p. 87.

Schmidt/Engel/Blümchen (Eds.)
Temporal Variations of the Cardiovascular System
© Springer-Verlag Berlin Heidelberg 1992

Table 1. Age-dependent means for 24-h blood pressure values

	20–29 years	30–39 years	40–49 years	50–59 years	60–69 years	70–79 years
BP systolic (mmHg)	120±3.1	117±3.9	121±3.9	124±3.7	122±4.6	126±4.4 n.s.
BP diastolic (mmHg)	70±2.3	71±3.0	74±3.4	78±2.2	73±3.2	72±2.4*

* $p < 0.01$; Kruskal-Wallis ANOVA by ranks.

Results

Mean 24-h Blood Pressure Values. The mean 24-h blood pressure values pooled for all subjects in each individual age decade showed that while the systolic mean values pooled for 24 h remain approximately unchanged, there is a tendency toward higher systolic mean values in the later age decades, which is, however, not statistically significant. The diastolic mean values, however, show typical age-dependent behavior: there is a rise in age decades III – VI from 70 to 78 mm Hg and a decrease to 72 mm Hg towards age decade VIII, both statistically significant (Table 1).

Sex-Dependent Diurnal Variability. As a whole, the systolic and diastolic mean values for women in all age decades are statistically significantly below those for men in the same age decades (Mantel-Haenszel-Pooling, $p < 0.01$). Even within-decade analysis showed a statistically significant difference in systolic and diastolic blood pressure values in some age groups (Fig. 1).

Age-Dependent Borderline Determination. The level of 90 mm Hg, mean diastolic value pooled over 24 h, is currently regarded as the cut-off between normotension

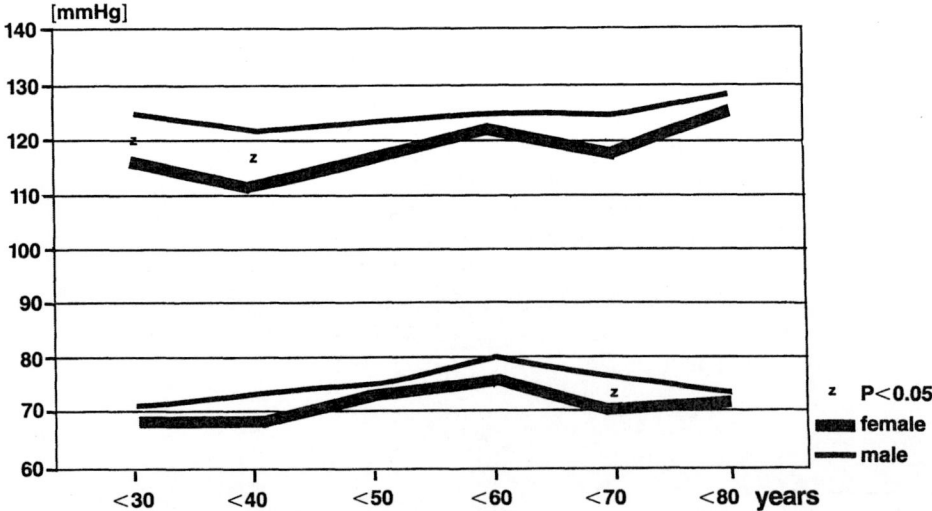

Fig. 1. Age- and sex-dependent diurnal variability

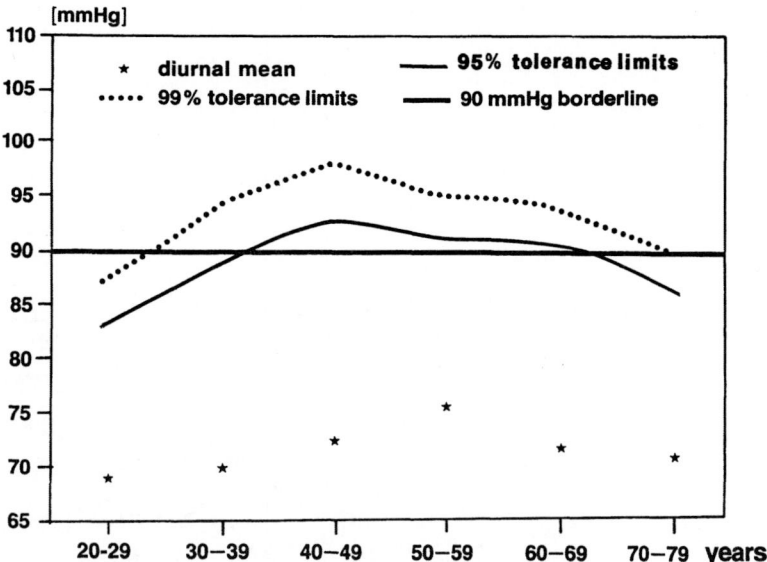

Fig. 2. Age-dependent borderline determination of diastolic blood pressure

and hypertension. Figure 2 shows the diastolic mean values and the 95% and 99% tolerance limits, calculated according to the Wald-Wolfowitz formula. If the 95% tolerance limit is considered, it can be seen that the middle-aged group is above the limit, but the younger and older age-groups are clearly below this limit. The significance of this for clinical trials is that in the middle-aged group normotensive subjects could be included, while in the younger and older age groups genuine hypertensives are exccluded. Thus in borderline determination an age-dependent corrective should be considered (Fig. 2).

Diurnal Blood Pressure Profile. The histograms of the hourly pooled mean values (Fig. 3) show the characteristic diurnal rhythmicity in each age decade. There is a rise in the morning, a plateau during the daytime, a decrease in the evening, and a nadir during the night. If the blood pressure profiles are superimposed, it can be seen that they diverge particularly in the sleeping phase and in the morning hours (Fig. 4). When comparing blood pressure profiles of age decades III–VI, it can be seen that the diastolic blood pressure in the older age group is considerably higher in the sleeping phase and in the morning hours, while the systolic blood pressure only rises slightly in the morning hours (Fig. 5). When comparing blood pressure profiles of age decades III and VIII, this is reversed; there is only a slight increase in diastolic blood pressure and a considerable increase in systolic blood pressure in the morning hours (Fig. 6).

Diurnal Time Interval Analysis. When analyzing the diurnal values measured at 6-h intervals, a statistically significant behavior in diastolic blood pressure can be seen for the time intervals 0000–0600 hours and 0600–1200 hours, again with a rise from age decades III to VI and a decrease toward age decade VIII. There is

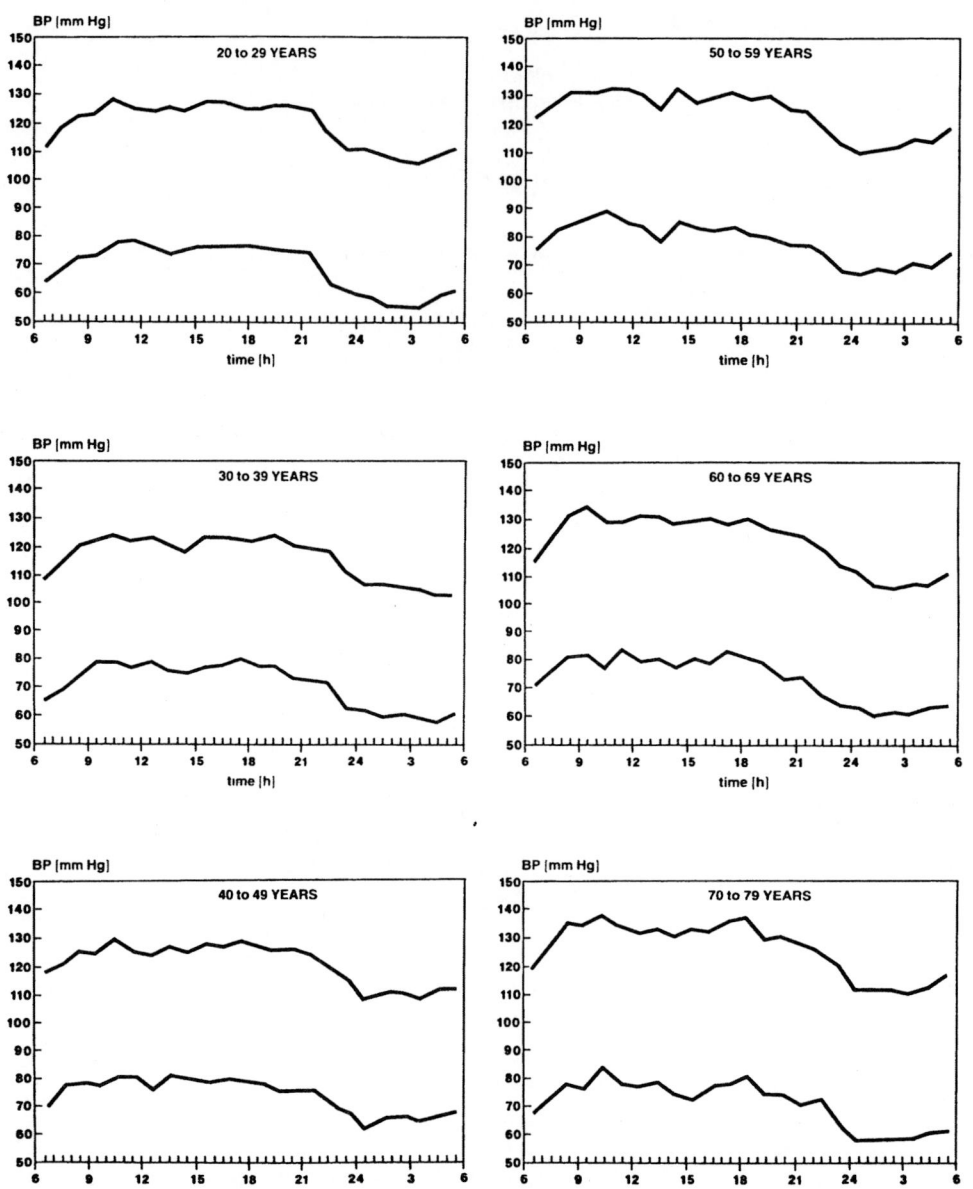

Fig. 3. Diurnal blood pressure profile in the six age decades

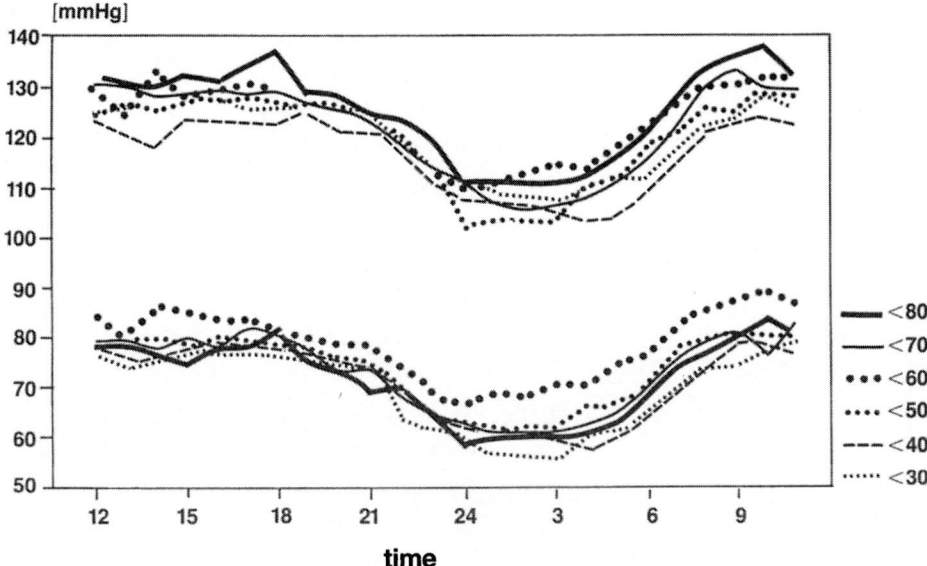

Fig. 4. Diurnal blood pressure profile in the six age decades, superimposed upon one another

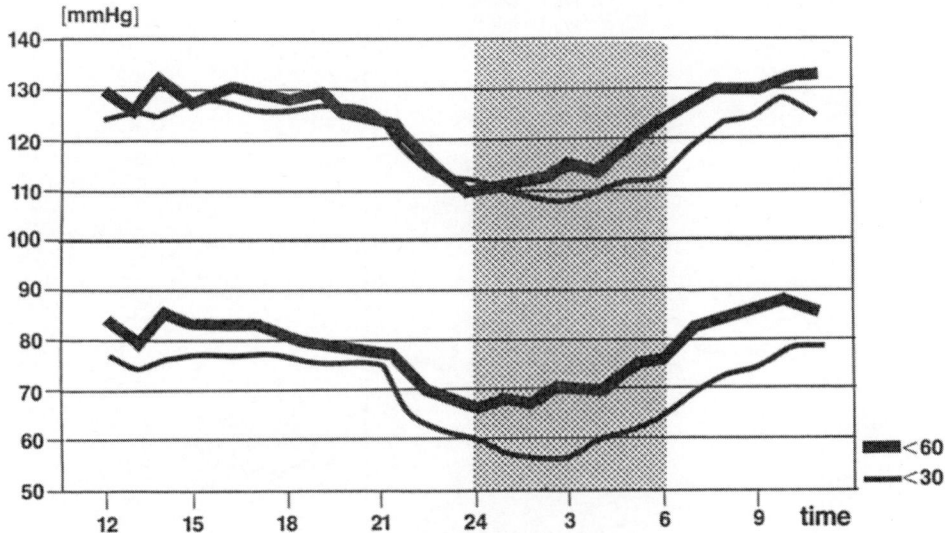

Fig. 5. Diurnal blood pressure profile in age decades III and VI

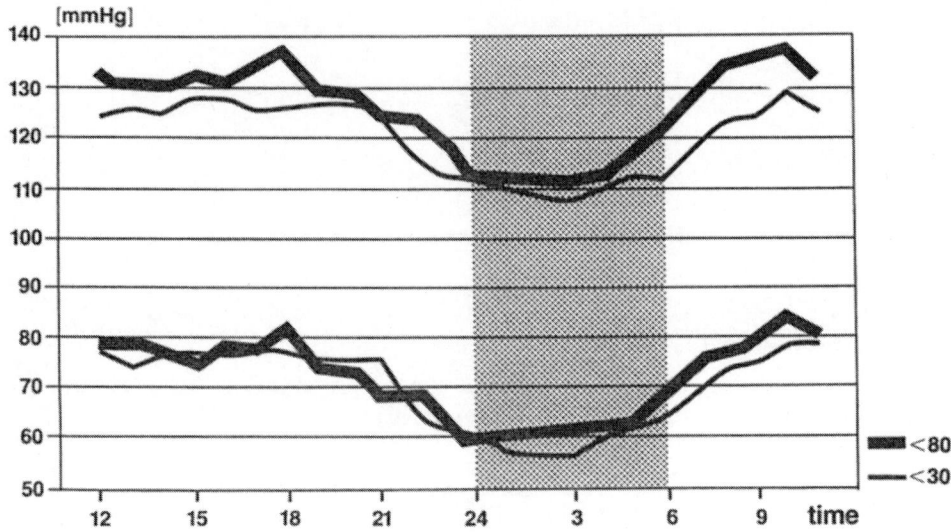

Fig. 6. Diurnal blood pressure profile in age decades III and VIII

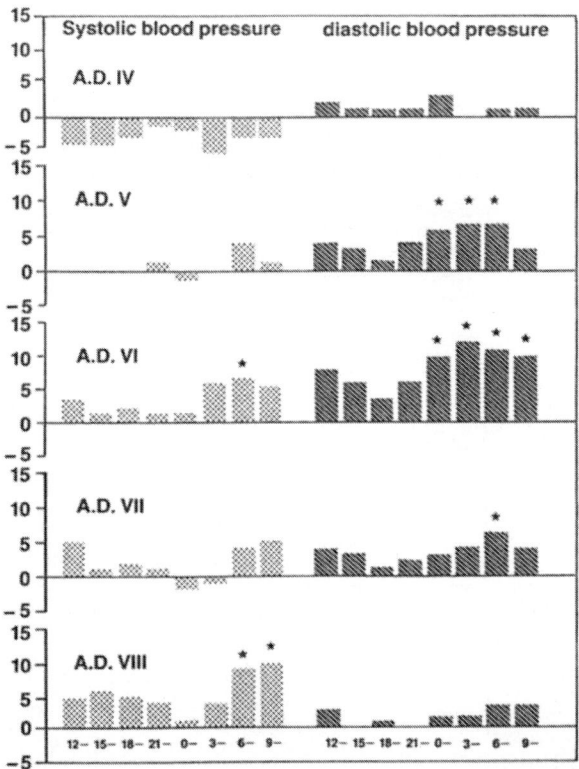

Fig. 7. Absolute differences in blood pressure mean values (mm Hg) for age decades (*A.D.*) IV– VIII compared to age decade III

Table 2. Age-dependent behavior of systolic and diastolic mean values at diurnal 6-h intervals

	1200–1800		1800–2400		0000–0600		0600–1200	
	Sys (mmHg)	Dia (mmHg)	Sys (mmHg)	Dia (mmHg)	Sys (mmHg)	Dia (mmHg)	Sys (mmHg)	Dia (mmHg)
20–29 years	126	76	122	72	110	58	123	73
30–39 years	122	77	121	73	106	60	120	74
40–49 years	127	80	123	74	110	65	125	78
50–59 years	129	83	124	76	114	70	129	84
60–69 years	129	79	124	73	108	62	127	78
70–79 years	132	78	127	73	112	61	133	78

also a statistically significant rise in systolic blood pressure in the morning hours in age decades IV–VIII (Table 2). To demonstrate this rhythmicity of diurnal time intervals even better, the absolute differences in blood pressure mean values for age decades IV–VIII compared to age decade III as a baseline are examined at 3-h intervals (Fig. 7). It can be seen that the highest diastolic blood pressure values are in age decade VI and the highest systolic blood pressure values in age decade VIII. With regard to the diastolic values there is again an increase toward age decade VI and a decrease toward age decade VIII, which is statistically significant in the time interval 0000–1200 hours. With regard to the systolic values there is a statistically significant increase from age decade V to age decade VIII, which is essentially restricted to the time interval 0600–1200 hours (Fig. 7). The nadir for diastolic blood pressure is in the evening hours between 1800 and 2100 hours, and for systolic blood pressure it is in the night between 0000 and 0300 hours (Fig. 7).

References

1. De Gaudemaris R, Mallion J-M, Battistella P, Battistella B, Siché J-P, Blatier J-F, Francois M (1987) Ambulatory blood pressure and variability by age and sex in 200 normotensive subjects: reference population values. J Hypertens 5 [Suppl 5]:429–430
2. Drayer J, Weber MA, Chard ER (1983) Non-invasive automated blood pressure monitoring in ambulatory normotensive men. In: Weber MA, Drayer JIM (eds) Ambulatory blood pressure monitoring. Steinkopff, Darmstadt, pp 129–135
3. Imai Y, Nakatsuka Abe H, Ikeda M, Nagai K, Munakata M, Sakuma H, Hashimoto J, Yoshinaga K (1990) A cross-sectional survey of home BP and ambulatory BP in a community in northern Japan. J Hypertens 8 [Suppl 3]:S89 (abstract)
4. Kennedy HL, Horan MJ, Sprague MK, Padgett NE, Shriver KK (1983) Ambulatory blood pressure in healthy normotensive males. Am Heart J 10:717–722
5. O'Brien E, Murphy J, Tyndall A, Atkins N, McCarthy G, O'Malley K (1990) 24-Hour ambulatory blood pressure in normotensive subjects. J Hypertens 8 [Suppl 3]:S87 (abstract)
6. Pagny J-Y, Delva R, Aouizerate M, Chatellier G, Battaglia C, Devriès C, Plouin PF, Corvol P, Ménard J (1987) La pression artérielle ambulatoire des sujets normotendus. Presse Méd 16:1621–1624
7. Tseng Y-Z, Lin L-J, Tseng C-D, Lo H-M, Chiang F-T, Hsu K-L, Wu T-L, Tseng W-P (1990) 24-Hour ambulatory blood pressure measurements in normal young adults. XIth World Congress of Cardiology. Phil J Cardiol 19 [Suppl 1]:411 (abstract)
8. Wallace JM, Thornton WE, Kennedy HL, Pickering TG, Harshfield GA, Frohlich ED, Messerli FH, Gifford RW, Bolen K (1984) Ambulatory blood pressure in 199 normal subjects, a collaborative study. In: Weber MA, Drayer JIM (eds) Ambulatory blood pressure monitoring. Steinkopff, Darmstadt, pp 117–127

Diurnal Variations
in Drug Actions

Recent Advances in the Chronopharmacology of Cardiovascular Active Drugs

B. Lemmer

Circadian rhythms in the functions of the cardiovascular system are now well established [1–4]. However, biological rhythms in heart rate and blood pressure were already described at the end of the eighteenth and during the nineteenth century by Falconer [5], Autenrieth [6], Wilhelm [7], Zadek [8], Knox [9], and others. Following these early reports, numerous more sophisticated studies have provided convincing evidence for circadian rhythms in heart rate and in blood pressure both in healthy subjects and in patients suffering from cardiovascular diseases. The development and use of automatic 24-h blood pressure monitoring devices has greatly contributed to our present knowledge about circadian rhythms in the cardiovascular system. While the rhythms in heart rate and blood pressure are the best known periodic functions in the cardiovascular system, other parameters have been shown to exhibit circadian variations as well, e.g., in blood flow, stroke volume, peripheral resistance, parameters of ECG recordings, in the plasma concentrations of pressor hormones such as noradrenaline, renin, angiotensin, aldosterone, in atrial natriuretic hormone, and plasma cAMP concentration, in blood viscosity, aggregability, and fibrinolytic activity. Some of these are relevant for an understanding of the chronopathology of cardiovascular disease and the chronopharmacokinetics and -dynamics of cardiovascular active drugs (for details see review articles mentioned above). In addition to circadian rhythms in physiological functions of the cardiovascular system, various clinical reports clearly indicate that the onset of cardiovascular diseases and symptoms exhibits pronounced temporal dependency [1–4]. These physiological and pathophysiological findings of circadian changes in the regulatory mechanisms and functions of the cardiovascular system clearly indicate that the effects (desired and undesired) as well as the pharmacokinetics of drugs used in the treatment of cardiovascular disorders are likely to exhibit circadian temporal dependencies as well. This has been convincingly demonstrated not only in animal experiments [10] but in human chronopharmacological studies [3, 4, 11]. Tables 1 and 2 list those drugs for which daily variations in their pharmacodynamics or in their pharmacokinetics have been reported in man [12].

This review concentrates on recent data with therapeutically relevant, cardiovascularly active drugs in man in whom simultaneously the pharmacokinetics and the hemodynamic drug effects were determined after drug application at different times of the day.

Schmidt/Engel/Blümchen (Eds.)
Temporal Variations of the Cardiovascular System
© Springer-Verlag Berlin Heidelberg 1992

Table 1. Cardiovascular active drugs: chronopharmacodynamics [12]

Beta-blockers	Calcium channel blockers
Acebutolol	Amlodipine
Atenolol	Nifedipine
Bevantolol	Nisoldipine
Bopindolol	Nitrendipine
Labetolol	Verapamil
Mepindolol	
Metoprolol	**ACE inhibitors**
Nadolol	Captopril
Oxprenolol	Enalapril
Pindolol	
Propranolol	**Others**
Sotalol	Clonidin
	Prazosin
Diuretics	Potassium chloride
Hydrochlorothiazide	
Indapamide	**Nitrates**
Piretanide	Glyceryl-trinitrate
Xipamide	Isosorbide-dinitrate
	Isosorbide-5-mononitrate

Table 2. Cardiovascular active drugs: chronopharmacokinetics [12]

Beta-blockers	Calcium channel blockers
Propranolol	Diltiazem
	Nifedipine
	Verapamil
Nitrates	
Isosorbide-dinitrate	
Isosorbide-5-mononitrate	
Immediate-release	
Sustained-release	
Glycosides	**Others**
Digoxin	Dipyridamol
Metildigoxin	Potassium chloride

Beta-receptor blocking drugs are still of great therapeutic value in the treatment of various cardiovascular disorders, e.g., coronary heart disease, hypertension, and arrhythmias. The various beta-receptor blocking drugs differ not only in their specific effects (receptor affinity and selectivity, intrinsic sympathomimetic activity) and in their nonspecific effects (related to lipophilicity of the compound), but they also differ greatly in their main routes of elimination (lipophilic ones: mainly hepatic biotransformation; hydrophilic ones: renal elimination). Various beta-receptor blocking drugs have been studied intensively in animal experiments [11, 13, 14] as well as in patients [2–4, 15] in relation to circadian time. However, detailed chronopharmacokinetic studies with different beta-blockers have only been performed in rats [11, 13–15]. In man the pharmacokinetics of only

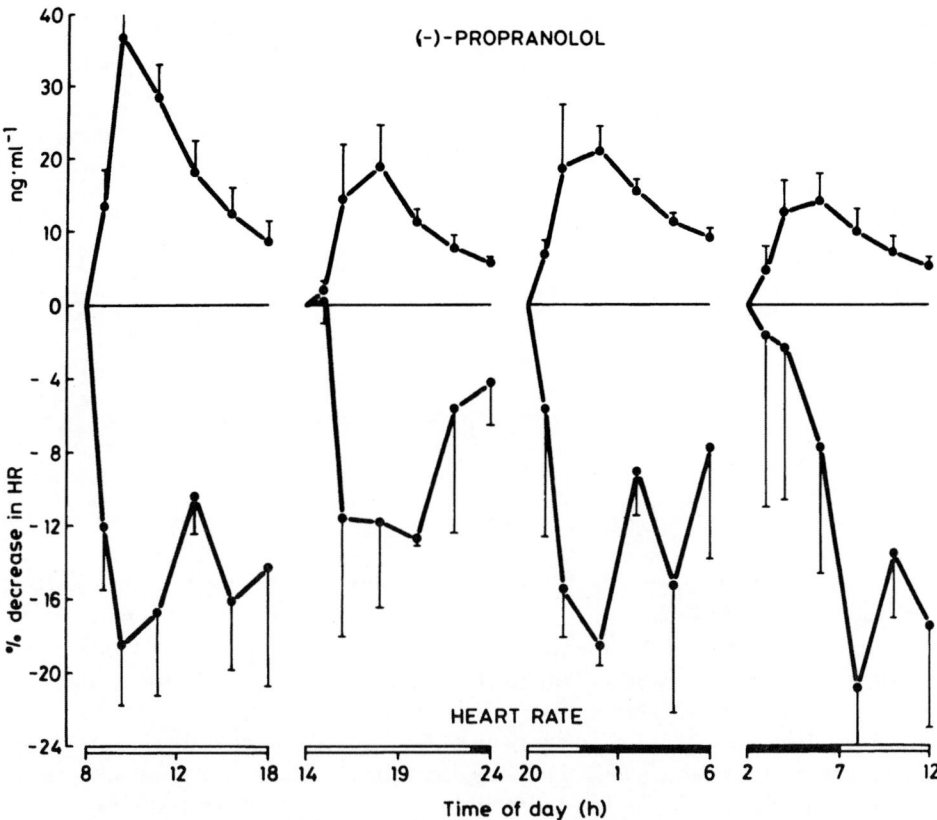

Fig. 1. Circadian phase dependency in the plasma concentrations of (−)-propranolol and in heart rate decrease as percentage of circadian control values after oral intake of 80 mg racemic propranolol by healthy volunteers at either 0800, 1400, 2000, or 0200 hours local time. Mean values ± SEM [17]

propranolol were investigated at different times of day [16, 17]. In our own study significant daily variations in peak drug concentration (C_{max}), area under the curve (AUC), and elimination half-life were found when racemic propranolol (Dociton) was administered at four circadian times (0800, 1400, 2000, 0200 hours) to healthy subjects (Fig. 1, Table 3). Trough values in C_{max} and AUC were found after drug application at 0200 hours and peak values in C_{max} and AUC were obtained at 0800 hours [17]. As has been shown for other lipophilic drugs, the absorption of propranolol was clearly circadian stage dependent, being greatest when ingested at 0800 hours (Table 3). At any time of drug intake the ratio of the plasma concentrations of (−)- to (+)-propranolol was about 1.5 [17]. Thus, the stereospecific metabolism of propranolol did not display a circadian phase dependency. Interestingly, in man shorter elimination half-lives of either (−)- or (+)-propranolol were found when the drug was given at 0800 hours rather than at 2000 hours [17]. Fig. 1 demonstrates that the changes in heart rate in relation to the respective circadian control values (hemodynamic functions always measured in

Table 3. Pharmacokinetic and hemodynamic parameters of propranolol (80 mg p. o.) administered at four different times in a day to four healthy volunteers [17]

	Time of propranolol administration			
	0800 hours	1400 hours	2000 hours	0200 hours
Pharmacokinetics				
C_{max} (ng/ml)	38.6 ± 11.2	20.0 ± 6.5	26.2 ± 5.3	18.4 ± 4.4 [a]
t_{max} (h)	2.5 ± 0.5	3.5 ± 0.5	3.0 ± 0.6	3.5 ± 1.0
AUC (ng ml^{-1} h^{-1})	169 ± 47	106 ± 30	140 ± 23	92 ± 22
$t_{1/2}\beta$ (h)	3.3 ± 0.4	4.2 ± 0.5	4.9 ± 0.2	4.4 ± 0.6 [b]
C_{max}/t_{max} (ng ml^{-1} h^{-1})	17.9 ± 6.4	7.5 ± 3.9	10.6 ± 3.7	7.1 ± 2.4 [a]
Hemodynamics (heart rate)				
E_{max} (b/min)	16.0 ± 2.4	11.7 ± 1.8	16.3 ± 1.5	15.3 ± 4.6
T_{max} (h)	2.3 ± 0.6	4.5 ± 1.0	6.5 ± 1.5	7.0 ± 1.0 [a]

[a] $p < 0.05$; ANOVA;
[b] $p < 0.01$; ANOVA.

the sitting position) were markedly different depending on the time of propranolol
ingestion. After administration of propranolol at 0200 hours the heart rate was
only slightly affected within the first 6 h after drug intake. However, 2 h later, at
the onset of the activity span when sympathetic tone was increasing again (as
demonstrated by the rhythm in plasma noradrenaline and cAMP), the heart rate
lowering effect was pronounced again and about equally to that found after drug
application at 0800 hours (Fig. 1). Thus, peak drug effects coincided with peak
drug concentrations only after propranolol intake at 0800 and 1400 hours and
were delayed after propranolol administration at 2000 and at 0200 hours (Table 3),
indicating a circadian time dependency in the dose-response relationship of
propranolol. Furthermore, these data clearly demonstrate that the chronopharmacokinetics of propranolol cannot mainly be responsible for the daily
variations in the drug's hemodynamic effects. The daily rhythm in the level of the
sympathetic tone seems mainly to determine the degree in beta-adrenoceptor
blockade and thus leading to more pronounced effects in the activity period of
humans during daytime hours, in which sympathetic tone is high.

As already described, the onset of angina pectoris and the frequency of angina
attacks exhibit a circadian rhythm, a finding which has been confirmed by many
authors [1–4]. Aside from the early report of Yasue et al. [18] that in patients
suffering from Prinzmetal angina pectoris nitroglycerin was more effective in the
morning than in the afternoon, no data are available on a possible chronopharmacology of oral nitrates. In several studies we have investigated in healthy
volunteers simultaneously the pharmacokinetics and the hemodynamic effects of
isosorbide dinitrate (ISDN) and of two formulations (immediate-release,
sustained-release) of isosorbide-5-mononitrate (IS-5-MN) [19–22]. In all of the
studies the hemodynamic effects were always measured after 3 min standing
upright, and drug effects were compared to the individual circadian control values
determined under the same experimental conditions. Due to its complex
metabolism into two active metabolites the chronopharmacokinetic situation is

Table 4. Pharmacokinetic parameters of ISDN (20 mg p. o.) administered at four different times of a day to six healthy volunteers [20, 22]

	Time of ISDN administration			
	0800 hours	1400 hours	2000 hours	0200 hours
C_{max} (ng/ml)	30.7 ±11.8	26.0 ±10.2	25.3 ±11.0	27.3 ±11.8
t_{max} (h)	0.62±0.12	0.53±0.20	0.63±0.20	0.51±0.21
AUC (ng ml^{-1} h^{-1})	33.9 ±6.9	24.8 ±3.7	25.4 ±4.5	34.1 ±4.1 [a]
$t_{1/2}\beta$ (h)	0.6 ±0.2	0.8 ±0.3	1.1 ±0.4	1.3 ±0.4 [b]

[a] $p < 0.01$, 0800 hours versus 1400 and 2000 hours, 0200 versus 1400 and 2000 hours; Neuman-Keuls;

[b] $p < 0.05$; ANOVA.

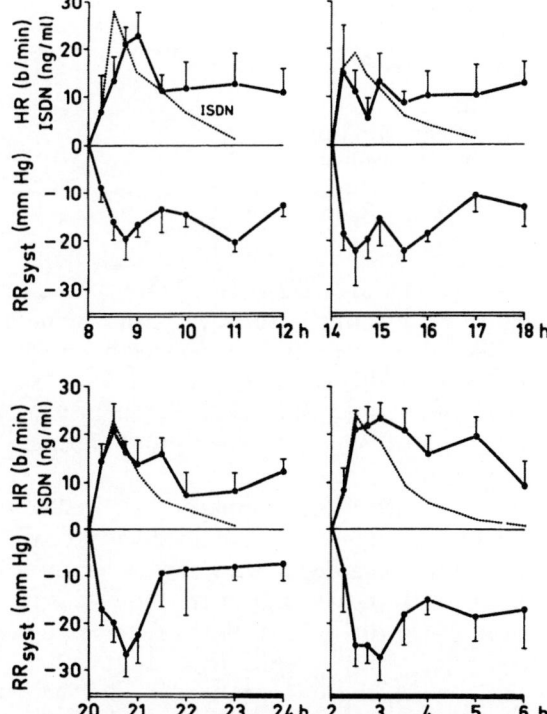

Fig. 2. Daily variations in the decrease in systolic blood pressure and increase in heart rate (3 min standing upright) after oral intake of 20 mg ISDN at either 0800, 1400, 2000, or 0200 hours local time. Data were calculated in relation to circadian control values. Dotted lines, ISDN mean plasma concentrations. Mean values ± SEM [20, 22]

Table 5. Pharmacokinetic and hemodynamic parameters of an immediate-release preparation of IS-5-MN (60 mg p.o.) administered at two different times of a day to eight healthy volunteers [19, 20]

	Time of i.r. IS-5-MN administration	
	0630 hours	1830 hours
Pharmacokinetics		
C_{max} (ng/ml)	1605 $\pm$175	1588 $\pm$173
t_{max} (h)	0.9$\pm$0.3	2.1$\pm$0.4 [a]
AUC (ng ml^{-1} h^{-1})	9539 $\pm$827	10959 $\pm$707
$t_{1/2}\beta$ (h)	4.6$\pm$0.4	4.2$\pm$0.4
Hemodynamics		
T_{max} BP_{sys} decrease (mm Hg)	0.7$\pm$0.1	1.1$\pm$0.1
T_{max} BP_{dia} decrease (mm Hg)	0.4$\pm$0.1	0.6$\pm$0.2
T_{max} HR increase (b/min)	0.8$\pm$0.3	0.9$\pm$0.2

Wilcoxon test: * $p < 0.01$;
[a] $p < 0.01$; Wilcoxon test.

complicated in the case of ISDN [20, 22]. Table 4 shows that daily variations in the pharmacokinetics of ISDN (Iso Mack) could nevertheless be observed in healthy subjects with about a 40% variation in bioavailability (AUC, Table 4). No circadian phase-dependent differences were found in C_{max} and t_{max} of ISDN or in the pharmacokinetics of the metabolites IS-2-MN and IS-5-MN, half-life of ISDN, however, was shorter during nightly hours than during daytime (Table 4). The latter finding was similar to that observed with oral propranolol (Table 3). Hemodynamic effects – mainly reflexly induced increase in heart rate – were most pronounced after ISDN application at 0200 hours (Fig. 2).

Interesting results were obtained with the two IS-5-MN preparations [19–22]. With the immediate-release preparation of IS-5-MN (IS-5-MN Stadapharm) clear-cut daily variations were found in regard to t_{max} being significantly shorter after morning (0.9$\pm$0.3 h) than after evening (2.1$\pm$0.4 h) application (Table 5). Most interestingly, time to peak drug effects in describing blood pressure and reflexly increasing heart rate coincided with t_{max} in pharmacokinetics in the morning but were in advance by about 1 h in the evening (Table 5). No daily variations were observed in the pharmacokinetics of the sustained-release formulation of IS-5-MN (Coleb-Duriles; Table 5 [21]). Figure 3 shows the daily variations in the mean control values in systolic and diastolic blood pressure and in heart rate after 3 min standing upright [21]. Rhythm (cosinor) analysis of the group mean data revealed significant rhythmic variations for the 24-h rhythms of systolic ($p < 0.00001$) and diastolic blood pressure ($p < 0.038$) and for the 12-h rhythm in heart rate ($p < 0.001$; Fig. 3 [21]). Rhythm-adjusted means for systolic, diastolic blood pressure and heart rate were 115.0$\pm$0.4 mm Hg, 82.4$\pm$0.4 mm Hg, and 80.8$\pm$0.5 beats/min, respectively. Peak values of rhythms

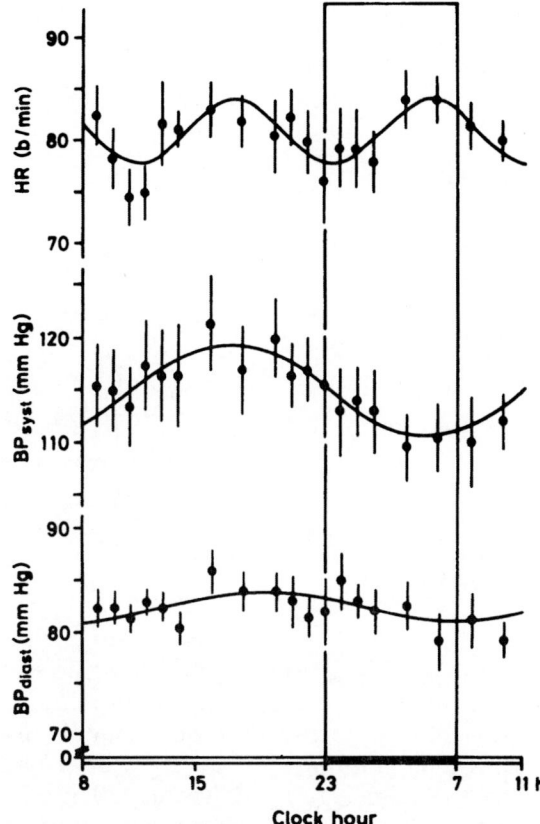

Fig. 3. Daily variations in heart rate, systolic and diastolic blood pressure after 3 min standing upright in ten healthy men. Cosinor analysis revealed a significant ($p < 0.01$) 12-h rhythm in heart rate and a 24-h rhythm in systolic ($p < 0.00001$) and diastolic ($p < 0.038$) blood pressure. Mean values $\pm$ SEM of ten subjects [21]

(acrophases) occurred at 17.23 ± 0.4 h (systolic blood pressure), at 18.98 ± 1.24 h (diastolic blood pressure) and at 17.58 ± 0.4 h and 5.58 ± 0.4 h (heart rate; see also Fig. 3). Thus, these hemodynamic data clearly demonstrate that significant daily variations are present also when hemodynamic functions are measured in the standing position throughout 24 h of a day. Peak drug effects in lowering blood pressure and increasing heart rate again coincided with t_{max} in the drug's pharmacokinetics (around 5 h) in the morning, but occurred about 2 h earlier after drug application in the evening (Table 6). This again points to daily variations in the dose response relationship of drugs as already mentioned before for propranolol and nifedipine (see below). In addition, the data obtained with the two different formulations of IS-5-MN indicate that also the kind of drug formulation may be of importance whether or not chronokinetics can be observed.

Recently, we were also able to demonstrate significant daily variations in the pharmacokinetics of an immediate-release preparation of nifedipine in healthy

Table 6. Pharmacokinetic and hemodynamic parameters of sustained release IS-5-MN (60 mg p. o.) administered at two different times of a day to ten healthy volunteers [21]

	Time of s. r. IS-5-MN administration	
	0800 hours	2000 hours
Pharmacokinetics		
C_{max} (ng/ml)	509 $\pm$ 31	530 $\pm$ 26
t_{max} (h)	5.2 $\pm$ 0.7	4.9 $\pm$ 0.3
AUC (ng ml^{-1} h^{-1})	6729 $\pm$ 375	6418 $\pm$ 199
$t_{1/2}$ (h)	6.4 $\pm$ 0.6	6.1 $\pm$ 0.5
Hemodynamics		
T_{max} BP_{sys} decrease (mm Hg)	5.0 $\pm$ 0.6	2.8 $\pm$ 0.5 [a]
T_{max} BP_{dia} decrease (mm Hg)	6.0 $\pm$ 0.7	2.9 $\pm$ 0.5 [b]
T_{max} HR increase (b/min)	5.2 $\pm$ 1.0	3.8 $\pm$ 0.6

[a] $p < 0.05$;
[b] $p < 0.005$.

subjects [23, 24]. In this study nifedipine (Cordicant Kapsel) was applied to healthy subjects at a dose of 10 mg either at 0800 or at 1900 hours. The pharmacokinetic analysis revealed that not only t_{max} was significantly longer after evening than morning application (37.5 versus 22.5 min), but that also C_{max} (45.7 versus 82.0 ng/ml), AUC (85 versus 130 ng ml^{-1} h^{-1}) and drug absorption (C_{max}/t_{max}: 1.5 versus 4.5 ng ml^{-1} h^{-1}) were significantly greater in the morning than in the evening. Thus, a significant daily variation in the bioavailability was found with a reduction in bioavailability of about 35% in the evening. Since the ratio in the AUC of the main nitropyridine metabolite to the parent compound was not significantly different at the two time points of drug application, it was assumed that the reduction in nifedipine bioavailability must mainly be due to a reduced absorption and/or an increased presystemic metabolism in the evening [23, 24]. Only minor daily variations were found in the cardiovascular effects in normotensive subjects of this nifedipine preparation [23, 24]. Thus it turned out that also the dose-response relationship of the calcium channel blocker nifedipine was different during daytime and during night. In a very recent study we could demonstrate that a retard formulation of nifedipine (Cordicant Retard) did not show significant daily variations in its pharmacokinetics when applied twice daily (20 mg at 0800 and at 1900 hours) for 7 days [25]. Time to peak drug effects on blood pressure decrease, however, was significantly shorter after evening than after morning administration whereas the duration in blood pressure decrease was slightly longer after morning drug application [25].

References

1. Smolensky MH, Tatar SE, Bergmann SA, Losmann JG, Barnard CN, Dacso CC, Kraft IA (1976) Circadian rhythmic aspects of human cardiovascular function: a review by chronobiologic statistical methods. Chronobiologia 3:337–371
2. Lemmer B (1989) Circadian variations in the effects of cardiovascular active drugs. In: Arnim von T, Maseri A (eds) Predisposing conditions for acute ischemic syndromes. Steinkopff, Darmstadt, pp 1–11
3. Lemmer B (1989) Temporal aspects of the effects of cardiovascular active drugs in humans. In: Lemmer B (ed) Chronopharmacology – cellular and biochemical interactions. Dekker, New York, pp 525–541
4. Lemmer B (1989) Circadian rhythms in the cardiovascular system. In: Arendt J, Minors DS, Waterhouse JM (eds) Biologigal rhythms in clinical practice. Butterworth, London, pp 51–70
5. Falconer W (1797) Beobachtungen über den Puls. Heinsius, Leipzig
6. Autenrieth JHF (1801) Handbuch der empirischen Physiologie, Teil 1. Heerbrandt, Tübingen
7. Wilhelm GT (1809) Unterhaltungen über den Menschen: dritter und letzter Band: von dem Körper und seinen Teilen und Funktionen insbesondere. Engelbrecht'sche Kunsthandlung, Augsburg
8. Zadek J (1881) Die Messung des Blutdrucks des Menschen mittels des Bach'schen Apparates. Z Klin Med 2:509–555
9. Knox R (1815) On the relation subsitsting between time of the day, and various functions of the human body; and on the manner in which the pulsation of the heart and the arteries are affected by muscular exertion. Edinburgh Med Surg J 11:52–65
10. Lemmer B (1989) Temporal aspects of the regulation of the sympathetic nervous system in the rat. In: Lemmer B (ed) Chronopharmacology – cellular and biochemical interactions. Dekker, New York, pp 477–508
11. Lemmer B (1989) Temporal aspects of the effects of cardiovascular active drugs in humans. In: Lemmer B (ed) Chronopharmacology – cellular and biochemical interactions. Dekker, New York, pp 525–541
12. Lemmer B, Scheidel B, Behne S (1991) Chronopharmacokinetics and chronopharmacodynamics of cardiovascular active drugs: propranolol, organic nitrates, nifedipine. Ann NY Acad Sci 618:166–181
13. Lemmer B, Bathe K (1982) Stereospecific and circadian-phase-dependent kinetic behaviour of d, l-, l- and d-propranolol in plasma, heart and brain of light-dark-sychronized rats. J Cardiovasc Pharmacol 4:635–644
14. Lemmer B, Winkler H, Ohm T, Fink M (1985) Chronopharmacokinetics of beta-receptor blocking drugs of different lipophilicity (propranolol, metoprolol, sotalol, atenolol) in plasma and tissues after single and multiple dosing in the rat. Naunyn-Schmiedebergs Arch Pharmacol 330:42–49
15. Lemmer B, Bathe K, Lang PH, Neumann G, Winkler H (1983) Chronopharmacology of β-adrenoceptor blocking drugs: pharmacokinetics and pharmacodynamic studies in rats. J Am Coll Toxicol 2:347–35
16. Semenowizc-Siuda K, Markiewicz A, Korczynska-Wardecka J (1984) Circadian bioavailability some effects of propranolol in healthy subjects and liver cirrhosis. Int. J Clin Pharmacol Ther Toxicol 22:653–658
17. Langner B, Lemmer B (1988) Circadian changes in the pharmacokinetics and cardiovascular effects of oral propranolol in healthy subjects. Eur J Clin Pharmacol 33:619–624
18. Yasue H, Omote S, Takizawa A, Nagao M, Miwa K, Tanaka S (1979) Circadian variation of exercise capacity in patients with Prinzmetal's variant angina: role of exercise-induced coronary arterial spasm. Circulation 59:938–948
19. Scheidel B, Lenhard G, Blume H, Becker HJ, Lemmer B (1989) Chronopharmacology of isosorbide-5-mononitrate (immediate release, retard formulation) in healthy subjects. Eur J Clin Pharmacol 36 [Suppl]:A177
20. Lemmer B, Scheidel B, Stenzhorn G, Blume H, Lenhard G, Grether D, Renczes J, Becker HJ (1989) Clinical chronopharmacology of oral nitrates. Z Kardiol 78 [Suppl 2]:61–63

21. Lemmer B, Scheidel B, Blume H, Becker H-J (1991) Clinical chronopharmacology of oral sustained-release isosorbide-5-mononitrate in healthy subjects. Eur J Clin Pharmacol 40:71–75
22. Scheidel B, Lemmer B, Blume H (1990) Influence of time of day on pharmacokinetics and hemodynamic effects of oral organic nitrates. In: Lemmer B, Hüller H (eds) Clinical chronopharmacology, Klinische Pharmakologie/clinical pharmacology, Vol 6. Zuckschwerdt, Munich pp 75–79
23. Lemmer B, Behne S, Becker HJ (1989) Chronopharmacology of oral nifedipine in healthy subjects. Eur J Clin Pharmacol 36 [Suppl]: A 177
24. Behne S, Becker H-J, Liefhold J, Lemmer B (1990) On the chronopharmacokinetics, effects on cardiovascular functions and plasma cAMP or oral nifedipine in healthy subjects. In: Lemmer B, Hüller H (eds) Clinical chronopharmacology, Klinische Pharmakologie/clinical pharmacology, vol. 6, Zuckschwerdt, Munich pp 59–63
25. Lemmer B, Nold G, Behne S, Becker H-J, Liefhold J, Kaiser R (1990) Chronopharmacology of oral nifedipine in healthy subjects and in hypertensive patients. Eur J Clin Pharmacol 183:521

Chronopharmacokinetic Aspects with Special Reference to Cardiovascular Drugs

B. Bruguerolle

Introduction

Some drugs have a narrow therapeutic range, and it has been shown for these drugs that therapeutic monitoring is necessary since there is a close relationship between the pharmacological effect and the blood level. This constitutes the basis for pharmacokinetic studies involving the study of the fate of drugs in the organism related to time, i.e., absorption, distribution, metabolism, and elimination processes. Mathematical models are used to simplify and summarize these processes and thus simulate concentrations of the drug in all parts of the organism. This concept underlies the search for a constant blood level of the drug thought to be necessary to obtain an effect as constant as possible. Obviously, the chronopharmacological data deny this concept, since the efficacy, toxicity and kinetics of drugs have been reported to depend on the moment of its administration (Reinberg and Halberg 1971), (Reinberg and Ghata 1990). Chronopharmacokinetics concerns the study of the temporal changes in absorption, distribution, metabolism, and elimination of a drug and thus the influence of time of administration on mathematical parameters that describe these different stages. The chronokinetics of more than 100 drugs has been reported in animal or in man, as reviewed by Reinberg and Smolensky (1982), Lemmer (1981 b), Bruguerolle (1983 a, b, 1987), and Levi et al. (1989).

We elaborate here on chronopharmacokinetics with special reference to cardiovascular drugs. We consider successively some chronobiological data involved in chronopharmacokinetics, the main experimental and clinical kinetic studies concerning cardiovascular drugs, the approach of some mechanisms, and finally a number of methodological problems.

Chronobiological Data Involved in Chronopharmacokinetics

A drug successively undergoes absorption, distribution, metabolisation, and finally excretion from the organism; each of these steps involves biological phenomena that obviously may vary with the time of day. Some of these factors are shown in Fig. 1. Circadian rhythms in human cardiovascular functions such as

Schmidt/Engel/Blümchen (Eds.)
Temporal Variations of the Cardiovascular System
© Springer-Verlag Berlin Heidelberg 1992

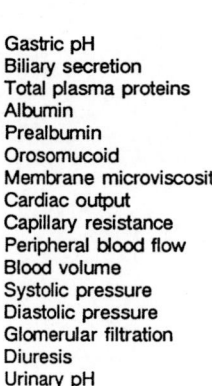
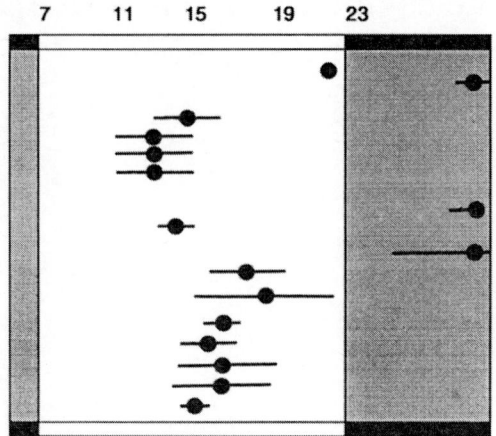

Fig. 1. Chronobiological data involved in chronokinetics

heart rate, blood flow, systolic and diastolic pressure, and blood volume may play an important role in the chronokinetics of cardiovascular drugs. One must notice that the acrophases of most of them are in the middle of the day. Also, as shown in Table 1, some plasma proteins involved in plasma drug protein binding vary over 24 h with a peak arround 1200 hours.

Main Experimental and Clinical Kinetic Studies Concerning Cardiovascular Drugs

The chronopharmacokinetics of cardiovascular drugs such as antiarrhythmics, cardiotonics, β-adrenergic blocking agents, and calcium blockers have been reported in animals or in man; the main findings of these studies are summarized in Tables 1 and 2. For example, the chronokinetics of procainamide were investigated in the rat after a single intramuscular dose administered at four different fixed time points of a 24-h period (Bruguerolle and Jadot 1985). When procainamide was given at 2200 hours, its elimination half-life was shorter than when given at 1000, 1600 or 0400 hours. Also, the kinetics of the main metabolite, N-acetylprocainamide (NAPA), varied over 24 h, indicating a maximal N-acetylation at 0400 hours. The chronokinetics of β-blocking agents were also studied intensively by Lemmer et al. in rats. They clearly demonstrated in rodents temporal variations in tissular and plasmatic levels of these agents. Thus the elimination half-life significantly decreases during the dark phase (i.e., the activity period). If one takes into account the opposition in phase of the mode of synchronization between rodents and humans, it is clear that these results agree well with data obtained in man (better bioavailability in the morning and shorter elimination half-life).

Table 1. Chronopharmacokinetic changes of cardiovascular drugs in man

Drugs	Subjects	Variables	Major observations	References
Digoxin	Elderly men	C_{max}, T_{max}, AUC	C_{max} higher at 0900 hours	Bruguerolle et al. 1988a
Dipyridamole	Adult healthy men	Plasma levels urinary excretion	Max. bioavailability at 0600 hours; min. urinary excretion between 1800 and 0200 hours	Markiewicz, Semenowicz, 1980
Isosorbide dinitrate	Adult healthy men	C_{max}, T_{max}, AUC C_{max}/T_{max},	Highest AUC at 0200 hours; no diff. with sustained-release form	Lemmer et al. 1989
Methyldigoxin	Adult patients	Plasma levels, AUC	Max. AUC at 1600 hours, second peak in morning	Carosella et al. 1979
Nifedipine	Adult healthy men	C_{max}, T_{max}, AUC	C_{max} lower and T_{max}, longer in the evening; max. AUC in morning	Lemmer et al. 1990
Nitrindipine	Adult healthy subjects (Sd)	C_{max}, T_{max}, $T_{1/2}\beta$, AUC	C_{max} higher at 0900 hours	Fujimura et al. 1989
Nitrindipine	Adult healthy subjects (8-day treatment)	Plasma levels	No significant differences	Lecocq et al. 1991
Procainamide	Adult men and women	Plasma levels	No significant differences	Fujimura et al. 1989a
Propranolol	Adult subjects	C_{max}, T_{max}, AUC C_{max}/T_{max}, $T_{1/2}$	C_{max}, AUC and C_{max}/T_{max} highest at 0800 hours; T_{max} and $T_{1/2}$ lowest at 0800 hours	Langner and Lemmer 1988
Verapamil	Adults with angina pectoris	C_{max}, T_{max}, AUC $T_{1/2}\beta$	Greater AUC and prolonged time to peak at 2200 hours	Jespersen et al. 1989

Sd, single dose; C_{max}, maximal plasma concentration; T_{max}, maximal time to reach C_{max}; $T_{1/2}\beta$, elimination half-life; AUC, area under plasma concentrations curve.

Approach of Chronopharmacokinetic Mechanisms

Temporal Variations in Drug Absorption

Circadian variations in gastrointestinal pH or motility, digestive secretions, intestinal blood flow, and membrane permeability may be involved in temporal variations of drug resorption. The chronopharmacokinetic effects have often been considered to depend only on oral absorption and have thus been considered to be strictly related to gastric or intestinal emptying. Obviously, food influences the

Table 2. Chronopharmacokinetic changes of cardiovascular drugs in animals

Drugs	Species	Variables	Major observations	References
Disopyramide	Mice	C_{max}, $T_{1/2}\beta$, Vd, Cl, AUC, protein binding	max. Vd, Cl at 2200 hours; max. AUC at 0400 hours; max. protein binding at 1600 hours	Bruguerolle 1984b
Lidocaine	Rat	Plasma and RBC levels	max. $T_{1/2}\beta$ at 1000 hours; max. AUC at 1600 hours; max. Vd at 0400 hours	Bruguerolle et al. 1982
Procainamide NAPA	Rat	Plasma levels	$T_{1/2}\beta$ shorter at 2200 hours; N-acetylation max. at 0400 hours	Bruguerolle 1984
Propranolol	Rat	Plasma, heart, brain levels	$T_{1/2}\beta$ shortest at night	Lemmer et al. 1985
Metoprolol, Sotalol, Atenolol	Rat	Plasma, heart, brain levels Sd and Rd	$T_{1/2}\beta$ shortest at night; no significant diff. after Rd	Lemmer et al. 1985

Sd, single dose; C_{max}, maximal plasma concentration; T_{max}, maximal time to reach C_{max}; $T_{1/2}\beta$, elimination half-life; Vd, volume of distribution; AUC, area under plasma concentrations curve.

rate of absorption of a drug; in the presence of food, a drug passes less rapidly through intestinal membranes than in fasting conditions. Galenic considerations may also be involved in drug absorption. Smolensky (1989) recently reviewed temporal variations in theophylline disposition and described differences in temporal changes of the absorption of the slow-release forms according to the galenic formulation. Circadian phase dependent differences in the pharmacokinetics were also reported for an immediate-release and a retard formulation of isosorbide-5-mononitrate (Lemmer et al. 1989). A more rapid absorption after morning drug administration than after evening intake was recently reported for propranolol (Langner and Lemmer 1988). Most lipophilic drugs seem to be faster absorbed in man when the drug is taken in the morning. The influence of posture is often adduced to explain temporal variations of the oral absorption of a drug. This factor must obviously be stricly controlled in chronokinetic studies since posture is a factor that can modify the pharmacokinetics of a drug by modifying local blood flow. Finally, it appears that while temporal variations of drug absorption do exist, these may be influenced by many factors such as food, posture, and galenic form of the drug (Bruguerolle 1989). Thus, future chronokinetic studies must consider and control all these factors.

Temporal Variations in Drug Distribution

The process of distribution of a drug involves its passage through biological membranes, its transport by plasma proteins or red blood cells, and its tissue binding.

Temporal Changes of Binding to Plasma Proteins. Drugs are transported from their site of administration to receptor sites by plasma proteins such as serum albumin, alpha-1 acid glycoprotein, globulins, and lipoproteins. Since only the unbound drug can diffuse through membranes and tissues (representing the active fraction of the drug), the protein binding of drugs has important pharmacological implications. We have reported circadian variations for free plasma drug level of basic (lidocaine, disopyramide) drugs. In rodents the lower free level (i.e., the highest protein binding) was located at 2200 hours for lidocaine (Bruguerolle et al. 1982) or disopyramide (Bruguerolle 1984b). Such variations provide at least in part explicative mechanisms for chronokinetics. Haen et al. (1985) reported circadian variations in propranolol plasma protein binding in rats with peaks at 1600 and 2400 hours. All these data may depend on temporal variations of different plasma proteins, as reported by Reinberg et al. (1977), Hecquet and Sucche 1986 or Bruguerolle et al. (1986b). We have studied the physiological circadian time structure of some plasma proteins in man and its alterations by age or by different disease states such as cancer (Bruguerolle et al. 1986b) and inflammatory diseases (Focan et al. 1988). Such changes are of important interest concerning the possible explanations of chronopharmacological effects or of chronokinetic mechanisms. But the practical question raised by temporal variations of plasma protein drug binding is also their clinical implications. It is generally admitted by pharmacologists that clinically significant consequences of drug binding changes are observed only for drugs which are highly bound (more than 80%); thus, temporal variations in plasma drug binding may have clinical implications only for drugs characterized by a high protein binding and a small apparent volume of distribution.

Temporal Aspects in Drug Binding to Erythrocytes and Membrane Permeability. Drugs may also be transported in the blood by red blood cells. Time dependency of drug binding to erythrocytes has not been reported, to our knowledge, with the exception of local anesthetics (lidocaine, bupivacaine, etidocaine, and mepivacaine) and indomethacin. We reported in rats the chronokinetics of lidocaine as well as the circadian variations of its passage into red blood cells (Bruguerolle and Jadot 1983). To assess the circadian time dependent passage into the erythrocytes, the ratio of drug concentration in erythrocytes to plasma concentrations was calculated; when the drug was given at 2200 hours, the ratio was 0.74 versus 0.48 at 10.00 hours (Bruguerolle and Jadot 1983). Time dependency of the passage of drugs into red blood cells provides a strong argument for temporal variations of the passage of drugs through biological membranes since red blood cells are often used as a model for the study of the passage of drugs through membranes.

Temporal Variations in Drug Metabolism

The main site of drug metabolism is the liver, but many other tissues may also be implicated, such as lungs, kidneys, blood, and digestive tract. Drug metabolism is generally assumed to depend on liver enzymes activity or hepatic blood flow; for some drugs such as lidocaine and propranolol (high hepatic coefficient of extraction) the metabolism depends on hepatic blood flow. For some others the biotransformations essentially depend on the enzymatic activity of the hepatocytes. Many factors may affect these biotransformations; temporal variations are of particular interest since they were described from many years and evoked to explain chronopharmacokinetic changes. Several chronobiological studies have been devoted to the study of temporal changes in liver enzymes activity by direct measurement or indirect evidence by measuring the chronokinetics of drugs and their metabolites.

Temporal Variations in Enzyme Activity. Circadian or ultradian rhythms of liver drug metabolism activity were demonstrated in vitro for the oxidative metabolism of drugs such as aminopyrine, *p*-nitro-anisol, hexobarbital (Radzialowsky and Bousquet 1968; Jori et al. 1971; Nair and Casper 1969) or 4-dimethylaminoazo-benzene (Radzialowsky and Bousquet 1968), with a peak located during the dark activity period. The oxidative reactions catalyzed by the cytochrome P-450 system are the major pathway involved in drug metabolism; the temporal changes in the hepatic P-450 system have been investigated by many authors and are reviewed by Belanger (1988). Many other rhythmic variations in enzymatic activity were documented and are reviewed by Belanger (1988) and Feuers and Scheving (1988). These circadian changes in metabolic pathways may be responsible for the variation in drug response. An interesting inverse relationship was found between the hepatic hexobarbital oxydase activity and the hexobarbital-induced sleep duration; the maximal hepatic hexobarbital activity (2200 hours) correspond to the minimal sleep duration in rats. This example is of particular interest since it underlines the temporal relationships between pharmacodynamic and pharmacokinetic parameters.

Temporal Variations in Hepatic Blood Flow. For drugs with a high extraction ratio (lidocaine, propranolol, etc.) the hepatic metabolism depends on hepatic blood flow. Circadian variations in hepatic blood flow induce modifications of liver perfusion and thus temporal variations in the clearance of drugs. To our knowledge, circadian variations of hepatic blood flow have not yet been documented in man; in rats, Dore et al. (1984) demonstrated circadian variations of hepatic blood flow which is maximal during the dark phase. To explain the temporal variations of lidocaine kinetics mentioned above (Bruguerolle et al. 1984), (Bruguerolle and Isnardon 1985) circadian variations in hepatic blood flow were evoked. Lemmer (1981) demonstrated temporal variations in propranolol plasma clearance (higher values at the end of the activity span). The clearance of propranolol depends upon the liver blood flow, which has been shown to be circadian phase dependent. Finally, it appears from studies of Belanger et al. (1981) that temporal variations in hepatic clearance may be detected for drugs having a high hepatic extraction ratio (paracetamol, antipyrine etc.) but not for those with a low ratio.

Indirect Evidence of Temporal Variations in Drug Metabolism. Numerous experimental or clinical chronopharmacological studies have documented chronokinetics. Some of these have indirectly investigated temporal variations in hepatic drug metabolism capacity by demonstrating chronokinetics of drugs and their metabolites; even if a metabolite is not pharmacologically active, its measurement indicates the rate of metabolizing capacity. For example, we reported chronokinetics of procainamide and its main metabolite, *N*-acetylprocainamide in rats (Bruguerolle and Jadot 1985); the elimination of these two compounds is circadian time dependent with maximal elimination during the dark activity phase. Elsewhere, these data have indicated a circadian rhythm of acetylation, which is maximal in the rat at 0400 hours.

Temporal Variations in Drug Excretion

Most drugs are eliminated by the renal route. Circadian rhythmicity of major renal functions, such as glomerular filtration, renal blood flow, urinary pH, and tubular resorption, have been documented by Cambar et al. (1979). Thus the urinary excretion of many drugs may depend on these rhythmic variations (Jones 1845). Physicochemical properties are of particular importance in this field since renal elimination depends partially on ionization of drugs and thus may be modified by temporal changes in urinary pH. Related to these variations, acidic drugs such as sodium salicylate (Reinberg et al. 1975) and sulfasymazine (Dettli and Spring 1966) exhibit a faster excretion after an evening than a morning administration. By contrast, renal excretion of sulfanilamide, another basic sulfamide (pKa = 10.5), does not vary over the 24-h scale (Dettli and Spring 1966).

Specific Methodological Aspects of Chronokinetics

Different specific methodological points must be underlined before starting a chronokinetic study. For instance, the state of patients (healthy or ill) participating in a chronokinetic study may influence the conclusions of the study. Temporal variations of biological rhythms in the organism are known to be modified by illness and thus may interfere with drug chronokinetics. We reported recently (Bruguerolle et al. 1986b, Focan et al. 1988) alterations of circadian time structure of plasma proteins in cancerous and inflammatory subjects; such variations may modify drug protein binding and thus have kinetic implications. To study the chronokinetics of a drug, several time points (dosing times) are needed. Choosing only two time points may lead one to ignore a temporal variation which exist in fact but may be detected only by choosing two more time points. If only two dosing times are possible, the choice of these time points must be determined according to a preliminary experiment or according to relevant reasons such as correspondance with peak or crest time of a biological marker (Reinberg et al.

1990). The importance of food intake on temporal variations of drug absorption has been discussed before and underlined by Reinberg et al. (1990). We would like to point out the necessity to control feeding habits in chronokinetics studies. Also, posture has been discussed as having a great importance in such studies since posture is obviously different in resting and activity conditions and may influence some factors involved in kinetic processes. For example, a 60% variation in hepatic blood flow has been demonstrated in man between standing and lying positions. Thus, posture must be also strictly controlled in kinetic studies.

Most chronokinetic studies have been carried out by comparing the kinetics of a drug taken at different time points after a single dose intake. One can argue that such variations may disappear when repeated doses are administered; some chronokinetic studies have been carried out with repeated doses (e.g., theophylline, diazepam, sodium valproate) and still demonstrated significant temporal variations. Drug delivery at a constant rate is thought to produce constant blood levels. Recent chronokinetic studies on anticancer agents (5-fluorouracil, adriamycin, vindesine); (Levi et al. 1986; Focan et al. 1989; Petit et al. 1988), antiinflammatory (ketoprofen; Decousus et al. 1987) heparin (Decousus et al. 1985), and local anesthetics (bupivacaine; Bruguerolle et al. 1988) demonstrated that continuous intravenous infusion does not lead to constant plasma levels but results in large-amplitude circadian changes. In spite of a continuous (36-h) constant rate infusion by peridural route, bupivacaine plasma clearance varied over 24-h with a maximum at 0600 hours (Bruguerolle et al. 1988 b). On the other hand, programmable implanted pumps allows one to vary the infusion rate in a sinusoidal fashion; such findings have been applied to anticancer drugs. Levi et al. (1989), for instance demonstrated that a constant delivery rate of adriamycin in patients suffering from advanced breast cancer resulted in temporal variations in adriamycin plasma concentrations. In contrast, when the same 24-h dosage was delivered by an infusion rate varying in a sinusoidal fashion, the temporal changes in plasma concentrations followed the pump delivery pattern. Thus it was possible to modulate the circadian rate infusion to give more drug when it was best tolerated.

Recent findings of Lemmer et al. on chronokinetics of nitrates (1989) and nifedipine (1990) have demonstrated the influence of galenic presentation in the detection and the amplitude of chronokinetic changes. Also, Smolensky (1989) has recently reviewed the main studies concerning chronokinetics of theophylline and particularly the influence of the galenic form (sustained-release forms).

As mentioned above the different steps in the fate of a drug in the organism are expressed as kinetic parameters by calculation of a theoretical mathematical model. The moment of administration of a drug is generally not taken into account in such models. Hecquet (1986) have proposed differents models integrating the moment of administration as a supplementary factor involved in kinetic processes. Temporal variations are responsible for nonlinearity of kinetics and thus must be taken into account, as must many other factors of nonlinearity. Finally, the interest of such chronokinetic studies is to control one factor (the moment of administration) among others, responsible for variations of drug kinetics but also to try to explain, at least in part some chronopharmacological effects. In most cases chronopharmacological effects are explained in part by chronokinetics, but there are also some examples describing the opposition in phase of chronopharmacodynamic and chronokinetic findings. Such correlations between effects and kinetics are, in any case, based upon a relationship between blood levels and pharmacological effect. This relationship depends on the time of administration of drugs.

References

Belanger PM (1988) Chronobiological variation in the hepatic elimination of drugs and toxic chemical agents. Annu Rev Chronopharmacol 4:1–46

Belanger PM, Labrecque G, Dore F (1981) Rate limiting steps in the temporal variations in the metabolism of selected drugs. Int J Chronobiol 7:208–215

Bruguerolle B (1983a) Influence de l'heure d'administration d'un médicament sur sa pharmacocinétique. Therapie 38:223–235

Bruguerolle B (1983b) Cycle menstruel et pharmacocinétique des médicaments. J Gynecol Obstet Biol Reprod (Paris) 12:825–827

Bruguerolle B (1984a) La chronopharmacologie. Ellipses, Paris

Bruguerolle B (1984b) Circadian phase dependent pharmacokinetics of disopyramide in mice. Chronobiol Int 1:267–271

Bruguerolle B (1987) Données récentes en chronopharmacocinétique. Pathol Biol (Paris) 35:925–934

Bruguerolle B (1989) Temporal aspects of drug absorption. In: Lemmer B (ed) Chronopharmacology cellular and biochemical interactions. Dekker, New York, pp 3–13

Bruguerolle B, Isnardon R (1985) Daily variations in plasma levels of lidocaine during local anaesthesia in dental practice. Ther Drug Monit 7:369–370

Bruguerolle B, Jadot G (1983) Influence of the hour of administration of lidocaine on its intraerythrocytic passage in the rat. Chronobiologia 10:295–297

Bruguerolle B, Jadot G (1985) Circadian changes in procainamide and N-acetylprocainamide kinetics in the rat. J Pharm Pharmacol 37:654–656

Bruguerolle B, Jadot G, Valli M, Bouyard L, Bouyard P (1982) Etude chronocinétique de la lidocaïne chez le rat. J Pharmacol (Paris) 13:65–76

Bruguerolle B, Barbeau G, Belanger P, Labrecque G (1986a) Chronokinetics of indomethacin in elderly subjects. Annu Rev Chronopharmacol 3:425–428

Bruguerolle B, Levi F, Arnaud C, Bouvenot G, Mechkouri M, Vannetzel J, Touitou Y (1986b) Alteration of physiologic circadian time structure of six plasma proteins in patients with advanced cancer. Annu Rev Chronopharmacol 3:207–210

Bruguerolle B, Bouvenot G, Bartolin R, Manolis J (1988a) Chronopharmacocinétique de la digoxine chez le sujet de plus de soixante dix ans. Thérapie 43:251–253

Bruguerolle B, Dupont M, Lebre P, Legre G (1988b) Bupivacaine chronokinetics in man after a peridural constant rate infusion. Annu Rev Chronopharmacol 5:223–226

Cambar J, Lemoigne F, Toussaint C (1979) Diurnal variations evidence of glomerular filtration in the rat. Experientia 35:1607–1608

Carosella L, Dinardo P, Bernabei R, Cocchi A, Carbonin P (1979) Chronopharmacokinetics of digitalis. Circadian variations of β-methyldigoxin serum levels after oral administration. In: Reinberg A, Halberg F (eds) Chronopharmacology. Pergamon, Oxford, p 125

Decousus H, Croze M, Levi F, Perpoint B, Jaubert J, Bonnadona JF, Reinberg A, Queneau P (1985) Circadian changes in anticoagulant effect of heparin infused at a constant rate. Br Med J 290:341–344

Decousus H, Ollagnier M, Cherrah Y, Perpoint B, Hocquart J, Queneau P (1987) Chronokinetics of ketoprofen infused intravenously at a constant rate. Annu Rev Chronopharmacol 3:321–324

Dettli L, Spring P (1966) Diurnal variations in the elimination rate of a sulfonamide in man. Helv Med Acta 4:921–926

Dore F, Belanger P, Labrecque G (1984) Distribution tissulaire de microsphères radioactives en fonction de l'heure du jour et de l'état nutritionel chez le rat. Union Med Can 38:964–966

Feuers RJ, Scheving LE (1988) Chronobiology of hepatic enzymes. Annu Rev Chronopharmacol 4:209–254

Focan C, Bruguerolle B, Arnaud C, Levi F, Mazy V, Focan-Henrard D, Bouvenot G (1988) Alteration of circadian time structure of plasma proteins in patients with inflammation. Annu Rev Chronopharmacol 5:21–24

Focan C, Doalto L, Mazy V, Levi F, Bruguerolle B, Cano JP, Rahmani R, Hecquet B (1989) Vindesine en perfusion continue de 48 heures (suivie de cisplatine) dans le cancer pulmonaire avancé. Données chronopharmacocinétiques et efficacité clinique. Bull Cancer (Paris) 76:909–912

Fujimura A, Kajiyama H, Kumagai Y, Nakashima H, Sugimoto K, Ebihara A (1989a) Chronopharmacokinetic studies of propanofen and procainamide. J Clin Pharmacol 29:786–790

Fujimura A, Ohashi K, Sugimoto K, Kumagai Y, Ebihara A (1989b) Chronopharmacokinetic study of nitrendipine in healthy subjects. J Clin Pharmacol 29:909–915

Haen E, Gerdsmeier W, Arbogast B (1985) Circadian variation in propranolol protein binding. Naunyn-Schmiedebergs Arch Pharmacol 329:393

Hecquet B (1986) Constant pharmacologic effect and chronopharmacology: theoretical aspects. Chronobiol Int 3:149–154

Hecquet B, Sucche M (1986) Theoretical study of the influence of the circadian rhythm of plasma protein binding on cisplatin area under the curve. J Pharmacokinet Biopharm 14:79–93

Jespersen CM, Frederiksen M, Fisher Hansen J, Kligaard NA, Sorum C (1989) Circadian variations in the pharmacokinetics of verapamil. Eur J Clin Pharmacol 37:613–615

Jones HB (1845) On the variations of the acidity of the urine in the state of health. Philos Trans R Soc (Lond) 135:335–349

Jori A, Di Salle E, Santini V (1971) Daily rhythmic variation and liver drug metabolism in rats. Biochem Pharmacol 20:2965–2969

Langner B, Lemmer B (1988) Circadian phase dependency in pharmacokinetics and cardio-vascular effects of oral propranolol in man. Annu Rev Chronopharmacol 5:335–338

Lecocq B, Jaillon P (1990) Influence de l'horaire de prise sur la pharmacocinetique de la nitrindipine chez le sujet sain. La lettre du Pharmacologue 4:3–4

Lemmer B, Nold G, Behne S, Becker HJ, Liefhold J, Kaiser R (1990) Chronopharmacokinetics and hemodynamic effects or oral nifedipine in healthy subjects and in hypertensive patients. Annu Rev Chronopharmacol 7:121–124

Lemmer B (1981a) Pharmacokinetics of beta-adrenoceptors blocking drugs of different polarity (propranolol, metoprolol, atenolol) in plasma and various organs of the light-dark synchronised rat. Naunyn-Schmidebergs Arch Pharmacol 316:R60

Lemmer B (1981b) Chronopharmacokinetics. In: Breimer D, Speiser P (eds) Topics in pharmaceutical sciences. Elsevier, Amsterdam, pp 49–68

Lemmer B, Winkler H, Ohm T, Fink M (1985) Chronopharmacokinetics of β-receptor blocking drugs of different lipophilicity (propranolol, metoprolol, sotalol, atenolol) in plasma and tissues after single and multiple dosing in rats. Naunyn-Schmiedebergs Arch Pharmacol 330:42–49

Lemmer B, Scheidel B, Stenzhorn G, Blume H, Lenhard G, Grether D, Renczes J, Becker HJ (1989) Clinical chronopharmacology of oral nitrates. Z Kardiol 78:61–63

Levi F, Metzger G, Bailleul F, Reinberg A, Mathe G (1986) Circadian varying plasma pharmacokinetics of doxorubicin (DOX) despite continuous infusion at a constant rate. Proc Am Assoc Cancer Res 27:175

Levi F, Bruguerolle B, Hecquet B (1989) Mecanismes et perspectives en chronopharmacocinetique clinique. Thérapie 44:313–321

Markiewicz A, Semenowicz K (1980) Does a rhythmicity of serum concentrations and urinary excretion of dipyridamole exist during long term treatment? Pol J Pharmacol Pharm 32:289–295

Nair V, Casper R (1969) The influence of light on daily rhythm in hepatic drug metabolising enzymes in rat. Life Sci 8:1291–1298

Petit E, Milano G, Levi F, Thyss A, Bailleul F, Schneider M (1988) Circadian rhythm-varying plasma concentration of 5-fluorouracil during a five day continuous venous infusion at an constant rate in cancer patients. Cancer Res 48:1676–1679

Radzialowski FM, Bousquet WF (1968) Daily rhythmic variation in hepatic drug metabolism in the rat and mouse. J Pharmacol Exp Ther 163:229–238

Reinberg A, Ghata J (1990) Les rythmes biologiques, 5th edn. Presses Universitaires de France, Paris

Reinberg A, Halberg F (1971) Circadian chronopharmacology. Annu Rev Pharmacol 11:455–492

Reinberg A, Smolensky MH (1982) Circadian changes of drug disposition in man. Clin Pharmacokinet 7:401–420

Reinberg A, Clench J, Ghata J, Halberg F, Abulker C, Dupont J, Zagula-Mally Z (1975) Rythmes circadiens des paramètres de l'excrétion urinaire du salycylate (chronopharmacocinétique) chez l'homme adulte sain. C R Acad Sci Paris 280:1697–1700

Reinberg A, Schuller E, Deslanerie N, Clench J, Helary M (1977) Rythmes circadiens et circannuels des leucocytes, proteines totales, immunoglobulines A, G et M. Etude chez neuf adultes jeunes et sains. Nouv Presse Med 6:3819–3823

Reinberg A, Levi F, Smolensky M, Labrecque G, Ollagnier M, Decousus H, Bruguerolle B (1990) Chronokinetics. In: Hansch C (ed) Comprehensive medicinal chemistry, vol 5. Pergamon, London, pp 279–296

Smolensky MH (1989) Chronopharmacology of theophylline and β-sympathomimetics. In: Lemmer B (ed) Chronopharmacology cellular and biochemical interactions. Dekker, New York, pp 65–114

Nocturnal Hemodynamic Effects of Commonly Used Cardiovascular Drugs: Possible Implications for Clinical and Pharmacological Management

M. I. Talan

In a number of experiments conducted in chaired monkeys (*Macaca mulatta*), instrumented for beat-by-beat recording of heart rate (HR), stroke volume (SV), systolic (SP), diastolic (DP), and central venous blood pressure (CVP), we have reported a stable diurnal pattern of hemodynamic parameters [8, 9]. This pattern (Fig. 1) consists of a monotonic decline in cardiac output (CO) during the night (light-off period) accompanied by an elevation in total peripheral resistance (TPR). The decline in CO was mediated by a reduction in HR because SV remained unchanged throughout the night. SP and DP were lower at night than during the day, but they did not show any nocturnal trend. CVP declined monotonically throughout the night, but contrary to CO and TPR, which returned to early evening values when the light came on, CVP continued to decline throughout the morning [9]. This hemodynamic pattern is indicative of a reduction in plasma volume since experiments with sympathetic blockade [9, 16] showed that the reduction in circulating volume was not related to redistribution of the blood into different vascular compartments.

We do not know yet what factors govern the nocturnal hemodynamic pattern:

1. a reduction in plasma volume, as a primary mechanism, that results in a decline of CO and CVP, while the rise in TPR is an adaptive response to maintain blood pressure; or
2. a rise in TPR, as a primary mechanism, that results from whole body autoregulation [5], while the reduction in plasma volume and related decline in CO is a compensatory mechanism to prevent blood pressure elevation.

Neither do we know what particular mechanism or mechanisms are responsible for the nocturnal decline in plasma volume: an active water and electrolyte regulating mechanism or simply a negative balance between water consumption and excretion. It is known that monkeys do not drink at night while urine formation is reduced but is not stopped [14]; at the same time the loss of water through respiration and perspiration continues throughout the night.

Figure 1 presents our findings on nocturnal water consumption in two animals. Despite differences between the animals in the volume of water consumed, the patterns were similar: most of the water consumed during the daytime is

Schmidt/Engel/Blümchen (Eds.)
Temporal Variations of the Cardiovascular System
© Springer-Verlag Berlin Heidelberg 1992

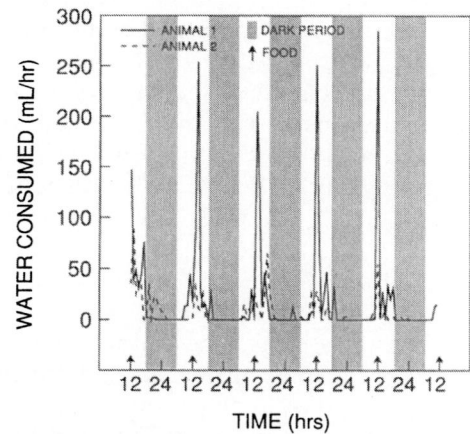

Fig. 1. Water consumption in two monkeys during five consecutive 24-h time periods. *Shaded areas*, time when light was off; *arrows*, time when food was provided

associated with food consumption. Reduction in total plasma volume throughout the night was also reported in humans [6, 7, 12].

What physiological significance could this nocturnal pattern have? We believe that the simplest and most likely answer is that the reduction in plasma volume during the night and the concomitant hemodynamic pattern is a mechanism for reduction in left ventricular work (LVW) without large reduction in blood pressure. When the nocturnal decline in HR was prevented from occurring by daily atrial demand pacing ([10, 17]; Engel, this volume), there was an elevation of LVW. One consequence of this persistent elevation of LVW was a reduction in cardiac performance. Thus, we believe that the nocturnal reduction in plasma volume and the related nocturnal reduction in heart work is a restorative mechanism. However, it is conceivable that in some conditions such a hemodynamic pattern may have adverse physiological effects. For instance, it is possible that the nightly, progressive reduction in plasma volume may reduce coronary perfusion and thus aggravate ischemic heart disease. In addition, a nightly increase in TPR reflects an increase in vascular tone and therefore may contribute to the pathophysiology of hypertension.

In the light of these findings and inferences, we monitored the effects of several commonly used antihypertensive drugs on nocturnal hemodynamic patterns:

1. atenolol, a β-adrenergic blocker commonly used in the treatment of angina pectoris and high blood pressure [3];
2. prazosin, an α-adrenergic blocker commonly used in antihypertensive therapy [15];
3. a combination of both, i.e., double sympathetic blockade, a conventional antihypertensive therapy [1];
4. verapamil, a calcium channel blocker, usually used to treat angina, cardiac arrhythmias, and mild hypertension [11]; and
5. captopril, an angiotensin converting enzyme (ACE) inhibitor and a very potent antihypertensive drug [2].

Experiments were conducted on normotensive monkeys (*Macaca mulatta*). Each weighed approximately 4 kg at the time of entry into the study. Each animal was chronically chaired and maintained in a primate booth throughout the duration of the study. A permanent magnet flow probe was implanted at the root of aorta and an arterial catheter was implanted into the abdominal aorta.

During diurnal testing the booth door was closed at 1700 hours and opened at 1200 hours the following day. Feeding was restricted to the period between 1200 and 1700 hours; filtered tap water was available at all times. The light-dark cycle was 12 h with the light off at 2000 hours. Data collection was started at 1800 hours and completed at 1200 hours each day. The computer collected HR, SV, SP, and DP data on a beat-by-beat basis. Every 60 s the data were reduced to means and stored for subsequent analyses. Hourly means were calculated for each of the four primary cardiovascular responses and for two derived indexes, CO and TPR. Observations were continued for about 20 consecutive days for a control period and each of the experimental drugs. All drugs were delivered intraarterially as a continuous infusion in a dose which greatly exceeded the usual therapeutic dose, i.e., in a dose which effectively blocked the relevant agonist.

The results presented below are averages of about 20 days of observation started 3–4 days after beginning drug infusion, i.e., they are steady-state effects, not acute effects of the drugs. Data were analyzed with the use of repeated measures analyses of variance. The results with all of the sympathetic blockers are based on the four animals; the verapamil results are based on three different animals; and the captopril results are based on four different animals.

The results are presented in Fig. 2. Infusion of atenolol decreased the overall level of CO because the small rise in SV was not sufficient to compensate for the marked decrease in HR. TPR was substantially elevated but not enough to prevent the fall in blood pressure. Therefore, the hypotensive effect of atenolol was a result of a reduction in arterial blood flow which may reflect a reduction in total plasma volume: β-blockers are known to inhibit renin-angiotensin activity and therefore to suppress the aldosterone-mediated sodium retention [4]. The nocturnal hemodynamic pattern was markedly exaggerated and characterized by a sharper overnight decline in CO and a steeper rise in TPR.

Infusion of prazosin resulted in an increase of the overall level of CO and reduction in SP. The level of TPR was decreased and the level of HR was unchanged. Prazosin resulted in a significantly sharper decline in CO, while the trend in TPR was not different from control.

During double sympathetic blockade, the overall level of HR was markedly reduced and SV was increased. Overall levels of CO and TPR did not change; however, the nighttime trends of CO and TPR were much more pronounced: CO fell more sharply toward morning hours and the TPR rate of rise was steeper than during control.

Infusion of captopril resulted in a reduction of the average levels of SP, DP, and CO while the levels of HR and TPR were not affected. The hemodynamic pattern of nocturnal decline of CO and rise in TPR was exacerbated. While during control, the nightly CO decrease was almost entirely a result of a reduction in HR during captopril infusion, the fall in CO early in the evening was mediated by a fall in HR; however, during most of the night, the reduction in CO was mediated by a fall in

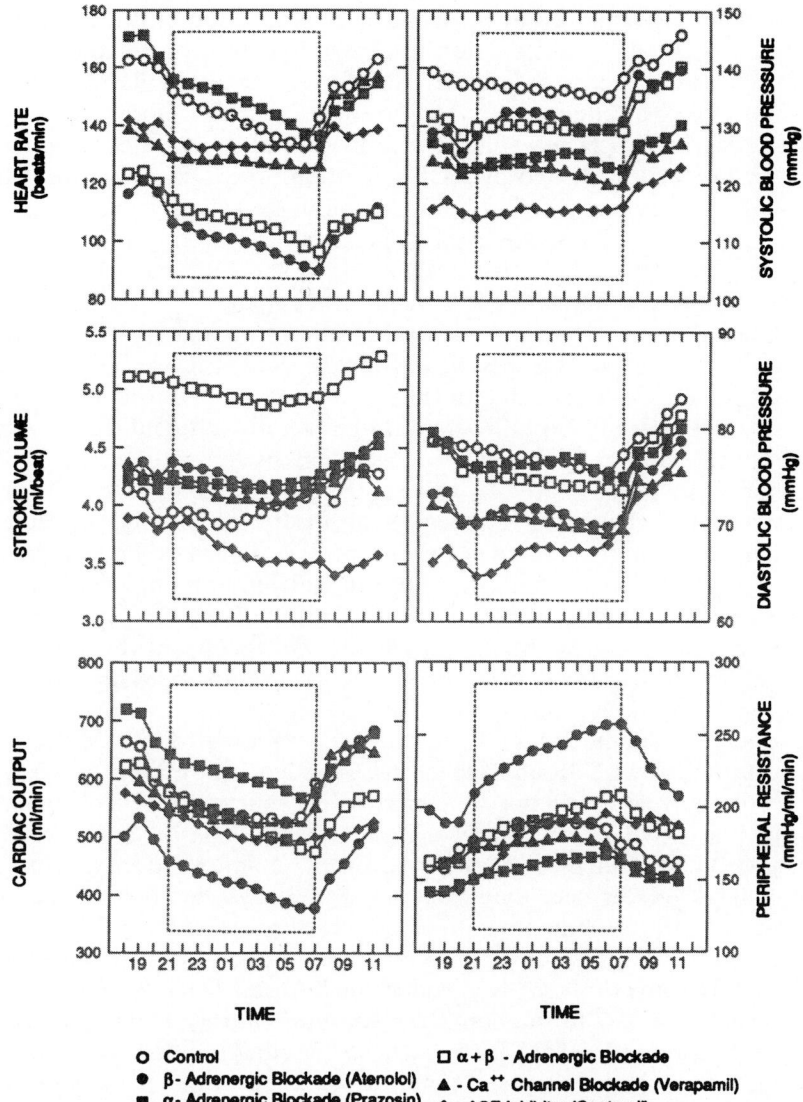

Fig. 2. Diurnal patterns of heart rate, stroke volume, cardiac output, systolic and diastolic blood pressure, and total peripheral resistance during control (*open circles*), and continuous infusion of: β-adrenergic blocker atenolol (*closed circles*); α-adrenergic blocker, prazosin (*closed squares*); combination of α- and β-adrenergic blockers (*open squares*); calcium channel blocker verapamil (*triangles*); and angiotensin-converting enzyme inhibitor captopril (*diamonds*). *Area inside the block*, time when light was off

SV while HR remained at the same level. Reduction in the angiotensin II level should bring about a reduction in aldosterone-mediated sodium retention and thus a decrease in plasma volume. The further decrease in plasma volume may also be a result of a reduction of vasopressin release. Therefore, the usual nocturnal reduction in the plasma volume may have been superimposed on an additional plasma reduction elicited by ACE inhibition. The excessive reduction in plasma volume probably resulted in an activation of the sympathetic system that limited the HR decline. Thus, captopril, which is a very potent antihypertensive agent, exacerbates the usual nocturnal trends of CO and TPR and may result in excessive reduction of plasma volume throughout the night.

During calcium channel blockade with verapamil, there was a significant reduction in the levels of HR, SP, DP, and TPR. The level of SV was elevated, and the level of CO was not significantly different from control. The patterns of CO, TPR, and both SP and DP were not significantly different from control. During verapamil, infusion HR declined overnight significantly less, and SV declined significantly more relative to control conditions. Thus, calcium entry blockade resulted in a change of the mechanism mediating the nightly decrease in CO. During control, the decline in CO was mediated primarily by a reduction in HR, while SV remained unchanged, but during calcium entry blockade this pattern was reversed. The decline in CO was mediated primarily by a reduction in SV, while the HR decline was substantially attenuated. We think that this reversal may have been a result of the negative inotropic effect of verapamil. The nocturnal trends of CO and TPR were not changed.

Therefore, all the drugs except verapamil exacerbated the nocturnal pattern of a monotonic rise in TPR and decline in CO (prazosin affects only CO). In the case of atenolol and captopril, this effect may reflect an additional nocturnal reduction in total plasma volume. For prazosin, it is a shift of blood from the arterial to the venous compartment, superimposed on the nocturnal decrease of total plasma volume. We infer here that while all these drugs clearly produce the clinically expected effects (reduction in blood pressure – prazosin, captopril, atenolol, verapamil – or reduction in LVW and thus cardiac oxygen demand – verapamil, atenolol), some of them also produce undesirable hemodynamic effects at night. Vascular tone rises throughout the night more sharply, and in the case of atenolol even the average level of TPR is much increased. It is difficult to understand how a drug that increases vascular tone can be useful for the treatment of a disease characterized by increased vascular tone. Reduction in plasma volume clearly reduces coronary flow. This undesirable effect obviously is compensated by decreased LVW, i.e., decreased demand. However, as a result of the additional reduction in plasma volume during early morning hours, thrombogenesis may be increased, thereby enhancing the probability of morning occlusive episodes. Verapamil was the only drug evaluated in this study which lowered blood pressure and LVW without modifying the nocturnal pattern of CO and TPR. Thus, on the basis of hemodynamic considerations, this form of drug therapy seems to be the most rational.

On the basis of these findings, we strongly recommend research on human hemodynamic patterns at night to determine whether specific drugs may produce adverse hemodynamic effects in patients with various cardiovascular disorders.

Finally, while this report has focused on the nocturnal hemodynamic effects of drugs used to treat cardiovascular disorders, it also should be noted that these findings may have broader implications. The nocturnal decline in plasma volume may be a mechanism responsible for the higher morning concentration of many drugs in the plasma [18, 19]. Could this nocturnal fall in plasma volume account for some of the reported cases of unexpected morning toxicities of medications [13]?

References

1. Ando G, Parrow A (1981) Prazosin – a Swedish multicentre study. In: Rawlins M, Lund-Johansen P, Lawrie T (eds) Prazosin Pharmacology, hypertension and congestive heart failure. Royal Society of Medicine, London; Academic, London; Grune and Stratton, New York, pp 105–113
2. Aono J, Koga T, Yamazaki T, Shiraki Y, Sakai K (1988) Antihypertensive action of a novel orally active angiotensin converting enzyme inhibitor altipril calcium (MC-838) in several hypertensive models of rats: comparison with captopril. Arch Int Pharmacodyn Ther 292:203–222
3. Brunner H (1977) Observations on the pharmacology of the beta-blockers. In: Kielholz P (ed) Beta-blockers and the central nervous system. Huber, Bern, pp 11–20
4. Buhler FR, Marbet G, Patel U, Burkart F (1975) Renin-suppressive potency of various beta-adrenergic blocking agents at supine rest and during upright exercise. Clin Sci Mol Med 48 [Suppl 2]:61–73
5. Cowley AW Jr, Hinojosa-Laborde C, Barber BJ, Harder DR, Lombard JH, Greene AS (1989) Short-term autoregulation of systemic blood flow and cardiac output. News Physiol Sci 4:219–225
6. Cranston WI (1964) Diurnal variation in plasma volume in normal and hypertensive subjects. Am Heart J 68:427–428
7. Cranston WI, Brown W (1963) Diurnal variation in plasma volume in normal and hypertensive subjects. Clin Sci 25:107–114
8. Engel BT, Talan MI (1987) Diurnal pattern of hemodynamic performance in nonhuman primates. Am J Physiol 253 (Regulatory Integrative Comp Physiol 22):R779–R785
9. Engel BT, Talan MI (1991) Diurnal variations in central pressure. Acta Physiol Scand 141:273–278
10. Engel BT, Talan MI, Chew P (1991) The effect of heart rate pacing on diurnal hemodynamic patterns (to be published)
11. Frishman WH, Sonnenblick EH (1986) The calcium antagonist. In: Hurst JW (ed) The heart, 6th edn. McGraw-Hill, New York, pp 1624–1639
12. Greenleaf JE (1984) Physiological responses to prolonged bed rest and fluid immersion in humans. J Appl Physiol 7 (Respiratory Environmental Exercise Physiol):619–633
13. Moore-Ede M (1973) Circadian rhythms of drug effectivness and toxicity. Clin Pharmacol Ther 14:925–935
14. Moore-Ede MC, Herd JA (1977) Renal electrolyte circadian rhythms: independence from feeding and activity patterns. Am J Physiol 232 (Renal Fluid Electrolyte Physiol): F128–F135
15. Rawlins MD, Lund-Johansen P, Lawrie TD (1981) Prazosin: pharmacology, hypertension and congestive heart failure. Royal Society of Medicine, London; Academic, London; Grune and Stratton, New York
16. Talan MI, Engel BT (1989) Effect of sympathetic blockade on diurnal variation of hemodynamic patterns. Am J Physiol 256 (Regulatory Integrative Comp Physiol 25):R778–R785
17. Talan MI, Engel BT, Chew P (1992) Systemic nocturnal demand pacing results in high output heart failure. J Appl Physiol (in press)
18. Ritschel WA (1984) Chronopharmacokinetics. Pharm Int 14:116–122
19. Reinberg A, Smolensky MH (1982) Circadian changes of drug disposition in man. Clin Pharmacokinet 7:401–420

Subject Index

abdominal aorta   384
ABP (ambulatory blood pressure)   259
– constitutional between-subject factors
   262
– and heart rate, self-reported, emotional
   strain   297ff.
– home vs. work   259
– measuring instrument   259
– mood effects   259, 260
– place   259
– posture   259
– racial differences   275
– renin-angiotensin-aldosterone system
   279
– social situation   259, 261
– work vs. nonwork day differences   260
ABPM (24-h indirect ambulatory blood
   pressure monitoring)   324
acclimatization, temperature   346
ACE (angiotensin converting enzyme)
   383
– inhibition   386
– inhibitor   213, 341, 362
– – captopril   216
– – cilazapril   339, 340
– – Portapres   183, 185, 220
acebutolol   362
activity   136, 272, 295, 307
– physical   160
– – 24-h recording, Portapres   191, 197,
   198, 201
– and sleeping periods   322
adolescents, black and white American
   277
adrenaline, plasma   242
African
– blacks in Africa   277
– normotensive   277
afternoon
– shift   319 – 322

– ST segment depression, coronary heart
   disease   159
age/aging
– decades   354 – 356
– rhythm parameter   26
age-dependent
– Borderline determination   352
– variation of diurnal blood pressure
   351ff.
airconditioned room   223
albumin   372
alcohol   285, 287, 333, 349
aldosteronism, primary   274, 275
– postsurgery   274
ambulatory
– blood pressure (see ABP)   259
– monitoring
– – occupational and domestic stress
   305ff.
– – ST segment depression, coronary
   heart disease   159
American
– blacks   277
– – adolescents   277
– – adults, normotensive   277
– – in America   277
– white adolescents   277
amlodipine   362
anesthetics, local   378
anger   136
angina
– attacks   364
– pectoris   159, 364, 383
– Prinzmetal's variant angina   160
– unstable, coronary thrombosis, theory
   of triggering   152
angiographic data, trigger onset   148
anticancer agents   378
antihypertensive
– drug   383

– medication, Portapres   219
– therapy   383
anxiety   136
aorta, abdominal   384
arousal   136, 307
– autonomic   314
arrhythmias, Portapres   188
arterial catheter   384
arterosclerotic plaque, ruptured   145
artery
– pulmonary, diastolic pressure   161
– tone of the epicardial coronary arteries   160
aspirin   145
atenolol   362, 374, 383, 384, 386
atherosclerotic plaque, coronary thrombosis, theory of triggering   152
atrial demand pacing   383
– nocturnal hemodynamic responses
   164ff.
– – cardiac output   165, 167, 168
– – central venous pressure   165, 167,
   168
– – diastolic pressure   167, 168
– – heart rate   165
– – peripheral resistance   167, 168
– – stroke volume   165, 167 – 169
– – systolic pressure   167, 168
– – week Starling curves   169
atropine   119, 236
autonomous rhythms   19
– external modifications of   42ff.
– from 24 h   17
– internal stabilization   25
autopsy, trigger onset   148
awakening   308
– and sleep, white, black, male and female   309

bainbridge   234
Barbadian, normotensive   277
baroreceptor   234, 294
– neurovegetative system   119
baroreflex   232
– blood pressure   243, 244
basic-independent rhythm   10
beat-to-beat blood pressure   256
bedrest   5, 8
behavior/behavioral   303
– activation, rhythmicity in the chronotropic cardiac control   109
– factors   198, 283ff.
– – blood pressure, throughout the day
   283ff.
– – Portapres   198
– heart rhythm   91
– moods, Portapres   185, 217

– variables   294
β-blockers   362, 384
β-adrenergic
– blocker   145, 383
– input   142
bevantolol   362
bicycle
– (bike), Portapres   186
– tolerance test   351
biliary secretion   372
biological marker   377
BIOPORT system   183
blacks
– adolescents, American   277
– adults   276
– – African in Africa   277
– – American in America   277
– – American, normotensive   277
– awake and sleep   309
– female   277
– male   277
– of hypertension   262
blockade (see also β-blockers)
– calcium entry blockade   386
– double sympathetic   383
– sympathetic   384
blood flow 8, 9
– extremities   9
– hepatic   376, 378
– peripheral   372
– redistribution within 24 hours   8, 10
– total forearm   223, 232
blood level/pharmacological drug effect,
   relationship   379
blood pressure   3, 5, 8, 361, 366–368,
   383
– beat-to-beat   256
– cilazapril   206, 207
– continuous noninvasive 24-h ambulatory finger blood pressure   173
– control, day vs. night, diurnal variations   240ff.
– day and night control   240ff.
– diastolic (DBP)   133, 254
– – sexual activity   188
– diurnal variations   171ff.
– field assessment   258ff.
– fluctuations   253
– invasive measurement   325
– measurement   4
– – fully automatic device   330
– – in man (see also Portapres)
– – at night   4
– – during sleep   5
– noninvasive measurement   325
– systolic (SBP)   133, 254
– transient   250

– variations of 344
– – diurnal, placebo 199
– – in hypertension 324ff.
blood viscosity, morning increase, myocardial infarction 150
blood volume 372
body
– core and shell of, distribution of blood 8, 9
– motility, gross 285
– temperature and heart rate 3, 6–8
bopindolol 362
boso oscillomat 330
bradykinin 121
brain stem 294
breath holding tests 210ff.
– Portapres 184, 185
breathing, sleep-related breathing disorders and nocturnal hypertension 332ff.
British white hypertensives 277

caffein 285, 287
calcium
– channel blocker 362, 383
– entry blockade 386
cAMP 364
cancer/cancerous
– anticancer agents 378
– inflammatory subjects, plasma proteins 377
capillary resistance 372
captopril 362, 383, 386
– ACE-inhibitor 216
– infusion 384
cardiac
– arrhythmias 383
– control, chronotropic, rhythmicity in 109, 111, 114
– death 145, 314
– – coronary thrombosis, theory of triggering 152
– output 164–166, 168, 232, 372
– – atrial demand pacing, nocturnal hemodynamic responses 165, 167, 168
– – dye dilution 237
– – (HZV) 6
– – Portapres 190
– oxygen demand 386
– rhythms
– – diurnal variations 85ff.
– – in rodents 87
– – – small mammals 87
– – – species-specific patterns 87
– transplantation 274
cardiologist 329
cardiopulmonary
– receptors 233

– reflex 22, 232
cardiovascular
– drugs 362
– – chronopharmocokinetic aspects 371
– – chronopharmacology 361
– – experimental and clinical kinetic studies 372
– measure, continuous 128
– mortality 349
– reactivity, measurement 128
– regulation, neural 256
– responses
– – active coping 127ff.
– – laboratory field 127ff.
– – – heart rate 131, 133
– – – pulse transit time 131
– system, Tupaias 93, 361
– variabilities, spectral analysis 125
catecholamines 162, 333
– levels 344
– release 161
catheter, arterial 384
cats 248
– sino-aortic denervated 248
central
– nervous activation 106
– venous pressure 164, 166, 233
– – atrial demand pacing, nocturnal hemodynamic responses 165, 167, 168
chest X-ray 351
children 302
chores 287
chronobiological data, chronopharmocokinetics 371
chronokinetic studies 378, 379
– methodological aspects 377
chronopathology 361
chronopharmacokinetics 362
– cardiovascular drugs 371
chronopharmacology, cardiovascular active drugs 361
chronotropic cardiac control, rhythmicity in 109, 111, 114
cigarette smoking 285
cilazapril 339, 340
– blood pressure and heart rate 206, 207, 210
– diurnal variation 198
– Portapres 183, 185
– vagal activation 216
circadian
– basic principles in human 15ff.
– rhythm 361
circulatory system, 24-h rhythm 5
cleaning, Portapres 186
climatic influences, heart rate 91

clinic/clinical populations, diurnal
  rhythm   272, 273
clock
– internal   6, 12, 322
– like disposition   11
– "the stomach is the best clock"   11
clonidin   362
CO   382, 384
coagulation, hypercoagulable state   145
cohabitation, harmonious   97
coitus, Portapres   188 – 190
colder periods   349
computation speed   16
concentration, morning   387
conductance   9
"constant routine"   6
constitutional
– between-subject factors, ABP   262
– determinants   344
contact plates   16
continuous cardiovascular measure   128
coping
– active   132
– – cardiovascular responses   127ff.
– hyperactive   132
copulation   94
core of the body   8, 9
coronary
– blood flow, morning increase, myocardial infarction   150
– heart disease, daily variations in ST
  segment depression   159ff.
– insufficiency   160
– perfusion   383
– thrombi   145
– thrombosis, theory of triggering (see
  also thrombosis)   151, 152
– vasoconstriction   145
cortisol   21
– free cortisol   16
– plasma   162, 242
– – morning increase, myocardial infarction   150
cosinar analysis   367
couple, harmonious   94, 98
CPAP, nCPAP therapy   334 – 336, 341
Cushing's syndrome   274, 275
CVP   382
cyclic order   295
cycling   222ff.
– Portapres   186, 189
cycloergometry, Portapres   176

daily variations in ST segment depression,
  coronary heart disease   159ff.
– afternoon   159
– morning hours   159

darkness, sleep in   7
day
– blood pressure, behavioral factors
  283ff.
– control of blood pressure   242
– heart rate   93
– time of diastolic blood pressure after
  removal of influence of behavioral factors   294
day-night variations   3ff.
– blood pressure   240ff.
days of the night-shift   320
DBP (diastolic blood pressure)   254
– white and black   278
death (see also cardiac death)   314
defecation   285
dependency, serial   128
depressants   333
desk work   285, 287
desynchronized rhythms, internal   32ff.,
  41, 62
– experiments   32ff.
– – locomotor activity   33
– – nap   33
– – night sleep   33
– – rectal temperature   33
– fractional   62
– spontaneous occurence of   35
diabetes   274
diary entries, methodological considerations   267, 268
diastolic blood pressure (DBP)   133, 161,
  254, 372
– atrial demand pacing, nocturnal hemodynamic responses   167, 168
– pulmonary artery   161
– sexual activity   188
diazepam   378
dietary habits   349
digoxin   362, 373
diltiazem   362
dinamap   259
dipyridamol   362, 373
disopyramide   374
diuresis   372
diuretics   362
diurnal
– animals, strictly   95, 98
– blood pressure   171ff., 322
– – age-dependent   351ff.
– – profile   353
– effect, work tolerance   160
– heart rate cycles   91
– pattern, Portapres   164, 219
– rhythms   7, 160, 273
– – of blood pressure   307
– – in clinical populations   273

– – 24-h day in a healthy young man for 14 successive days   15
– – intra-arterial blood pressure   241
– time interval analysis   353
– variation
– – of blood pressure   272
– – and triggers of onset   145ff.
– – in cardiac rhythms   85ff.
– – drug actions   359ff.
diving tests   210ff.
– Portapres   184
domestic
– and occupational stress   305ff.
– stress   313, 314
dominance
– fight for   95
– relation   98
dose-response relationship   364
DP   384
drinking alc or caffein   285, 287
drinks, Portapres   186
driving a car   285, 287
drug
– absorption   378
– actions, diurnal variations   359ff.
– distribution, temporal variations   375
– excretion   377
– infusion   384
– metabolism   376
– – indirect evidence of temporal variations   3776
dye dilution   236
– cardiac output   237

early morning
– hours   386
– rise   307
eating   285, 287
– Portapres   186
ECG   223, 224, 351
echocardiography   351
EEG   334
elderly patient   67, 68, 274
– light-dark alternations   67, 78
electrolyte regulating mechanism   382
EMG   334
– of the left thigh, Portapres   183
– normotensive, Portapres   191
emotion/emotional   295
– exited situations   98
– neutrality   307
– strain   303
– – self-reported and ABP and heart rate   297ff.
employees, university employees   286
enalapril   362
endocrine mechanisms   333

environmental
– determinants   344
– events, Portapres   185
– factors, Portapres   198
enzyme activity   376
EOG   334
epicardial coronary arteries, tone of   160
epinephrine
– excretion, urinary   314
– plasma, morning increase, myocardial infarction   150
erythrocytes   375
essential hypertension   273
evening   273
– pulse   4
excretion   382
exercise   3
– programs   161
– stress test   159
experimental units   19
external
– and internal factors   162
– measured blood pressure and heart rate   289
– time triggers   322
extrapyramidal-cerebellar system   295
extremities, blood flow   9

female
– managers   314
– workers, awake and sleep   309
fibrinolytic activity   162
field
– assessment of blood pressure   258ff.
– – variability and methodological considerations   258ff.
– of laboratory
– – hyperreactors   142
– – hyporeactors   142
– psychological and physiological processes   140
fight   95
– for dominance   95
finapres (see also Portapres)   173, 208
finger
– blood pressure   173, 189, 190
– – continuous noninvasive 24-h ambulatory   173
– – Portapres   189, 190
– switching between cuffed fingers, Portapres   175
– venous congestion in the finger, Portapres   175
flights, transmeridian   322
food intake   3, 378
free cortisol   16
frustration   136

gastric pH   372
geographically temperature   346
getting up, propper timing   3
glomerular filtration   372
glyceril-trinitrate   362
glycosides   362
guinea pig, heart rate reaction   90

harmonious couple   94, 98
healthy, 24-h day in a healthy young
  man   15
heart
– beats, Portapres   188, 190
– nocturnal   98
– rate   6, 8, 361, 367
– – atrial demand pacing, nocturnal hemodynamic responses   165
– – and body temperature   3, 7
– – cilazapril   206, 207
– – climatic influences   91
– – day heart rate   93
– – fluctuations   98
– – laboratory field   131, 133
– – lower   98
– – mental stress   100, 105, 108
– – morning increase, myocardial infarction   150
– – night heart rate   93
– – pattern
– – – harmoniously cohabiting   97
– – – 0,1 Hz   114
– – Portapres   183, 188, 190
– – prolonged confrontation   96
– – ranges, 100 bpm to 650 bpm   98
– – reaction   90
– – – guinea pig   90
– – – rabbit   90
– – – tree shrew   90, 94
– – R-R interval   103, 107, 109, 110,
  113
– – Raven test   111
– – rhythmicity, autonomic tone   112
– – self-reported, emotional strain
  297ff.
– – species-specific   91
– – spectral analysis, state of activity
  99ff.
– – /stress in real life, relationship   135
– – /time structure, relationship during
  102
– – – mental stress   102
– – – physical rest   102
– – – physical work   102
– rhythm
– – behavioral   91
– – hormonal   91
– work   383

heat
– balance, averages of   9
– loss   8
– production   8
– transfer   9
HEIGHT (height signal, Portapres)   174,
  177
hemodynamic
– conditions   223
– effects, nocturnal   164, 387
– function   164
– pattern   383
heparin   378
hepatic blood flow   376, 378
heteronomous rhythms   44
– jet lag simulation   52
– light-dark alternations   44, 49, 54
– pecularities in
– – an elderly subject   67
– – in an ill patient   46
HF (high-frequency)   253
history, medical   351
Holter tape recorder, portable   124
home   313
– environments   272
– vs. work, ABP   259
hormonal heart rhythm   91
house (broom), Portapres   186
household chores   285
HR   383, 384
hydrochłorothiazide   362
hypercapnia   333
hypercoagulable state   145
hypertension   383
– blood pressure variations in   324ff.
– /bradycarda, relationship   250
– control of   324
– essential   273
– secondary   274
– substained   313
– /tachycardia, relationship   250
hypertensive
– and normotensive individuals   273
– status   262
hypnotics   333
hyporeactive subject   132
hypoxemia   333
HZV (cardiac output)   6

ill patient, light-dark alternations   46, 78
immediate-release   362
inactivity   272
indapamide   362
infarction (see also myocardial infarction)
inflammatory subjects, cancerous, plasma
  proteins   377
information as a Zeitgeber   69

instruments, methodological considerations 266
internal
– clock 6, 322
– conductance 8, 10
– desynchronized rhythms (see also desychronized) 32ff.
– and external factors 162
– measured blood pressure and heart rate 289
– phase relationships 23
– stabilization of autonomous rhythms 25
– synchronized rhythms (see also synchronized) 19ff.
intrabrachial arterial pressure 223
– Portapres 177 – 179
– – ambulatory continuous noninvasive 173, 182
– – – finger blood pressure 173
IS-5-Mn 364, 366
– hemodynamics 366, 368
– immediate release 366
– pharmacokinetics 366, 368
– sustained release 366
ischemic heart disease 383
ISDN 364 – 365
– pharmacokinetics 365
isolation, station constructed for experience under temporal isolation 18
isosorbide dinitrate 362, 364, 373
isosorbide-5-mononitrate 362, 364

jet lag
– light-dark alternations 80
– stimulation, heteronomous rhythms 52
job strain 312
– high-strain jobs 313

Korotkoff methods 325 – 327
– invasive 326
– oscillometric 326
– sounds or oscillations 325

labetolol 362
laboratory
– field, cardiovascular responses 127ff.
– hyperreactors 142
– psychological and physiological processes 140
– reactivity 263
– reactors, low and high 138, 140
– screening 351
– stressors 130
left ventricular
– mass 312

– work 168 – 383
LF (low-frequency) 253
lidocaine 374
light
– bright light as a zeitgeber 69
– cycle 95
light-dark alternations
– absolute 54
– – with bright light 54
– – Zeitgeber period 62, 71
– bright-light 76
– – Zeitgeber vs. information Zeitgeber 78
– constant periods, Zeitgeber period 52
– external modifications, Zeitgeber period 59
– heteronomous rhythms 44, 52, 54, 59, 62, 71, 73, 76
– melatonin effects 82
– peculiarities
– – in an elderly patient 67, 78
– – in an ill patient 46, 78
– – to jet lag 80
– – to shift workers 79
– phase shifts, Zeitgeber period 52
– pure 44
– relative 44
– – by regular request cues 49
– – with bright light 73
light-dark cycle 384
local anesthetics 378
locomotor activity 16, 20
longterm variation in blood pressure, seasonal and environmental temperature 344ff.
low-frequency (LF) 253
LVW 386

macaca mulatta (monkeys) 382, 384
male
– awake and sleep 309
– managers 314
"Man-Clock" 4
manager
– female 314
– male 314
marker, biological 377
married 313
masking 4 – 6
– effect, internal interactions 38
meal-independent rhythm 10
meals 5, 295
–, standardized 5
measurement, cardiovascular reactivity 128
meat 349
medical history 351

meeting   285, 287
melatonin   21, 82
membrane
– microviscosity   372
– permeability   375
mental
– arithmetic analysis, R-R variability
   124
– stress
– – coronary thrombosis, theory of triggering   152
– – heart rate   100, 105, 108
– – – spectral analysis   100
---/time structure, relationship during
   102
– – R-R interval   113
– triggers   145
mephentermine   236
mepindolol   362
mercury sphygmomanometer   259
methodological considerations
– diary entries   267, 268
– instruments   266
– posture   266
– potentially confounding variables   265,
   267
– reliability   265
methodological determinants   344
methoxamine   236
methyldigoxin   373
metildigoxin   362
metoprolol   339, 340, 362, 374
MF (mid-frequency)   253
micturation   285
midmorning   273
mild hypertension (MH)   383
monitoring, ambulatory, ST segment depression, coronary heart disease   159
monkeys (macaca mulatta)   382, 384
mood   307
– effects, ABP   259, 260
moon, speed of   4
morning
– activities, trigger onset   146
– concentration   387
– early morning
– – hours   386
– – rise   307
– hours   314
– – ST segment depression, coronary
   heart disease   159
– – – early morning hours   159
– increase, myocardial infarction   149,
   150
– – blood viscosity   150
– – coronary blood flow   150
– – heart rate   150

– – plasma cortisol   150
– – plasma epinephrine   150
– – tpA activity   150
– pulse   4
– shift   319 – 322
– toxicities   387
mortality, cardiovascular   349
motility   295
motor components, neurovegetative system   125
multioscillator concept   37
muscules   8
music, listening to, Portapres   186
myocardial infarction   145, 147, 314
– acute   159
– coronary thrombosis, theory of triggering   152
– morning increase   149, 150
– prevention   151
– trigger onset   148
myocardial ischemia, transient   145, 147

nadolol   362
nature   130
nCPAP therapy   334 – 336, 341
neocortical-limbic system   295
nervous activity, sympathetic   233, 272,
   314, 344
neural cardiovascular regulation   246ff.,
   256
– blood pressure   246ff.
– pulse interval variability   246ff.
neurovegetative system   117ff.
– α blockers   118
– baroreceptors   119
– internal and external environments
   117
– motor, visceral and verbal components   125
– no block   118
– rest   121
– strech of the aorta, pressor and heart
   rate responses   118
– TILT   121
– vagal afferents   119
nifedipine   160, 362, 368, 373, 378
– immediate release   367
– retard formulation   368
night   383, 386
– control of blood pressure   242
– day-night variations   3ff.
– – blood pressure   240ff.
– heart rate   93
– shift   319 – 322
nisoldipine   362
nitrates   362, 378
nitrendipine   362, 373

nitroglycerin   122, 364
nocturnal
– decline in BP   275
– fall in output   164
– heart   98
– hemodynamic effects   387
– – atrial demand pacing   164ff.
– – clinical and pharmacolocial manage-
    ment   382ff.
– hypertension, sleep-related breathing
    disorders   332ff.
noise, Portapres   218
non-REM sleep   334, 337
noradrenaline, plasma   242, 364
normotensive and hypertensive indivi-
    duals   273

occupational stress   305ff.
– on blood pressure   310, 311, 313
– and domestic stress   305ff.
orgasm, measuring after orgasm, Por-
    tapres   188
orosomucoid   372
oscillomat, boso oscillomat   330
oscillometric method   326, 327
oxprenolol   362
oxygen uptake (V_{01})   6

pacemaker   165 – 168
pacing, atrial demand   383
– nocturnal hemodynamic responses
    164ff.
peak
– heart rate   134
– response   128
peripheral
– blood flow   372
– resistance 165
– – atrial demand pacing, nocturnal he-
    modynamic responses   167, 168
– – changes upon stand-up compared to
    those upon tilt-up   222ff.
– – total and forearm   229, 231
pH
– gastric   372
– urinary   372
pharmacological conditions   223
pharmacological/blood level, drug effect,
    relationship   379
pharmacology, chronopharmacology, car-
    diovasculary active drugs   361
pharmacotherapy of arterial hypertension,
    sleep apnea   338
phase, internal phase relationships   23
phentolamine   119
pheochromacytoma   273, 274
physical

– examination, age-dependent diurnal
    blood pressure   351
– and psychological demands   272
physiological processes, laboratory and
    field   140
pindolol   362
piretanide   362
place, ABP   259
placebo, blood pressure variation, diur-
    nal   199
plaque
– atherosclerotic, coronary thrombosis,
    theory of triggering   152
– rupture   145
– – coronary thrombosis, theory of trig-
    gering   152
plasma
– proteins   375
– – in cancerous inflammatory subjects
    377
– – total   372
– volume   164 – 166, 169, 386, 387
platelet aggregation   162
plethysmograph, venous occlusion   224
PORTAP (height signal, Portapres)   177
– intrabrachial pressure   177 – 179
Portapres
– ACE-inhibitor   183, 185, 220
– ambulatory continuous noninvasive
    173, 181
– – intrabrachial pressure   173, 182
– antihypertensive medication   219
– arrhythmias   188
– behavioral factors   185, 198, 217
– bike (bicycle)   186
– breath holding test   184, 185
– cardiac output   190
– cilazapril   183, 185
– coitus   188 – 190
– cold water   185
– continuous noninvasive 24-h ambulato-
    ry finger blood pressure   173
– cycling   186, 189
– cycloergometry   176
– diurnal pattern   219
– diving test   184
– EMG
– – as a measure of physical activity
    183
– – normotensive   191
– environmental events   185, 198
– exposure to cold   182
– field study   176
– Finapres   208, 217
– finger
– – blood pressure   189, 190
– – switching   175, 182

– – switching between two cuffed
    fingers   175
– heart beats   190
– heart rate   183, 188, 190
– height signal (HEIGHT)   174
– – height correction   174, 182
– house (broom)   186
– hydrostatic pressure   182
– measuring after orgasm   188
– multiple regression analysis   195
– music, listening to   186
– noise   218
– physical activtiy   191, 197, 198, 201
– physical exercise   184
– positions   186
– prelude   188
– prototype   174
– – size, weight and power   174
– psychosocial stimuli   198
– pulse contour method   188
– reaction time   184
– rest (sitting)   184
– restrictions   217
– rucksack   182, 218
– sleep   198, 218
– stroke volume   188, 190
– switching between two cuffed fingers
    175
– toilet   186
– urinating   186
– venous congestion in the finger   175
posture   295, 378
– ABP   259
– methodological considerations   266
potassium   21, 278
– chloride   362
prazosin   362, 383, 386
prealbumin   372
pressure
– on behavior   284
– compartments   233
prevention of myocardial infarction   151
primigravida   274
Prinzmetal's variant angina   160
procainamide   373
– NAPA   374
propranolol   119, 362–364, 373
– administration   363, 364
– hemodynamics   364
– metabolism   363
– pharmacokinetics   364
– plasma concentration   363
psychiatric disorders   349
psychological
– disorders   349
– and physical demands   272
– processes, laboratory and field   140

psychosocial stimuli   198
psychosomatic disorders   349
pulmonary artery, diastolic pressure   161
pulse   3
– contour formula   237
– contour method, Portapres   188
– in the evening (faster)   4
– interval changes   250
– – frequency fluctuations   254
– measurements   4
– in the morning (slower)   4
– rate   3, 5
– transit time, laboratory field   131
-/ watch, physicians   3

R-R interval, heart rate   103, 107, 109,
    110, 113
– mental stress   113
– physical rest   113
– physical work   113
– variability and rhythmicity   107
rabbit, heart rate reaction   90
race (blacks prevalence of hypertension)
    262
racial differences in ABP patterns   275
Raven test   111
reading   285, 287
rectal, temperature   10, 16, 20, 21
relaxants   333
relaxing   285, 287
REM   23
– sleep   334, 337, 341
renin-angiotensin activity   384
– plasma   242
renin-angiotensin-aldosterone system
    333
– and ABP patterns   279
repeatability   228
reproducibility   301
respiration   124
rest and activity   307
restrictions, Portapres   217
retire   11
rhythmicity in the chronotropic cardiac
    control, behavioral activation   109
rhythms
– autonomous   19, 25, 42ff.
– – external modifications of   42ff.
– – internal stabilization   25
– diurnal   7
– heteronomous   44
– internally
– – desynchronized rhythms (see also
    desynchronized)   32ff.
– – synchronized rhythms (see also
    synchronized)   19ff.
– parameters   24ff.

– – age   26
– – intercorrelation among   29
– – reliabilities   24
– – sex   26
rodents, cardiac rhythms   87
room temperature   344
rucksack, Portapres   182, 218
ruptured arterosclerotic plaque   145

salt   349
SBP (systolic blood pressure)   254
– white and black   278
seasonal variations   344
– temperature   349
sedatives   333
self-reported, emotional strain, ABP and
    heart rate   297ff.
– methodological problems   303
sequence analysis, transient blood pres-
    sure and pulse interval changes   250
sex, rhythm parameter   26
sex-dependent diurnal variability   352
sexual
– activity, diastolic blood pressure   188
– following   94
– intercourse   285
shell of the body   8–10
shift workers   273, 319
– light-dark alternations   79
single   313
skin
– blood   8
– temperature   8
sleep/sleeping   3, 6, 287
– and activity periods   322
– and awake, white, black, male and fe-
    male   309
– apnea   332 – 334
– – pharmacotherapy of arterial hyper-
    tension   338
– in darkness   7, 11
– deprivation   5
– intra-arterial blood pressure   241
– non-REM sleep   334, 337
– onset of   9, 10, 12
– periods   313
– Portapres   189, 218
– REM sleep   334, 337, 341
– sleep-independent rhythm   10
– sleep-related breating disorders and
    nocturnal hypertension   332ff.
– sleep-wakefulness cycle   295, 333
– and working phases   318ff.
smoking cigarettes   285
social
– situation, ABP   259, 261
– stress   92

sodium   278
– valproate   378
sotalol   362, 374
SP   384
spacelab   259, 330
species-specific heart rate   91
spectral analysis, heart rate   99ff.
– mental stress   100
– physical rest   100
– physical work   100
sphygmomanometer, mercury   259
sphygmomanometric method   326
spring and late summer   344
ST segment elevations   160
– coronary heart disease, daily varia-
    tions   159ff.
stand-up   222ff.
Starling curves, week to week, atrial de-
    mand pacing, nocturnal hemodynamic
    responses   166, 169
stomach, "the stomach is the best
    clock"   11
stress   136
– and cardiovascular disease   309
– differs, perception of   303
– domestic   313, 314
– exercise stress test   159
– mental
– – coronary thrombosis, theory of trig-
    gering   152
– – heart rate, spectral analysis   100
---/ time structure, relationship during
    102
– – R-R interval   113
– occupational   310, 311, 313
– – and domestic   305ff.
– physical, coronary thrombosis, theory
    of triggering   152
– in real life/heart rate, relationship   135
– severe stress   98
– social   92
stretch receptors   233
stroke   145, 314
– volume 8, 164–166, 168
– – atrial demand pacing, nocturnal he-
    modynamic responses   165, 167-169
– – Portapres   188, 190
14 successive days   15
summer   348
– spring and late summer   344
sustained-release   362
SV   384
sympathic/sympathetic
– activities   123
– blockade, double sympathetic   383
– blockers   384
– nervous

– – activity   314, 344
– – control   233
– – system   272
synchronized rhythms, internally   19ff.
– experiments   20ff.
– – cortisol, urinary   20
– – melatonin, urinary   20
– – potassium, urinary   20
– – rectal temperature   21
– sleep-wake   20
– – urine volume   21
– – wake-sleep   21
syndrome
– Cushing's   274, 275
– syndrome X   161
systolic blood pressure (SBP)   133, 254,
   372
– atrial demand pacing, nocturnal hemodynamic responses   167, 168

talking   285, 287
tape recorder, portable, Holter   124
TEAC   183
telemetric equipment   124
telephoning   287
television, watching   285
temperature   344ff.
– acclimatization   346
– colder periods   349
– daytime   346
– dependent BP variation   347
– geographically   346
– rectal   6, 10, 16, 20, 21
– room   344
– seasonal differences   349
– skin   8, 10
tests
– bicycle tolerance test   351
– breath holding tests   210ff.
– – Portapres   184, 185
– diving tests   210ff.
– – Portapres   184
– exercise stress test   159
– Raven test   111
theophylline   378
therapy   273
– antihypertensive   383
– nCPAP   334 – 336, 341
"thermal conductance"   8
thrombi, coronary   145
thrombogenesis   386
thrombosis, coronary, theory of triggering   151
– angina, unstable   152
– atherosclerotic plaque   152
– cardiac death   152
– myocardial infarction   152

– plaque   152
– – atherosclerotic   152
– – rupture   152
– stress   152
– – mental   152
– – physical   152
tilt-up   222ff.
time
– consuming questionaire   303
– of day (hours)   294, 311
– to retire   11
– to rise   4
– pressure   136
– structure/heart rate, relationship during
   (see heart rate)   102
tone of the epicardial coronary arteries
   160
total peripheral resistance   see TPR
– plasma proteins   372
toxicities, morning   387
tpA activity, morning increase, myocardial
   infarction   150
TPR   164, 166, 382, 384
– pulse contour   222ff.
– – during coitus   190
tranquilizers   333
transient blood pressure   250
transmeridian flights   322
transplantation, cardiac   274
tree shrew, heart rate reaction   90, 94
– long-term changes   92ff.
triggers   314
– coronary thrombosis   151
– external time   322
– mental   145
– morning activities   146
– of onset   145ff.
– physical   145
trimethaphan   119
TRP   232ff.
Tupaias, cardiovascular system   93
24-hours
– day in a healthy young man   15
– rhythm, circulatory system   5
– routine   16

university employees   286
UPPP (uvulo-palato-pharyngoplasty)
   333
urinary
– epinephrine excretion   314
– pH   372

vagal
– activities   123
– – cilazapril   216
– afferents, neurovegetative system   119

valsalva effects   232
vascular tone   383, 386
vasoconstriction   160
– coronary   145
vasodilation   191
vena cava   234
venous
– congestion in the finger, Portapres
   175
– occlusion, plethysmograph   224
– pressure   6
ventricular pressure   161
verapamil   362, 373, 383, 384, 386
verbal components, neurovegetative system   125
visceral
– components, neurovegetative system
   125
– nervous system   121

wake   21
-/ sleep cycle   333
wakefulness-sleep cycle   295
walking   285, 287
watching TV   285, 287
water consumption   382, 383
water and electrolyte regulating mechanism   382
white
– adolescents, American   277
– awake and sleep   309

– female   277
– hypertensives, British   277
winter   348
work/working   272, 285, 287
– ABP, home vs. work   259
– afternoon shift   322
– desk work   285, 287
– morning shift   319 – 322
– night shift   319 – 322
– physical
– – heart rate   100, 106
– – – spectral analysis   100
– – – time structure, relationship dur-
      ing   102
– – , R-R interval   113
– shift workers   273, 319
– and sleeping phases   318ff.
– vs. nonwork day differences, ABP
   260
workdays   311
workloads   160

X-ray, chest   351
xipamide   362

Zeitgeber period
– heteronomous rhythms, light-dark alterations   44, 52, 59, 62, 71
– information as a Zeitgeber   69
– – bright light   71